# Jonas & Kovner's
# HEALTH CARE
# DELIVERY IN THE
# UNITED STATES

## 8th Edition

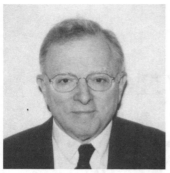

**Anthony R. Kovner, PhD,** is Professor of Health Policy and Management at the Robert F. Wagner Graduate School of Public Service at New York University, in New York City. He is trained in organizational behavior, health services management, and social and economic development. He received bachelor's and master's degrees from Cornell University, and his doctorate in public administration from the University of Pittsburgh.

Dr. Kovner is an experienced health care manager, having served as CEO of a community hospital, senior health care consultant for a large union, manager of a group practice, of a nursing home, and of a large neighborhood health center. He is a board member of the Lutheran Medical Center, Augustana Nursing Home, and Health Plus, of Brooklyn, NY.

He has several funded research projects, most recently on Factors Associated with use of Management Research in Health Systems. He is the author or editor of 9 books and the author of 43 journal articles and 24 case studies. He has carried out several national demonstration programs funded by major foundations. Dr. Kovner was the fourth recipient, in 1999, of the Gary L. Filerman prize for Educational Leadership, from the Association of University Programs in Health Administration.

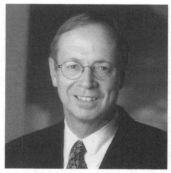

**James R. Knickman, PhD,** is Vice President for Research and Evaluation at The Robert Wood Johnson Foundation. At RWJF, Dr. Knickman has responsibility for external evaluations of national initiatives supported by the Foundation. He and his staff also take lead roles in developing research initiatives supported by the Foundation and conducting internal analysis related to the grant-making priorities of the Foundation. At various times during his tenure at the Foundation, Dr. Knickman also has led grant-making teams in three areas: clinical care for the chronically ill, supportive services, and population health. Prior to joining the RWJF staff in 1992, Dr. Knickman was on the faculty at New York University and directed the University's Health Research Program, where he conducted research on a range of issues related to health care delivery. In addition to his position at RWJF, Dr. Knickman is currently Chair of the Board of Directors for The Robert Wood Johnson University Hospital. Dr. Knickman received a BA degree from Fordham University and a PhD in Public Policy Analysis from the University of Pennsylvania.

# Jonas & Kovner's
# HEALTH CARE
# DELIVERY IN THE
# UNITED STATES

## 8th Edition

**Anthony R. Kovner, PhD**
**James R. Knickman, PhD**
Editors

**Steven Jonas, MD, MPH, MS**
Founding Editor

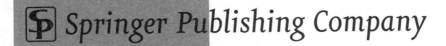 Springer Publishing Company

Springer Publishing Company, Inc.
11 West 42nd St.
New York, NY 10036

*Acquisitions Editor: Sheri W. Sussman*
*Production Editor: Pamela Lankas*
*Cover and page design by Reyman Studio*

05 06 07 08 09/5 4 3 2 1

**Library of Congress Cataloging-in-Publication Data**

Jonas and Kovner's health care delivery in the United States / [edited by] Anthony R.
Kovner & James R. Knickman — 8th ed.
    p. cm.
    Includes bibliographical references and indexes.
Summary: "How do we understand and also assess the health care of America?
Where is health care provided? What are the characteristics of those institutions
that provide it? Over the short term, how are changes in health care provisions
affecting the health of the population, the cost of care, and access to care?" These
core issues regarding our health policy are answered in this text. This is a textbook
for course work in health care, the handbook for administration and policy makers,
and the standard for in-service training programs.—Provided by the Publisher.
    ISBN 0-8261-2087-3 (hard cover) — ISBN 0-8261-2088-1 (soft cover)
    1. Medical Care—United States.
    [DNLM: 1. Delivery of Health Care—United States. 2. Health Policy—United
States. 3. Health Services—United States. 4. Quality of Health Care—United
States. W84 AA1 J68 2005] I. Title: Health care delivery in the United States. II.
Jonas, Steven. III. Kovner, Anthony R. IV. Knickman, James.
RA395.A3J656 2005
362.1'0973—dc22

2005006979

Printed in the United States of America by Victor Graphics.

# CONTENTS

## III: SYSTEM PERFORMANCE

## IV: FUTURES

## V: APPENDICES

# FOREWORD

## By Steven A. Schroeder

THE FIELD OF health care delivery is concerned with the way we convert medical knowledge into services that actually help people get healthy when ill or stay healthy before they get ill. The potential of health care to improve the lives of all Americans is enormous.

Health care as a service industry represents a large part of our economy, accounting for 14.9% of the U.S. gross domestic product and 7% of all jobs. This crucial service sector has been growing consistently during the last 4 decades. As medical knowledge and medical technology expanded during the last half of the 20th century, the task of managing the delivery of health care became more complex.

*Health Care Delivery in the United States*, 8th edition, offers excellent introduction to the many issues involved in the delivery of health care. The 18 chapters that comprise the book are written by some of the leading thinkers and practitioners in the field. Each chapter introduces the reader to issues related to a distinct aspect of the challenge of delivering health services.

The effort to understand the social and organizational dimensions of health care delivery is an important undertaking. It is not enough for a nation to have excellent medical know-how. In addition, we need to understand how to get services to people as well as the social responsibilities and organizational challenges involved in delivering services.

This book properly focuses attention—in almost every one of its chapters—on the core challenges of the delivery of health care: how to achieve quality, efficiency, value, fairness, and universal access. Currently, our delivery system is good in most of these dimensions, but not good enough. Given the large share of our national resources devoted to this endeavor, quality should be greater and more consistent, resources should be used more efficiently to create more valuable services, and perhaps most important, every American should have access to the health care services they need.

The current edition of this book also recognizes the important balance in the health care endeavor between medical interventions to restore health and the social, behavioral, and public health interventions that prevent illness and avoid the need for expensive medical care. The current system focuses most of its resources on the medical intervention side, but there is increasing evidence that investments in the prevention side actually have greater impacts on overall population health. Therefore, it is time to integrate management and policy strategies so that we better coordinate our efforts to improve both medical care and the public health interventions that address social, behavioral, and environmental determinants of health and well-being.

The challenge for the next generation of health care leaders is to make our health care delivery and public health systems fairer, more efficient, and better able to assure quality. The field needs new thinkers and new leaders to find the solutions that will achieve a better health care delivery system than we developed by the end of the 20th century. We need to sort out the roles of the public sector, the private sector, and the nonprofit sector in the health care delivery system. We need to understand how better to train, organize, and motivate the large and dedicated workforce that delivers services every day to millions of Americans. We need to acquire better management skills and systems that will allow us to run a delivery system that gets more complex every day. We need to design strategies to make the delivery system and the financing system less complex and less cumbersome.

These are the challenges for people entering the field today. There are endless opportunities to harness creativity, technical expertise, and social commitment to make a difference in how we deliver medical services, manage our public's health, and make the most of the many new advances in health-promoting technologies that will emerge in the coming years. *Health Care Delivery in the United States* offers a comprehensive introduction to the many dimensions of the health system that need to be understood if we hope to make progress in improving the health of all Americans.

# ORGANIZATION OF THIS BOOK

This book, *Health Care Delivery in the United States*, 8th edition, is organized into four parts: I—"Perspectives," II—"Providing Health Care," III—"System Performance," and IV—"Futures" (see figure below). The titles of these four parts can be formulated as answers to the following questions: How do we understand and assess the health care sector of our economy? Where and how is health care provided? How well does the health care system perform? Where is the health care sector going in terms of the health of the people, the cost of care, access to care, and quality of care?

Part I, "Perspectives," is divided into an introduction and chapters on measurement, financing, public health, the role of government in health care, and a comparative analysis of health systems in wealthy countries. Part II, "Providing Health Care," con-

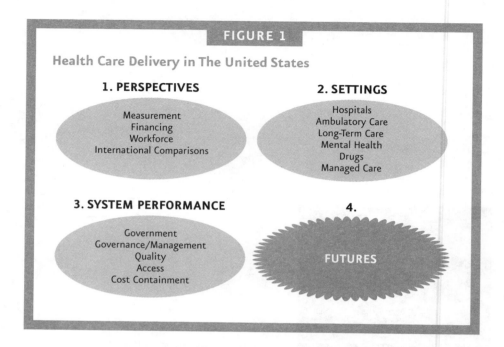

FIGURE 1

Health Care Delivery in The United States

**1. PERSPECTIVES**

Measurement
Financing
Workforce
International Comparisons

**2. SETTINGS**

Hospitals
Ambulatory Care
Long-Term Care
Mental Health
Drugs
Managed Care

**3. SYSTEM PERFORMANCE**

Government
Governance/Management
Quality
Access
Cost Containment

**4.**

FUTURES

tains seven chapters, including acute care, chronic care, long-term care, health-related behaviors, pharmaceuticals and medical devices, the health care workforce, and information management. Part III, "System Performance," is divided into four chapters, on governance, management and accountability, the complexity of health care quality, access to care, and cost containment. Finally, in Part IV, "Futures," the last chapter projects what health care in the United States will look like over the short term. There are three appendices—a glossary, a guide to sources of data, and a listing of useful health care Web sites.

Each of the 18 chapters contains learning objectives, a topical outline, a list of key words, a case study, and questions for further analysis and discussion.

# ACKNOWLEDGMENTS

So you want to write a book? A few years ago, the editors of the 8th edition of this textbook faced the following tasks: Selecting a new co-editor and working out responsibilities, reviewing the 7th edition as to topics and authors (this includes reviewing competitive textbooks), recruiting new authors and specifying deadlines and formats, working with the publisher regarding contracts and deadlines, developing the *Instructor's Guide* and writing our own chapters. Then there was the long editorial process in front of us, involving 18 chapter authors, three appendices authors, and the tireless nagging that goes on between publishers and editors and between editors and chapter authors. We guess another word for "nagging" is "encouragement."

We wish to acknowledge here the considerable help we have received, focusing on the 8th edition (rather than on those who have helped us achieve everything we have accomplished in our lives). These individuals (and there are many) fall into the following groups: (a) those who have helped us with the production process, (b) those who came before (the other seven editions), and (c) those who support and help us so that we can do this kind of work. First, above all others in the (a) group is Debbie Malloy, whose management of the texts and of the editors, has been peerless. Second is the wonderful group of book people at Springer Publishing, to include the indefatigable Ursula Springer; the utterly reliable no-nonsense Sheri Sussman; her capable assistant, Janet Picknally; Pam Lankas (whom we have never met); and the mercurial Matt Fenton. Preeminent among those who have "come before" (a category often omitted in these kinds of enterprises) is Steve Jonas, the ebullient triathaloner, sole editor of the first edition, and progenitor of everything that has come "après moi," a most generous and compassionate spirit. Then there are all the chapter authors who have come before, but there are too many to name here. In the third group we wish to thank the chief executives in the organizations within which we work, who encourage the kind of scholarly activity that this book represents—Risa Lavizzo-Mourey, President, the Robert Wood Johnson Foundation, and Ellen Schall, Dean of NYU's Wagner School of Public Service. Next we wish to thank the chief executives of our lives, Terry Clark and Chris Kovner, and the next generation of chief executives in our lives, (we can dream, can't we?) Annie Knickman, Sarah Kovner, and Anna Kovner.

We take sole responsibility for all the shortcomings of this text. We regard Health Care Delivery in the United States, as a work in progress, to be continued, we hope, by ourselves and eventually by others.

# CONTRIBUTORS

**Gerard F. Anderson, PhD,** is the National Program Director for the Robert Wood Johnson Foundation sponsored program "Partnership for Solutions: Better Lives for People with Chronic Conditions." Dr. Anderson is a professor of health policy and management and international health at the Johns Hopkins University Bloomberg School of Public Health, professor of medicine at the Johns Hopkins University School of Medicine, director of the Johns Hopkins Center for Hospital Finance and Management, and co-director of the Johns Hopkins Program for Medical Technology and Practice Assessment.

Dr. Anderson is currently conducting research on chronic conditions, comparative insurance systems in developing countries, medical education, hospital payment reform, and technology diffusion. Prior to his arrival at Johns Hopkins in 1983, Anderson held various positions in the Office of the Secretary, U.S. Department of Health and Human Services, where he helped to develop Medicare prospective payment legislation. He has authored two books on health care payment policy, has published over 180 peer reviewed articles, testified in Congress over 25 times as an individual witness, and serves on multiple editorial committees.

**John C. Billings, JD,** Associate Professor of Health Policy and Public Service Research, who teaches in the area of health policy. He is principal investigator on numerous projects to assess the performance of the safety net for vulnerable populations and to understand the nature and extent of barriers to optimal health for vulnerable populations. Much of his work has involved analysis of patterns of hospital admission and emergency room visits as a mechanism to evaluate access barriers to outpatient care and to assess the performance of the ambulatory care delivery system. He has also examined the characteristics of high cost Medicaid patients to help in designing interventions to improve care and outcomes for these patients. As a founding member of the Foundation for Informed Decision Making, Professor Billings is helping to provide patients with a clearer mechanism for understanding and making informed decisions about a variety of available treatments. Professor Billings received his JD from the University of California (Berkeley).

**Carol S. Brewer, PhD,** is an Associate Professor at the University at Buffalo School of Nursing and Director of Nursing at the New York State Area Health Education Center Statewide System. She has conducted nursing workforce research for over 10 years, and published and presented widely. Her current research involves developing a model of workforce participation for registered nurses that accounts for Metropolitan Statistical Area differences, and attitudes such as satisfaction and work family conflict. Past research has utilized both secondary and primary data collection to examine a variety of nursing workforce issues. She has also conducted research focusing on the New York State supply of nurses and is responsible for the strategic planning for nursing workforce programs for the NYS AHEC Statewide System. The NYS AHEC Statewide System focuses on recruiting, educating, and retaining the health care workforce for rural and underserved populations. Brewer also teaches graduate students about health care systems, policies and ethics. She received a Masters degree in Nursing from the University of Knoxville, a Masters degree in Applied Economics from the University of Michigan, and a PhD in Nursing Systems from the University of Michigan.

**Joel C. Cantor, ScD,** is the Director of the Center for State Health Policy and Professor of Public Policy at the Edward J. Bloustein School of Planning and Public Policy at Rutgers, The State University of New Jersey. Dr. Cantor's research focuses on issues of health care financing and delivery at the state and local levels. His recent work includes studies of health insurance market regulation, access to care for low-income and minority populations, the health care safety net, and the supply of physicians providing care to underserved populations. Dr. Cantor has published widely on health policy topics, and serves on the editorial board of the policy journal *Inquiry*. Dr. Cantor frequently serves as an advisor to New Jersey government on health care policy. Most recently, he was appointed to the State's Mandated Health Benefits Advisory Commission by Governor McGreevey and serves as chair of that panel. Prior to joining the faculty at Rutgers, Dr. Cantor served as director of research at the United Hospital Fund of New York and director of evaluation research at the Robert Wood Johnson Foundation. He received his doctorate in health policy and management from the Johns Hopkins University School of Hygiene and Public Health in 1988, and was elected a Fellow of the Academy of Health (formerly the Academy for Health Services Research and Health Policy) in 1996.

**Carol A. Caronna, PhD,** is an Assistant Professor in the Department of Sociology, Anthropology, and Criminal Justice at Towson University. She did her graduate work in sociology at Stanford University and, from 2000–2002, was a Robert Wood Johnson Foundation Scholar in Health Policy Research at the University of California at Berkeley School of Public Health, in collaboration with the University of California at San Francisco. Her work focuses on issues of organizational identity and institutional theory, with specific projects on the organizational identity of Kaiser Permanente, the multi-layered identities of Catholic hospitals, and the development and evolution of physician and administrator relations in integrated health care systems. She is the co-author of Institutional Change and Healthcare Organizations: From Professional Dominance to Managed Care (2000), as well as author of several articles and book chapters.

**Elaine F. Cassidy, PhD,** is a Program Officer in Research and Evaluation at the Robert Wood Johnson Foundation, where she has worked on programs related to Addiction Prevention and Treatment, Childhood Obesity, Vulnerable Populations, and Pioneering. She formerly held research, administrative, and teaching positions at the University of Pennsylvania. At the University of Pennsylvania, she managed a study of obesity and psychosocial health among school-aged children in an urban public school. She also managed a within-school, anti-aggression program for children and adolescents in the remedial disciplinary system in a large urban area. She is a certified school psychologist and a trained mental health clinician, who has provided therapeutic care to children and families in outpatient and acute partial hospitalization settings. Dr. Cassidy earned a BA in Psychology and Liberal Studies from the University of Notre Dame, an MSEd in Psychological Services from the University of Pennsylvania, and a PhD in School, Community, and Child-Clinical Psychology from the University of Pennsylvania.

**Mary Ann Chiasson, DrPH,** is an epidemiologist who joined Medical and Health Research Association of New York City (MHRA) in 1999 as Vice-President for research and evaluation. She oversees all research and evaluation activities at MHRA, a not-for-profit organization that provides health and health-related services, conducts demonstration and research programs, and offers management services in order to improve community health and strengthen health policy. Before joining MHRA, Dr. Chiasson served for nine years as an Assistant Commissioner of health at the New York City Department of Health with scientific and administrative responsibility for AIDS Surveillance, AIDS Research and Vital Statistics and Epidemiology. Her research focuses on the epidemiology of HIV (particularly risk factors for sexual transmission and gynecologic manifestations of HIV), women's reproductive health, and infant mortality. Dr. Chiasson is also an Associate Professor of Clinical Epidemiology (in Medicine) at the Mailman School of Public Health, Columbia University.

**Penny Hollander Feldman, PhD,** is Vice President for Research and Evaluation at the Visiting Nurse Service of New York (VNSNY) and Director of the Center for Home Care Policy and Research. Prior to joining VNSNY, Dr. Feldman served on the faculties of the Kennedy School of Government and the Department of Health Policy and Management at the Harvard School of Public Health, where she continued as Visiting Lecturer through June 2003. At the Center for Home Care Policy and Research, she directs projects focused on improving the quality, outcomes and cost-effectiveness of home-based care, supporting informed policy-making by long-term care decision-makers, and helping communities promote the health, well-being and independence of people with chronic illness or disability. Dr. Feldman has served on the Institute of Medicine's Committee on Improving Quality in Long-Term Care, the Home Healthcare Steering Committee of the National Quality Forum, the National Commission on Nursing Workforce for Long-Term Care, and the Advisory Committee on Designing a Long-Term Care System for the Future of the National Academy of Social Insurance. She earned her PhD in Political Science from Harvard University.

**Steven A. Finkler, PhD, CPA,** is Professor of Public and Health Administration, Accounting, and Financial Management at New York University's Robert F. Wagner Graduate School of Public Service. At NYU he is also the Director of the Specialization in Healthcare Financial Management. An award winning teacher and author, Dr. Finkler is currently engaged in a variety of research topics in the areas of health care economics and accounting. His most recent awards are the 2002 Pioneering Spirit Award from the American Association of Critical-Care Nurses (AACN), and the 2003 Sigma Theta Tau International Research Award.

Among his publications are sixteen books. Several of them are *Finance and Accounting for Nonfinancial Managers*, 3rd Ed., *Financial Management for Public, Health, and Not-for-Profit Organizations*, 2nd Ed., *Budgeting Concepts for Nurse Managers*, 3rd Ed., and *Cost Accounting for Health Care Organizations: Concepts and Applications*, 2nd Ed. (1999, with David Ward).

He received a BS in Economics (Summa Cum Laude) and MS in Accounting from the Wharton School at the University of Pennsylvania. His MA in Economics and PhD in Business Administration were awarded by Stanford University. Dr. Finkler, who is also a CPA, worked for several years as an auditor with Ernst and Young and was on the faculty of the Wharton School before joining NYU. He serves on the editorial boards of *Health Care Management Review and Research in Healthcare Financial Management*. He is the former Editor of *Hospital Cost Management and Accounting*, and served on the editorial board of Health Services Research.

**Ron Geigle** is the founding partner of Polidais LLC, a policy analysis and public affairs consulting firm in Washington, DC. The firm provides research, policy analysis, policy positioning, and communications services for clients in the fields of health care, science, and technological innovation. Mr. Geigle specializes in medical technology and pharmaceutical issues, particularly evidence-based medicine, health care outcomes, and health economics. He has spent more than 20 years in the medical technology industry, first as Vice President of policy and communications for the industry's leading trade association and then as an independent consultant working with device and pharmaceutical firms. Mr. Geigle also spent a decade working in policy and public affairs positions in Congress and the Executive Branch. He is a graduate of Harvard University.

**Marc N. Gourevitch, MD, MPH,** is Professor of Medicine at the New York University (NYU) School of Medicine, where he is Director of the Division of General Internal Medicine. His research interests center on health service utilization, medication adherence, and clinical epidemiology among drug users and other underserved populations; pharmacologic treatments for opioid dependence; and effective strategies for fostering behavior change among patients and clinicians. Prior to joining NYU, Dr. Gourevitch was Director of Addiction Medicine at Montefiore Medical Center and Albert Einstein College of Medicine, in the Bronx, New York. There, he implemented a system of integrated on-site primary care and psychiatric services in a network of methadone maintenance treatment programs. Dr. Gourevitch received his medical degree from Harvard Medical School and completed his internship and residency in primary care internal medicine at Bellevue Hospital and the NYU School of Medicine.

**Michal D. Gursen, MPH, MS,** is a Research Analyst at the Center for Home Care Policy and Research at the Visiting Nurse Service of

New York (VNSNY). At the Center, Ms. Gursen works primarily on three projects: the AdvantAge Initiative, Information Brokering for Long-Term Care, and Livable Communities for Adults with Disabilities. Before coming to the Center, Ms. Gursen worked at the New York State Psychiatric Institute where she studied psychoeducational interventions for people with mental illness. Prior to that, Ms. Gursen worked at Mount Sinai School of Medicine where she researched psychosocial pathways leading to drug use. Ms. Gursen received her MPH in Health Policy and Management with a concentration in Effectiveness and Outcomes Research, and MS in Social Work from Columbia University. She holds a BA in Psychology from Barnard College.

**Kelly Hunt, MPP,** is a research officer at RWJF and a member of the Disparities Team. Her research activities at the Foundation have focused on long-term care, emergency department overcrowding, and racial and ethnic disparities in health care. Her work on the Disparities Team reflects her interest in data collection and measurement of the issue of unequal treatment. Before joining the Foundation in August, 2000, Hunt held several consulting positions at Towers Perrin and KPMG. At Towers Perrin, she assisted Fortune 500 companies in designing their health and welfare benefit packages. While at KPMG, Hunt worked on employee health benefit surveys and published annual reports and peer-reviewed articles reflecting changes in the health care system. Hunt earned an MPP from Georgetown University and a BA from Villanova University.

**Kelli Hurdle** graduated from Villanova University with a Bachelor of Science in Economics and is currently pursuing her Masters of Public Administration in Health Policy and Management at New York University's Wagner School. She is a Research Assistant at the Center for Health and Public Service Research, where she works on the national evaluation of the Robert Wood Johnson's Urban Health Initiative. Prior to starting work at NYU Wagner, Kelli provided technical assistance to a variety of health care organizations around New York City in the areas of building clinic capacity, improving patient satisfaction, and integrating HIV services.

**Steven Jonas, MD, MPH, MS,** is Professor of Preventive Medicine, School of Medicine and Professor, Graduate Program in Public

xxiv  ||  HEALTH CARE DELIVERY IN THE UNITED STATES

Health, at Stony Brook University (NY). He is a Fellow of the American College of Preventive Medicine, the New York Academy of Medicine, and the New York Academy of Sciences, and Editor-in-Chief of the *American Medical Athletics Association Journal*, and Associate Editor of *Preventive Medicine*. Over the course of his academic career, which began in 1971, his research has focused on preventive medicine, public health, and health care delivery systems analysis. He has authored, co-authored, edited, and co-edited over 20 books, and published more than 135 articles in scientific journals, as well as numerous articles in the popular literature. It was in the mid-70s that, with the strong support of Dr. Ursula Springer, he created *Health Care Delivery in the United States*. Having been actively involved with the first seven editions, he is proud to continue to have his name associated with the book, which for this 8th edition has been so beautifully renewed and reinvigorated by Dr. Kovner and his new co-editor, Dr. James Knickman.

**Gary Kalkut, MD,** is the VP and Medical Director of Montefiore Medical Center in the Bronx, New York. As Medical Director of a three-hospital system with over 1,000 beds, he directs clinical information systems for quality improvement, network throughput, the medical staff office, and supervises a residency training program with 865 houseofficers that is one of the largest in the country. He has a particular interest in the impact of health care financing on clinical practice and teaching programs. Dr. Kalkut is an internist and practicing infectious diseases physician.

**Roger Kropf, PhD,** is a Professor in the Health Policy and Management Program at New York University's Robert F. Wagner Graduate School of Public Service, where he teaches courses to physicians, nurses, and other health care professionals on health care management information systems. Dr. Kropf has also been a Visiting Professor since 1997 at the University of Colorado at Denver, where he teaches in the Executive MBA Program in Health Administration. The Executive Program uses faculty from the Network for Healthcare Management, an educational collective consisting of fourteen universities across the United States. One of his principal interests is in helping health care professionals to use strategic planning and management information systems to achieve their organizations' goals and objectives. This is the major subject of his book, *Strategic Analysis for Hospital Management*, written with

James Greenberg, PhD in 1984. Dr. Kropf has conducted research on how computer and telecommunications systems can be used in innovative ways in the strategic management of health-care services, and in improving patient and physician satisfaction.

**Laura C. Leviton, PhD,** has been a Senior Program Officer of the Robert Wood Johnson Foundation in Princeton, NJ since 1999. She came to the Foundation from the University of Alabama at Birmingham (UAB), where she served for 5 years as a Professor, Department of Health Behavior, School of Public Health. Prior to her appointment at UAB, she was an Associate Professor of Public Health at the University of Pittsburgh. Dr. Leviton has served and continues to serve in numerous professional and scientific societies, and was President of the American Evaluation Association in the year 2000. She was a member of the Institute of Medicine committee that developed *Preparing for Terrorism*, a framework to evaluate DHHS' Metropolitan Medical Response System. She served on the CDC's National Advisory Committee on HIV/STD Prevention and served on both NIMH and NIH study sections on HIV prevention, as well as chairing such a study section for the University of California system's research awards on HIV prevention. She received the 1993 award from the American Psychological Association for Distinguished Contributions to Psychology in the Public Interest, for her work in HIV prevention and health promotion at the workplace. She was awarded a W.K. Kellogg National Fellowship, and has received several other awards. Dr. Leviton earned a Bachelor's degree in Psychology at Reed College, Portland, Oregon; a Master's degree and PhD in Psychology at the University of Kansas; and was a Postdoctoral Fellow in the Methodology and Evaluation Research Program, and Center for Health Services and Policy Research, at Northwestern University.

**John R. Lumpkin, MD, MPH,** is the Senior Vice President for the Health Care Group of the Robert Wood Johnson Foundation (RWJF). Prior to joining RWJF, he was the first African American to hold the position of Public Health Director in the state of Illinois. He served the second longest tenure of any director since the present agency structure was created in 1917. As director of the Illinois Department of Public Health (IDPH), Dr. Lumpkin oversaw an agency of 1,300 employees located in Springfield, Chicago, seven regional offices and three laboratories who share primary responsibility for the quality of life in the state. Dr. Lumpkin's career in public health began with his appointment in 1985 as associate director of IDPH's Office of Health Care Regulations. He has overseen improvements to programs dealing with women's and men's health, information technology, emergency and biopreparedness, infectious disease prevention and control, immunization, local health department coverage, and the state's laboratory services.

Dr. Lumpkin received his medical degree in 1974 from Northwestern University Medical School. He trained in Emergency Medicine at the University of Chicago and earned his M.P.H. from the University of Illinois at Chicago, School of Public Health. Since 1996, Lumpkin has served as chairman of the National Committee on Vital and Health Statistics. He was elected to membership in the Institute of Medicine of the National Academies. He is past president of the Association of State and Territorial Health Officials (ASTHO), a former member of the Board of Trustees of the Foundation for Accountability, a former Commissioner of the Pew Commission on Environmental Health, a former board member of the National Forum for Health Care Quality Measurement and Reporting, a past board member of the American College of Emergency Physicians and past president of the Society of Teachers of Emergency Medicine. Lumpkin has also been the recipient of the Bill B. Smiley Award, Alan Donaldson Award, African American History Maker, and Public Health Worker of the Year.

**Pamela Nadash** is a Senior Research Associate at the Medstat Group, currently assessing the feasibility of and helping to design a demonstration of a consumer-directed Medicare home health benefit. Ms. Nadash is also working toward her PhD at Columbia University, earning a joint degree between the Mailman School of Public Health and the Political Science department. Her dissertation focuses on managed long-term care.

Prior to working at Medstat, Ms. Nadash worked at the Center for Home Care Policy and Research at the Visiting Nurse Service of New York, conducting research on VNSNY's managed long-term care program, VNS CHOICE, and promoting research on long-term care through the Information Brokering for Long Term Care project (supported by The Robert Wood Johnson Foundation.) Prior to that, she worked at the National Council on the Aging as Director of the National Institute on Consumer-Directed Long-Term Services, sitting on the management team of the Cash and Counseling Demonstration and Evaluation and also supporting the National Program Office of The Robert Wood Johnson–funded Independent Choices grants program. Ms. Nadash has also conducted research on the experience of children with special health care needs in managed care. While working at the Policy Studies Institute in London, she acted as co-investigator for a major study of cash payments for personal care services in the UK. Ms. Nadash earned her BA from Bryn Mawr College and a BPhil (a master's degree) in political theory from Oxford University.

**Jennifer A. Nelson, MPH,** is a Research Associate in the Research and Evaluation Unit at Medical and Health Research Association of New York City, Inc. She is a graduate of the Center for Population and Family Health at the Joseph L. Mailman School of Public Health of Columbia University. Before joining MHRA in 2000, she worked on policy research at the National Center for Children in Poverty. Previously, she provided reproductive health education and clinical assistance at a Planned Parenthood clinic, and, as a Peace Corps Volunteer at a rural health clinic in West Africa, she provided growth monitoring services, nutritional counseling, and family planning education. Recent research projects have focused on issues related to childhood obesity, reproductive health, and maternal and child health.

**C. Tracy Orleans, PhD,** is a Senior Scientist at the Robert Wood Johnson Foundation, where she works in several areas—Tobacco, Health and Behavior, Health Care Quality, Childhood Obesity, and Research and Evaluation. Her work has a common theme of promoting the translation of clinical and behavioral research into practice and policy and improving health care quality for the prevention and management of chronic disease. She has played a leading role in developing the Foundation's grant-making strategies in the areas of tobacco dependence treatment, chronic disease prevention and management, and the adoption of healthy behaviors, including physical activity promotion (active living) and childhood obesity prevention. Dr. Orleans remains active in behavioral medicine and public health research and publication, has authored or co-authored over 175 publications, and serves on a number of journal editorial boards, national scientific panels and advisory groups (e.g., Institute of Medicine, AHRQ-CDC National Commission on Prevention Priorities, the Interagency Committee on Smoking and

Health Subcommittee on Tobacco Cessation, American Legacy Foundation, Society of Behavioral Medicine). She is a past member of the U.S. Preventive Services Task Force, past president of the Society of Behavior Medicine, and recipient of the Society's Distinguished Service Award. She also has received the Joseph Cullen Tobacco Control Research Award of the American Society of Preventive Oncology. Dr. Orleans earned a BA from Wellesley College in Massachusetts and a PhD from the University of Maryland.

**Scott D. Rhodes, MPH, PhD,** is Assistant Professor at Wake Forest University School of Medicine, Department of Public Health Sciences. He has an MPH from the University of South Carolina and a PhD from the University of Alabama at Birmingham. He completed a 2-year postdoctoral fellowship with the W. K. Kellogg Community Health Scholars Program at the University of North Carolina at Chapel Hill. He is currently PI for the CDC-funded project, HoMBReS: Hombres Manteniendo Bienestar y Relaciones Saludables (Men Maintaining Wellness and Healthy Relationships) to reduce the risk of sexually transmitted disease infection among Latino migrant and seasonal farmworkers in central North Carolina.

**Victor G. Rodwin, PhD, MPA,** Professor of Health Policy and Management, teaches courses on community health and medical care, comparative analysis of health care systems and international perspectives on health care reform. Professor Rodwin is the recipient of a 3-year Robert Wood Johnson Foundation Health Policy Investigator Award on "Megacities and Health: New York, London, Paris and Tokyo." He is the author of numerous articles and books, including *The Health Planning Predicament: France, Quebec, England, and the United States* (University of California, 1984); *The End of an Illusion: The Future of Health Policy in Western Industrialized Nations* (with J. de Kervasdoué and J. Kimberly, University of California, 1984); *Public Hospitals in New York and Paris* (with C. Brecher, D. Jolly, and R. Baxter), New York University Press, 1992); and *Japan's Universal and Affordable Health Care: Lessons for the US.?* (Japan Society, 1994). His most recent book (edited with Michael Gusmano), *Growing Older in Four World Cities: New York, London, Paris and Tokyo*, will be published by Vanderbilt University Press. Recent journal articles have appeared in *Journal of Urban Health*, Indicators, and the *American Journal of Public Health*. Professor Rodwin directs the World Cities Project, a collaborative venture between the Wagner School and the

International Longevity Center-USA, which examines the impact of population aging and longevity on New York, London, Paris, and Tokyo. He has consulted with the World Bank, the UN, the French National Health Insurance Fund, and other international organizations. Professor Rodwin earned his doctorate in city and regional planning, and his MPH in public health, at the University of California at Berkeley.

**Steven A. Schroeder, MD,** is Distinguished Professor of Health and Health Care, Division of General Internal Medicine, Department of Medicine, UCSF, where he also heads the Smoking Cessation Leadership Center. The Center, funded by the Robert Wood Johnson Foundation, works with leaders of American health professional organizations and health care institutions to increase the rate at which patients who smoke are offered help to quit.

Between 1990 and 2002 he was President and CEO, the Robert Wood Johnson Foundation. During his term of office the Foundation made grant expenditures of almost $4 billion in pursuit of its mission of improving the health and health care of the American people.

Dr. Schroeder graduated from Stanford University and Harvard Medical School, and trained in internal medicine at the Harvard Medical Service of Boston City Hospital and in epidemiology as an EIS Officer of the CDC. He has published extensively in the fields of clinical medicine, health care financing and organization, prevention, public health, and the work force, with over 250 publications. He currently serves as chairman of the American Legacy Foundation and of the International Review Committee of the Ben Gurion School of Medicine, and is a member of the editorial board of the *New England Journal of Medicine*, the Harvard Overseers, the James Irvine Foundation, the Save Ellis Island Foundation, and the Council of the Institute of Medicine, National Academy of Sciences.

**Michael S. Sparer, PhD, JD,** is a Professor of Health Policy at the Joseph L. Mailman School of Public Health at Columbia University. He received a doctorate in political science from Brandeis University and a JD from Rutgers School of Law (Newark). Dr. Sparer spent 7 years as a litigator for the New York City Law Department, specializing in intergovernmental social welfare litigation. He now studies and writes about the politics of care. He is the author of

Medicaid and the *Limits of State Health Reform* (Temple University Press, 1996) as well as numerous articles and book chapters.

**Robin Strongin,** a partner with the Washington, DC-based health care consulting firm, Polidais LLC, has been specializing in the areas of health policy and communications (media strategy, message development, placement, and writing for educational campaigns) for the past 20 years.

Prior to joining Polidais LLC, Ms. Strongin was a Senior Research Associate with George Washington University's National Health Policy Forum. While at the Forum, she developed educational seminars for Capitol Hill and executive branch staff, directed the Forum's corporate sponsorship activities, and assisted with grant writing and foundation reporting requirements.

Prior to consulting, Ms. Strongin was the Acting Executive Director and Director of Research Programs for the Health Care Technology Institute, a privately funded organization dedicated to the support of public policy research and analysis of issues related to health care technology.

Ms. Strongin has served as staff to the National Leadership Coalition on Health Care, the Prospective Payment Assessment Commission (now the Medicare Payment Advisory Commission), and was selected as a Presidential Management Intern where she served in the Office of Legislation and Policy in the Health Care Financing Administration (now the Centers for Medicare and Medicaid Services), as well as in the office of Congressman James J. Florio (D-NJ) and the Council of State Governments.

Ms. Strongin graduated *magna cum laude* with a BA in psychology from the State University of New York at Albany and attended C.W. Post College on a full scholarship, where she graduated *summa cum laude* with an MPA and a specialization in health administration. She was elected to the *Pi Alpha Alpha* Honor Society and the *Signum Laudis* Honor Society.

**Bonnie J. Wakefield, PhD, RN,** is a Department of Veterans Affairs Health Services Research and Development Service (VA HSR&D) Advanced Career Development awardee and investigator in the VA HSR&D Center for Implementation of Innovative Strategies in Practice (CRIISP) at the Iowa City VA Medical Center. She holds an appointment as Clinical Associate Professor at the University of Iowa College of Nursing. Dr. Wakefield's research interests focus on assessment and improvement of outcomes in older patients; the professional culture surrounding patient safety issues; and application of innovative telemedicine strategies to improve health care delivery.

**Douglas S. Wakefield, PhD,** is Professor and Head of the Department of Health Management and Policy at the University of Iowa, College of Public Health. His research interests are in patient care, quality and safety. Dr. Wakefield's research has been funded from a variety of sources including, AHCPR, HRSA, The Robert Wood Johnson Foundation, Northwest Area Foundation, John Deere Health Foundation, and the Veterans Administration.

# PART I
# PERSPECTIVES

# 1

# OVERVIEW: The State of Health Care Delivery in the United States

Anthony R. Kovner and
James R. Knickman

- Understand defining characteristics of the American health care delivery system.
- Identify issues and concerns with the current system.
- Understand the causes of current issues and concerns.
- Analyze stakeholder interests in the delivery of care.
- Identify goals for health care delivery which are realistic and politically feasible.

☐ Defining characteristics of the American health care delivery system
☐ Issues and concerns
☐ Stakeholder interests in health care delivery
☐ Goals for health care delivery

Health care delivery, life expectancy, infant mortality, quality of care, chronic care, health care providers, Medicare, national health insurance, stakeholders, comprehensive coverage, universal health insurance, access

---

IN THIS OVERVIEW we present defining characteristics of the American health care delivery system, raise major issues and concerns, and make recommendations for changing health care delivery in this country. Health care is costly, highly technological, yet of irregular quality and inaccessible for millions of Americans. As early as 1932, a presidential commission studied the American health care system and pointed out that the United States had the economic resources to provide satisfactory medical service to all of its people and meet the associated costs (Committee on the Costs of Medical Care, 1970, p. 2). Now, more than 70 years later, we face the same predicament. So why do we still have a health care system that does not better serve all Americans? Unless Americans can satisfactorily explain why this system looks the way it does today, it is unlikely that we can make realistic recommendations for reforming it.

## DEFINING CHARACTERISTICS OF THE AMERICAN HEALTH CARE SYSTEM

Americans spend large sums of money on health care—over $5,440 per capita per year, exceeding health care expenditures in all 30 developed countries. At the same time, over forty-four million Americans (16%) lack insurance coverage for basic health care services, again a much higher percentage than is found in any developed country. The quality of care in the U.S. is uneven as well. For example, the majority of people suffering from high blood pressure are unaware that they have the condition, and the majority of people coping with depression do not receive the types of medicines known to be effective. Yet, the United States has the most highly developed medical technology, the most expensive and well-equipped hospitals, and the most highly paid doctors in the world. Thus, at least the Americans who can afford health insurance, or who are well insured, can get the best care that medical technology can offer. Even so, the most expensive care is often fragmented or insufficient, and may not restore the patient to health or adequate functioning. The kind of access to care that most Americans lack has been cited by Berwick (2002) as follows:

> ... self care strongly supported and unequivocally encouraged; group visits of patients with like needs, with or without professionals involved; Internet use for access to scientific and popular information; e-mail care between patients and clinicians; and well-managed chat rooms, electronic and real, for patients and significant others who face common challenges. (p. 43)

## MAJOR ISSUES AND CONCERNS

What value do we, as a population, get for what we spend on health care? Is the health of Americans better overall than that of people in other developed countries? Apparently not. For example, among the world's developed countries, the United States is not a leader in life expectancy at birth (U.S. Census Bureau, Table 1352), nor are we among the leaders in low infant-mortality rates. We lead the rest of the world in only one health statistic: life expectancy beyond the age of 80, for two possible reasons. This age group may have a better underlying health status, or have better access to high-technology health care, funded mainly through Medicare, which provides health insurance coverage to almost all of America's elderly.

There are other distressing aspects of our health care delivery system beyond excessive cost, undesirable outcomes, and inaccessibility. The quality of care and service is uneven. Too much money is spent on administration, in large part because the financing of health care is so extraordinarily complex. Hence, too little money is spent on chronic care, though nearly 50% of the U.S. population has at least one chronic health condition. This compromise on quality occurs partly because of the complexity of the financing system, especially the extensive, cumbersome regulation of health care providers by government and insurers. By the late 1990s, Mayo Clinic officials had counted more than 130,000 pages of legal requirements for Medicare, compared to 10,000 for the U.S. Internal Revenue Service (Lawrence, 2002). Additionally, millions of Americans have poor health practices: for example, those who use tobacco, those who drink excess alcohol, those who eat a poor diet, and those who do not exercise. (Consider the prevalence of obesity, now recognized as a major U.S. health problem.) There are also those who engage in acts of violence, with easy access to firearms or who use illicit substances creating another demand on the health care system. In addition, millions of poor and illiterate Americans lack knowledge of good health practices and how to gain access to services.

No doubt another part of the health care problem is that millions of Americans are ambivalent about health behaviors, such as what constitutes best health practices and how to lead healthier lives. Americans want to look and feel healthy, but are not always willing to change their behaviors in order to get enough sleep and proper exercise, eat well, or to stop abusing tobacco or alcohol.

## WHAT MOST AMERICANS CAN AGREE ON

Broad reform of the national health care system was not a top priority issue in the 2004 presidential election. Rather it focused on specific issues like prescription drug benefits for seniors. Nonetheless, we think that most Americans agree on the following principles: (a) all Americans should have access to basic health care services of adequate quality, (b) the United States can afford to provide all Americans with such access, and (c) the U.S. government should more effectively hold the health sector accountable for providing better value for the dollars spent on care and services. But in the legislative arena, health care is not dealt with in principle. With regard to specific legislation, those interests who benefit from the status quo simply do not want to make changes, or if they do, they support those designed to further their interests rather than those of the consumer and taxpayer. However, Americans do not agree on how we should pay to provide access to everyone for basic health services of adequate quality, nor do we agree on what "basic health services" are or what "adequate quality" is.

## WHY WE HAVE THE SYSTEM THAT WE DO

Opinions differ as to why we have the health care delivery system we do and how we should go about changing it. Some argue that the means for getting enough value for the dollars that we spend on health care and for insuring all of us is in the creation of a national governmental health insurance system that assures basic health benefits to all Americans. Such universal coverage could be achieved, though at considerable cost, by expanding Medicare and Medicaid. Others argue that the private sector of the health care system needs to be strengthened and that approaches to assuring

### TABLE 1.1

#### Stakeholder Interests in Health Care Delivery

| GROUPS STAKEHOLDER | POLICIES THEY FAVOR | POLICY THEY OPPOSE |
|---|---|---|
| Taxpayers | Limits on provider payment | Higher taxes |
| Patients | Comprehensive coverage<br>Quality of care<br>Lower out-of-pocket costs | Limited access to care<br>Higher patient payments |
| Providers | Income maintenance<br>Autonomy<br>Comprehensive coverage | Limits on provider payment |
| Vendors and suppliers | Comprehensive coverage<br>Research funding | Limits on provider payment |
| Employers and (payers) | Cost containment<br>Administrative simplification<br>Elimination of cost shifting | Governmental regulation |
| Regulators (government) | Disclosure and reporting by providers<br>Cost containment<br>Access to care<br>Quality of care | Provider autonomy |

access should be built on the existing private system. Before reaching a particular conclusion about how to change the system, we must recognize that many stakeholders in the health care delivery system prefer the system much the way it is now, and would only be in favor of change if it were more favorable to their interests. Stakeholders are groups who can influence or who are influenced by the current health care system as categorized in TABLE 1.1.

Table 1.1 certainly oversimplifies a complex political economy. But stakeholders in the health care system have diverse needs and interests. Patients who require chronic care have different interests than those who are basically healthy; nurses have interests that differ from those of physicians; generalist physicians have different priorities than do specialists; and the interests of insurers, educators, consultants, researchers, and unions and trade organizations (vendors and suppliers in Table 1.1) differ according to the health care issue. Table 1.1 also classifies the public by two different categories, taxpayers and patients, because when people are healthy, they and their families have different priorities regarding coverage and costs than when they are sick.

What we learn from Table 1.1 is that there are stakeholders who favor comprehensive coverage (patients, vendors and suppliers, and providers), while other stakeholders favor limits on payments to health care providers (taxpayers, and employers/payers).

## WHAT CAN BE DONE

Let us assume that Americans agree on the desirability of achieving (a) access to basic health care of adequate quality for all Americans, (b) universal health insurance coverage for all Americans, and (c) more effective governmental regulation of providers. What must we do then to attain these goals? First, we must define in measurable terms what we mean by these three goals. For example, how should basic health care and adequate quality be defined? We could define basic health care as what is covered by a typical employer's benefit plan, or in a typical plan for government employees. But there is much disagreement even here. For example, to what extent should nursing home and home health care be covered? If there is a gap between best and simply adequate health care practice, how can we finance closing the gap? But we have to start somewhere and make choices. We Americans have the health care system that we have because of the choices that we have made, through the political process and through our market. We can have whatever specific coverages are politically preferable, but Americans cannot cover everything unless the taxpayers are willing to pay the price.

Second, Americans have to measure how well the system is performing today with regard to the issues we have discussed. For example, who does not have access to basic health care or has uneven quality of care, and what are the consequences for those involved, and for the rest of us paying for their subsequent care?

Third, we need an acceptable plan to implement the recommendations. For example, to finance additional coverage, we either have to provide narrower coverage with lower payments to providers, or raise additional revenues from other sources. These and other issues are discussed in depth in the chapters that follow, including health care financing, cost containment, quality management, access, and futures.

## JOINING THE EFFORT

Every reader of this text is a stakeholder in the American health care delivery system. We believe that after you have read this book, you will want the American health care delivery system to move faster toward providing greater access, improved quality, universal health insurance, more effective (but not more) governmental regulation, and increased efficiency.

We hope our text will provide you with data and perspectives so that you can seek further information to form your own conclusions about America's health care delivery system. Through our own work on this complex topic, we have been fascinated by the difficulty of finding satisfactory solutions to the imbalance and high cost of our present health care system. We have been inspired by the tremendous pace of change in health care in terms of new technologies and therapies, new demands and consumer preferences, and new ways of organizing services and training the health care workforce. At the same time, the underlying problems of uneven quality of care, fragmentation of services, high cost, and lack of access for millions of Americans remain virtually unresolved.

The journey of understanding and changing the world's most complicated, expensive, and often dysfunctional—or at least wasteful—health care delivery system has been both exhilarating and exhausting. Even so, we hope that you will work with us to improve our system.

## CASE STUDY

Politicians have suggested extending Medicare to the rest of the American population. They intend to pay for increasing the population eligible for these benefits by increasing payroll taxes and premiums. Discuss which groups or interests in American society are likely to favor or oppose such legislation for what reasons.

## DISCUSSION QUESTIONS

1. What are the characteristics of the American health care delivery system?
2. What are the problems and issues associated with these characteristics?
3. What are the reasons for these problems and issues?
4. What are some suggestions to overcome the opposition of certain interest groups to national health insurance for all Americans?
5. What is likely to be the response from these interests to your suggestions?

## REFERENCES

Berwick, D. (2002). *Escape fire: Lessons for the future of health care.* New York: The Commonwealth Fund.

Committee on the Costs of Medical Care. (1970). *Medical care for the American people.* Chicago: University of Chicago Press. Washington, DC: USD-HEW. (Original work published 1932)

Lawrence, D. (2002). *From chaos to care: The promise of team-based medicine.* Cambridge, MA: Perseus.

U.S. Census Bureau. (1999). *Statistical abstract of the United States: 1999* (119th ed.). Washington, DC.

# 2

# MEASURING HEALTH STATUS

Mary Ann Chiasson and
Steven Jonas

## LEARNING OBJECTIVES

- List and characterize the major categories of data used to describe the people served *and not served* by the health care delivery system.
- List and characterize the major categories of data used to describe the health care delivery system and its activities.
- Describe the principal sources of health and health services data and state how and where to find them (using Appendix B as well as this chapter).
- To be able to define the key words listed below.

## TOPICAL OUTLINE

- Data for health and health services: What are they? *Why are they collected?*
- How are health and health services data commonly organized and presented? What are the primary sources for the common data?
- Numbers and rates
- Primary defining characteristics of the U.S. population
- Vital statistics
- Morbidity and mortality
- Health status and health-related behaviors
- Utilization of health services

## KEY WORDS

Data, census, vital statistics, surveillance, demographic characteristics, rates, numerator, denominator, morbidity, mortality, natality, infant mortality, crude and specific rates, age-adjusted and age-standardized rates, incidence, prevalence, health status, provider- and patient-perspective utilization, ambulatory services, hospitalization, health services utilization, program planning

QUANTITATIVE DESCRIPTION AND analysis provide the basic means for understanding both the nature and health status of the population the health care delivery system is meant to serve and to show how the system operates. Data are used to describe the population and its health, to plan for and target services and interventions, and to measure the delivery of services and the outcomes of interventions. Commonly used data can be divided into five broad categories: census data, vital statistics data (births, deaths, marriages, and divorces), surveillance data, administrative data, and survey research data.

Data useful in describing the health of a community can be obtained from a variety of sources and collected for a variety of purposes. Data collected through surveillance—defined as the ongoing, systematic collection of information by established, often legally-mandated reporting systems—directly monitor the health of the public (communicable diseases, cancer registries). Health-related data also may be collected as an adjunct to a civil registration procedure (births and deaths), data may be collected by health care providers (health services utilization) and governmental and non-governmental insurers, or they may be collected through population-based health and behavior interview surveys.

None of the data presented in this chapter are current given the lapse between data gathering and the book's publication. Thus, the utility of the statistics presented is not to be found in their description of the current reality; rather, the data presented are to be viewed as examples of *how* numbers are and can be used to better understand the health care delivery system, those it serves, and those outside the system.

The explosion in information technology has certainly revolutionized our access to data. Virtually all the numbers presented in this chapter are from national surveys and data collection systems; summaries of these data are available on the Internet, in addition to being published on a regular, usually annual, basis. (See Appendix B for descriptions of the principal data sources.) Thus, the most recent numbers available for many data categories of interest can be found online at the time they are needed. It is important to note, however, that because data collection and analysis are lengthy processes, the most recent available data are still usually several years old.

Despite this technological revolution, not all important data categories are regularly (or ever) collected or reported. Most routinely used population and health data come from data collection systems that monitor conditions of public health importance as mandated by federal, state, or local law. Because publicly supported data systems are traditionally under-funded, health care financing must balance the need for these systems, and the information they provide on the part of public officials, health care providers, health planners, researchers, and the public, with the need for treatment and prevention programs.

Mortality data serve as one example of how public health officials have attempted to maximize data collection while minimizing cost. Cause of death (e.g., heart disease, cancer, diabetes) is usually easily determined by diagnosis and regularly reported on the death certificate, while underlying risk factors (e.g., lifestyle, obesity, cigarette smoking) are not. As an inexpensive way of increasing the collection of this important information, some jurisdictions have added items to the death certificate related to the decedent's history of smoking and alcohol use. However, these efforts have had limited success because this information is difficult to obtain. Therefore, one often must look beyond the traditional vital statistics reports to gain an understanding of the causes of morbidity and mortality.

Population-based surveys can provide this additional data. Such surveys are routinely used to collect more detailed, risk-related information from a relatively small sample of individuals chosen to be representative of the population. Data from interview surveys have been invaluable in linking behaviors to health outcomes and in describing the underlying prevalence of these behaviors at the national level.

Unfortunately, findings from national surveys usually cannot be extrapolated to the state or local level since neither health-related behaviors nor illnesses are randomly distributed in the population, and the number of individuals in any single sociodemographic subgroup is likely to be too small to provide reliable information at the state or local level. In recent years, statewide surveys have become more common, but, again, the findings usually cannot be generalized to the local level. Thus, while many characteristics of the population of a given geographic area can be described using readily accessible sources like census and vital statistics data, all too often health officials, health planners, and researchers can obtain only imprecise estimates of the incidence and prevalence of chronic diseases and health-related behaviors in the specific populations of interest to them.

Therefore, this chapter focuses primarily on national data. The principal sources of the data presented are the *National Vital Statistics Reports*,[1] *Vital Statistics of the United States*, and special studies published in the NCHS publication *Vital and Health Statistics*, Series 20.

1 Until the appearance of Vol. 47, No. 1 in 1988, this publication was known as the Monthly Vital Statistics Report. With the change of name came some changes in the ways that and the frequency with which the relevant data are reported, but it is still the primary, regularly and frequently published source for vital statistics data for the United States.

Some of these data are also published regularly in the *Statistical Abstract of the United States* and the regular publication *Health, United States*. Detailed state and local vital statistics data are available from each state health department. Data from the many surveys and data collection systems of the Department of Health and Human Services, including those from the National Center for Health Statistics and the National Center for Chronic Disease Prevention and Health Promotion, are also used. Some of these surveys, particularly the Behavioral Risk Factor Surveillance System, collect state-specific data. (See Appendix B for descriptions of each of these sources as well as the website addresses where they can be accessed.)

## QUANTITATIVE PERSPECTIVES

### Purposes
There are three major purposes for characterizing a population's health and health care status quantitatively: description, program planning and evaluation, and performance measurement.

### *Description*
There are three quantitative perspectives that can be used for description: the size and demographic characteristics of the population, direct measures of health and ill health status, and utilization of health services. First, quantification *describes* the population being served using simply the *numbers* of people and their "demographic" (the Greek for "describing the people") characteristics. Among the important demographic indices are age, sex, race, birthplace, geographic location, and such social characteristics as marital status, income, educational attainment, and employment. Demographic characteristics such as geographic location (Do many people live near standing water inhabited by mosquitoes carrying West Nile Virus?) and age distribution (Are there many infants and/or people older than 65?) by themselves may well provide some indication of the population's relative disease risks.

Second are the *direct measures of health and ill health* in a population. Given the current level of sophistication of data gathering and analysis, it is much easier to characterize the latter than the former. The ill-health status of the population is described by measures of mortality (death) and morbidity (sickness). Mortality and morbidity may be counted for the population as a whole—referred to as *crude* rates; or mortality and morbidity may be counted by cause, or by demographic characteristics used to describe segments of the population (e.g., age, sex)—also called *specific* rates.

Disease-specific mortality and morbidity rates highlight the major clinically apparent health and illness problems in the population. The infant mortality rate gives some indication of both general health levels and the availability of medical care. The distribution of crude and disease-specific mortality and morbidity rates by place, age, sex, ethnic group, and social class shows which population subgroups are being affected by which diseases. The prevalence of behavioral risk factors like smoking, sedentary lifestyle, and sun exposure in the population suggests the level and kinds of interventions needed and projects future health care needs.

The third quantitative perspective for viewing a population in terms of health and ill health is the *utilization and quality of its health services*: which kinds of services are offered, who provides them, who uses how many of which kinds of services, when, and where, and what the patient outcome is. Utilization can be measured quantitatively and qualitatively from three points of view: that of the consumer, that of the provider, and that of an accrediting organization. For example, physician-patient encounters can be reported in terms of how many visits the average patient makes to the physician each year. The same set of events can be reported in terms of how many patient visits the average physician provides each year. The type and frequency of the visits themselves and the outcomes of the medical procedures can also be compared to national standards.

Patient-perspective utilization data can provide some idea of the possible differential (over- or under-) utilization of health services by social class, ethnicity, and geography. It is also important to include measures of health status when examining utilization rates since older, sicker patients would obviously use more services than healthier patients. Provider-perspective utilization data can tell us, for example, about physician and hospital workloads, in terms of provider characteristics (credentials, size, location, services offered, etc.). Taken together, these two perspectives can identify barriers to health care access at the individual and institutional level, while the findings of accrediting organizations depict the types and quality of services being provided.

In summary, health status and services quantification describes how many of which kinds of people are at risk, which kinds of diseases and ill-health conditions they have, how those problems are distributed in the population, who goes where for how many of which kinds of health services, delivered by which types of providers, and, in some cases, what the outcome is of these services. These descriptive data can also be used for the following purposes.

### Program Planning and Evaluation

The second purpose of quantification in health care delivery is *program planning and evaluation*. It may be done, for example, by a private physician, a hospital, a health services network, a city or state health services administration, or a federal government agency. Descriptive data can reveal the existence of health or health services problems and can be used to help design solutions to identified problems or unmet needs. Since not everyone who is in need of a specific service will utilize it, data-based utilization projections are essential for estimating costs as well as service needs. Once new programs are under way, having data on them is necessary if they are to be evaluated. It is essential to know whether the program, once it is operational, is being used by those for whom it was intended.

It must be remembered, however, that data alone are not sufficient for effective and useful planning. Before data can have any real meaning for planning, the agencies and institutions in charge must first make a policy decision to actually engage in the process. They must also agree to make their planning data-based. (Too often in the real world, program planning, even if it is done, is not data-based.) Further, to make the planning process work, the policy makers who have authorized it must also have decided that once arrived at, a suitable plan will be implemented. Some of the data-based questions to be asked in any health services planning exercise are listed:

1. How many people live in the proposed service area, where are they located, and what forms of transportation are available?
2. What are the age, sex, and marital status distributions?
3. What are the education levels, income, ethnicity, and languages spoken?
4. What is the sickness and health profile?
5. How is the population size and composition changing over time?
6. What are the financial resources of the target population and what sorts of health insurance coverage do they have?

7. What are the existing health care resources, where are they, and how are they used?
8. What do existing providers see as their needs? How do they view the new facility, and how will they relate to it?

### Performance Measures

With the advent of managed care and the increasing need to control health care costs, interest in what health care does and how well it does it has intensified as has competition among providers and plans. The NCQA (National Committee for Quality Assurance) HEDIS (Health Plan Employer Data and Information Set) clinical measures have been developed to assess managed care quality and the HEDIS CAHPS (Consumer Assessment of Health Plans) composite measures, which include patient satisfaction measures as well as health care and health care provider ratings, serve as important indicators of the industry's overall performance (National Committee for Quality Assurance [NCQA] *State of Managed Care Quality*, Report 2004).

Numerous forms of health plan report cards (see **FIGURE 2.1**) have been developed to help consumers (formerly patients) and

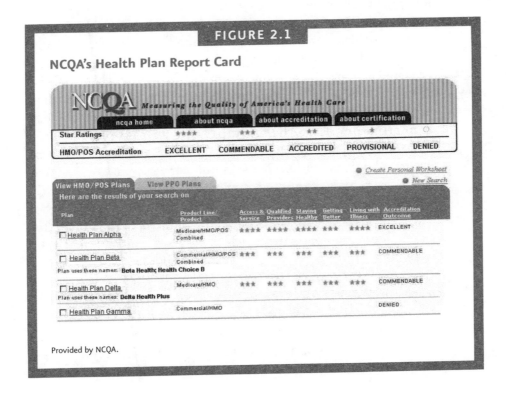

**FIGURE 2.1**

**NCQA's Health Plan Report Card**

Provided by NCQA.

health care purchasers compare health plans and make informed choices. NCQA includes information about a health plan's performance in five key areas: access and service, qualified providers, staying healthy (immunization and screening programs), getting better, and living with illness. While interpreting report cards can sometimes be a difficult task for consumers, there are likely to be many benefits beyond choosing the appropriate health plan. Never have the practice patterns of health care providers been under such public scrutiny, though the overall level of care is likely to improve as a result of this monitoring and feedback.

## NUMBERS AND RATES

Population, health status, and utilization data all can be presented in two forms: numbers and rates. A *number* is simply a count of conditions, individuals, or events. A *rate* has two parts: a numerator and a denominator. The numerator is the number of conditions, individuals, or events counted. The denominator is (usually) a larger group of persons, conditions, or events from among which the subset described by the numerator data is drawn. For example, for 1997, the crude death rate for the United States was 8.6 per 1,000 population (U.S. Census Bureau [USCB], 1999, Table 130).

It is customary to present a rate as applying during a particular time period. For example, one could determine that 1,000 deaths occurred in a particular population during a year. This *number* of deaths would be the numerator of a *rate*. Let's say that the whole population in which those deaths occurred numbers 100,000 (the denominator). Then the mortality *rate* for that population is 1,000/100,000 per year. Then the rate per thousand (in this case, 10), or any other formulation that is useful, per year, can be calculated.

The magnitude of the denominator is usually chosen to make the rate a number of reasonable size with a numerator of one or higher. Thus, the less frequent the event being counted by the numerator, the larger the denominator needs to be. For example, crude death rates for a whole population, all causes, are usually given as per-thousand population. Cause-specific mortality rates are usually presented as per 100,000, or even as per 1,000,000 population, depending upon the frequency of the event to which the rate refers.

Both denominators and numerators can be quite specific, as can their units. For example, in describing deaths from lung cancer that are caused by cigarette smoking, an age/cause-specific rate could be the number of deaths per year from lung cancer in males over age 45 who have smoked 2 or more packs of cigarettes per day for 20 years or more (the numerator), divided by the number of *all* males over 45 who have smoked 2 or more packs of cigarettes per day for 20 years or more (the denominator). The units of the numerator and the denominator in health indices can also be different. For example, in cause-specific mortality rates, the unit for the numerator is deaths by cause, while the unit for the denominator is the total number of persons in the population being served.

Although rates are usually fractions (as in a crude death rate of 8.6 per 1,000), occasionally they will be whole numbers. For example, in measuring total morbidity in a population, one may find that the number of diagnosed disease conditions is greater than the number of people. The rate then is usually given with a denominator of 1, for example, "In the population of a central African city there are 2.5 diseases per person." This usage also occurs in utilization rates, for example, "The annual physician-visit rate in the United States is about 6 per person." Rates are especially useful for measuring and describing changes over time, in everything from deaths to per capita health care expenditures. It is important to keep in mind, however, that there are no hard and fast rules for data presentation, and it is always crucial to be aware of the size of the denominator.

Health service utilization rates constitute a special group of rates. Usually they do not have customary numerators and denominators. For example, hospital-specific admission rates are commonly presented simply as a number per unit of time, as follows: "In 1997, the admission rate for hospital Y was 1,000 per month." One reason for using this formulation is that the sizes of the populations served by both institutional and individual providers are generally not known. These data generally refer to events not to individuals, i.e., one patient can have multiple admissions.

Now let us consider certain classes of data in some detail.

## CENSUS DATA

### Numbers

The Constitution of the United States requires that a census of the nation be taken at least once every 10 years (U.S. Census Bureau [USCB], 2003, p. 1). The original purpose of the census was to provide the basis for the apportionment among the states of seats in the U.S. House of Representatives. A census has been carried out every 10 years since 1790. Although every effort is made for completeness, the Census Bureau has estimated that in 1990 it undercounted by between 1 and 2%, ranging from 5.0% for Hispanics through 4.4% for Blacks to 0.7% for non-Hispanics Whites (USCB, 1999, p. 1). The Census Bureau has not yet published a report on the accuracy of the 2000 census count, although the current estimate is a net national overcount of 1.3 million persons (New York City Department of City Planning, 2004).

In addition to carrying out the decennial censuses, the Census Bureau makes interim population estimates on various parameters, based on information gathered from samples and a variety of other sources. The estimated U.S. resident population is over 294 million (see U.S. Census Bureau: http://www.census.gov).

Births, deaths, immigration, and emigration are the four factors producing change in population size. During the 1970s and 1980s, the population growth rate in the U.S. averaged about 1.0% per year (USCB, 1999, Tables 2 and 4). During the 1960s the population had grown at the rate of about 1.3% per year. The decline in rate of growth resulted primarily from a decrease in the birth rate. It is projected that population growth will likely decline further, to 0.7% per year by 2050.

Nevertheless, the "mid-range" U.S. population size projection for that year is still about 420 million, an increase of about 49% over the 2000 population. Even without taking into account the accompanying changes in the age composition of a population growing ever older, as well as growing in size, the bearing of such factors as simple population size and growth rate on health services need and utilization is obvious.

### Demographic Characteristics

By 2000, 80.3% of the U.S. population lived in what are called *metropolitan statistical areas* (MSAs, variously referred to, with slightly different definitions, as standard metropolitan statistical areas [SMSAs] and consolidated metropolitan statistical areas [CMSAs]) (USCB, 2003, Table 25). The figures for 1960 and 1980 were 63% and 78%, respectively, suggesting an increasingly urban population. (The definitions of "metropolitan statistical area" and its variants have varied over time. See the current edition of the *Statistical Abstract of the United States* for the current definitions.)

As of 2002, it was estimated that the U.S. population was 49.1% male, 87.3% non-Black, and had a median age of 35.7 (34.4 for males, 37.0 for females), up considerably from 30 in 1980 (USCB, 2003, Tables 11 and 13). In 2002, 12.3% of the population was age 65 and over, an increase from 11.3% in 1980. In 2002, about 61% of males and 62% of females 18 and over were married, contrasting with 69% and 63%, respectively, in 1980 (USCB, 1999, Table 62 and USCB, 2003, Table 62). At the end of 2003, over 2 million Americans were imprisoned (U.S. Department of Justice).

During the next 50 years, the population is expected to age dramatically, which is likely to have a profound impact, not only on health and health care delivery in the United States, but on society itself. In 1995, there were 34 million people ages 65 and older representing 13% of the population. Mid-range projections for 2050 indicate that there will be 87 million people ages 65 and older, representing 20% (one fifth!) of the population. Within this group of older Americans, the proportion of those 85 and over is growing the fastest and is projected to more than double from nearly 4 million (1.4% of the population) in 1995 to over 8 million (2.3%) in 2025, then to more than double again in size to 21 million (5%) from 2025 to 2050. The effects on the need for health care and social services are likely to be staggering (USCB, 2003, Table 12).

Other realized and anticipated changes in the demographic composition of the United States are likely to have important but less dramatic effects. Educational attainment continues to rise, and in March 1995, 82% of adults ages 25 and over had completed at least high school and 23% had earned a bachelor's degree. Attainment varied by race/ethnicity, however, with 83% of Whites, 74% of Blacks, and 53% of Hispanics having at least a high school degree (USCB, 1997).

Another change that will affect the U.S. linguistically, culturally, and socially is the increase in the number and proportion of foreign born in the population. Foreign born declined from a high of 14.7% in 1910 to a low of 4.8% in 1970 and increased steadily to 9.7% of the total population in 1997—nearly one in ten. The majority were born in Latin America (50.7%), Asia (27.1%), and Europe (16.1%) (USBOC, 1997). Since the foreign born tend to live in central cities within a metropolitan area, cultural competence within health care delivery systems in these areas will be essential in the twenty-first century.

In addition to sources cited, the information presented so far in this chapter comes primarily from the "Population" section of the

*Statistical Abstract of the United States: 2003* (USCB). Additional information necessary to develop a comprehensive profile of the population is contained in the "Vital Statistics," "Education," "Social Insurance and Human Services," "Labor Force, Employment, and Earnings," and "Income Expenditures, and Wealth" sections of the same publication and on the U.S. Census Bureau Web site: (www.census.gov).

## VITAL STATISTICS

### What They Are and How They Are Collected

In public health, "vital statistics" include data on births, deaths, fetal deaths, marriages, and divorces available from the National Center for Health Statistics (NCHS). Birth and death data, in particular, are probably the most widely studied and reported on indicators of the health status of a community. In the United States, the state has the primary responsibility for collecting these data. In addition to the 50 states, the District of Columbia and New York City are independent vital registration areas. Vital registration systems are operated by the state government (or local for New York City and the District of Columbia) and are usually a function of the state department of health or its equivalent. These agencies in turn frequently delegate power to county or local health departments or local registrars to receive and process birth and death certificates. Not all states collect all categories of data although all states have collected birth and death data since 1933.

The first vital statistic to be collected in the United States on an annual basis was mortality. While there is no Constitutional requirement for states to participate, in 1900, 10 states and the District of Columbia voluntarily became the first "death registration states," carrying out that task and forwarding the results to the federal government. Beginning in 1915, 10 states and the District of Columbia formed a "birth registration area," collecting birth data on an annual basis. Fetal deaths have been counted annually since 1922. Since 1933, the birth and death registration area has included all of the states and the District of Columbia. A "marriage registration area" was first formed in 1957. By 1999, it included 42 states and the District of Columbia. The "divorce registration area" was established in 1958. By 1999, it covered 31 states and the Virgin Islands (USCB, 1999, p. 73).

Until 1946, the Census Bureau assembled and reported on vital statistics at the national level. From 1946 to 1960, the work was performed by the Bureau of State Services of the U.S. Public Health Service, but since 1960, the National Center for Health Statistics (NCHS), the Centers for Disease Control and Prevention (CDC), and the U.S. Department of Health and Human Services (USDHHS) have carried out this function. NCHS shares the costs incurred by the states in providing vital statistics data for national use. Through cooperative activities of the states and NCHS, standard forms for data collection and model procedures for the uniform registration of vital events are developed and recommended for state use. All states model their birth and death certificates after the U.S. standard certificates of live birth and death. Certified copies of birth and death certificates are legal documents: the original certificates remain on file with the state.

Although the process varies slightly from state to state, in general, the birth certificate is used to legally register births occurring in that state by collecting information on the newborn's name, date, time, and place of birth and the mother and father's name, address, date, and place of birth. This information is included on the copy of the birth certificate the state provides to the mother. A confidential portion of the original certificate filed by the hospital of birth contains extensive demographic and medical information on the mother and newborn, which may include a chronology of the birth, maternal medical (e.g., gestational diabetes) and behavioral (e.g., smoking) risk factors in the pregnancy, birth weight, abnormal conditions and congenital anomalies of the newborn. The hospital or other facility where the birth occurs is required to complete and file the birth certificate with the state. Thus, the health care system bears the actual responsibility for collecting and reporting birth data.

In a similar manner, death certificates are used to register every death in the state where it occurs. Although there is variation from state to state, the certificate collects extensive information about the decedent including date, time, and place of death; name, age, sex, race/ethnicity, birthplace, usual occupation, and marital status. The certificate also provides a format for reporting causes of death. Generally, a licensed physician must pronounce death and certify the cause. The conditions reported on the certificate are coded by the state health department through the use of a classification structure and selection and modification rules contained in the applicable revision of the International Classification of Diseases (ICD) published by the World Health Organization (WHO) (as discussed below). These coding rules provide a template for the international standardization of mortality data and improve its usefulness by systematically selecting a single cause of death from the reported sequence of conditions. The single cause selected through this procedure is called the *underlying cause of death*, while the combination of the underlying cause of death and all other causes listed on the certificate is designated the multiple causes of death. Unless otherwise specified, mortality statistics refer to the underlying cause of death. (See **FIGURE 2.2** for a copy of the U.S. Standard Certificate of Death.)

NCHS calculates the national vital statistics rates. The population denominators, both by total and by numerous demographic subgroups, are based on the actual number of persons counted by the Census Bureau on April 1 of each decennial year, as well as on the midyear estimates made for other years. As discussed above, the cause of death is classified according to the *International Classification of Diseases (ICD), 10th Revision, Adapted for Use in the United States* (NCHS, 1979a [www.cdc.gov/nchs/about/major/dvs/icd/des.htm]).[2]

## Natality

Natality data refer only to live births. In 2002, about 4 million births were registered in the United States, somewhat fewer than the 4.1 million births in 1990 (Sutton & Matthews, 2004). The birth rate was 13.9 per 1,000 population, the lowest rate ever recorded and well below the highest rate recorded in recent years, 16.7% in 1990. The birth rate has been steadily dropping from a post–World War II high of 25, reached in 1955, the peak of the so-called "baby boom" (Ventura, Martin, Curtain, Matthews, & Park, 2000).

The "fertility rate" is defined as the number of births per 1,000 women aged 15 to 44 (women of childbearing age). For 2002, it continued a downward trend to 64.8, down from the post–World War II high of 123 reached in 1957 (USCB, 1999, Table 93) (Sutton et al., 2004).

---

2 ICD classification is also used in other coding schemes. The ICD-10-Clinical Modification (ICD-10-CM) is an extension of the ICD-10 that is used to code and classify morbidity data from inpatient and outpatient records, physician offices, and most NCHS surveys. All hospitals in the U.S. receiving federal funds are required to use this classification system. ICD is revised periodically to incorporate changes in medicine: ICD-10 was implemented by NCHS on January 1, 1999. The most important effect of ICD revisions is a discontinuity of trends in causes of death. (See footnote 3.)

FIGURE 2.2

## U.S. Standard Certificate of Death

LOCAL FILE NO. STATE FILE NO.

NAME OF DECEDENT_______
For use by physician or institution

**To Be Completed/Verified By: FUNERAL DIRECTOR**

1. DECEDENT'S LEGAL NAME (Include AKA's if any) (First, Middle, Last)
2. SEX
3. SOCIAL SECURITY NUMBER
4a. AGE-Last Birthday (Years)
4b. UNDER 1 YEAR — Months / Days
4c. UNDER 1 DAY — Hours / Minutes
5. DATE OF BIRTH (Mo/Day/Yr)
6. BIRTHPLACE (City and State or Foreign Country)
7a. RESIDENCE-STATE
7b. COUNTY
7c. CITY OR TOWN
7d. STREET AND NUMBER
7e. APT. NO.
7f. ZIP CODE
7g. INSIDE CITY LIMITS? • Yes • No
8. EVER IN US ARMED FORCES? • Yes • No
9. MARITAL STATUS AT TIME OF DEATH • Married • Married, but separated • Widowed • Divorced • Never Married • Unknown
10. SURVIVING SPOUSE'S NAME (If wife, give name prior to first marriage)
11. FATHER'S NAME (First, Middle, Last)
12. MOTHER'S NAME PRIOR TO FIRST MARRIAGE (First, Middle, Last)
13a. INFORMANT'S NAME
13b. RELATIONSHIP TO DECEDENT
13c. MAILING ADDRESS (Street and Number, City, State, Zip Code)
14. PLACE OF DEATH (Check only one: see instructions)
IF DEATH OCCURRED IN A HOSPITAL: • Inpatient • Emergency Room/Outpatient • Dead on Arrival
IF DEATH OCCURRED SOMEWHERE OTHER THAN A HOSPITAL: • Hospice facility • Nursing home/Long term care facility • Decedent's home • Other (Specify):
15. FACILITY NAME (If not institution, give street & number)
16. CITY OR TOWN, STATE, AND ZIP CODE
17. COUNTY OF DEATH
18. METHOD OF DISPOSITION: • Burial • Cremation • Donation • Entombment • Removal from State • Other (Specify):
19. PLACE OF DISPOSITION (Name of cemetery, crematory, other place)
20. LOCATION-CITY, TOWN, AND STATE
21. NAME AND COMPLETE ADDRESS OF FUNERAL FACILITY
22. SIGNATURE OF FUNERAL SERVICE LICENSEE OR OTHER AGENT
23. LICENSE NUMBER (Of Licensee)

**To Be Completed By: MEDICAL CERTIFIER**

**ITEMS 24-28 MUST BE COMPLETED BY PERSON WHO PRONOUNCES OR CERTIFIES DEATH**
24. DATE PRONOUNCED DEAD (Mo/Day/Yr)
25. TIME PRONOUNCED DEAD
26. SIGNATURE OF PERSON PRONOUNCING DEATH (Only when applicable)
27. LICENSE NUMBER
28. DATE SIGNED (Mo/Day/Yr)
29. ACTUAL OR PRESUMED DATE OF DEATH (Mo/Day/Yr) (Spell Month)
30. ACTUAL OR PRESUMED TIME OF DEATH
31. WAS MEDICAL EXAMINER OR CORONER CONTACTED? • Yes • No

**CAUSE OF DEATH (See instructions and examples)**

32. **PART I.** Enter the chain of events--diseases, injuries, or complications--that directly caused the death. DO NOT enter terminal events such as cardiac arrest, respiratory arrest, or ventricular fibrillation without showing the etiology. DO NOT ABBREVIATE. Enter only one cause on a line. Add additional lines if necessary.

Approximate interval: Onset to death

IMMEDIATE CAUSE (Final disease or condition ------> resulting in death) a.____
Due to (or as a consequence of):
Sequentially list conditions, if any, leading to the cause listed on line a. Enter the **UNDERLYING CAUSE** (disease or injury that initiated the events resulting in death) **LAST** b.____
Due to (or as a consequence of):
c.____
Due to (or as a consequence of):
d.____

**PART II.** Enter other significant conditions contributing to death but not resulting in the underlying cause given in PART I.

33. WAS AN AUTOPSY PERFORMED? • Yes • No
34. WERE AUTOPSY FINDINGS AVAILABLE TO COMPLETE THE CAUSE OF DEATH? • Yes • No
35. DID TOBACCO USE CONTRIBUTE TO DEATH? • Yes • Probably • No • Unknown
36. IF FEMALE: • Not pregnant within past year • Pregnant at time of death • Not pregnant, but pregnant within 42 days of death • Not pregnant, but pregnant 43 days to 1 year before death • Unknown if pregnant within the past year
37. MANNER OF DEATH • Natural • Homicide • Accident • Pending Investigation • Suicide • Could not be determined
38. DATE OF INJURY (Mo/Day/Yr) (Spell Month)
39. TIME OF INJURY
40. PLACE OF INJURY (e.g., Decedent's home; construction site; restaurant; wooded area)
41. INJURY AT WORK? • Yes • No
42. LOCATION OF INJURY: State: City or Town: Street & Number: Apartment No.: Zip Code:
43. DESCRIBE HOW INJURY OCCURRED:
44. IF TRANSPORTATION INJURY, SPECIFY: • Driver/Operator • Passenger • Pedestrian • Other (Specify)
45. CERTIFIER (Check only one):
• Certifying physician-To the best of my knowledge, death occurred due to the cause(s) and manner stated.
• Pronouncing & Certifying physician-To the best of my knowledge, death occurred at the time, date, and place, and due to the cause(s) and manner stated.
• Medical Examiner/Coroner-On the basis of examination, and/or investigation, in my opinion, death occurred at the time, date, and place, and due to the cause(s) and manner stated.
Signature of certifier:____
46. NAME, ADDRESS, AND ZIP CODE OF PERSON COMPLETING CAUSE OF DEATH (Item 32)
47. TITLE OF CERTIFIER
48. LICENSE NUMBER
49. DATE CERTIFIED (Mo/Day/Yr)
50. **FOR REGISTRAR ONLY**- DATE FILED (Mo/Day/Yr)

**To Be Completed By: FUNERAL DIRECTOR**

51. DECEDENT'S EDUCATION-Check the box that best describes the highest degree or level of school completed at the time of death.
• 8th grade or less
• 9th - 12th grade; no diploma
• High school graduate or GED completed
• Some college credit, but no degree
• Associate degree (e.g., AA, AS)
• Bachelor's degree (e.g., BA, AB, BS)
• Master's degree (e.g., MA, MS, MEng, MEd, MSW, MBA)
• Doctorate (e.g., PhD, EdD) or Professional degree (e.g., MD, DDS, DVM, LLB, JD)

52. DECEDENT OF HISPANIC ORIGIN? Check the box that best describes whether the decedent is Spanish/Hispanic/Latino. Check the "No" box if decedent is not Spanish/Hispanic/Latino.
• No, not Spanish/Hispanic/Latino
• Yes, Mexican, Mexican American, Chicano
• Yes, Puerto Rican
• Yes, Cuban
• Yes, other Spanish/Hispanic/Latino (Specify)____

53. DECEDENT'S RACE (Check one or more races to indicate what the decedent considered himself or herself to be)
• White
• Black or African American
• American Indian or Alaska Native (Name of the enrolled or principal tribe)____
• Asian Indian
• Chinese
• Filipino
• Japanese
• Korean
• Vietnamese
• Other Asian (Specify)____
• Native Hawaiian
• Guamanian or Chamorro
• Samoan
• Other Pacific Islander (Specify)____
• Other (Specify)____

54. DECEDENT'S USUAL OCCUPATION (Indicate type of work done during most of working life. DO NOT USE RETIRED).
55. KIND OF BUSINESS/INDUSTRY

SOURCES : The Centers for Disease Control and Prevention, National Center for Health Statistics. http://www.cdc.gov/nchs/data/dvs/DEATH11-03final-ACC.pdf

## Mortality

### Crude Death Rates

Mortality data are reported rather neatly. Death is a well-defined event. As noted, there is one primary reporting authority for deaths, usually the local health department or registrar. Since both hospitals and funeral directors are legally required to report all deaths, we can assume that almost all deaths are reported.

For 2002, the crude death rate (total deaths per 100,000 population) in the United States was 848.9 (Kochanek & Smith, 2004), essentially the same as the 2001 rate. There were about 2.5 million deaths in each of the two years. Mortality varies considerably by age and sex. It is relatively high during the first year of life, drops by increasing age group to a relatively low level until the mid-40s, and then begins to climb again (USCB, 1999, Tables 129 and 131). Males have a higher mortality rate than females, at all ages. Data on differential death rates by the basic demographic variables of age, ethnicity, and sex can be found in the *National Vital Statistics Reports, Vital Statistics of the United States*, special studies published in the NCHS publication *Vital and Health Statistics*, Series 20, as well as the *Statistical Abstract* (again, refer to Appendix B).

### Age-Adjusted Death Rates

In addition to crude death rates, age-adjusted (standardized) death rates are also commonly used to compare relative mortality risk across groups over time. These constructed rates eliminate variability due to differences in the age composition of various populations. Differences in age composition may have a large impact on the crude rate because of the widely differing mortality rates experienced by different age groups. Statistically, an age-adjusted death rate is a weighted average of the age-specific death rates in which the weights are fixed population proportions by age. For the past 50 years, the existing standard was based on the 1940 U.S. population, but beginning with the 1999 death data, a new standard, based on the year 2000 population, was put in place (Anderson & Rosenberg, 1998). This change was made because the age composition of the 1940 population no longer reflects the increasing proportion of the U.S. population in the older age groups with higher death rates.

Although the discussion of crude versus age-adjusted death rates may appear to be of interest only to statisticians, the following example will help to illustrate the kinds of interpretation errors that can be made when mortality data are viewed by only one measure. The crude death rate for the U.S. *rose* 3.2% from 852.2 per 100,000 population in 1979 to 880.0 in 1995. In contrast, during this time period, the age-adjusted death rate *dropped* 12.7% from 577.0 per 100,000 U.S. standard population (1940) to 503.9, showing that the increase in the crude rate was due to the increasing proportion of the population in older age groups with higher death rates, not to a higher death rate by age group (Anderson & Rosenberg, 1998).

## Disease-Specific Mortality

Disease-specific causes of death are used to monitor prevention and treatment practices and programs. Determination of the disease-specific cause of death in a given case can present some problems. In most cases it is the responsibility of a physician to certify that a patient is dead and to determine the underlying cause of death. However, physicians have varying diagnostic styles, perspectives, and abilities and may have little or no first hand knowledge of the patient's medical history. Furthermore, there have been changes in the medical understanding and technical definitions of causes of death over time.[3] As an example of the potential difficulty, consider the following question: In a patient who dies from a heart attack that resulted from the complications of diabetes, is the cause of death diabetes or coronary artery disease? It is up to the physician to determine the immediate cause of death (most would say heart attack) and then to sequentially list conditions leading to the immediate cause, entering the underlying cause (disease or injury) that initiated the chain of events leading to death last. Ultimately, physicians are responsible for cause of death coding. Most physicians follow NCHS coding instructions but some do not.

In 2002, the 10 leading causes of death by disease-specific diagnostic category were heart disease, cancer, stroke, chronic obstructive pulmonary disease, accidents (unintentional injuries), diabetes mellitus, influenza and pneumonia, Alzheimer's disease, kidney disease, and septicemia (infection of the blood stream) (Kochanek et al., 2004). With a few notable exceptions, the leading causes were similar in 1990: The top three, heart disease, cancer and stroke, remained the same followed by personal injury, chronic obstructive pulmonary disease, pneumonia and influenza, diabetes

---

3 For a detailed discussion of this problem, see "Estimates of Selected Comparability Ratios Based on Dual Coding of 1976 Death Certificates by the eighth and ninth revisions of the International Classification of Diseases," Monthly Vital Statistics Report, 28(11), (Suppl.) February 1980.

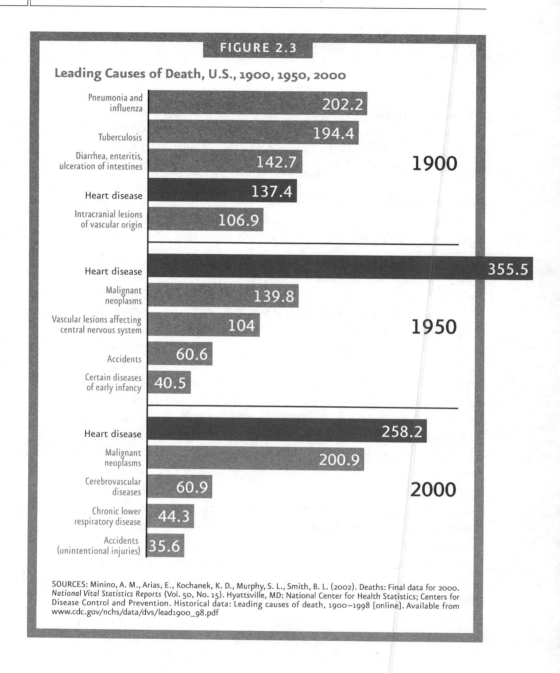

FIGURE 2.3

Leading Causes of Death, U.S., 1900, 1950, 2000

**1900**

| Cause | Value |
|---|---|
| Pneumonia and influenza | 202.2 |
| Tuberculosis | 194.4 |
| Diarrhea, enteritis, ulceration of intestines | 142.7 |
| Heart disease | 137.4 |
| Intracranial lesions of vascular origin | 106.9 |

**1950**

| Cause | Value |
|---|---|
| Heart disease | 355.5 |
| Malignant neoplasms | 139.8 |
| Vascular lesions affecting central nervous system | 104 |
| Accidents | 60.6 |
| Certain diseases of early infancy | 40.5 |

**2000**

| Cause | Value |
|---|---|
| Heart disease | 258.2 |
| Malignant neoplasms | 200.9 |
| Cerebrovascular diseases | 60.9 |
| Chronic lower respiratory disease | 44.3 |
| Accidents (unintentional injuries) | 35.6 |

SOURCES: Minino, A. M., Arias, E., Kochanek, K. D., Murphy, S. L., Smith, B. L. (2002). Deaths: Final data for 2000. *National Vital Statistics Reports* (Vol. 50, No. 15). Hyattsville, MD: National Center for Health Statistics; Centers for Disease Control and Prevention. Historical data: Leading causes of death, 1900–1998 [online]. Available from www.cdc.gov/nchs/data/dvs/lead1900_98.pdf

mellitus, suicide, liver disease, and other infectious and parasitic diseases (predominantly human immunodeficiency virus and AIDS) (USCB, 1999, Table 137). FIGURE 2.3 illustrates the changing causes of death since 1900. Heart disease is the only cause that has been in the top five since 1900.

Most changes in the leading causes of death occur gradually but there have been several important changes in the past decade. AIDS no longer appears because of the dramatic decline in deaths due to AIDS following the introduction of effective therapy in 1996. Alzheimer's disease, on the other hand, unexpectedly appeared as a leading cause of death in 1999. Over 10,000 additional deaths were attributed to this cause in 1999 compared to 1998, suggesting an "epidemic." A closer examination of the data, however, shows that the increase in these deaths resulted from reclassifying deaths due to presenile dementia from being a separate category in the ICD-9 to inclusion with Alzheimer's disease in the ICD-10 (Anderson, Minino, Hoyert, & Rosenberg, 2001). This illustrates once again how easy it is to make a serious mistake in data interpretation in the absence of a thorough understanding of the database used.

### Risk Factor-Specific Mortality

In the United States today, most deaths are caused by chronic diseases or conditions (such as personal injury) in which environmental and personal risk factors play a major causative role. To make the mortality data picture more useful for understanding what is truly going on in matters of health status and for program planning, McGinnis and Foege (1993) took a different approach to characterizing the causes of death in the United States.

They went beyond the classic lists of death-associated, disease-specific diagnoses to the identification of the major external (non-genetic) factors known to be causally associated with death. After an exhaustive review of the literature covering the period 1977–1993, McGinnis and Foege attributed approximately half of all deaths occurring in 1990 to the following 10 risk factors: tobacco use (400,000 deaths annually), diet and activity patterns (300,000), alcohol use (100,000), microbial agents (90,000), toxic agents (60,000), firearms (35,000), sexual behaviors (30,000), motor vehicle use (25,000), and use of "illicit drugs," primarily heroin and cocaine (20,000).

Using a method similar to that pioneered by McGinnis and Foege, investigators from the Centers for Disease Control and Prevention identified the actual causes of death in the U.S. in 2000. While smoking remained the leading cause of mortality at 18.1% of all deaths, poor diet and lack of physical activity were a close second at 16.6% and may soon overtake smoking as the leading cause of death (Mokdad, Stroup, & Gerberding, 2004).

The picture arising from these analyses is particularly helpful in planning public health programs to prolong life, especially healthy life. Using it, one can focus on changeable/modifiable human behaviors, for example, cigarette smoking, eating patterns, and physical activity rather than on classic, disease-specific prevention for such conditions as heart disease, cancer, and stroke, treatment for hypertension. The former, focusing on lifestyle change, have even more potential to reduce mortality than do the latter, which treat diseases or conditions that have already developed (McGinnis & Foege, 1993).

### Infant Mortality

The infant mortality rate is the number of deaths under the age of one year among children born alive, divided by the number of live births in that year. A nation's infant mortality rate is related to a variety of socioeconomic, environmental, and health care factors and is considered a fairly sensitive indicator of general health levels in a population. In 2001, the infant mortality rate in the United States was 6.8 per 1,000 live births, the lowest ever recorded in the United States (Matthews, Menacker, & MacDorman, 2003). The rate has been declining steadily since 1940, when it was 47. In fact, the infant mortality rate has been falling since it was first recorded in this country at 99.9 in 1915 (Grove & Hetzel, 1968, Table 38).

The most striking feature of the U.S. infant mortality rate is that while it has consistently declined over the years, the rate for Blacks has consistently remained about double the rate for Whites (USCB, 1999, Table 133). Detailed examinations of the relationships among ethnicity, other factors, and infant mortality are contained in *Vital and Health Statistics* (NCHS, 1992).

### Marriage and Divorce

In 2003 the marriage rate stood at 7.5 per 1,000 population (Munson & Sutton, 2004), down from 10.6 in 1980 (USCB, 1999, Table 155). The divorce rate, which was at a high of 5.2 per 1,000 population in 1980 (USCB, 1999, Table 155), was down to 3.8 in 2003 (Munson & Sutton, 2004). Both the marriage and divorce rates have dropped over time (phenomena that may be related). Current detailed analyses of birth, marriage, and divorce statistics can be found in the *Vital and Health Statistics* Series 23, "Data from the National Survey of Family Growth," as well as in the *National Vital Statistics Reports*.

# MORBIDITY

## Definitions

Morbidity refers to sickness and disease. Like mortality, morbidity data can be expressed in both numbers and rates. Like other data, morbidity data can be cross-tabulated with the broad range of demographic characteristics. Morbidity data are extremely important in characterizing the health status of a population. Since many widely prevalent diseases and conditions of ill health do not appear in mortality figures, by themselves, the latter are not adequate for health status characterization. This is particularly so in a country like the United States, in which communicable diseases, with a few notable exceptions such as AIDS, pneumonia, and influenza, are major causes of morbidity but not mortality.

Morbidity data can be reported in terms of both incidence and prevalence. Incidence is the number of new cases of the disease in question occurring during a particular time period, usually a year. For example, in 2002 there were about 42,000 new cases of AIDS reported in the United States (Centers for Disease Control and Prevention [CDC], 2004). Prevalence is the total number of cases existing in a population during a time period, or at one point in time (in which case it is known as point-prevalence). For example, in 2002, the estimated total number of cases of AIDS (both living and dead) reported in the United States since the first known case-report was made, was 857,516 (CDC, 2004). The prevalence of living AIDS cases in 2002 was 384,906.

The list of significant nonfatal causes of ill health in the United States includes: arthritis, low-back pain, the common cold, influenza, nonfatal injuries, dermatitis, and mild emotional and sexual problems (NCHS, 1999a, p. 5). There are other diseases that may kill but do so rarely in relation to their prevalence. Included in this category are sexually transmitted diseases (STD) other than AIDS; duodenal ulcer, and gall bladder disease. Morbidity data highlight not only the important diseases and the patterns of their distribution in the population but also illustrate disease-related limitations of activity.

Counting and reporting morbidity are not nearly as simple as reporting mortality; however, consider the following questions. What is meant by the term "sickness," and just when is a person "sick"? Who decides? The physician? The patient? Furthermore, while state law requires that all deaths be reported, only one category of sickness, the infectious diseases, are reportable in every state.

Until the advent of antibiotics and vaccines, death and disability caused by infectious diseases posed the greatest risk to the U.S. population. After several decades of complacency, the emergence of new threats (e.g., AIDS, hantavirus, *E. coli* 0157:H7, Hepatitis C) and the resurgence of old threats (e.g., tuberculosis) together with concerns about pathogen resistance to antibiotics and the risk of bioterrorism have reignited interest in and funding for infectious disease surveillance.

As of December 31, 2002, more than 50 infectious diseases were designated as notifiable at the national level. "A notifiable disease is one for which regular, frequent, and timely information regarding individual cases is considered necessary for the prevention and control of the disease" (CDC, 2002, p. 2). States voluntarily report cases, and the incidence of infectious diseases appears in a weekly publication of the Centers for Disease Control and Prevention of the United States Public Health Service, called the *Morbidity and Mortality Weekly Report*. An annual summary of notifiable diseases in the U.S., and individual disease (AIDS) and disease category summaries (e.g., sexually transmitted diseases), are also published by the CDC.

Surveillance for infectious diseases is both passive (health departments wait for reports from physicians) and active (laboratory logs and hospital and clinic charts are routinely reviewed for new cases) for more serious diseases like AIDS. In general, however, surveillance relies on physicians, and it is well known that some physicians fail to report certain diseases, even when legally required to do so. There are many reasons why physicians fail to report, including the time it takes to complete the required paperwork. Some physicians will not report sexually transmitted diseases in private patients, on the grounds of "avoiding embarrassment." Physicians may not report tuberculosis because of possible economic consequences for the patient in terms of maintaining employment. Many physicians fail to report cases of common childhood viral infections because these infections are considered "inconsequential," even though they may have serious sequelae and may signal incomplete coverage by immunization programs.

Surveillance for several classes of infectious diseases (tuberculosis, sexually transmitted diseases, and AIDS), which involves reporting individual cases by name to local and state health departments, generated considerable controversy during the twentieth century. An intense debate surrounding named reporting of HIV infection continues today, fueled by fear of discrimination and the potential for breaches of confidentiality (Bayer & Fairchild, 2000). This debate highlights the importance of privacy and confidentiality protections for all surveillance systems, in particular, and medical records in general. Although most surveillance systems are protected by state law, and the names of individuals with infectious diseases are retained by the state and not included in reports sent to federal agencies, many people support federal regulation of surveillance systems.

Other diseases, events, and conditions of public health significance are reportable in at least some states, including, among others, cancer, injuries, lead poisoning, childhood asthma, and congenital malformations. In recognition of cancer's rank as the second leading cause of death in the United States, Congress responded to the need for cancer surveillance by establishing the National Program of Cancer Registries in 1992 (Cancer Registries Amendment Act, Public Law 102–515), which provides support to either enhance existing registries or to implement them in 45 states, 3 territories, and the District of Columbia. There are, however, no mandatory reporting requirements for many disease categories that are equally important, such as heart disease, diabetes, and stroke, to say nothing of very common, sometimes crippling but usually nonfatal conditions like arthritis and osteoporosis, as well as such negative health conditions as sedentary lifestyle, obesity, and cigarette smoking.

## Data on Morbidity and Mortality

Turning to the data itself, for mortality there is only one possible source—and it isn't the patient. For morbidity, it is obvious that both providers and patients can be data sources and, as a result, quite different pictures of the same reality can be obtained. Providers can report morbidity by diagnostic categories and by patient chief complaints—that is, what the patient reports to the physician as being the problem.

However, most patients don't usually come to a physician saying "I think I've got diabetes mellitus, Doctor," but rather something like, "Doctor, I've been feeling kind of weak, I'm drinking a great deal of water and urinating a lot. Do you think maybe something's wrong?" It is up to the physician to characterize the problem and make a diagnosis that he or she then can report. Patients can also report chief complaints directly to data gatherers, as in a population survey.

A partial picture of morbidity patterns can be drawn from a chief complaint profile for a population obtained from either source. One advantage of deriving information directly from a population sample is that certain people with certain types of illnesses will never come to medical attention. Thus, morbidity surveys that gather information only from providers will not give a complete picture.

In the United States, morbidity data are published on a regular basis by the National Center for Health Statistics (NCHS) and, as noted, for the reportable communicable diseases, the Centers for Disease Control and Prevention (in the *Morbidity and Mortality Weekly Report*). From the NCHS, the data sources include the National Health and Nutrition Examination Survey (NHANES), the National Health Interview Survey (NHIS), the National Hospital Discharge Survey (NHDS), the National Ambulatory Medical Care Survey (NAMCS), and the National Hospital Ambulatory Medical Care Survey (NHAMCS).

The results of these surveys are published periodically in both *Vital and Health Statistics* and *Advance Data*. Together these activities constitute the National Health Care Survey (NHCS). Series 1 of *Vital and Health Statistics* contains the general methodological and historical accounts of the whole endeavor. Detailed descriptions of all the surveys can be found in Appendix I of *Health, United States 1999* (NCHS, 1999b).

Considering some examples of morbidity data, in 1996 the incidence of acute conditions was 164 per 100 persons per year, down a bit from 174 per 100 in 1995 (NCHS, 1999a, p. 3). Most common were respiratory conditions, including the common cold and influenza (79 per 100), injuries (22 per 100), infective and parasitic diseases (21 per 100), and digestive system conditions (6.7 per 100).

Persons sought medical attention for these conditions about two thirds of the time. Acute conditions were associated with about 624 days of restricted activity per 100 persons per year, leading to about 272 days in bed due to illness and 297 school-loss days per 100 persons 5–17 years of age, and for persons 18 and over, about 284 work-loss days per 100.

About 14.4% of the population experienced limitation in all activity due to chronic conditions (NCHS, 1999a, p. 5). The major chronic conditions causing limitations in activity in 1996 were (in descending order of frequency) arthritis, sinusitis, deformity or orthopedic impairment, hypertension, and hay fever or allergic rhinitis, hearing impairment, and heart disease (NCHS, 1999a, p. 4).

An example of provider-perspective data, the National Hospital Discharge Survey (NHDS) reports on hospital utilization by age and sex of patients, their lengths of stay, and their diagnoses and surgical and nonsurgical procedures, which afford a rather accurate illness profile of hospitalized patients (Hall & DeFrances, 2003). It must be remembered, however, that the overwhelming majority of ill persons do not require hospitalization. Thus, the morbidity profile of the population as a whole does not match that seen in hospitals. The results of the NHDS are published in *Vital and Health Statistics*, Series 13, and in *Advance Data* from *Vital and Health Statistics*, published on an irregular basis. Selected results are also published periodically in *Health, United States*.

The National Ambulatory Medical Care Survey (NCHS, 1974a, 1974b) was developed in the 1970s as a component of the National Health Survey. It is a continuing survey of private, nonfederally employed, office-based physicians practicing in the United States (Cherry, Burt, & Woodwell, 2003). The data are collected using a stratified random sample of all office-based physicians (both allopathic and osteopathic) in the contiguous United States, excluding anesthesiologists, pathologists, radiologists, and physicians engaged primarily in teaching, research, and administration. In the early 1990s, these data were being reported primarily by physician specialty.

In the NAMCS, morbidity data are collected from both the patient's and the physician's perspectives. For example, in 2001 the five leading groups of symptoms causing patients to come to a physician's office were referable to the musculoskeletal system; respiratory system; eyes and ears; skin, hair and nails; and genitourinary system (Cherry et al., 2003, Table 8). The seven leading physician's diagnoses were essential hypertension; arthropathies (joint problems); acute upper respiratory infections, excluding pharyngitis; diabetes mellitus; spinal disorders; rheumatism, excluding back; and normal pregnancy (Cherry et al., Table 13).

## HEALTH STATUS AND HEALTH-RELATED BEHAVIORS

In 1979, the Office of the Assistant Secretary for Health (OASH) of the U.S. Department of Health and Human Services published the first national health status report, *Healthy People: The Surgeon General's Report on Health Promotion and Disease Prevention* (OASH). Subsequently, the Office of Disease Prevention and Health Promotion (ODPHP), part of OASH, published *Promoting Health and Preventing Disease: Objectives for the Nation* (ODPHP, 1980, 1986). In it, 216 objectives were established for dealing with 15 major diseases and conditions that can be prevented using existing knowledge and techniques.

The 15 major diseases and conditions were grouped into three sets of five; conditions were grouped according to the appropriate prevention strategy. For example, high blood pressure and sexually transmitted diseases were grouped in "Preventive Health Services"; such problems as toxic agent control and occupational safety and health were in "Health Protective Services"; and such conditions as cigarette smoking and sedentary lifestyle were grouped in "Health Promotion Programs."

In 1991, the U.S. Public Health Service (USPHS) published the next comprehensive update for the program *Healthy People 2000*, in which three broad goals were identified that focus on increasing the span of healthy life, reducing health disparities, and achieving access to preventive services for everyone In 1995, the *Healthy People 2000: Midcourse Review* was published (USDHHS), and the project expanded its scope to set National Health Promotion and Disease Prevention Objectives for dealing with 22 diseases, conditions, and health-related behaviors (and the means for tracking them) (USDHHS, 1995, Appendix A), including physical activity and fitness, nutrition, tobacco use, substance abuse (alcohol and other drugs), family planning, mental health and mental disorders, violent and abusive behavior, educational and community-based programs, unintentional injuries, occupational safety and health, environmental health, food and drug safety, oral health, maternal and infant health, heart disease and stroke, cancer, diabetes and chronic disabling conditions, HIV infection, sexually transmitted diseases, immunization and infectious diseases, clinically preventive services, and surveillance and data systems. Objectives were also established for educational and community-based programs, clinical preventive services, and surveillance and data systems. For the 22 designated areas, a total of 520 objectives and subobjectives were established.

Then in 2000, the next decennial iteration, *Healthy People 2010* (USDHHS), appeared, which is designed to achieve two overarch-

ing goals: increase the quality and years of healthy life; and eliminate health disparities by gender, race/ethnicity, income and education, disability, geography, and sexual orientation. The 2010
objectives were consolidated from 520 to 467 and are being tracked
by 190 data sources.

In support of the "Healthy People" efforts, beginning in 1985 the
National Center for Health Statistics carried out a Health Promo-
tion/Disease Prevention (HPDP) Survey as part of the ongoing NHIS
(NCHS, 1988). The HPDP Survey was repeated in 1990 and 1995 and
subsequently questions have been incorporated into the NHIS and
other surveys. Results are published in *Vital and Health Statistics
Series 10, Advance Data*, and the *Morbidity and Mortality Weekly Report*
(reporting data from the related Behavioral Risk Factor Surveillance System).

Key findings of the survey show that, as of 1995, 24.7% of persons
18 or older regularly smoked cigarettes, about 19% of persons
between 20 and 74 years of age had an elevated serum cholesterol,
about 23% of persons had hypertension, close to 35% of the population between 20 and 74 could be classified as overweight, and as of
1990, of the 72% of men and 51% of women who drank alcohol, 13.6%
of the men and 3.4% of the women could be classified as "heavier"
drinkers (NCHS, 1999b, Tables 61–71). Note that this "risk factor"
approach to morbidity has much in common with the McGinnis-
Foege approach to classification of actual causes of death.

Since data from national surveys generally cannot be analyzed
by state, all states and the District of Columbia began participating in the Behavioral Risk Factor Surveillance System (BRFSS) in
1994. These telephone surveys monitor the state-level prevalence
of personal health behaviors like smoking that play a major role in
premature morbidity and mortality. Data from BRFSS and the
Youth Risk Behavior Surveillance System (YRBS), which samples
high school students, complement the data from the NHIS. The
National Center for Chronic Disease Prevention and Health Promotion at the CDC is responsible for the BRFSS and YRBS. (See USD-
HHS, *Healthy People 2010*, Vol. 2, for a complete discussion of data
sources used for tracking their progress.)

# UTILIZATION OF HEALTH CARE SERVICES

## Introduction

We come now to the third quantitative perspective for viewing a population in terms of health and ill health: how the population utilizes the health care delivery system. We have pointed out that in quantifying the utilization of health services, the same series of events can be counted from either the patient's or the provider's perspective. The results of the two types of counts are not always the same. Thus, when discussing utilization one has to be careful to distinguish between the two approaches.

It should be noted that reliable utilization data is regularly reported primarily for services provided by licensed M.D.s and D.O.s (doctors of osteopathic medicine) in licensed allopathic (M.D. staffed) and osteopathic hospitals, and by licensed dentists. In the United States there is an unknown amount of "alternative therapy" provided by such healing disciplines as chiropractic, naturopathy, homeopathy, acupuncture/acupressure therapy and its variants, and by other "holistic health practitioners." These practitioners do not report utilization, they are not surveyed, and payment for much of their service is only sporadically reimbursed by insurance companies.

However, while regular utilization statistics are not collected, a one-time sampling survey estimated that over 40% of all adults in the U.S. use at least one alternative therapy, with an average annual visit rate among users of 7.6 (Eisenberg et al., 1998). In 1997, as in 1990, there were more visits made to alternative therapists (629 million) than to primary care physicians (485 million).

## Ambulatory Services

As we have noted, the NHIS provides patient-perspective data for the utilization of ambulatory services. According to the NHIS, in 1996 there were about 5.9 physician contacts per person (NCHS, 1999a, Table 71). Of these, about 54% took place in a physician's office, 12% in a hospital (primarily in the outpatient department including the emergency department), 12% on the telephone, with the balance at home and in other locations. Females averaged 6.9 visits per year, while males averaged 5.2. Whites averaged 6.1 visits, while Blacks averaged 5.4. Persons in families with an annual income of $10,000 or less averaged 8.4 visits per year, while persons in families with an annual income of $35,000 or more averaged 5.4

visits per year. Persons in the Southern geographic region averaged the most visits, 6.3. All of these numbers were down somewhat from 1994.

There are several sources of provider data on the utilization of ambulatory services. The most comprehensive one is the National Ambulatory Medical Care Survey, described briefly above, which is reported upon most commonly in *Advance Data*. In addition to morbidity data, the NAMCS provides data on visits by age, race, sex, geographic region, metropolitan/nonmetropolitan living area, type of physician, and duration of visit. The other major source of provider perspective ambulatory service utilization data is the American Hospital Association's (AHA) annual publication *Hospital Statistics*, published each summer. It reports hospital clinic and emergency department visits by such variables as number of beds, ownership, type, geographical region, and medical school affiliation.

## Utilization of Hospital In-Patient Services

Turning to utilization of hospital in-patient services, from the patient-perspective the National Health Interview Survey reported that in 1996 there were about 26.8 million discharges from short-stay hospitals, including about 3.5 million deliveries (down from 31.1 million discharges in 1991). These patients used about 142 million in-patient days of care with an average length of stay of 5.9 days (down from 199 million days in 1991) (NCHS, 1999a, Table 77). Other classes of data provided by the NHIS are utilization according to various hospital characteristics, morbidity (discussed previously), and an analysis of surgery.

The NCHS also provides provider-perspective hospital utilization data through the National Hospital Discharge Survey (*Advance Data*). The NCHS points out that because of "differences in collection procedures, population sampled, and definitions," the results from the NHIS and the NHDS are not entirely consistent (NCHS, 1979b, p. 1, and footnotes, NCHS, 1999b, Tables 89 and 90). For example, for 1996, the NHIS reported significantly fewer discharges from short-stay hospitals than did the NHDS: 82.4 per 1,000 population for the former compared with 102.3 per 1,000 for the latter (NCHS, 1999b, Tables 8 and 90).

Hospital utilization data are also published in the AHA's *Hospital Statistics*. For AHA-registered hospitals, it presents much data on bed size, admissions, occupancy rate, average daily census, and fiscal parameters, according to hospital type, size, ownership, and geographical location. Certain provider-perspective hospital utilization data also appear in *Health, United States*.

Data are also available on the quality of health care utilization events. The most widely used measures are the NCQA HEDIS clinical measures that focus on some of the nation's most serious and prevalent diseases and conditions. In addition, patient outcomes, including survival, can be measured for specific medical procedures. For example, New York State has taken a leadership role in setting standards for cardiac surgery services, monitoring outcomes and sharing performance data with patients hospitals and physicians (New York State Department of Health, 2000). Mortality rates have plummeted since the publication of the first survey in 1989.

## CONCLUSIONS

As we have seen in this chapter, an abundance of data concerning the U.S. population, its health, and how it uses the health care delivery system are collected and published in print and available on the Internet. Such ready access to data from multiple sources should not lull the reader into a less critical approach to using and interpreting these data. The reliability of the source of the data together with data collection methods must always be assessed. Additionally, although data sources may be reliable, not all data are consistent with one another as noted in the previous discussion of the differing hospital utilization rates obtained by NHIS and NHDS. This lack of consistency results in part from a lack of coordination of data collection efforts: even such seemingly standard information as race/ethnicity is recorded in different ways on different surveys and administrative data bases. Furthermore, there is the obvious gap between the provider-perspective and the patient-perspective on the counts, content, and quality of events.

There have been criticisms of the federal statistical collection, reporting, and analysis systems over a period of many years. A 1979 study by the Office of Technology Assessment [OTA] found "federal data collection activities . . . to be overlapping, fragmented, and often duplicative" (p. iii).[4] In brief, the report recommended that

---

4 This report will still be valuable to students of the federal data system and its users. It not only described data collection activities and the way they were organized and supervised, but also presented and analyzed all of the statutory authorities that establish those existing at the time (which happens to be almost all of those still in use).

a "strengthened coordinating and planning unit within HHS" be
established that "would embody three basic characteristics: sufficient authority to impose decisions on agencies; the necessary statistical and analytical capabilities to conduct activities requiring
technical expertise and judgement; and adequate resources to build
a viable core effort" (OTA, p. 55).

The USDHHS Data Council (http://aspe.hhs.gov/datacncl/index.
htm), established in 1995, is the current iteration of a department-
wide information systems committee. Not only does its charge
embody the recommendations of the 1979 OTA report, but it has
been expanded to encompass electronic information policy including data standards, privacy, telemedicine, and enhanced health
information for consumers.

Near universal access to the Internet and the widespread availability of high-speed computing capabilities have made the Council's tasks more difficult in some areas and easier in others. The
electronic information advances of the 1990s have greatly improved
communication at all levels and expanded access to databases and
the capacity to link multiple databases. This has been a boon to
health planners and researchers but has raised serious public concerns about protecting the privacy of health-related information.
In response to these concerns, Congress passed the Health Insurance Portability and Accountability Act (HIPPA) of 1996 (P. L.
104–191), the administrative simplification provisions of which will
ultimately reshape the way the health care industry collects,
processes, stores, protects and exchanges patient records. For the
first time, national standards are mandated to protect the privacy
of personal health records and common standards are set for electronic transmission of patient information within the health care
industry. Implementation by the USDHHS Data Council occurred
in 2001, with full compliance required by April 14, 2003.

Privacy concerns are likely to hold center stage among the many
policy issues related to data collection and use, but other issues of
importance include the utility and application of clinical trials
methodology to the study of health outcomes; health services malpractice and malpractice litigation; technological and ethical matters arising from the use of electronic data collection and analysis;
the relationship between data collected and data actually used; the
decision-making process governing what is counted and what data
are disseminated; cost/benefit analysis of health services interventions; government data collection requirements, utilization

## CASE STUDY

As Director of Human Resources for a large private university, you would like to tell the President what the University is getting for the money it spends on health services for its employees and their dependents. Right now you receive only the total dollar amount spent on claims each month. What other kinds of information about theses claims would you ask the health insurance companies to provide you, and why do you suppose the University doesn't get such information now?

and costs; the impact of the Internet on health data requirements and availability; what to do when we have too much or too little data; and what is changing and will change about health care data collection, publication, and analysis.

There will always be gaps in our data collection systems. Nevertheless, we know a great deal about health, disease, and illness in the United States, and about the functioning of the U.S. health care delivery system. Further, given whatever problems there may or may not be with the available health and health care data, we need to remember above all that data mean little unless they are put to proper use.

## DISCUSSION QUESTIONS

1. What are the uses of health data?
2. What are the uses of health services data?
3. How do health and health services data relate to each other?
4. How should data be used in the health and health services planning process?
5. What are the similarities and differences between disease-specific and risk-factor-specific health and illness data?
6. What impact has the Internet had on health and health services data utilization and dissemination in the United States?

# REFERENCES

Anderson, R. N., & Rosenberg, H. M. (1998). Age standardization of death rates: Implementation of the year 2000 standard. *National Vital Statistics Reports* (Vol. 47, No. 3). Hyattsville, MD: National Center for Health Statistics.

Anderson, R. N., Minino, A. M., Hoyert, D. L., & Rosenberg, H. M. (2001). Comparability of cause of death between ICD-9 and ICD-10: Preliminary estimates. *National Vital Statistics Reports* (Vol. 49, No. 2). Hyattsville, MD: National Center for Health Statistics.

Bayer, R., & Fairchild, A. L. (2000). Surveillance and privacy. *Science, 290*, 1898–1899.

Cancer Registries Amendment Act, Pub. L. No. 102–515 (1992).

Centers for Disease Control and Prevention. (2002). Summary of notifiable diseases, United States, 2002. *Morbidity and Mortality Weekly Report, 51*(53), 1–84.

Centers for Disease Control and Prevention. (2004). HIV/AIDS surveillance report 2002. *Morbidity and Mortality Weekly Report, 14*, 1–40.

Cherry, D. K., Burt, C. W., & Woodwell, D. A. (2003). National Ambulatory Medical Care Survey: 2001 summary. Advance data from *Vital and Health Statistics* No. 337. Hyattsville, MD: National Center for Health Statistics.

Eisenberg, D. M., Davis, R. B., Ettner, S. L., et al. (1998). Trends in alternative medicine use in the United States, 1990–97. *Journal of the American Medical Association, 280*, 1569–1575.

Grove, R. D., & Hetzel, A. M. (1968). *Vital statistics rates for the United States: 1940–1960.* Washington, DC: National Center for Health Statistics.

Hall, M. J., & DeFrances, C. J. (2003). 2001 National Hospital Discharge Survey. Advance data from *Vital and Health Statistics*, No 332. Hyattsville, MD: National Center for Health Statistics.

Health Insurance Portability and Accountability Act of 1996, Pub. L. No. 104–191, Title II, Subtitle F, 261–264 (1996).

Kochanek, K. D., & Smith, B. L. (2004). Deaths: Preliminary data for 2002. *National Vital Statistics Reports* (Vol. 52, No. 13). Hyattsville, MD: National Center for Health Statistics.

Matthews, T. J., Menacker, F., & MacDorman, M. F. (2003). Infant mortality statistics from the 2001 period linked birth/infant death data set. *National Vital Statistics Reports* (Vol. 52, No. 2). Hyattsville, MD: National Center for Health Statistics.

McGinnis, J. M., & Foege, W. H. (1993). Actual causes of death in the United States. *Journal of the American Medical Association, 270*, 2207–2212.

Mokdad, A. H., Marks, J. S., Stroup, D. F., & Gerberding, J. L. (2004). Actual causes of death in the United States, 2000. *Journal of the American Medical Association, 291*, 1238–1245.

Munson, M. L., & Sutton, P. D. (2004). Births, marriages, divorces, and deaths: Provisional data for 2003. *National Vital Statistics Reports* (Vol. 52, No. 22). Hyattsville, MD:; National Center for Health Statistics.

Murphy, S. L. (2000). Deaths: Final data for 1998. *National Vital Statistics Reports* (Vol. 48, No. 11). Hyattsville, MD: National Center for Health Statistics.

National Center for Health Statistics. (1974a). National Ambulatory Medical Care Survey: Background and methodology: United States, 1967–1972. *Vital and Health Statistics*, Series 2, No. 61.

National Center for Health Statistics. (1974b). The National Ambulatory Medical Care Survey: Symptom classification. *Vital and Health Statistics*, Series 2, No. 63.

National Center for Health Statistics. (1979a). *International classification of diseases, tenth revision, adapted for use in the United States.* Hyattsville, MD: U.S. Government Printing Office.

National Center for Health Statistics. (1979b). *Health resources statistics: Health manpower and health facilities, 1976–1977* (DHEW Publication. No. PHS 79–1509). Hyattsville, MD: U.S. Government Printing Office.

National Center for Health Statistics. (1985). Health promotion and disease prevention, U.S., 1985. *Vital and Health Statistics*, Series 10, No. 163.

National Center for Health Statistics. (1992). Infant mortality rates: Socioeconomic factors. *Vital and Health Statistics*, Series 22, No. 14.

National Center for Health Statistics. (1993). *Health United States 1992 and Healthy people 2000 review* (DHHS Pub. No. PHS 93–1232). Hyattsville, MD: U.S. Public Health Service.

National Center for Health Statistics. (1999a). Current Estimates from the National Health Survey, 1994. *Vital and Health Statistics*, Series 10, No. 200.

National Center for Health Statistics. (1997). *Health United States 1996–97 and injury chartbook* (DHHS Pub. No. [PHS] 97–1232). Hyattsville, MD: Centers for Disease Control and Prevention.

National Center for Health Statistics. (1999b, September). *Health United States 1999, health and aging chartbook* (DHHS Pub. No. [PHS] 99–1232). Hyattsville, MD: Centers for Disease Control and Prevention.

National Committee for Quality Assurance. (2003). *The state of managed care quality, Report 2004.* Washington, DC: National Committee for Quality Assurance. Available online: http://www.kaisernetwork.org/health_cast/hcast_index.cfm?display=details&hc=1266

New York City Department of City Planning. (2004). http://www.nyc.gov.html/dcp/html/census/pop2000.html

New York State Department of Health. (2000, September). *Coronary artery bypass surgery in New York State 1995–1997.*

Office of the Assistant Secretary for Health. (1979). *Healthy people: The surgeon general's report on health promotion and disease prevention* (DHEW

Pub. No. [PHS] 70–55071). Washington, DC: U.S. Government Printing Office.

Office of Disease Prevention and Health Promotion. (1980). *Promoting health/preventing disease: Objectives for the nation*. Washington, DC: U.S. Government Printing Office.

Office of Disease Prevention and Health Promotion. (1986). *The 1990 health objectives for the nation*. Washington, DC: U.S. Government Printing Office.

Office of Technology Assessment. (1979). *Selected topics in federal health statistics*. Washington, DC: U.S. Government Printing Office. Sutton, P. D., & Matthews, T. J. (2004). Trends in characteristics of births by state: United States, 1990, 1995, and 2000–2002. *National Vital Statistics Reports* (Vol. 52, No. 19). Hyattsville, MD: National Center for Health Statistics.

U.S. Census Bureau. (1971). *Statistical abstract of the United States: 1971*. Washington, DC.

U.S. Census Bureau. (1997, March). *How we're changing. Demographic state of the nation: 1997. Current Population Reports Special Studies*, Series P23–193.

U.S. Census Bureau. (1999). *Statistical abstract of the United States: 1999* (119th ed.). Washington, DC: U.S. Government Printing Office.

U.S. Census Bureau. (2003). *Statistical abstract of the United States: 2003* (123rd ed.). Washington, DC: U.S. Government Printing Office.

U.S. Department of Health and Human Services. (1995). *Healthy people 2000: Midcourse review and 1995 revisions*. Washington, DC: U.S. Government Printing Office.

U.S. Department of Health and Human Services. (2000, January). *Healthy people 2010* (Conference edition in two volumes). Washington, DC: U.S. Government Printing Office.

U.S. Department of Justice. (2003). *Office of Justice Programs. Bureau of Justice Statistics. Prison Statistics*. Available: http://www.ojp.usdoj.gov/bjs/prisons.htm

U.S. Public Health Service. (1991). *Healthy people 2000: National health promotion and disease prevention objectives* (DHHS Publication. No. PHS 91–50213). Washington, DC: U.S. Government Printing Office.

Ventura, S. J., Martin, J. A., Curtin, S. C., Matthews, T. J., & Park, M. M. (2000). Births: Final data for 1998. *National Vital Statistics Reports* (Vol. 48, No. 3). Hyattsville, MD: National Center for Health Statistics.

# 3

# FINANCING FOR HEALTH CARE

Kelly A. Hunt and
James R. Knickman

- Quantify health care spending in the United States over time.
- Describe the major sources of health care spending.
- List and tabulate the major categories of services purchased.
- Differentiate between public and private spending and purchasing in addition to the categories of health plan types within the public and private system.
- Demonstrate an understanding of the extent to which health care spending is rising and the factors that contribute to such growth.
- Describe the major reimbursement mechanisms for health care services.
- Explain current policy issues in health care financing.

KEY WORDS

Health care spending, sources and uses of health care funds, managed care, capitation, uninsured, public insurance, private insurance, quality, long-term care, physician payment rates, DRGs

---

HEALTH CARE IS a complex set of services, and thus it is not surprising that the way we pay for health care is so complicated. However, because so many people think of health care as a social good, it is sometimes surprising how technical the American approach to paying for health care services has become.

At the heart of approaches to paying for health care are the complications caused by insurance (Culver & Newhouse, 2000). For most goods and services in our economy, simple prices can be set by suppliers—usually as dictated by market forces—and then consumers can choose whether or not to purchase a good or service at the offered price. Then there is a moment when a "transaction" occurs between the supplier and the purchaser, and the money changes hands. Insurance takes away this direct link between the supplier and purchaser of health care services, however, because in effect consumers pay for much of their health care with a fixed, annual payment to insurers who then must negotiate the price they will pay to providers when an insured person uses a service during the year. Establishing the payments to be made to providers in this environment depends on many factors: market power, political considerations (since government in essence is a major insurer), and concepts of fairness.

Many industrialized countries around the world rely on a public financing system to pay for most health care. For example, Great Britain has its well-known National Health Service subsidized by the national government. Canada also has a national health insurance system to pay for most health services. In America, however, we have chosen to rely much more on private financing mechanisms to pay for health care and on government financing to fill in the gaps where private financing does not work. An ongoing debate in American politics continues to focus on whether what we do currently with private financing works adequately and fairly (see for example Blendon et al., 2002; Blendon, Young, & DesRoches, 1999; Davis & Schoen, 2003; Reinhardt, 2003).

The American health care financing system has been evolving continually since the large public financing programs Medicare and Medicaid were implemented in the late 1960s. The costs of health care began to increase rapidly in the 1970s—partly because of the expanding public and private insurance systems and partly because of emerging, expensive health care technology—and so most insurers began to seek more and more technical and complex approaches for reimbursing hospitals, physicians, and other health care providers.

Almost always, the drive for innovations in health care payment systems comes from concerns about cost and efficiency. However, in recent years, many payers have also begun to change their reimbursement systems to encourage providers to improve the quality of health care (see chapter 15 by the Wakefields in this volume). Therefore, a well-grounded understanding of health care financing is essential for people interested in many aspects of health care improvement: improving quality, improving efficiency, improving fairness, improving access, and improving the viability of health care delivery organizations.

To explain how the American health care financing system operates, this chapter focuses on (a) what the money devoted to health care buys, (b) where the money comes from, (c) how health care providers are paid, and (d) current policy issues in financing.

## GENERAL OVERVIEW OF COSTS

The Centers for Medicare & Medicaid Services (CMS) tracks national health care expenditures and is part of the U.S. Department of Health and Human Services (USDHHS). CMS is responsible for the administration and oversight of Medicare, and it works with the states to administer Medicaid and the State Children's Health Insurance Program (SCHIP). In addition, CMS has some regulatory responsibilities. Formerly the Health Care Financing Administration (HCFA), the agency was renamed CMS by HHS Secretary Tommy Thompson in 2001. The renaming of the agency was part of a larger reform process that emphasized its commitment to beneficiaries and providers as well as to quality improvement (Centers for Medicare & Medicaid Services [CMS], 2004a).

According to CMS, national health expenditures were $1.6 trillion in 2002, constituting nearly 15% of GDP in 2002 (see **TABLE 3.1** and **FIGURE 3.1**). These expenditures represent $5,440 per year of health spending for each individual in the United States. Health expenditures have grown dramatically since the United States began tracking these costs. During the early part of the twentieth century, national health represented less than 5% of GDP. By 1970, national health expenditures were $73.1 billion, or 7% of GDP, and they increased at a quick pace over that decade, due in part to the implementation of Medicare and Medicaid. Thirty years later, costs are exponentially higher (Levit, Smith, Cowan, Sensenig, Catlin, & the Health Accounts Team, 2004; CMS, 2004c).

Figure 3.1 shows the rapid growth in health spending as a share of the United States GDP. As a percentage of GDP, health care spending has steadily increased since 1980 and has typically been higher than the rate of general inflation. The rate of spending slowed briefly during the early 1980s, which was related to reimbursement mechanisms for providers. It actually stabilized in the early 1990s with the evolution of managed care plans in the private sector. In fact, in 1996, the U.S. experienced its lowest annual increase in health care spending since 1960, with a growth rate of only 5%. However, the rate of health care spending has steadily increased since 1996, as the grip of managed care loosened and

## TABLE 3.1

Aggregate and Per Capita National Health Expenditures, by Source of Funds and Percentage of Gross Domestic Product, Select Calendar Years, 1929–2013

| CALENDAR YEAR | TOTAL GDP, in billions | TOTAL HEALTH EXPENDITURES | | |
| | | AMOUNT in billions | PER CAPITA | PERCENTAGE OF GDP |
|---|---|---|---|---|
| 1929 | 103.3* | $3.6 | $29 | 3.5%* |
| 1935 | 72.2* | 2.9 | 23 | 4.0* |
| 1940 | 99.7* | 4.0 | 30 | 4.0* |
| 1960 | 503.7* | 26.9 | 146 | 5.3* |
| 1970 | 1,040 | 73.1 | 348 | 7.0 |
| 1980 | 2,796 | 245.8 | 1,067 | 8.8 |
| 1988 | 5,108 | 558.1 | 2,243 | 10.9 |
| 1993 | 6,642 | 888.1 | 3,381 | 13.4 |
| 1997 | 8,318 | 1,092.8 | 4,007 | 13.1 |
| 2000 | 9,825 | 1,309.4 | 4,670 | 13.3 |
| 2001 | 10,082 | 1,420.7 | 5,021 | 14.1 |
| 2002 | 10,446 | 1,553.0 | 5,440 | 14.9 |
| 2005a | 12,219 | 1,920.8 | 6,547 | 15.7 |
| 2013a | 18,243 | 3,358.1 | 10,709 | 18.4 |

* Gross national product
a Projected

health insurance underwriting cycles caught up (Levit et al., 2004; CMS, 2004c).

Indeed, U.S. spending on health care is among the highest in the world. The U.S. leads nation members of the Organization for Economic Cooperation and Development (OECD) in terms of per capita health spending, but it is unclear how this high level of spending is related to the capacity and quality of the system. It is also unclear whether this high amount of spending leads to better health outcomes than in other nations (Anderson, Reinhardt, Hussey, & Petrosyan, 2003; Reinhardt, Hussey, & Anderson, 2004;

| PRIVATE HEALTH EXPENDITURES | | | PUBLIC HEALTH EXPENDITURES | | |
|---|---|---|---|---|---|
| **AMOUNT** in billions | **PER CAPITA** | **PERCENTAGE OF TOTAL** | **AMOUNT** in billions | **PER CAPITA** | **PERCENTAGE OF GDP** |
| $3.2 | $25 | 86.4 | $0.5 | $4 | 13.6%* |
| 2.4 | 18 | 80.8 | 0.6 | 4 | 19.2* |
| 3.2 | 24 | 79.7 | 0.8 | 6 | 20.3* |
| 20.3 | 110 | 75.3 | 6.6 | 36 | 24.7* |
| 45.4 | 216 | 62.1 | 27.6 | 131 | 2.7 |
| 140.9 | 612 | 57.3 | 104.8 | 455 | 3.7 |
| 331.7 | 1,333 | 59.4 | 226.4 | 910 | 4.4 |
| 497.7 | 1,895 | 56.0 | 390.4 | 1,487 | 5.9 |
| 589.2 | 2,161 | 53.9 | 503.6 | 1,847 | 6.1 |
| 714.9 | 2,550 | 54.6 | 594.6 | 2,121 | 6.1 |
| 768.4 | 2,716 | 54.1 | 652.3 | 2,306 | 6.5 |
| 839.6 | 2,941 | 54.1 | 713.4 | 2,499 | 6.8 |
| 1,056.6 | 3,606 | 55.0 | 864.2 | 2,949 | 7.1 |
| 1,806.0 | 5,752 | 53.8 | 1552.1 | 4,943 | 8.5 |

SOURCES: 1929–1960: Thorpe, K.E. & Knickman, J.R. (2002). Financing for health care. In Kovner, A.R. & Jonas, S., eds. Health Care Delivery in the United States." New York: Springer Publishing Company. 1970-2002: Levit, K., Smith, C., Cowan, C., Sensenig, A., Catlin, A, & the Health Accounts Team. (2004) Health spending rebound continues in 2002. Health Affairs, 23(1): 147–159. 2005–2013: Hefler, S., Smith, S., Keehan, S., Clemens, M.K., Zezza, M., & Truffer, C. (2004) Health spending projections through 2013. Health Affairs, Web Exclusive:W4-79-W4-93. Accessed July 22, 2004 at: *http://content.healthaffairs.org/cgi/content/full/hlthaff.w4.79v1/DC1.*

Hussey, 2004). For example, in 2001, the OECD countries Switzerland, Luxembourg, Norway, Canada, and the U.S. led per capita health care spending. Despite the fact that the U.S. spent about $2,000 more per capita than these comparison countries, it ranked lower than these countries on key health indicators. For example, infant mortality rates remained high at 6.8 deaths per 1,000 live births, compared with 5.0 deaths per 1,000 live births—the average rate for the other three countries (Organization for Economic Cooperation and Development [OECD], 2004). U.S. health spending projections are also troubling. Figure 3.1 shows the steep incline pre-

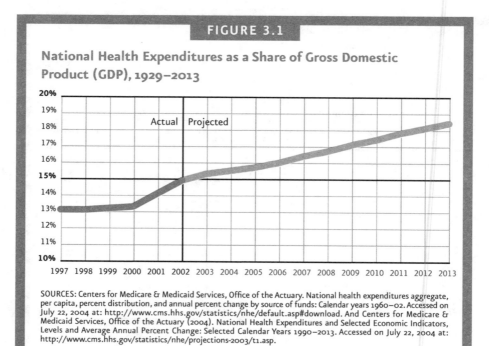

### FIGURE 3.1

**National Health Expenditures as a Share of Gross Domestic Product (GDP), 1929–2013**

SOURCES: Centers for Medicare & Medicaid Services, Office of the Actuary. National health expenditures aggregate, per capita, percent distribution, and annual percent change by source of funds: Calendar years 1960–02. Accessed on July 22, 2004 at: http://www.cms.hhs.gov/statistics/nhe/default.asp#download. And Centers for Medicare & Medicaid Services, Office of the Actuary (2004). National Health Expenditures and Selected Economic Indicators, Levels and Average Annual Percent Change: Selected Calendar Years 1990–2013. Accessed on July 22, 2004 at: http://www.cms.hhs.gov/statistics/nhe/projections-2003/t1.asp.

dicted by CMS actuaries. Unless any major system overhauls are implemented, researchers project a spending level of $3.4 trillion by 2013. In other words, almost 20% of our GDP will go towards health care expenditures (Hefler, Smith, Keehan, Clemens, Zezza, & Truffer, 2004).

## WHAT THE MONEY BUYS

CMS breaks health care spending into two major categories: health services and supplies, and investment (see TABLE 3.2 and FIGURE 3.2). Of health services and supplies, personal health care expenses traditionally constitute the bulk of costs, representing $1.3 trillion in 2002. CMS projects personal health expenses will reach $2.9 trillion by 2013. Within personal health expenses, the largest spending categories are for hospital care, physician and clinical services, nursing home care, and prescription drugs. These four categories of spending account for over 80% of personal health care spending.

Hospital services claim the largest share of total national health

## TABLE 3.2

### Aggregate and Per Capita Amount and Percentage Distribution of National Health Expenditures, Selected Calendar Years, 1970–2013

| TYPE OF EXPENDITURE | AGGREGATE AMOUNT ($BILLIONS) | | | | | | | |
|---|---|---|---|---|---|---|---|---|
| | 1970 | 1980 | 1993 | 1997 | 2000 | 2002 | 2005* | 2013* |
| Hospital Care | $27.6 | $101.5 | $320.0 | $367.6 | $413.2 | $486.5 | $585.8 | $934.3 |
| Physician and Clinical Services | 14.0 | 47.1 | 201.2 | 241.0 | 290.3 | 339.5 | 412.0 | 700.9 |
| Dental Services | 4.7 | 13.3 | 38.9 | 50.2 | 60.7 | 70.3 | 82.3 | 126.3 |
| Other Professional Services | 0.7 | 3.6 | 24.5 | 33.4 | 38.8 | 45.9 | 54.2 | 92.8 |
| Other Personal Health Care | 1.3 | 3.3 | 16.1 | 27.7 | 36.7 | 45.8 | 62.6 | 155.9 |
| Home Health Care | 0.2 | 2.4 | 21.9 | 34.5 | 31.7 | 36.1 | 43.2 | 73.4 |
| Nursing Home Care | 4.2 | 17.7 | 65.7 | 85.1 | 93.8 | 103.2 | 116.9 | 184.8 |
| Prescription Drugs | 5.5 | 12.0 | 51.3 | 75.7 | 121.5 | 162.4 | 233.6 | 519.8 |
| Durable Medical Equipment | 1.6 | 3.9 | 12.8 | 16.2 | 17.7 | 18.8 | 21.5 | 32.6 |
| Other Nondurable Medical Products | 3.3 | 9.8 | 23.4 | 27.9 | 30.8 | 31.7 | 39.3 | 60.5 |
| A. Subtotal: Personal Health Care | $63.2 | $214.6 | $775.8 | $959.2 | $1,135.3 | $1,340.2 | $1,651.5 | $2,881.2 |
| Program Administration and Net Cost of Private Health Insurance | $2.8 | $12.1 | $53.3 | $60.9 | $80.3 | $105.0 | $134.7 | $233.7 |
| Government Public Health Activities | 1.4 | 6.7 | 27.2 | 35.4 | 45.8 | 51.2 | 66.8 | 127.1 |
| B. Subtotal: Administration and Public Health | $4.2 | $18.8 | $80.5 | $96.3 | $126.1 | $156.2 | $201.5 | $360.8 |
| C. Total Health Services and Supplies (A+B) | $67.3 | $233.5 | $856.3 | $1,055.5 | $1,261.4 | $1,496.3 | $1,853.0 | $3,241.9 |
| Research | $2.0 | $5.5 | $15.6 | $18.7 | $28.8 | $34.3 | $41.5 | $75.4 |
| Construction | 3.8 | 6.8 | 16.2 | 18.5 | 19.2 | 22.4 | 26.3 | 40.8 |
| D. Total Investment | $5.8 | $12.3 | $31.8 | $37.2 | $48.0 | $56.7 | $67.8 | $116.1 |
| Grand Total: NHE (C+D) | $73.1 | $245.8 | $888.1 | $1,092.8 | $1,309.4 | $1,553.0 | $1,920.8 | $3,358.1 |

\* Projected
Numbers may not add to totals due to rounding.
SOURCES: 1970–2002: Levit, K., Smith, C., Cowan, C., Sensenig, A., Catlin, A, & the Health Accounts Team. (2004) Health spending rebound continues in 2002. Health Affairs, 23(1): 147–159. 2005–2013: Hefler, S., Smith, S., Keehan, S., Clemens, M.K., Zezza, M., & Truffer, C. (2004) Health spending projections through 2013. Health Affairs, Web Exclusive: W4-79-W4-93. Accessed July 22, 2004 at: http://content.healthaffairs.org/cgi/content/full/hlthaff.w4.79v1/DC1.

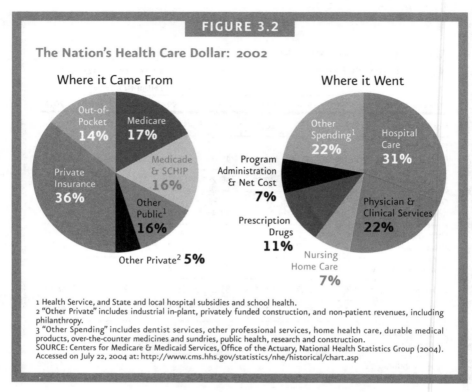

## FIGURE 3.2

### The Nation's Health Care Dollar: 2002

#### Where it Came From

- Out-of-Pocket **14%**
- Medicare **17%**
- Medicade & SCHIP **16%**
- Private Insurance **36%**
- Other Public[1] **16%**
- Other Private[2] **5%**

#### Where it Went

- Other Spending[1] **22%**
- Hospital Care **31%**
- Program Administration & Net Cost **7%**
- Physician & Clinical Services **22%**
- Prescription Drugs **11%**
- Nursing Home Care **7%**

1 Health Service, and State and local hospital subsidies and school health.
2 "Other Private" includes industrial in-plant, privately funded construction, and non-patient revenues, including philanthropy.
3 "Other Spending" includes dentist services, other professional services, home health care, durable medical products, over-the-counter medicines and sundries, public health, research and construction.
SOURCE: Centers for Medicare & Medicaid Services, Office of the Actuary, National Health Statistics Group (2004). Accessed on July 22, 2004 at: http://www.cms.hhs.gov/statistics/nhe/historical/chart.asp

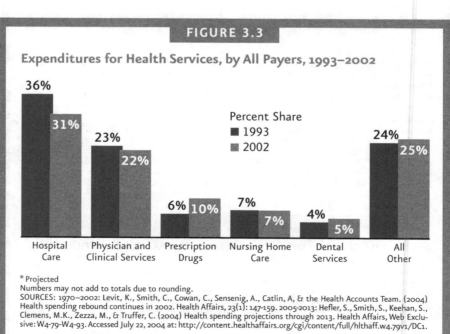

## FIGURE 3.3

### Expenditures for Health Services, by All Payers, 1993–2002

Percent Share
■ 1993
■ 2002

| | Hospital Care | Physician and Clinical Services | Prescription Drugs | Nursing Home Care | Dental Services | All Other |
|---|---|---|---|---|---|---|
| 1993 | 36% | 23% | 6% | 7% | 4% | 24% |
| 2002 | 31% | 22% | 10% | 7% | 5% | 25% |

* Projected
Numbers may not add to totals due to rounding.
SOURCES: 1970–2002: Levit, K., Smith, C., Cowan, C., Sensenig, A., Catlin, A, & the Health Accounts Team. (2004) Health spending rebound continues in 2002. Health Affairs, 23(1): 147-159. 2005-2013: Hefler, S., Smith, S., Keehan, S., Clemens, M.K., Zezza, M., & Truffer, C. (2004) Health spending projections through 2013. Health Affairs, Web Exclusive: W4-79-W4-93. Accessed July 22, 2004 at: http://content.healthaffairs.org/cgi/content/full/hlthaff.w4.79v1/DC1.

expenditures, although it has declined somewhat over the past decade (see FIGURE 3.3). Prescription drugs represent the most rapidly expanding category of spending. Spending on prescription drugs constituted 10% of total NHE in 2002, up from 5.8% in 1993. In fact, spending in this category is growing at the fastest pace (Levit et al., 2004; CMS, 2004c).

The share of personal health expenditures contributed by public sources has actually increased in recent years. This trend is driven by increases in Medicaid expenditures towards rising drug costs and expansions in benefits (Kaiser Commission on Medicaid and the Uninsured, 2003b).

## HOW WE PAY FOR HEALTH CARE

The American approach to paying for health care is a hybrid system that relies to some extent on direct payments by consumers, to a large extent on payments by private insurers and independent health plans, and—in the case of the poor, the elderly, the military, and some disabled Americans or war veterans—by payments from the public sector. Private insurance is financed in part by payments by individuals and in part by payments by employers. The approach varies firm by firm and individual by individual. The approach is complicated from both the provider perspective and the consumer perspective.

In 2002, private funds represented just over half of all national health expenditures (54%), with the bulk of private payments coming from private insurance ($549.6 billion representing 65% of all private payments) (Levit et al., 2004). Public funds represent 46% of all health care spending, and the majority of public funds are spent on Medicare.

### Publicly Financed Health Care

In 2002, 44% of personal health expenditures were financed by the public sector (Levit et al., 2004). This number has increased greatly over time, especially since 1965, and is largely a result of greater federal expenditures. Proportionately, state and local outlays have remained rather constant over time. Medicare and Medicaid programs, Titles XVIII and XIX of the Social Security Act, account for the significant rise in federal spending.

*Medicaid*

Medicaid, begun in 1966, originally targeted recipients of public assistance, primarily single parent families and the aged, blind, and disabled. Over the years, Medicaid has expanded to additional groups so that it now targets poor children in single- and two-parent households, parents of poor children, the disabled, pregnant women, and very poor adults (including 65 and over). The only exception to these expansions was the passage of the Personal Responsibility and Work Opportunity Reconciliation Act of 1996 (PRWORA, P.L. 104–193, 1996), which changed eligibility for legal/illegal immigrants.

Medicaid is administered by the states, and both the states and the federal government finance the program. Although this allows states the flexibility to implement and administer Medicaid benefits in a way that they believe meets the needs of their residents—with the exception of minimum mandatory benefits, there are many, seemingly arbitrary differences in benefits across the states (CMS, 2004e). For example, while many states cover emergency dental treatment and dental care for children, fewer than half of the states cover yearly dental exams and cleaning (Kaiser Commission on Medicaid and the Uninsured, 2003b; American Dental Association, 2001). Another problematic issue with this structure is that bleak economic times often cause states to contract Medicaid eligibility, enrollment standards, and benefits in order to reduce their budgets (see, for example, Boyd, 2003; Holahan, Wiener, & Lutzky, 2002).

Some suggest that Medicaid is limited in terms of its reach because it leaves many gaps in coverage for nonelderly, middle-class Americans. In addition, many individuals who are eligible for the program either do not know they are eligible, view it as a program with a stigma attached to it because it is means-tested, or are put off by complicated enrollment procedures.

Four million individuals were enrolled in Medicaid during its first year of implementation, 1966 (Klemm, 2000; Institute for Medicaid Management, 1978). By December 2002, 39.6 million people were enrolled in Medicaid programs (Kaiser Commission on Medicaid and the Uninsured, 2003a). In 2002, the states and the federal government expended $250.4 billion on Medicaid—most of which was directed towards its elderly, blind, or disabled participants. FIGURE 3.4 illustrates this spending phenomenon, using the most recent enrollment data available. Elderly and disabled par-

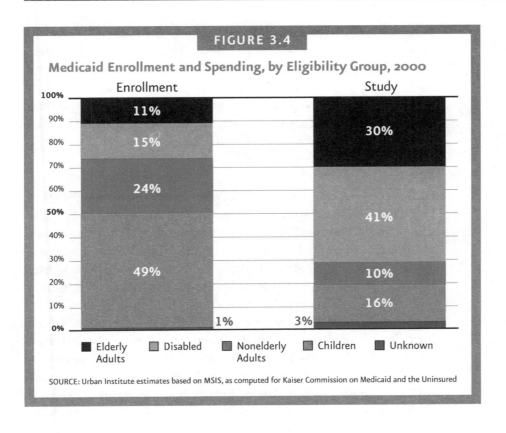

**FIGURE 3.4**

**Medicaid Enrollment and Spending, by Eligibility Group, 2000**

SOURCE: Urban Institute estimates based on MSIS, as computed for Kaiser Commission on Medicaid and the Uninsured

ticipants comprised about one quarter of the Medicaid rolls, yet the program expends almost three quarters of all funds on this group (Holahan & Bruen, 2003).

A major legislative change to the infrastructure of our public coverage system occurred in 1996 when welfare reform de-linked welfare from Medicaid as a result of the Personal Responsibility and Work Opportunity Reconciliation Act (PRWORA, P.L. 104–193, 1996). Prior to this legislation, eligibility for cash assistance was linked to eligibility for Medicaid. Temporary Assistance for Needy Families (TANF) replaced Aid to Families with Dependent Children (AFDC), however, and eligibility for TANF does not guarantee Medicaid benefits (Ellwood & Ku, 1998).

Another major change in the Medicaid program was its move towards managed care in the early 1990s. Proponents hoped that enrolling more individuals in managed care plans would achieve greater savings for the program. A number of issues challenged the amount of savings that could really be achieved. First, Medicaid payers already paid providers rates below the commercial level. Second, safety net providers received a large proportion of their funds through Medicaid support—any savings extracted from them would jeopardize financial viability. Finally, although most Medicaid spending is directed towards the elderly and disabled, efforts to target managed care enrollment were directed at low-income women and children. (Hurley & Somers, 2003).

## SCHIP

Congress passed the State Children's Health Insurance Program (SCHIP) with the Balanced Budget Act (BBA) of 1997 (BBA, P.L. 105–33, 1997). Under SCHIP, the federal government provides money to the states to expand coverage programs to children at higher eligibility levels than those afforded by Medicaid. SCHIP is also jointly financed at the state and federal levels, but the federal government pays a higher percentage of the cost of this program compared to Medicaid. It is a voluntary program on the part of the states, which have flexibility in the way they implement and administer it, similar to Medicaid. Some states introduce SCHIP as a stand-alone program, separate from Medicaid, while others blend the two together into a seamless program. Under federal law, the states may enroll children in families with incomes up to 200% of the (federally determined) "poverty" level, or they may enroll children in families with incomes up to 50 percentage points above the level currently determining Medicaid eligibility (CMS, 2004d).

## Medicare

The Medicare program was also created in 1965 as part of the Social Security Act and is administered by the federal government (Social Security Act, P.L. 89–97, 1965). This program originally targeted the elderly (65 and over) and was quickly expanded to cover individuals with disabilities and severe kidney disease. To qualify, an individual had to be a resident of the U.S. for a specified number of years and pay into the social security system. For individuals who did not meet the latter requirement, this entitlement was expanded in 1972 to allow them to pay a premium for coverage.

Medicare has two parts—Part A, which is hospital insurance, and Part B, which is supplemental medical insurance (SMI). When an individual turns 65, he or she is automatically enrolled in Medicare Part A. Individuals who want SMI must voluntarily enroll and pay a premium, which is heavily subsidized. Medicare and Social Security, combined together, have provided the U.S. elderly with a means for basic economic security. In 1970, 20.5 million individuals were enrolled in the Medicare program; by 2002, this number was 40.5 million (CMS, 2004b). The federal government expended $267.1 billion through the Medicare program, in 2002, compared to $7.7 billion in 1970 (Levit et al., 2004). This makes the federal government the single largest payer of health care expenses in the American system (Iglehart, 2001).

The Balanced Budget Act (BBA) of 1997 brought the Medicare+ Choice program into existence. This legislation was designed to build on existing Medicare managed care programs and expand the health options available to seniors under Part B, or "Medigap" coverage. In addition to introducing more choice into the Medicare marketplace, it was supposed to introduce savings to the program. Enrollment in Medicare managed care programs was actually more rapid prior to passage of the legislation, although it continued to grow steadily until about 1999. This uptick in enrollment was due in large part to the low or zero premiums offered to seniors by these plans, who could afford it given the government payments to Medicare+Choice plans at the time. In addition, many of these plans covered expensive benefits such as outpatient drugs and even vision care. However, enrollment started to decline after 1999. First, a natural market phenomenon occurred—many plans ceased offering this plan choice because they could not or did not want to compete effectively. Second, government payments to these plans were reduced, which translated into increasing premiums and out-of-pocket costs borne by seniors. Many managed care plans eventually pulled out of entire health care markets because it just was not profitable business for them (Gold, 2001, 2003).

In the 1980s and 1990s, the Medicare program experienced a series of changes to its payment mechanisms, which is reflected in the dips in the overall growth rate of national health expenditures. In the 1980s, Medicare first moved to prospective payment for hospitals. By the 1990s, it had moved to relative value scale payments for physicians. The only other major change to the program before 2004 was the Medicare Catastrophic Act (1988), which was repealed within two years of its passage because it was unpopular with seniors and interest groups. This legislation was designed to provide catastrophic financial protection to senior citizens, but many of the individuals the law was intended to protect already had supplemental insurance for catastrophic illness and were unwilling to accept a new tax to finance such coverage for the entire Medicare population. In addition, many elderly did not understand the legislation, feared deductibles and coinsurance, and were satisfied with their current private insurance policies (Rice, Desmond, & Gabel, 1990).

Any chances for Medicare reform were minimized for a number of years as a result of the Medicare Catastrophic Coverage Act repeal. The issue finally came back onto the political radar screen when George W. Bush based part of his first presidential campaign on a promise to add drug coverage for senior citizens to Medicare. The right policy forces were in place; the Congress passed and the President signed into law the Medicare Modernization Act in December 2003. The Congressional Budget Office estimates the cost of this legislation at $395 billion the first 10 years, and over $1 trillion per subsequent decade (Holtz-Eakin, 2004).

Indeed, the most notable change to Medicare resulting from this legislation is the addition of a prescription drug benefit. The other major change this legislation adopts is heavy subsidization of managed care plans to expand the availability of private insurance options to seniors. On the surface, this bill would seem to improve the benefits and choices of senior citizens. However, the bill has many critics on both sides of the political spectrum. Two key issues that are debated by critics are directly related to the drug coverage and the subsidization of private insurance options. First, although the bill does add prescription drug coverage to Medicare, it leaves huge gaps in coverage that the poorest and sickest beneficiaries will not be able to afford. Millions of these individuals are actually worse off than under the old Medicare coverage because they will not be able to afford the drugs they previously could, and in some cases, the drugs they need may not be covered (Park & Greenstein, 2003). Second, the subsidies afforded to private managed care plans are actually quite substantial, which creates an uneven playing field for traditional FFS Medicare (Park, Nathanson, Greenstein, & Springer, 2003; Butler & Moffitt, 2003). Because of these subsidies, managed care plans will be able to fill the gap in drug coverage and offer better cost-sharing options. This will essentially force many beneficiaries off traditional fee-for-service Medicare coverage and into a managed care option. The ultimate goal ought to be cost reduction, but the large subsidies paid out to private managed care plans will actually increase the overall costs of the program.

Critics also cite problems with the changes in tax policy introduced by this legislation, which are regressive in nature. Many find
the cost containment measures embedded in the legislation and its
overall long-term cost implications troubling. Senior citizens and
their interest groups are clearly a powerful political force—a
power strong enough to demand the repeal of the Medicare Catastrophic Act. Only time will tell if Congress will repeat the mistakes
of its past with the Medicare Modernization Act of 2003.

### Public Health

The U.S. spent $51.2 billion on the public health system during 2002,
accounting for less than 4% of national health spending. It must be
noted, however, that while federal prevention and disease control
operations are included in this figure, excluded are funds expended
at the state and local levels by departments other than health, for
air and water pollution control, sanitation and sewage treatment
(Letsch, Levit, & Waldo, 1988). In addition, private expenditures on
public health by employers and individuals are not accounted for
in the $51.2 billion figure. Projections for public health spending
suggest that this level of spending will be maintained. The relatively
low level of government funding for public health activities relative to health insurance payments deserves special attention, particularly in light of the lack of state and local preparedness for
bioterrorism threats (Trust for America's Health, 2003).

### Other Public Programs

In addition to Medicaid, SCHIP, and Medicare, the United States
has a patchwork of other public programs that administer health
care to special populations. These programs constitute only 12% of
overall health care spending in the U.S. (Centers for Medicare &
Medicaid Services, 2004c). Eligible groups include both active and
retired military personnel, Native Americans, and injured and disabled workers.

Coverage for active and military personnel has changed significantly over the past 10 years. Administered by the Department of
Defense (DoD), the Civilian Health and Medical Program of the Uni-
formed Services (CHAMPUS) was established in 1956 to expand coverage to military retirees and families of active duty personnel.
Prior to CHAMPUS, the health care option available to this group
was military facilities, which were inadequate to meet demand. In
the 1990s, the DoD overhauled the CHAMPUS program in order to

control costs and improve access. It was renamed TRICARE and represented the military's effort to introduce managed care into the system. Eligible groups include military personnel, retirees, and their dependents and survivors. TRICARE is currently responsible for administering health benefits to more than eight million military personnel, family of military personnel, retirees, retirees' family members, survivors, and other eligible beneficiaries (Congressional Budget Office, 2003). Two major complaints about the system are that the TRICARE network of providers is inadequate and that provider reimbursement rates are too low (Landers, 2003). Another issue that is especially evident in current times is that TRICARE benefits are less generous in comparison to employer-sponsored benefits. Since members of the National Guard and reservists rely on TRICARE benefits when called to active duty, it is a difficult transition for the families.

TRICARE spending almost doubled from 1988 to 2003, rising from $14.6 billion to $27.2 billion. Since the DoD cut the size of the active-duty force by 38% over that same period, medical spending per active-duty service member nearly tripled, rising from $6,600 to $19,600. The same issues affecting the nation at large are affecting this growth in spending—greater use of technology, changes in the utilization of health care services, and higher medical prices. Two other factors specific to the DoD influence this rise in costs—a shift to accrual budgeting (where the cost of deferred compensation is reflected during a participant's working years) and a shift in the covered population towards more retirees. Spending projections suggest a growth of $40 to 52 billion for TRICARE by 2020 (Congressional Budget Office [CBO], 2003).

The Veterans Health Administration (VHA), led by the Acting Under Secretary for Health, operates the largest integrated health care system in America. The VHA provides primary care, specialized care, and related medical and social support services to U.S. veterans (Veterans Administration, 2004). In 2002, the Veterans Health Administration spent $25.9 billion on health care, treating 4.5 million veterans in 163 hospitals and 859 clinics across the nation (Haugh, 2003). During the past decade, the VA has worked at health care reform by establishing 22 regional, integrated service-delivery networks, reducing the number of open hospital beds, and concentrating on guaranteeing access to high-quality primary care (Fisher, 2003). One result of these efforts is that the VHA seems to be spending less to deliver higher quality care, noting reduced patient stays and improved patient health. A major element of quality improvement for the VHA has been widespread implementation of information technology. Over the past few years they have spent hundreds of millions of dollars on an electronic medical record system, bar-coded medication administration, and computerized physician order entry. The Veteran's Administration estimates that enrollment in its health care program has increased from 2.9 million in 1996 to 6.8 million today, due in part to relaxed eligibility requirements set by Congress in 1996. These relaxed requirements combined with the recent quality improvement efforts have increased demand for VHA health care services, sometimes causing waits of six months or more, although this number fluctuates (Haugh, 2003).

Funds for health services specific to the Native American population were established as part of the Snyder Act in 1921. Known today as the Indian Health Service (IHS), this program is administered by the Department of Health and Human Services (DHHS). Its budget is approximately $3.5 billion annually. Eligible individuals include members of federally recognized Indian tribes and their descendants. This program covers approximately 1.6 million of the nation's estimated 2.6 million American Indians and Alaskan natives (USDHHS, 2004).

Worker's compensation is an insurance system operated by the states, each with its own law and program that provides covered workers with some protection against the costs of medical care and loss of income resulting from work-related injury and, in some cases, sickness (Congressional Research Service, 1976; Price, 1979a, 1979b; U.S. National Commission on State Workmen's Compensation Laws, 1973). The first worker's compensation law was enacted in New York in 1910; by 1948 all states had enacted such laws. The theory underlying worker's compensation is that all accidents, irrespective of fault, must be regarded as the result of the risks of working in industry, and that the employer and employee shall share the burden of loss.

## Privately Financed Health Care

The nonpublic share of health care expenditures has been declining since the 1960s and even since the late 1980s with the growth of Medicare, Medicaid, and other public sources of payments. In 2002, the private share of the health care dollar was 54% or $840 billion. "Third party payers"—mostly insurance companies—

accounted for $479 billion of these private dollars with the balance coming from out-of-pocket payments by patients at the time they get services. The share of payments made by private insurers increased steadily over most of the twentieth century. Even in 1978, private insurance accounted for 21% of all payments compared to 54% in 2002.

What is the logic of private insurance and why has it come to play such a large role in the payment system? Essentially, insurance is a mechanism for sharing the risk of uncertain events across a wider population of people who each face approximately the same risk. In the early twentieth century, when health care did not cost very much, insurance was not necessary. However, as the cost of care exploded during the latter part of the twentieth century with the growth of technology and medical knowledge, it became more and more logical to purchase an insurance policy at a fixed annual payment to avoid the risk of very large medical bills if and when one became ill.

The typical nonelderly person in America who is unlucky enough to need to be hospitalized at least one time during a given year accounts for health expenditures that average over $9,400. But, this only happens to 6% of the nonelderly (Agency for Healthcare Research and Quality [AHRQ], 2004). Most Americans could not afford such a large bill, but they can afford a smaller annual insurance payment that effectively spreads the 6% risk of needing hospital care across the population. In essence, we all help one another pay for expensive medical events through private insurance.

### Employer-Sponsored versus Individual Health Insurance

The concept of medical care insurance began during the Great Depression when hospitals found that most Americans could not afford to pay for their hospital bills (Starr, 1982). The hospital industry, through the American Hospital Association, supported the growth of the first major insurers: the Blue Cross plans in each state that pay for hospital care and the Blue Shield plans that pay for physician and other outpatient services. These nonprofit insurers over time had to compete with for-profit insurance companies that began to emerge mostly during the Second World War when unions began to lobby strenuously to have employers pay for the cost of medical insurance as part of workers' benefits packages. In some ways, growth in the health insurance market was fueled by wage and price controls during the war, which made enhancements to benefits packages a key way unions and employees in general could secure increased total compensation. However, the growing costs of health care would have led to increased private or public insurance over time even if the war-related wage controls had not occurred. In the history of the emergence of health insurance, the fact is that the dominant type of private insurance became employer-based rather than a service purchased directly by employees. And, the emergence of employer-based insurance perhaps dampened efforts to consider publicly-financed national health insurance.

Although employer-based insurance dominates the health insurance sector, there remains a significant market for individual private insurance. The Employee Benefit Research Institute estimates that in 2002, more than 160 million (64%) nonelderly Americans were covered by employment-based health benefits, but about 17 million nonelderly Americans (7%) purchased insurance coverage for themselves and family members in the individual market (Fronstin, 2003).[1] In addition, many individuals who receive coverage from their employer still have to pay some or all of the costs of this insurance directly rather than receive the coverage as part of a total compensation package. In both 2002 and 2003, 66% of all employers offered at least one health plan to their employees. This is a slight drop from 68% in 2001 (Claxton et al., 2003). Among covered workers, 76% pay a share of the insurance costs for single coverage and 92% pay a share of the costs for family coverage (Kaiser Family Foundation/HRET, 2003).

Some people either work for an employer who does not offer insurance, or are between jobs, ineligible for public insurance, or are self-employed. These are the individuals who need to rely on the market for individual (vs. employer) insurance. The individual market is characterized by high premiums and less than generous benefits. Employers are able to secure lower premiums and better benefits for their employees because employed individuals tend to be in better health than others, reducing the risk and thus the cost to the insurer. In addition, marketing and administrative costs are lower when an entire group purchases the same insurance as negotiated by an employer. Risk is also spread out across the group, rather than concentrated in one individual.

---

[1]These numbers may vary slightly from other cited sources (such as Claxton et al., 2003) as they do not include the few insured, working elderly, or a selection of individuals who use multiple forms of health insurance.

## COBRA

COBRA stands for the Consolidated Omnibus Budget Reconciliation Act of 1985. This act amended the Employee Retirement Income Security Act (ERISA), the Internal Revenue Code, and the Public Health Service Act. COBRA became law in 1986 as an attempt to reduce gaps in insurance coverage for individuals between jobs, by requiring employers to extend their health insurance benefits for up to 18 months to former employees. Depending on qualifying circumstances, coverage benefits may also be extended up to a total of 36 months for a spouse or dependent children. Employees generally pay the entire premium for coverage up to 102% of the cost of the plan (100% plus a possible 2% administrative fee) (U.S. Department of Labor [USDOL], 2004; CMS, 2004b). Although this cost is often high, it is still much less expensive than comparable insurance coverage purchased in the individual market.

### Managed Care

The biggest change in the privately financed portion of the U.S. health care system over the last three decades is the shift in the health plan offerings of employers towards "managed care" that started in the late 1980s and took hold by the mid-1990s. Large businesses were at the helm of this shift towards managed care, which was driven by their desire to achieve cost savings. In 1988, almost three quarters of workers were enrolled in conventional, fee-for-service health insurance plans. By 2003, this number was down to only 5%. The balance of workers is enrolled in managed care plans, which have evolved over the past decade.

Managed care plans introduced a different way of structuring and reimbursing care from providers. Very strict managed care plans, like health maintenance organizations (HMOs), used the capitated payment model for their network of providers. They also introduced the concept of primary care physician as gatekeeper to other types of coverage. About a quarter of workers are enrolled in HMOs as of 2003, and this proportion has only declined modestly since the mid-1990s (see TABLE 3.3). HMOs set up provider networks within their plan offerings. And, within these networks, they offered providers capitated, or fixed payments, for services, or negotiated discount payments. The capitated payments were meant to be a mechanism for controlling costs because they essentially gave providers a budget within which to work. The attraction of grouping providers into networks was the potential for increased

| TABLE 3.3 |
|:---:|

**Health Plan Enrollment for Covered Workers, by Plan Type, 1988–2003**

| | PERCENTAGE OF ENROLLMENT | | | | | | | | |
|---|---|---|---|---|---|---|---|---|---|
| **PLAN TYPE** | **1988** | **1993** | **1996** | **1998** | **1999** | **2000** | **2001** | **2002** | **2003** |
| **Conventional FFS** | 73% | 46% | 27% | 14% | 10% | 8% | 7% | 4% | 5% |
| **HMO** | 16% | 21% | 31% | 27% | 28% | 29% | 24% | 27% | 24% |
| **PPO** | 11% | 26% | 28% | 35% | 39% | 42% | 46% | 52% | 54% |
| **POS** | N/A | 7% | 14% | 24% | 24% | 21% | 23% | 18% | 17% |

SOURCES: 1988–96: KPMG Survey of Employer-Sponsored Health Benefits. 1998–2003: Kaiser/HRET Survey of Employer-Sponsored Health Benefits

patient flow as directed by the plans. In return for giving up free-dom to choose any physician or any hospital for service, consumers often receive care that is more organized and referrals to specialists who can coordinate their care better with primary care physicians.

HMOs are designed in several different ways and have varying relationships with their hospitals. They generally act as both the insurer and the provider of services. All HMOs have at the very least a network of physicians and gatekeeping requirements. Group models are the most restrictive type of HMOs. Kaiser Permanente is an example of a group model HMO. It owns its hospitals and has a defined network of providers within those walls that participants must use or face high out-of-pocket payments. Staff model HMOs, on the other hand, contract with a network of physicians, but they do not own their hospitals. Both models may use capitated or fee-for-service payment arrangements.

While research generally finds that HMOs deliver efficient, lower cost, and higher quality care (Luft, 1978), most consumers in most markets do not choose to enroll in these plans. Only in California and, to a lesser extent, the other West Coast states do HMOs represent a significant share of the insurance and delivery mar-ket. And, in many areas of the country—including most of the Eastern half of the country—HMOs do not exist.

Point-of-Service (POS) plans are a slightly more liberal health plan offering than HMO plans. These plans allow individuals to leave the provider network, unlike HMOs. However, plan members who choose to go out of network for care are faced with high out-of-network costs. At the other end of the managed care spectrum are Preferred Provider Organizations (PPOs). PPOs negotiate discounts with a list of physicians and encourage plan members to use these physicians for care. Plan members who use preferred providers pay lower out-of-pocket costs than if they choose nondiscounted providers.

In recent years, PPOs have grown rapidly both in terms of what employers are offering as well as in the proportion of workers enrolled. In 1998, only 11% of workers were enrolled in a PPO plan. By 2003, more than half were enrolled, giving PPO plans the largest market share among employer-sponsored offerings. PPOs grew in popularity from about 1998 onward as a reaction to the managed care backlash. These plans afforded workers more flexibility in where they received their health care.

PPO plans are characterized by their lack of network care requirements. These plans encourage participants to use providers from a list, offering economic incentives achieved by negotiating discounts with providers. Thus plan participants who use other providers face higher deductibles and copays or coinsurance than if they go to a discounted provider. Patients who don't go to a discounted provider often must pay the difference between the insurer's negotiated reimbursement rate and the rate the physician decides to charge if the physician is not on the preferred list.

Managed care as a mechanism for reducing costs was very effective during the mid to late 1990s. A managed care backlash emerged, however, just as costs were stabilizing. Individuals felt constrained by provider networks and gatekeepers as well as other "hassle factors" and demanded more choice in their plan options. Employers began to introduce less stringent plans to their mix of offerings in an attempt to streamline some of the traditional approaches to "managing" care. The growth in PPO plan enrollments highlights this switch. By 2003, more than half of workers were enrolled in a PPO plan, and POS plans had completely disappeared (Kaiser Family Foundation/HRET, 2003).

### Consumer-Driven Health Care

An emerging issue in the private insurance market is that of consumer-driven health care. This is a strategy that seems to be gaining momentum in an effort to both allow employees more choice in their health care decisions as well as to stabilize health care costs. The design of consumer-driven plans varies, but essentially employers provide employees with a "personal care account," which is a fixed amount and offered in the form of a voucher, refundable tax credit, higher wages, or some other transfer of funds (Gabel, Lo Sasso, & Rice, 2002; Christianson, Parente, & Taylor, 2002; Martin, 2002). Employees may choose their own services and providers, as well as manage their annual spending. If an employee uses up all the funds in their personal care accounts, they are responsible for expenses up to a "deductible," at which point wraparound or catastrophic coverage starts. A deductible places a minimum amount at which major medical expenses will be covered (e.g., $1,000).

Typically, employees can use this fixed sum to purchase health care through an employer-sponsored intermediary. They may do so through intermediaries or, theoretically, on their own, though we know of no individually-administered plans to date. Some intermediaries, such as Internet-based companies that give employees flexibility in choosing physicians and services, take on some of the sponsorship duties formerly borne by employers. They contract with networks of providers just like a PPO plan would; members can select providers who are in- or out-of-network. Other intermediaries allow employees to design their plans at a much more detailed level; employees select copayments and doctors to form a personalized "network."

Consumer-driven health care is still in its infancy, and, until recently, skeptics have doubted that it would take off among employers. However, in many industries the demand for labor has decreased since the late nineties, and employers no longer need to compete on health benefits. And, the Internal Revenue Service has ruled to ease restrictions on tax-exempt health spending accounts funded by employers, allowing employees to roll over the unused portion of their spending account and maintain it with their employer even after leaving the company. These developments make cost-saving new health care financing models very attractive.

## The Uninsured

The U.S. system of private and public health insurance is quite extensive, but gaps in coverage remain. The most recent Current Population Survey estimated that nearly 45 million Americans were uninsured in 2003 (U.S. Census Bureau, 2004). Almost one

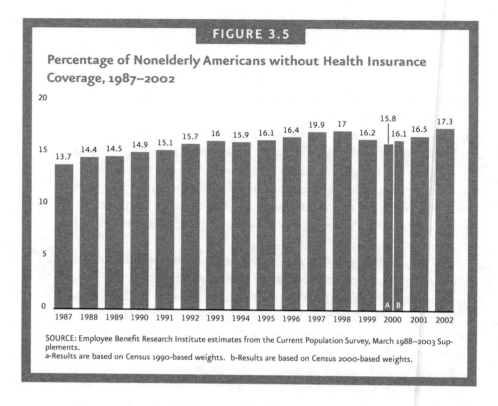

## FIGURE 3.5

### Percentage of Nonelderly Americans without Health Insurance Coverage, 1987–2002

SOURCE: Employee Benefit Research Institute estimates from the Current Population Survey, March 1988–2003 Supplements.
a-Results are based on Census 1990-based weights.  b-Results are based on Census 2000-based weights.

fifth—17.3% of the nonelderly population—are uninsured (see FIG-URE 3.5). Many of these individuals are from families where the head of household works on a full-year, full-time basis (26 million)[2] and many of these individuals are children (9 million) (Fronstin, 2003). While the percentage of uninsured dropped slightly in 1999 and 2000, during the high point of our economy, it started to creep up again by 2001. A stunning reality about these statistics is that even at the height of our economy, the percentage of uninsured dropped only ever so slightly.

Because the uninsured have no formal means for getting care, they tend to rely on our "safety net" system, which includes feder-

2 The number of full-year, full-time working adults without health insurance is provided by the Employee Benefits Research Institute (EBRI) based on the March 2002 Current Population Survey (CPS) data. EBRI adjusts the raw number because CPS enables people to report more than one type of coverage. EBRI's final number (26.2 million), represents all nonelderly. Although the number of uninsured, working elderly is extremely small, we still note the possible discrepancy with other sources that may cite slightly higher numbers.

ally qualified health centers and the emergency departments of hospitals. Some experts have attempted to estimate how much medical care the uninsured use and who pays for it. Hadley and Holahan (2003) estimated that, in 2001, individuals who were uninsured for at least part of the year received $98.9 billion in care, of which about a third was uncompensated (i.e., not paid for out of pocket or by a private or public insurance source).

Finally, it is important to understand the concept of "under-insurance." While over 80% of Americans had some form of insurance in 2002, some of these individuals have bare-bones policies that do not cover basic things such as a general physical exam, well woman visit, or other preventive services. Where an individual works determines many of these differences; individuals who work for larger firms tend to have more extensive coverage than individuals who work for smaller firms (Bundorf, 2002; Kaiser Family Foundation/HRET, 2003; Williams & Lee, 2002; General Accounting Office [GAO], 2001).

## Insurance for Specialized Services

Another form of uninsurance is lack of coverage for some specific types of health-related care. The most significant services that generally are excluded from regular health insurance are long-term care services for the frail and disabled, prescription drug coverage, dental care, and vision care. Long-term care is not covered in most insurance policies because it is generally considered a social service as much as a health care service. Even the Medicare program—specifically designed for the elderly who are at highest risk of needing long-term care—excludes most forms of long-term care from the benefit package. Dental care and vision care traditionally are not the domain of medical care providers (i.e., physicians or hospitals) and were left out of historical processes for developing the insurance market. Prescription drugs is the most curious exclusion from insurance coverage since pharmaceutical interventions are such an integral part of the service regimen for so many health problems. However, 60 years ago when insurance was being designed, prescription drugs were much less central to treatments and they generally were not very expensive.

In recent years, the insurance market has developed special policies that cover each of these four types of services, and such policies are sold separately from basic health care coverage. Medicare recently added a prescription drug benefit—as discussed earlier—

and many employers now offer some form of prescription drug, dental, and vision care coverage, but generally with high coinsurance rates.

Private long-term care insurance products also are widely available as long as people purchase them before they start to become frail or at high risk of becoming frail. Long-term care insurance, however, is not prevalent; just 6 million of the elderly are covered by these plans, and a much smaller percentage of the nonelderly are covered by the plans (Potter, 2003). Long-term care insurance has not spread widely, mostly because it is expensive relative to the resources of many elderly. A policy purchased at age 65 can cost $3,000 per year for one person or $6,000 to cover a married couple. Annual premiums are lower if a person starts to pay for coverage at an earlier age, but people rarely think about the need for this type of coverage before their mid-fifties.

Many people decide to take their chances and not purchase long-term care insurance because they know that in most states, they can qualify for Medicaid coverage if their savings and income are not adequate to pay for care: after spending down most of one's assets and any monthly income, the Medicaid program generally pays for the balance of long-term care services. Because of this, some people look at long-term care insurance as a means of protecting inheritances more than a means to assure access to long-term care. However, in recent years state governments—which pay a large share of Medicaid costs—have been seeking ways to reduce their liabilities to pay for the long-term care of people who could have purchased private coverage.

Researchers project that the percentage of individuals who depend on Medicaid coverage for the catastrophic service needs that necessitate long-term care will decline over the next 25 years (Knickman, Hunt, Snell, Alecxih, & Kennell, 2003). At the same time, the group of financially independent individuals who would be able to afford most long-term care expenses with current income and savings will grow. The proportion of individuals who tend to spend down to Medicaid levels if they have a catastrophic health event—"tweeners"—will actually grow over this period, if these projections play out over time. Thus, policymakers should consider programs that educate tweeners about long-term care financing and insurance coverage.

## REIMBURSEMENT APPROACHES

Given the complexity of how we pay for health care in the United States, it should come as no surprise that our reimbursement approaches are somewhat complicated as well. Reimbursements come from both the private and public side, and when one side changes its approach, it has implications for the other. Fortunately, the analytical abilities of federal staff to understand the implications of reimbursement policies have improved markedly in recent years.

One item that is noticeably lacking in most physician and hospital reimbursement approaches is a link to quality. Payment is determined based on delivery of services, but not necessarily the right services for any given patient situation. Much debate has been given to this subject, and some health plans are only just beginning to experiment with incentive payment programs towards improving quality (Strunk & Hurley, 2004; Wakefield & Wakefield, this volume).

### How Doctors Are Paid

Spending for physician services is a huge component of our national health care bill; over one fifth of all health care spending is for physician services. The way physicians are reimbursed in the United States, and their relative autonomy in making patient care decisions has an impact not only on how much we spend directly on physician services, but, through referrals, on how much we spend for many other diagnostic and therapeutic health services. Two key factors are important to understand related to physician reimbursement. First, physicians typically work for themselves or in group practices rather than as salaried employees in hospitals, laboratories, or other health care delivery institutions. Thus costs incurred and payments to these institutions generally do not affect or determine physicians' incomes. Second, with the exception of the rise and fall of managed care, physicians have had a great deal of independence in making decisions related to patient care. It is the doctor who is in the driver's seat when prescribing drugs, ordering tests, suggesting procedures/operations, etc.

The way health plans and Medicare and Medicaid reimburse physicians for care, however, has changed a great deal in the past couple of decades. These third party payers are largely trying to create incentives to reduce waste in spending and increase quality.

Capitated payments were an attempt to place budget constraints on providers.

The traditional mechanism for paying physicians was a fee-for-service arrangement. In a nutshell, physicians set their price and the patient or insurer paid that price. This unregulated system is often blamed for some of the health care cost inflation since the 1960s. Physicians set rates that often were paid by insurers (who passed the costs along to employers). This system left nobody with an incentive to keep prices down. Consumers did not pressure for lower prices since they did not pay directly for care, and insurers and employers lacked a framework for intervening. The fast inflation in health care prices led to managed care on the one hand and to government regulation of reimbursement rates for Medicare and Medicaid on the other.

### Government Regulation of Physician Payment Rates

The federal Medicare program responded to price inflation by developing a complicated set of fixed rates for a large number of very specific physician services using a system called the Resource-Based Relative Value Scale (Hsiao et al., 1988a; Hsiao, Braun, Dunn, & Becker, 1988b; Hsiao, 1988c). Specific rates were set by measuring the expected time inputs and other types of resource inputs that physicians needed to use to deliver a specific service. These rates were set based on detailed research and with the guidance of a national advisory committee—now called the Medicare Payment Commission—that reports to Congress. Physicians are free to accept or reject these rates, but they cannot deliver services to any patients covered by Medicare if they do not accept the rate structures. Most physicians accept the rates since Medicare patients represent such a substantial share of physician services.

Each state Medicaid program also developed physician reimbursement rates, but most followed the federal approach of establishing "take it or leave it" fee schedules. However, the Medicaid fee schedules are often much lower than the Medicare fee levels for the same services, so many physicians choose to avoid caring for Medicaid patients because they feel the rates are less than the costs incurred by the physician (Zuckerman, McFeeters, Cunningham, & Nichols, 2004; Cunningham, 2002; Marquis, 1999). Based on results from the 2001 Community Tracking Study, 85.4% of physicians were serving Medicaid patients (Cunningham, 2002). However, only 54% of primary care physicians were accepting most or all new Medicaid patients (Zuckerman et al., 2004).

### Managed Care

Since the early 1990s, the concept of "managed care," which was discussed earlier, has been the dominant paradigm for setting physician (and hospital) reimbursement rates among private insurers. Currently, the most common approach for an insurer that attempts to manage care is to develop a PPO comprised of physicians who agree to accept discounted fee-for-service rates for the privilege of being able to take care of that insurer's covered population. In most markets, the preferred provider lists for each insurer include a majority of practicing physicians, but not all of them.

### How Hospitals Are Paid

Approaches to paying hospitals are similar in principle to the approaches used to reimburse physicians. Medicare and Medicaid offer "take it or leave it" rates often established based on complicated formulas while private insurers negotiate rates with hospitals one by one. In the case of managed care, insurers often let individuals use only selected hospitals in a market. The current system has evolved substantially from the initial days of insurance when insurers, including the Medicare program, generally paid hospitals whatever their costs were as long as costs were vaguely in line with reasonableness criteria. This unregulated approach—especially in an era when technology and new treatments were emerging rapidly—fueled hospital cost inflation.

### Diagnostic Related Groups and Prospective Payment

In 1983, the federal government introduced a new hospital reimbursement system that dramatically altered the way it paid for hospital care received by Medicare enrollees. The Diagnostic Related Groups (DRGs) System set rates prospectively rather than retrospectively after a hospital determined its actual costs for a patient's care. In effect, the DRG system was an actual "price" system rather than a cost accounting system that reimbursed actual costs. From an economic perspective, the unusual aspect of the DRG system was that it was a set of prices announced by a "purchaser" rather than a "supplier," and the prices were not set by market forces but rather by technical and sometimes political considerations.

DRG prices vary depending on the medical problem and the

treatments required for a patient admitted to a hospital (i.e., the "intensity" of care required). However, the prices do not vary for every patient; rather, patients are "grouped" in a way that combines patients who have similar conditions and medical needs; a price is set that is considered the prospectively determined, average cost for that group of patients. Over time, however, DRG prices have been adjusted and updated based as much on political, bureaucratic, and federal budgetary considerations as on considerations of actual costs to the hospital. Each hospital receives DRG prices that are based on the same formula but which can vary somewhat from hospital to hospital, depending on local wage and cost conditions as well as selected other factors.

An important feature of the DRG prices is that they pay the hospital a fixed amount for an entire hospital stay. Traditional hospital reimbursement approaches pay hospitals for each day of care provided. Thus, the DRG system creates strong incentives for hospitals to increase efficiency and to reduce the number of days it takes to restore a patient's health. Exceptions—called outlier payments—are made in the DRG system for patients who have unusually long hospital stays due to unexpected problems that make that patient understandably different from the average patient in a DRG group.

### Per Diem Hospital Reimbursement

DRG payment approaches have not spread widely among private insurers or among state Medicaid programs. Instead, hospitals continue to negotiate rates with these payers that pay per diem amounts for hospital care. State-based Medicaid programs often set rates prospectively and force hospitals to accept these rates. But in the case of private insurance, at least in most parts of the country, there are intense negotiations between insurers and hospitals about what rates will be paid for hospital services. Both insurers and hospitals use their market power to influence favorable rates. Insurers—especially if they cover a substantial share of a hospital's potential patient pool—have market power in that they may be able to keep their covered patients from using the hospital if favorable rates are not set. Hospitals have market power because many employers will not purchase insurance for their employees if high quality hospitals in the local area are not part of the insurer's "network" of providers.

This negotiation environment more closely mirrors how prices get set in many markets involving large purchasers and large producers (e.g., the market linking automobile manufacturers with the many companies that make parts for automobiles). When the market is working smoothly, both parties will come to rate agreements that push efficiency but which leave the supplier—the hospital in the health care case—with high enough rates that they can produce high quality care and stay financially viable.

## CURRENT POLICY ISSUES IN FINANCING

Most of this chapter is devoted to explaining how much the U.S. spends on health care, where the money goes, and how it is paid out. We highlight what seems like an exorbitant amount of public and private funds devoted to this one aspect of the GDP. If left unchecked, U.S. health care expenditures are projected to constitute 17% of GDP by the year 2011 (CMS, 2004c). This statistic sounds terribly daunting, but some experts wonder if it is really all that bad. The policy question is: Can the United States afford these rapid expenditure increases? At issue is whether we can afford to continue to purchase desired nonhealth care goods and services in light of increasing health care costs. Speaking in purely economic terms, if the portion of dollars spent on health care is rising, this indicates a rising demand for health care services. Nevertheless, it is important to consider the value gained for dollars expended towards health care—are we really gaining anything?

Some economists argue that the U.S. can afford to spend more on health care if it places relatively more value on these services compared to foregone nonhealth care service purchases (Chernew, Hirth, & Cutler, 2003). Chernew et al. estimate that spending on nonhealth care goods and services would continue to rise over a long period of time, although the share of income growth devoted to health care would be larger than it has been historically. This estimate assumes that real per capita national health spending rises one percentage point faster than real per capita GDP. If they assume a higher rate of growth in real per capita national health spending, spending on nonhealth care goods and services would drop, rendering health care spending "unaffordable."

These estimates bring up some important issues, which Chernew et al. as well as others point out. If health care spending increases were unsustainable, the United States would have to find a way to cut spending. If we are simply unwilling to sustain the health care spending increases, it suggests that we feel a tradeoff in value for health care versus value for nonhealth care spending. These researchers also point out some key issues: the ability of individuals to afford health care in a climate of increased spending, and the fact that some of the spending on health care is due to wasteful practices.

Other economists argue that allowing health care spending to increase unfettered is not desirable, even if we are able to sustain these increases (Altman, Tompkins, Eilat, & Glavin, 2003). Altman et al. highlight the cyclical swings in U.S. health care spending patterns and argue that some growth in spending is often desirable, but that the way we spend it is often wasteful and inefficient. In addition, wide swings in health care spending growth rates have an impact on the surrounding economy. And, growth in health care spending has a huge impact on employer-based coverage. As prices increase, employers cut back on benefits or shift much of the cost towards employees.

### Rethinking the Structure of Health Insurance

Earlier, we described the public-private nature of the health care system. With health care consuming an ever-growing share of GDP, it is important to think about the implications of increasing costs on the structure of the health insurance market—public, employment-based, and individual.

If health care costs continue to grow unabated, public insurers will be faced with tradeoff decisions because their budgets come from the state and federal government. Regardless of our ability to afford increases in costs, the states and the federal government have many competing budget line items. Increases in health care costs will inevitably put public programs on legislators' agendas. This scenario opens up the potential for states to scale back eligibility or enrollment procedures for public coverage programs like Medicaid and SCHIP. Two things can result from such a scenario— individuals covered by public programs receive benefits that are of lower value, and the number of uninsured may potentially increase, taxing the safety net.

When employers are faced with higher costs, this generally means scaling back benefit packages, shifting more costs to employees, or declining to offer health insurance altogether. In fact, the annual Kaiser Family Foundation/Health Research and Educational Trust survey (2003) of employers has found that employers have increased employee deductibles, copayments or coinsurance, and out-of-pocket payments over the past few years. In addition, employee contributions towards their premiums have also increased in the past few years (Claxton et al., 2003). These changes reduce the generosity and value of these benefit packages. Nichols stated the issue of health insurance value very clearly in testimony to the House Committee on Ways and Means: "Insurance differs in terms of the kind of financial protection it offers, in the potential for improvement to health it offers, and the humanity of the treatment when you contact the healthcare system" (2004, p. 4).

Very large employers also have the ability to revise the design of their insurance packages and tend to do so when faced with rapidly increasing costs. The managed care revolution of the 1990s is testimony to this fact. In the early part of the twenty-first century, employers are starting to tinker with a new offering called "consumer-driven health plans"—discussed earlier—which are characterized by their reimbursement arrangements (Martin, 2002). These plans raise a number of issues, however, not the least of which is the lack of information on the quality of care available to consumers today as well as the complexity of health service costs.

## Variations in Costs Across Areas

Clearly, the increasing share of GDP that health care costs take up has huge implications for the structure of the U.S. health insurance market. The changes that could result from rapidly increasing costs should motivate policymakers to really understand what is driving these costs and how to get them under control. For example, it is perhaps not a widely enough known fact that there are large, unwarranted variations in the use and payment for health care services across local health care markets. Wennberg, Fisher, and Skinner (2000) have published numerous articles on this issue. In a 2002 article, they cite cardiac bypass surgery rates (CABG), which vary by up to four times in different health care markets, from 3 per 1,000 in Albuquerque, New Mexico, to more than 11 per 1,000 in Redding, California (Wennberg et al., 2002). These variations are closely associated with the number of cardiac catheterization labs in these health care markets, rather than the incidence of heart attacks.

More recently, researchers have been learning that "more is not better" in the context of these variations in utilization and spending. Importantly, Fisher and colleagues (2003a, 2003b) found that in regions that spent more on health care, Medicare enrollees did not experience better quality of care or access to care. They also did not have better health outcomes or higher levels of satisfaction with their care. These findings highlight the wasteful spending that is apparent in the U.S. health care system. Some of the increases in health care costs that we are experiencing are likely due to variations in spending that are unwarranted and clearly not adding value. If addressed, money that is typically wasted could be saved and re-allocated to other areas.

## Creating Reimbursement Incentives for Quality

Finally, we cannot talk about the implications of increases in health care spending without addressing the issue of quality of care. In 1999, The Institute of Medicine published a high profile report—*To Err Is Human: Building a Safer Health System*—that described the failings of the U.S. health care system and outlined a strategy to improve the quality of care (Kohn, Corrigan, & Donaldson, 1999). One of the striking statistics from this report was the number of individuals who die due to medical error, estimated to be between 44,000 and 98,000.

Experts recommend that health care purchasers demand quality by paying for it. Though paying for quality sounds fairly straightforward, there is much debate over how to measure quality, and appropriate reimbursement mechanisms have yet to be developed. The Center for Studying Health System Change (HSC) recently reported case studies of health plans designing payment incentives from their site visit-based research (Strunk & Hurley, 2004). In 7 of the 12 communities HSC visits regularly, they found signs of a burgeoning movement on the part of health plans towards paying providers for high quality health care. These researchers note that there is little standardization in the way plans measure quality, but the structure of their quality payment programs took one of two forms. Some plans base increased payments for quality on a bonus system, while others base them on an increase in the share of a provider's regular payment over a multi-year contract.

Another issue that experts are attempting to address is the business case for quality (Leatherman et al., 2003), which means an actual financial return achieved from purchasing better quality care on behalf of beneficiaries. It is very easy to explain the social case for quality, but much more complex to calculate savings achieved within a reasonable time frame.

## CONCLUSIONS

The American approach to financing medical care services has evolved steadily as the health care delivery system itself has evolved into what essentially is the largest service industry in the nation. While this evolution has in part been shaped by a sense that "health care is different" from other services, in essence America has taken a very market-oriented approach to shaping and financing health care delivery even as the public sector expanded its involvement to pay for the care of many Americans who otherwise would have difficulty affording services.

Does the financing system work? Should it be dramatically reshaped? On one level, it is possible to say the system does work: millions and millions of service transactions occur each year across the country, and for the most part, providers receive reimbursements that keep them financially viable and individuals receive effective, required services. Based on other criteria, however, there are many shortcomings to our health care financing system.

Health care expenditures continue to increase at rates that most payers are not comfortable with, even if some of the expenditure inflation is for buying new technology that is extending life and improving well-being. There is a sense that the financial incentives in the health sector are not adequate to, on the one hand, force efficiency, but on the other hand, encourage improved quality and the diffusion of effective new technology and treatments.

The current financing system also leaves 45 million Americans without any form of health care insurance, putting these people at great risk in that they do not have adequate access to services. While the system compensates for this gap in health insurance coverage by providing "charity" care in many cases, this ad hoc approach to assuring access causes substantial financial problems for institutions in low income neighborhoods and certainly reduces the health and well-being of the millions of uninsured Americans who struggle to get services (Nichols, 2004).

From a provider perspective, the current financing approach also seems far from ideal. Physicians believe that they are receiving rates that are not adequate to fund their increasingly complex practices. From a macro perspective, it is true that in recent years, physician net incomes have decreased for many specialties and have grown slowly if at all for most other specialties and for primary care physicians. However, medical schools continue to recruit highly qualified candidates for the profession, and major physician shortages—which might be expected if reimbursements are inadequate—have not occurred.

Hospitals have had somewhat more ability to influence the rates paid by private insurers, probably because they have more market power since each community only has one or a small number of hospitals. Insurers can usually not afford to eliminate a key local hospital from its networks without being at risk of losing customers among local employers. Interestingly, physicians have not begun to organize into larger group practices in most areas of the country even though this organizational approach might give them increased market power to negotiate better rates.

Hospitals and physicians also complain about the administrative burden of the current financing system because rates are continuously changing and substantial administrative resources are required to document costs, interact with payers, and fight to receive actual payments due. Some research suggests that the total administrative costs (over and above the service costs) to run the American health system far exceeds that paid into systems for instance in Canada and Great Britain (Himmelstein, Woolhandler, & Wolfe, 2004).

A key point in the debate on the future of health care financing is whether to fix the problems through marginal improvements,

## CASE STUDY

Managed care took hold in the early 1990s largely because employers were searching for ways to reduce costs. The utilization management and gatekeeping aspects of managed care held promise for reducing health care costs, and employers realized these savings. However, the private sector has retracted from purchasing restrictive managed care plans since the late 1990s given the consumer backlash to plan requirements and restrictions. At the same time, health insurance costs have climbed. Employers are now experimenting with new health plan types in search of savings, namely consumer-driven health care plans.

What impact does consumer driven health care have on the ability of the private sector to get health care costs under control and then sustain these savings; access to care for the chronically ill; and quality of care?

working on one at a time, or if the current health care financing system needs to be abandoned and replaced by an entirely different one? This is a debate that needs to engage new thinkers, new leaders, and new researchers in the years to come.

## DISCUSSION QUESTIONS

1. What processes would be effective or desirable to reduce the variation in health care spending across the country?
2. The biggest change in Medicaid in the past decade was the introduction of the State Children's Health Insurance Program (SCHIP). What are the implications for this program given the rising costs of health insurance and the current economic environment?
3. Some may view increases in health care spending as a response to consumer demand while others see it as wasteful spending. When other industry sectors assume a rising share of GDP, it is viewed positively rather than a problem. Should we be concerned about the rising costs of health care and its share of GDP? What types of spending might be classified as valuable? What types of spending might be classified as wasteful?

## ACKNOWLEDGMENT

We are grateful for the research assistance of Kathryn Muessig. The interpretations and opinions are those of the authors and may not necessarily reflect those of The Robert Wood Johnson Foundation.

## REFERENCES

Agency for Healthcare Research and Quality. (2004). *Research findings #21: Health care expenses in the United States, 2000*. Rockville, MD. Retrieved July 21, 2004, from http://www.meps.ahrq.gov/papers/rf21 04--0022/rf21.htm

Altman, S. H., Tompkins, C. P., Eilat, E., & Glavin, M. P. V. (2003). Escalating health care spending: Is it desirable or inevitable? *Health Affairs*, Web Exclusives, January 8, 2003, W3–1 to W3–7.

American Dental Association. (2001). *2000 survey of state dental programs in Medicaid*. Catalog Code #5M00. Chicago.

Anderson, G., Reinhardt, U., Hussey, P., & Petrosyan, V. (2003). It's the prices stupid: Why the United States is so different from other countries. *Health Affairs, 22*(3), 89–105.

Balanced Budget Act of 1997, Pub. L. No. 105–33. Subtitle J, State Children's

Health Insurance Program. (1997). Retrieved June 15, 2004, from http://www.cms.hhs.gov/schip/legislation/kidssum.asp

Blendon, R. J., Schoen, C., DesRoches, C. M., Osborn, R., Scoles, K. L., & Zapert, K. (2002). Inequities in health care: A five-country survey. *Health Affairs, 21*(3), 182–191.

Blendon, R. J., Young, J. T., & DesRoches, C. M. (1999). The uninsured, the working uninsured, and the public. *Health Affairs, 18*(6), 203–211.

Boyd, D. (2003). The bursting state fiscal bubble and state Medicaid budgets. *Health Affairs, 22*(1), 46–61.

Bundorf, M. K. (2002). Employee demand for health insurance and employer health plan choices. *Journal of Health Economics, 21*(1), 65.

Butler, S., & Moffit, R. (2003). Time to rethink the disastrous Medicare legislation. *Web Memo No. 370.* Washington, DC: The Heritage Foundation. Retrieved June 4, 2004, from http://www.heritage.org/Research/HealthCare/wm370.cfm

Centers for Medicare & Medicaid Services. (2004a). Retrieved April 23, 2004, from http://www.cms.hhs.gov/about/reorg.asp

Centers for Medicare & Medicaid Services. (2004b). Medicare enrollment: National trends 1966–2002: Medicare aged and disabled enrollees by type of coverage. Retrieved June 17, 2004, from http://www.cms.hhs.gov/statistics/enrollment/natltrends/hi_smi.asp

Centers for Medicare & Medicaid Services, Office of the Actuary. (2004c). *2002 Data from the National Health Statistics Group.* Baltimore, MD.

Centers for Medicare & Medicaid Services. (2004d). State Children's Health Insurance Program. Welcome to the State Children's Health Insurance Program. Retrieved June 17, 2004, from http://www.cms.hhs.gov/schip/about-SCHIP.asp

Centers for Medicare & Medicaid Services. (2004e). Medicaid: A brief summary. Retrieved June 17, 2004, from http://www.cms.hhs.gov/publications/overview-medicare-medicaid/default4.asp

Centers for Medicare & Medicaid Services. (2004). How COBRA coverage works. Retrieved June 22, 2004, from http://www.cms.hhs.gov/hipaa/hipaa1/cobra/coverage.asp

Centers for Medicare & Medicaid Services. (2004). "CMS/HCFA History" Health Care Financing Administration. Retrieved June 17, 2004, from http://www.cms.hhs.gov/about/history/

Chernew, M. E., Hirth, R. A., & Cutler, D. M. (2003). Increased spending on health care: How much can the United States afford? *Health Affairs, 22*(4), 15–25.

Christianson, J. B., Parente, S. T., & Taylor, R. (2002). Defined-contribution health insurance products: Developments and prospects. *Health Affairs, 21*(1), 49–64.

Claxton, G., Holve, E., Finder, B., Gobel, J., Pickveign, J., Whitmore, H., et al. (2003). Employer health benefits: 2003 annual survey. Menlo

Park, CA & Chicago, IL: Kaiser Family Foundation/Health Research and Educational Trust (HRET).

Congressional Budget Office. (2003, September). *Growth in medical spending by the Department of Defense.* Retrieved June 16, 2004, from http://www.cbo.gov/showdoc.cfm?index=4520&sequence=0

Congressional Research Service. (1976). *Workmen's compensation: Role of the federal government* (IB75054). Washington, DC: Library of Congress.

Culver, A. J., & Newhouse, J. P. (2000). *Handbook of health economics.* Amsterdam, NY: Elsevier.

Cunningham, P. (2002, December). Mounting pressures: Physicians serving Medicaid patients and the uninsured, 1997–2001. Tracking Report No. 6. Available at: www.hschange.org/CONTENT/505/505.pdf (10 May 2004)

Davis, K., & Schoen, C. (2003). Creating consensus on coverage choices. *Health Affairs.* Web Exclusive, April 23, 2003, W3–199 to W3–211.

Ellwood, M. R., & Ku, L. (1998). Welfare and immigration reforms: Unintended side effects for Medicaid. *Health Affairs, 17*(3), 137–151.

Fisher, E. S., Wennberg, D. E., Stukel, T. A., Gottlieb, D. J., Lucas, F. L., & Pinder, E. L. (2003a). The implications of regional variations in Medicare spending. Part 1: The content, quality, and accessibility of care. *Annals of Internal Medicine, 138,* 273–287.

Fisher, E. s., Wennberg, D. E., Stukel, T. A., Gottlieb, D. J., Lucas, F. L., & Pinder, E. L. (2003b). The implications of regional variations in Medicare spending. Part 2: Health outcomes and satisfaction with care. *Annals of Internal Medicine, 138,* 288–298.

Fronstin, P. (2003, December). Sources of health insurance and characteristics of the uninsured: Analysis of the March 2003 Current Population Survey. *Employee Benefit Research Institute,* Issue Brief 264.

Gabel, J. R., Lo Sasso, A. T., & Rice, T. (2002). Consumer-driven health plans: Are they more than talk now? *Health Affairs.* Web Exclusive. Retrieved July 20, 2004, from http://content.healthaffairs.org/cgi/content/full/hlthaff.w2.395v1/DC1

General Accounting Office. (2001). *Private health insurance: Small employers continue to face challenges in providing coverage.* Washington, DC: GAO-02–8.

Gold, M. (2001). Medicare+Choice: An interim report card. *Health Affairs, 20*(4), 120–138.

Gold, M. (2003). Can managed care and competition control Medicare costs? *Health Affairs,* Web Exclusives, April 2, 2003, W176–188.

Hadley, J., & Holahan, J. (2003). How much care do the uninsured use, and who pays for it? *Health Affairs,* Web Exclusives, February 12, 2003, W66–81.

Haugh, R. (2003). Reinventing the VA. *Hospitals & Health Networks, 77*(12), 50–54.

Hefler, S., Smith, S., Keehan, S., Clemens, M. K., Zezza, M., & Truffer, C.

(2004). Health spending projections through 2013. *Health Affairs*, Web Exclusive: W4–79–W4–93. Retrieved July 22, 2004, from http://content.healthaffairs.org/cgi/content/full/hlthaff.w4.79v1/DC1

Himmelstein, D. U., Woolhandler, S., & Wolfe, S. M. (2004). Administrative waste in the U.S. health care system in 2003: The cost to the nation, the states, and the District of Columbia, with state-specific estimates of potential savings. *International Journal of Health Services, 34*(1), 79–86.

Holahan, J., & Bruen, B. (2003, September). *Medicaid spending: What factors contributed to the growth between 2000 and 2002?* Washington, DC: Kaiser Commission on Medicaid and the Uninsured, the Kaiser Family Foundation.

Holahan, J., Wiener, J., & Lutzky, A. (2002). Health policy for low-income people: States' responses to new challenges. *Health Affairs*, Web Exclusives, May 22, 2002, W187–218.

Holtz-Eakin, D. (2004). CBO testimony estimating the cost of the Medicare Modernization Act. Retrieved May 27, 2004, from http://www.cbo.gov/showdoc.cfm?index=5252&sequence=0

Hsiao, W. C., Braun, P., Dunn, D., Becker, E. R., Chen, S. P., Couch, N. P., et al. (1988a). A national study of resource-based relative value scales for physician services: Final report to the Health Care Financing Administration. Publication 17-C-98795/1–03. Boston: Harvard University School of Public Health.

Hsiao, W. C., Braun, P., Dunn, D., & Becker, E. R. (1988b). Resources-based relative values: An overview. *Journal of the American Medical Association, 260*(16), 2347–2353.

Hsiao, W. C., Braun, P., Dunn, D., Becker, E. R., De Nicola, M., & Ketchum, T. R. (1988c). Results and policy implications of the resource-based relative-value study. *New England Journal of Medicine, 319*(13), 881–888.

Hurley, R., & Somers, S. (2003). Medicaid and managed care: A lasting relationship? *Health Affairs, 22*(1), 77–88.

Hussey, P., et al. (2004). How does the quality of care compare in five countries? *Health Affairs, 23*(3), 89–99.

Iglehart, J. (2001). The Centers for Medicare & Medicaid Services. *New England Journal of Medicine, 345*(26), 1920–1924.

Institute for Medicaid Management. (1978). *Data on the Medicaid program: Eligibility/services/expenditures fiscal years 1966–78 (rev.) data from U.S. Department of Health, Education, and Welfare/Health Care Financing Administration, Medicaid Bureau, 1978.* As cited in Medicaid spending: A brief history. John Klemm. (2000, Fall). *Health Care Financing Review, 22*(1), 105–112.

Kaiser Commission on Medicaid and the Uninsured. (2003a, December). *Medicaid enrollment in 50 states: December 2002 data update.* Washington, DC: Kaiser Family Foundation.

Kaiser Commission on Medicaid and the Uninsured. (2003b, January).

*Medicaid benefits: Services covered, limits, copayments and reimbursement methodologies for 50 states, District of Columbia and the territories (as of January 2003). Dental Services.* Retrieved June 17, 2004, from http://www.kff.org/medicaidbenefits/dentalservices.cfm

Kaiser Family Foundation Health Research and Educational Trust (HRET). (2003, May). *Trends and indicators in the changing health care marketplace, 2003.* Menlo Park, CA: Kaiser Family Foundation.

Klemm, J. D. (2000). Medicaid spending: A brief history. *Health Care Financing Review, 22*(1), 105–112.

Knickman, J. R., Hunt, K. A., Snell, E. K., Alecxih, L. M. B., & Kennell, D. L. (2003). Wealth patterns among elderly Americans: Implications for health care affordability. *Health Affairs, 22*(3), 168–174.

Kohn, L. T., Corrigan J. M., Donaldson, M. S., & Committee on Quality Health Care (IOM). (Eds.). (1999). *To err is human: Building a safer health care system.* Washington, DC: National Academies Press.

Landers, P. (2003, March 31). Health care as war casualty: Reservists' families give up employer-paid insurance for coverage with big gaps. *Wall Street Journal,* B1.

Leatherman, S., et al. (2003). The business case for quality: Case studies and an analysis. *Health Affairs, 22*(2), 17–30.

Letsch, S., Levit, K., & Waldo, D. (1988). National health expenditures, 1987. *Health Care Financing Review, 10*(2), 109–123.

Levit, K., Smith, C., Cowan, C., Sensenig, A., Catlin, A., & the Health Accounts Team. (2004). Health spending rebound continues in 2002. *Health Affairs, 23*(1), 147–159.

Luft, H. S. (1978). How do health-maintenance organizations achieve their "savings"? Rhetoric and evidence. *New England Journal of Medicine, 298*(24), 1336–1343.

Marquis, M. S. (1999). Effects of changing Medicaid fees on physician participation and enrollee access. *Inquiry, 36*(3), 265–279.

Martin, K. E. (2002). *Shifting responsibilities: Models of defined contribution.* Washington, DC: AcademyHealth.

Nichols, L. M. (2004, March 9). Myths about the uninsured. Testimony prepared for a hearing on the uninsured before the U.S. House of Representatives Committee on Ways and Means Health Subcommittee.

Organization for Economic Cooperation and Development (OECD). (2004). *2004 health data.* Table 2: Infant mortality, Deaths per 1000 live births, Table 9: Total expenditure on health, per capita US$ PPP; Table 10: Total expenditure on health, %GDP. Retrieved June 18, 2004, from http://www.oecd.org/document/16/0,2340,en_2649_34631_2085200_119699_1_1_1,00.html

Park, E., & Greenstein, R. (2003). *Medicare agreement would make substantial numbers of seniors and people with disabilities worse off than under current law.* Washington, DC: Center on Budget and Policy Priorities.

Retrieved June 4, 2004, from http://www.cbpp.org/11–18–-03health.pdf

Park, E., Nathanson, M., Greenstein, R., & Springer, J. (2003). *The troubling medicare legislation*. Washington, DC: Center on Budget and Policy Priorities. Retrieved June 4, 2004, from http://www.cbpp.org/11–18–03health2.pdf

Personal Responsibility and Work Opportunity Reconciliation Act of 1996 (PRWORA), Pub. L. No. 104–193. (1996, August). Retrieved June 15, 2004, from http://www.acf.dhhs.gov/programs/opa/facts/prwora96.htm

Potter, A. (2003). *The evolution of long-term care insurance*. Windsor, CT: LIMRA International.

Price, D. (1979a). Workers' compensation programs in the 1970s. *Social Security Bulletin, 42*(5), 3.

Price, D. (1979b). Workers' compensation coverage, payments and costs, 1977. *Social Security Bulletin, 42*(10).

Reinhardt, U. (2003). The Medicare world from both sides: A conversation with Tom Scully. *Health Affairs, 22*(6), 167–174.

Reinhardt, U., Hussey, P., & Anderson, G. (2004). U.S. health care spending in an international context. *Health Affairs, 23*(3), 10–25.

Rice, T., Desmond, K., & Gabel, J. (1990). The Medicare Catastrophic Coverage Act: A post-mortem. *Health Affairs, 9*(3), 75–87.

Social Security Act of 1965, Medicare program, Pub. L. 89–97 (1965). H.R. 6675.

Starr, P. (1982). *The social transformation of American medicine: The rise of a sovereign profession and the making of a vast industry*. New York: Basic Books.

Strunk, B. C., & Hurley, R. E. (2004). Paying for quality: Health plans try carrots instead of sticks. *Issue Brief No. 82*. Washington, DC: Center for Studying Health System Change. Retrieved June 16, 2004, from http://www.hschange.org/CONTENT/675/

Trust for America's Health. (2003, December). *Ready or not? Protecting the public's health in the age of bioterrorism*. Washington, DC: Trust for America's Health.

U.S. Census Bureau. *Health insurance coverage: 2003*. Retrieved September 16, 2004, from http://www.census.gov/hhes/hlthins/hlthin03/hlth03asc.html#3

U.S. Department of Health and Human Services. (2004). Indian Health Service. *Fact sheet*. Retrieved June 16, 2004, from http://www.ihs.gov/PublicInfo/PublicAffairs/Welcome_Info/ThisFacts.asp

U.S. Department of Labor, Employee Benefits Administration. (2004). *Fact sheet: Consolidated Omnibus Budget Reconciliation Act of 1985*. Retrieved June 22, 2004, from http://www.dol.gov/ebsa/newsroom/fscobra.html

U.S. National Commission on State Workmen's Compensation Laws. (1973). *Report*. Washington, DC: U.S. Government Printing Office.

Veterans Administration, Veterans Health Administration. Health benefits and services: General information. Retrieved June 22, 2004, from http://www1.va.gov/health_benefits/page.cfm?pg=1

Wakefield & Wakefield this volume.

Wennberg, J. E., Fisher, E. S., & Skinner, J. S. (2002). Geography and the debate over Medicare reform. *Health Affairs*, Web Exclusives, February 13, 2004, W96–114.

Williams, C., & Lee, J. (2002). Are health insurance premiums higher for small firms? *Research synthesis report No. 2*. Retrieved June 16, 2004, from http://www.rwjf.org/publications/synthesis/reports_and_briefs/pdf/no2_researchreport.pdf

Zuckerman, S., McFeeters, J., Cunningham, P., & Nichols, L. (2004). Trends: Changes in Medicaid physician fees, 1998–2003: Implications for physician participation. *Health Affairs* Web Exclusive, June 23, 2004, W4–374 to W4–384.

# 4

# PUBLIC HEALTH: Policy, Practice, and Perceptions

Laura C. Leviton and
Scott D. Rhodes

---

IN THIS CHAPTER we introduce the policies, programs, and practices that constitute public health in the United States. The first section describes the distinctive goals and activities of public health. A report by the Institute of Medicine (1988) defined public health as "organized community efforts aimed at the prevention of disease and promotion of health" (p. 41). It focuses "on society as a whole, the community, and the aim of optimal health status" (p. 39).

We then describe the complex network of laws, regulation, authority, and services that comprise public health. State, federal, and local government agencies, often called the *infrastructure*, are responsible for the core public health functions (Institute of Medicine, 2003b). The United States has always provided legal and regulatory authority at each level of government to protect the health of populations (Duffy, 1992; Gostin, 2000). In addition, a wide variety of other public, private, and nonprofit organizations carry out responsibilities for public health.

Public health is in trouble. Health experts have warned about the system's "disarray" for close to 20 years (Institute of Medicine, 1988, 2003b). However, some very positive new developments show a better road ahead for public health. The challenges we face include the political and economic dominance of medical care and the fragmented responsibility for carrying out public health goals. The nation has consensus on many of these goals, but they are largely ignored and often misunderstood. Also, certain issues highlight a clash of values and can even be flashpoints for conflict in society.

## PUBLIC HEALTH EVERY DAY

Imagine waking up and going through your morning routine. You slept eight hours for a change, because health experts claim that lack of sleep causes stress and other health problems. You do wonder, though, whether the experts will claim something different next month. You wander into the bathroom and brush your teeth, which are still in your mouth thanks to adequate nutrition, the fluoride in your water system, routine dental visits, though not the dental hygiene you learned in school, but rather the fear of bad breath. You rinse your mouth with water from the faucet knowing that it is safe to drink; when you flushed the toilet, you were confident that the waste would not get into the water supply and kill you. Before the water ever reached your faucet, it was checked for heavy metals such as lead (which causes lower intelligence in children) and chemicals such as polychlorinated biphenyls (PCBs), which cause cancer. You get your children ready for school; so far, they've all survived, never having had measles, diphtheria, polio, or other diseases that killed and maimed so many children in bygone days. The kids' breakfast includes cereal and pure pasteurized milk. (The kids talked you into buying the cereal they saw on television, although you looked at the nutritional label and thought the ingredients were okay.)

Your sister calls to announce she's going to have a baby! She's able to have children because she never got infected with a sexually transmitted disease (STD), which can cause infertility. She is not aware that the toast she is eating is fortified with folic acid, the B vitamin that prevents birth defects. You and your sister also discuss your father. Both of you are worried about him because he is overweight, still smokes, and never exercises. Is a heart attack, diabetes, or stroke in his future? The odds are not in Dad's favor. Quit-smoking programs are available in the community without charge, so you agree that Dad's doctor should try suggesting them again. Too bad there are no sidewalks in Dad's neighborhood; he loves to walk but hates the traffic. Does the senior center have an exercise program that might appeal to him? You buckle the kids into their safety belts, confident that the car will likely protect you from injury. When you get to your job, you see the new sign: "607 days without an accident at this worksite."

Public health affects the lives of Americans profoundly, but invisibly. This scenario, an adaptation of a brochure for state legislators, makes this very clear (Hooker & Speisseger, 2002). **TABLE 4.1** lists some of the organizations, public policies, and activities that underlie the protections described in this scenario.

## WHO IS IN CHARGE OF PUBLIC HEALTH?

The responsibility for public health is diffuse and fragmented. Table 4.1 illustrates this point, although a comprehensive list of protections would consume the rest of this chapter. Public health law, regulation, and organizational practice are like snowballs, gathering new layers over time. The authority for assuring public health is also complex: federal, state, and local governmental agencies all have a role to play, as do professional associations, private and nonprofit organizations.

There are at least three general reasons for this complexity and diffuse responsibility. The first is our decentralized government, in which states have constitutional responsibility for public health except where specified by federal law. Local responsibility varies a great deal across and within states, and rests with diverse agencies, boards of health, and municipal codes.

The second cause for diffused responsibility for public health is the distinctive American tendency, first recognized in 1839, to design laws, policies, and associations that are issue-specific (de Tocqueville, 2001). For example, individual diseases receive special legal attention, so new federal bureaus are created to deal with them. Widely separated federal departments deal with such health problems as assuring pure food and drugs, monitoring and controlling infectious diseases, providing guidance to prevent chronic diseases, improving traffic safety, and assuring a healthy place to work. Political interests also cause fragmented responsibility. For example, in response to the meat lobby, the United States Department of Agriculture (USDA) inspects meat products while the Food

## TABLE 4.1

### Public Health Protection Every Day

#### GUIDANCE AND EDUCATION

| PUBLIC HEALTH ISSUE | FEDERAL RESPONSIBILITY | OTHER RESPONSIBILITY |
|---|---|---|
| Sleep (1) | NIH, CDC, SAMHSA, OSHA (shift workers) | Popular press, medical care providers, schools |
| Nutrition (2) | FDA, USDA, ODPHP | chools, medical care, nutritionists & dieticians |
| Dental hygiene (3) | CDC, NIH, Surgeon General | State & local health departments, schools, dental and medical care |
| Healthy weight (2) | ODPHP, NIH, CDC | Popular press, medical care, state & local health departments, American Heart Association, AARP |
| Smoking (2) | ODPHP, NIH, CDC | Popular press, medical care, state & local health departments, the courts, American Heart Association, American Lung Association |
| Physical activity (2) | ODPHP, NIH, CDC | Popular press, medical care, state & local health departments, American Heart Association, AARP, urban planners, YMCA, YWCA, Sierra Club |
| Seat belts (2) | ODPHP, CDC, NHTSA | tate & local health departments, schools, medical care, popular press |

#### LAW AND REGULATION

| PUBLIC HEALTH ISSUE | FEDERAL RESPONSIBILITY | OTHER RESPONSIBILITY |
|---|---|---|
| Fluoridation (1) | | State law, county and municipal codes |
| Drinking water (4) | EPA, FEMA | State and local health departments, state and local departments of environment, municipal water authority/sanitary districts |
| Childhood immunization (2) | DHHS regulation (standing orders to immunize) | State health codes (reportable disease) and immunization requirements |
| Food Labeling (2), Pure milk (5) | FDA, EPA | State inspection programs (some) |
| Reproductive health— STD control (6) | | State health codes (reportable diseases) |
| Folic acid (7) | FDA | |
| Seat belts (2, 8) | | All state transportation laws |
| Car safety (8) | NHTSA, other U.S. Dept. Transportation | State laws |
| Safety at work | OHSA | State laws and agencies |

(Continued)

## TABLE 4.1 (Continued)

### Public Health Protection Every Day

| | SERVICES | |
|---|---|---|
| PUBLIC HEALTH ISSUE | FEDERAL RESPONSIBILITY | OTHER RESPONSIBILITY |
| Nutrition (2, 3) | USDA, HHS (various) | State agencies, school districts, food pantries |
| Dental Care (3) | CMS, HRSA | State agencies, school districts, dentists |
| Immunization (2) | CMS, HRSA | State agencies, local health departments, school districts, medical providers |
| Reproductive health— STD control (6) | CDC (training, guidance, lab oversight) | State and local health departments, medical care, family planning and other non-profit organizations, medical care, pharmacies (condoms) |
| Folic acid (7) | USDA (WIC) | State and local health departments, medical care, pharmacies |
| Healthy weight (2) | | Medical care, private & nonprofit organizations (e.g., Weight WatchersTM) |
| Smoking (2) | HHS (various) | American Cancer Society, American Heart Association, American Lung Association, state & local health departments, medical care, private orgs. (SmokeEndersTM, pharmacies (nicotine replacement) |
| Physical activity (2) | | Senior centers, American Heart Association, AARP, YMCA, YWCA, parks and recreation department, Sierra Club |

SOURCES:
1. National Institute of Neurological Disorders and Stroke, 2003
2. USDHHS, 2000
3. Office of the Surgeon General, 2000
4. EPA, 2003
5. FDA, 1998
6. Institute of Medicine, 1997
7. March of Dimes, 2004
8. NHTSA, 1997

and Drug Administration (FDA) inspects most other foods; the USDA inspects frozen lasagna if it has meat in it, but the FDA inspects vegetarian lasagna.

Also distinctively American is our heavy reliance on nonprofit organizations, rather than the state, to achieve public health goals. Yet nonprofit organizations in the United States also tend to be issue specific because they arose to meet a specific need (e.g., the American Heart Association, the Planned Parenthood Federation of America, the Environmental Defense Fund, and local AIDS service organizations).

The third cause of diffused responsibility for public health lies in the definition of health goals and debates about what should be done to achieve them. The World Health Organization (WHO) defines health as more than the absence of disease. Health is "a state of complete mental, physical and social well-being" (1978, WHO charter at www.who.int). Well-being is achieved, for example, when children perform well in school and do not fear violence in their communities. It is seen when physical and mental functioning is maintained well into old age, and when people have a better quality of life due to their state of health. Social, behavioral, and environmental forces have by far the largest role to play in determining health status. But where, then, do we draw the line between a health goal and other societal goals? Should we draw such a line? Who has responsibility, and for which goals? There is no correct answer to these questions, but there are superior ways for public health leadership to meet their challenge.

## DEFINING CHARACTERISTICS OF PUBLIC HEALTH

Three key assumptions distinguish public health from the health care delivery systems discussed in this book: (a) a healthy population is in the public interest, (b) health is strongly determined by community and societal-level forces, and (c) working at a collective or community level, these forces can be changed to improve a population's health.

### A Healthy Population Is in the Public Interest

#### The Health of Populations

The health status of entire populations, as opposed to individuals, is the focus of public health. It concerns the prevalence, incidence, and distribution of health problems, as described in chapter 2. In using these indicators, public health aims to identify health problems and improve them through action at a community or collective level. This aim is well justified by past success. Most of the increased life expectancy seen in the twentieth century was not caused by curative medical care, but mainly by pervasive public health improvements in the areas of sanitation and nutrition (Institute of Medicine, 1988). Many other achievements at the collective level have improved health since then.

The focus on populations discards the idea that sick people need care and other people can be ignored. Rather, there is a continuum of risk for many diseases and injuries in the population as a whole (Institute of Medicine, 2003b). For example, most Americans have an increased risk of heart disease compared to other societies, due to high cholesterol, inactivity, smoking, high blood pressure, and overweight (USDHHS, 2000a). In the same way, the average American has a 1 in 3 chance of a serious motor vehicle accident in his or her lifetime (National Highway Traffic Safety Administration [NHTSA], 1997). Public health focuses not only on people at highest risk of disease or injury, but on the whole distribution of people at risk.

### The Public Interest Justification

Since ancient times, people have sought to protect themselves at a community or collective level when faced with plague, famine, and environmental problems (Fee & Fox, 1988; Rosen, 1993). Prevention became increasingly effective through science and technology in the nineteenth century, when bacteriology emerged as a discipline and cities created clean water and sanitation systems (Duffy, 1992). In that era, public health was justified mostly on utilitarian grounds: the greatest good for the greatest number. Healthy people were a more productive workforce and were better able to defend the nation (Rosen, 1993).

However, this justification has changed. In its Alma-Ata Declaration, the WHO (1978) formally redefined health as a human right, and public health as a means to achieve social justice. Some Americans question whether social justice is a legitimate public health concern. In truth, a blend of utilitarian and social justice arguments support most public health services. Too much attention to the one can obscure the other. For example, many health departments are medical care providers to the poor. But is this strictly a social justice issue? It is also utilitarian if it produces a healthy workforce. Even as a medical care provider, the health department is also promoting health and preventing disease, for example, when it immunizes children and promotes healthy pregnancies. These services benefit all of society in the long run.

Some writers also challenge the utilitarian focus, questioning whether collective action and community benefit will jeopardize individual liberty (Leviton, Needleman, & Shapiro, 1997). Public health policy and practice are usually a balance between individual liberty and collective benefit. For example, health departments have police powers to control infectious disease, but they need to do so confidentially and with restraint.

Finally, some may question whether public health is a good use of tax money. Public health agencies at all levels of government reflect the mixed economy of the United States. They address some market failures of both curative and preventive care. A case in point is the treatment and prevention of STDs, which are highly infectious, widespread, and dangerous. Chlamydia and gonorrhea are especially dangerous for women and often have no symptoms (Eng & Butler, 1997). Many private providers do not routinely screen for STDs and greatly under-diagnose STDs. Private providers have neither authority nor resources to identify and treat the patient's sexual partners, an important step to prevent reinfection, and one that is essential to control STDs at a population level. Because STDs are a clear and present danger to the community, health departments can require treatment and will confidentially notify the sexual partners. Some may find this topic distasteful, but health departments have to take responsibility for these dangerous diseases in a realistic, objective way. The health care market place cannot handle this problem. Public health services are often a job no one else wants (Institute of Medicine, 2003c).

## Health Is Strongly Determined by Community and Societal-Level Forces

### Determinants of Health

McGinnis and Foege (1993) established that behavioral and environmental forces cause 70% of avoidable mortality. Health care, by comparison, makes a fairly small contribution. Yet it is estimated that health care accounts for 95% of federal expenditures on health in the United States (Institute of Medicine, 2003b). Public health interventions, provided they are effective, are likely to have more pervasive impact on health than will curative medical care (McGinnis, Williams-Russo, & Knickman, 2002). "It then follows that the nation's heavy investment in the personal health care system is a limited future strategy for promoting health" (Institute of Medicine, 2003b, p. 21).

FIGURE 4.1 portrays the range of health determinants. Some writers describe a chain of events influencing health, in which "upstream" forces such as policies and environmental conditions

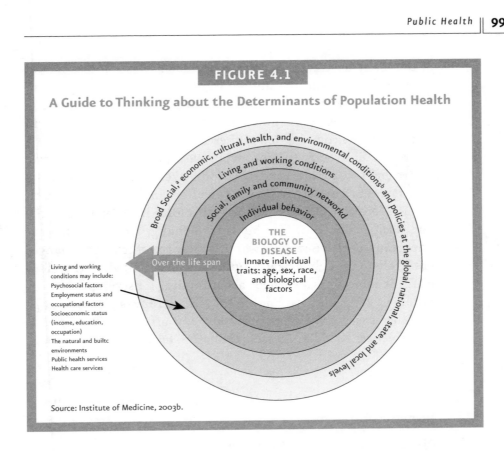

**FIGURE 4.1**

A Guide to Thinking about the Determinants of Population Health

Broad Social,ᵃ economic, cultural, health, and environmental conditionsᵇ and policies at the global, national, state, and local levels

Living and working conditions

Social, family and community networkᵈ

Individual behavior

THE BIOLOGY OF DISEASE
Innate individual traits: age, sex, race, and biological factors

Over the life span

Living and working conditions may include:
Psychosocial factors
Employment status and occupational factors
Socioeconomic status (income, education, occupation)
The natural and builtᶜ environments
Public health services
Health care services

Source: Institute of Medicine, 2003b.

can affect "midstream" forces, such as behaviors and other precursors of disease. Although it can address upstream and midstream determinants, medical treatment is primarily a "downstream" force, immediately and directly affecting a health condition. Public health often seeks strategies to affect upstream and midstream determinants. Kreuter and Lezin (2001) note,

> Both a focus on the individual and a focus on populations are important in order to achieve improvements in health. A population health approach stimulates us to consider a different and broader set of options for improving and sustaining health—not to replace a focus on individuals, but to complement and support it. (p. 4)

### Challenges for Public Health Policy
A focus on these broader determinants raises several questions. How far upstream should the public health mission extend? Which

of the many upstream, midstream, or downstream forces should be the focus? Should the intervention consist of law, regulation, partnerships with community leaders, collaboration with other private or nonprofit organizations, specific services, guidance and education, or a combination of these?

Green and Kreuter (1999) provide a useful framework to decide where and how to intervene. Decision-makers need to consider the *importance* of these forces (How big an effect do they have on health status?), *prevalence* (How common is this force in the population?), and *modifiability* (How feasible is it to change this force?). Most important, decision-makers want to know *how effective* the changes are likely to be. Public health funds are very limited, so therefore difficult choices must be made about funding for services. Yet with notable exceptions, the public health field was slow to adopt evidence-based practice or the analysis of effectiveness and cost-effectiveness (Haddix, Teutsch, & Shaffer, 1996; Leviton & Guinan, 2003).

## Community and Collective-Level Interventions Will Improve Health

### Disease Prevention and Health Promotion

At the *individual* level, the focus of prevention is on probabilities: reducing one's chances (risk) of disease. At a *population* level, the reduced risk for individuals translates into percentages or proportions: a lower rate of preventable diseases and injuries. The reduced burden of disease and injury is the nation's return on its investment in prevention.

The U.S. Preventive Services Task Force (1996) uses three long-accepted categories:

- *Primary prevention*, avoiding the onset of a health condition
- *Secondary prevention*, identifying and treating people who have developed risk factors or preclinical disease
- *Tertiary prevention*, treating established disease in order to restore the highest functioning, minimize negative impact, and prevent complications from disease

These categories obviously spill over into individual medical care delivery, but at a systems level, they are public health issues. Providers need guidance and support to carry them out. For example, primary prevention of cardiovascular disease involves maintaining a healthy weight, being physically active, and not smoking, all issues that primary care physicians should raise with patients. Secondary prevention of cardiovascular disease includes regular checkups for detection and treatment of high blood pressure, elevated cholesterol, and other risk factors (USDHHS, 2000a). Tertiary prevention of cardiovascular disease means avoiding death and loss of function through: widespread awareness of heart attack and stroke symptoms and the need to seek help quickly; rapid emergency services that will save the heart muscle or prevent stroke complications; treatment of atherosclerosis (blockages of the arteries); and cardiac rehabilitation and medication to restore function and prevent recurrence (National Heart, Lung and Blood Institute, 2004).

Notice that successful individual prevention depends on the availability of widespread prevention services at a *population* level. In this sense, even the rapid deployment of ambulances becomes a public health issue. Planning and development of prevention services requires a public health problem solving approach, one we describe in the next section.

Health promotion works to achieve the WHO definition of health as being more than the absence of disease. It is defined as "the combination of educational and environmental supports for actions and conditions of living conducive to health" (Green & Kreuter, 1999). Health promotion often focuses on prevalent behaviors, termed *behavioral risk factors* or *lifestyle factors* that promote or impair health (see chapter 10 and USDHHS, 2000a).

Risks that are preventable and unhealthful behaviors that can be changed are called *modifiable risk factors*. An important resource for public health, *Healthy People 2010* provides a comprehensive review of modifiable risk factors, effective strategies, and public health objectives for the nation (USDHHS, 2000a). The priority areas for these public health objectives are presented in EXHIBIT 4.1.

Strategies to prevent disease and injury vary in their effectiveness, cost-effectiveness, and public acceptability. Disease prevention and health promotion are rarely 100% effective because there are no "magic bullets" for most health problems. A residual group will continue to fall ill. For example, heart attacks will still occur, no matter how effective our primary and secondary prevention strategies become.

Together, several strategies can have a cumulative benefit. Motor

## EXHIBIT 4.1

### Healthy People 2010: Goals and Focus Areas

**What Is Healthy People 2010?**
Healthy People 2010 is a comprehensive set of disease prevention and health promotion objectives for the Nation to achieve over the first decade of the new century. Created by scientists both inside and outside of Government, it identifies a wide range of public health priorities and specific, measurable objectives.

**Overarching Goals:**
1. Increase quality and years of healthy life
2. Eliminate health disparities

**Focus Areas**

| | |
|---|---|
| 1. Access to Quality Health Services | 15. Injury and Violence Prevention |
| 2. Arthritis, Osteoporosis, and Chronic Back Conditions | 16. Maternal, Infant, and Child Health |
| | 17. Medical Product Safety |
| 3. Cancer | 18. Mental Health and Mental Disorders |
| 4. Chronic Kidney Disease | 19. Nutrition and Overweight |
| 5. Diabetes | 20. Occupational Safety and Health |
| 6. Disability and Secondary Conditions | 21. Oral Health |
| 7. Educational and Community-Based Programs | 22. Physical Activity and Fitness |
| | 23. Public Health Infrastructure |
| 8. Environmental Health | 24. Respiratory Diseases |
| 9. Family Planning | 25. Sexually Transmitted Diseases |
| 10. Food Safety | 26. Substance Abuse |
| 11. Health Communication | 27. Tobacco Use |
| 12. Heart Disease and Stroke | 28. Vision and Hearing |
| 13. HIV | |
| 14. Immunization and Infectious Diseases | |

**Healthy People 2010**
http://www.healthypeople.gov
Healthy People Information line: 1 (800) 367-4725

**healthfinders**
http://www.healthfinder.gov

**Office of Disease Prevention and Health Promotion**
http://odphp.osophs.dhhs.gov

SOURCE: USDHHS, 2000.

vehicle injury presents a case in point: safer roads and cars helped to reduce the rate of injury and deaths, but air bags still made a major, additional contribution (Warner, 1983). And even with these protections, using safety belts still prevents an additional 45% of fatalities, 50% of severe injuries (60% in light trucks), and 16% of minor injuries (NHTSA, 1997). At first, the auto industry opposed requiring air bags because they anticipated higher cost and reduced sales of new cars. The industry mounted a campaign to encourage seat belt use instead (Warner, 1983). However, many people will not use seat belts, finding them uncomfortable, or mistakenly believing that a seat belt will trap them inside a car. Education by itself was not effective, but together with laws to enforce seat belt use, it increased the percentage of people who buckle up (NHTSA, 1997). All states passed seat belt laws after major debates about individual liberty and societal cost. The laws substantially increased the percentage of people using seat belts. In 1998, 79% of people reported using seat belts "all of the time," although 10% also admitted they went without a seat belt at least once in the previous week (NHTSA, 2000). Both education and state laws can still be improved (see http://www.nhtsa.dot.gov/people/outreach/safesobr/0Planner/protection/lawskey.html).

### Universal and Targeted Prevention

Universal prevention means that everyone receives the interventions equally, while targeted prevention means identifying and serving people at higher risk of disease and injury. Where they are available, universal approaches are often more effective to improve the health of populations. The case of traffic safety illustrates these approaches. Targeting drunk driving has improved everyone's safety on the road (NHTSA, 1997). Those who drive while intoxicated are clearly at highest risk of accidents and endanger others. However, universal protections such as seat belts, air bags, and better vehicles contribute much more to reducing traffic fatalities and injuries (NHTSA, 1997).

People at the highest risk of disease or injury are an important focus for public health when the risk is prevalent and when there are effective means to identify and treat them. For example, a national campaign in the 1970s led to improved identification and treatment of people with high blood pressure. This, in turn, greatly reduced premature death and disability from cardiovascular disease (CDC, 1999). However, an initial goal was to make sure that providers screened *all* their patients for high blood pressure, a population focus.

In many cases, targeting those at highest risk can also reduce the overall burden of disease and injury in the population. For example, prevention of Autoimmune Deficiency Syndrome (AIDS) has shifted from creating awareness in the entire population, to a three-tiered approach. First priority is to identify individuals that are already infected with the human immunodeficiency virus (HIV), in order to give them early treatment, reduce their viral load to forestall progression to AIDS, and help them to avoid infecting others. Second priority goes to people whose behavior puts them at high risk of HIV infection through unprotected sex or sharing needles and other equipment to inject illegal drugs. Third priority goes to continued awareness of the need for prevention in the population at large (Janssen, Holtgrave, Valdiserri, Shepherd, & Gayle, 2001).

## CORE FUNCTIONS OF PUBLIC HEALTH

The other defining characteristic of public health is its distinctive approach to problem solving for population-level health issues. This approach involves three core functions: assessment of health problems, policy development to take action on those problems, and assurance that the proposed actions are taken (Institute of Medicine, 1988).

### Definition of Core Functions

#### Assessment

The basic tools of public health assessment were described in chapter 2. This chapter, by contrast, describes what decision-makers and practitioners do with these indicators to improve the public's health. Public health agencies are primarily responsible for surveillance of health status in their communities, monitoring of disease trends, and analysis of the causes of those trends. However, they do not carry out this function by themselves. They are highly dependent on people and institutions that provide the information. For example, health care providers are required by law to report new cases of certain infectious diseases. However, maintaining a high level of cooperation for reportable diseases is essential. Data collection on health status is undergoing profound changes in light of the need for rapid responses to potential bioterrorism, localized outbreaks of infectious diseases, and containment of emerging new infectious diseases such as avian flu and Severe Acute Respiratory Syndrome (SARS) (Institute of Medicine, 2003b, 2003c).

### Policy Development

The second core function is to create and advocate for solutions to achieve public health goals. Policy development activities can be formal or informal. Formal policy development includes devising laws and regulations to protect the public, as in the case of environmental protection; funding and reimbursement for specific services, such as child immunizations; and setting guidelines or standards for services, such as laboratory testing for infectious diseases. However, the informal policy development process is also important, because public health organizations have neither the legal authority, financial capability, nor personnel to address all health problems by themselves. Realistically, public health agencies need to engage other organizations, community leaders, and professionals in planning and problem solving.

### Assurance

This third core function involves enforcement of policy, as in the case of sanitation inspections in restaurants or nursing homes; ensuring good implementation of necessary services, as in the supervision of home visits to new mothers in disadvantaged communities; and adequate response to crises, such as preparedness for biological terrorist attack. Again, however, public health organizations have limited capacity to assure all the relevant activities, by themselves. For example, local health departments are helped a great deal by voluntary compliance with health and safety codes. At the national level, OSHA cannot protect workplace safety everywhere, constantly. OSHA inspections and prosecution of violators are costly, labor intensive, and not very frequent for the most part, making voluntary compliance essential. The USDA cannot thoroughly inspect every last chicken for salmonella and other problems—resources are too limited and legal challenges are too easy (Institute of Medicine, 2003a). By engaging others in the process, public health's effectiveness for the assurance functions can be greatly multiplied.

## Illustration of Public Health Problem-Solving

The following case of a birth defect illustrates the public health problem-solving approach. As shown in FIGURE 4.2, it is a cycle of activities (USDHHS, 2001) that begins with defining a health problem, its magnitude and nature; then identifying causes and protective factors; developing and testing intervention strategies; implementing the interventions; evaluating the impact of the interventions; and revisiting these activities (redefining the problem, reevaluating causes, and refining interventions).

*Assessment.* Spina bifida is a neural tube defect that in its most severe form leads to leg paralysis, bowel and bladder control problems, and without treatment, can lead to mental retardation. Spina bifida affects between 1,500 to 2,500 babies in the United States every year, or one in every 2,000 live births. *Policy development.* The March of Dimes (2004) projects that up to 70% of cases can be prevented if women take enough folic acid before and during pregnancy. Folic acid has the most benefit for neural tube development before pregnancy and during the critical first weeks. For this reason, the March of Dimes recommends that even before they become pregnant, women take a multivitamin with 400 mg of folic acid

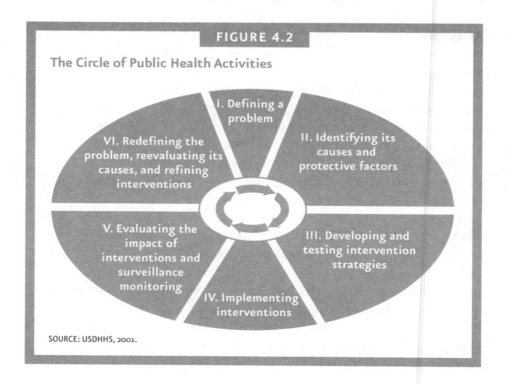

### FIGURE 4.2

The Circle of Public Health Activities

I. Defining a problem

VI. Redefining the problem, reevaluating its causes, and refining interventions

II. Identifying its causes and protective factors

V. Evaluating the impact of interventions and surveillance monitoring

III. Developing and testing intervention strategies

IV. Implementing interventions

SOURCE: USDHHS, 2001.

every day, and eat foods rich in folic acid. *Assessment.* Unfortunately, women may not be able to follow the guideline. Women may
not know they are pregnant until it is too late and the defect has
developed. Also, foods that naturally contain folic acid may not be
readily available to the poor. *Policy development:* One alternative is
to fortify common foods with folic acid. *Assurance:* Since 1998,
enriched cereal, pasta, flour, and bread products have been
required to include folic acid. *Assessment:* After this requirement
was introduced, one study found a decrease of 19% in neural tube
defects (March of Dimes, 2004). *Policy development:* Many scientists
believe that the amount of folic acid in grain products is not
enough and want to change the regulation to increase it (March of
Dimes, 2004).

## Core Functions: Overlap of Roles and Responsibilities

The public health focus on populations and prevention overlaps
and complements the focus of health care delivery systems. This
happens in several ways. First, health care delivery systems often
deal with individual-level prevention. Also, a large variety of public, private, and nonprofit organizations adopt a public health
focus when they recommend, require, or train providers to deliver
more widespread prevention. A second area of overlap is that
health departments can sometimes serve as the medical provider of
last resort, providing curative medical care as well as prevention.

A third way that health delivery systems overlap public health is
when they use population health indicators. For example, an insurance company may study the health status of the "lives" it covers
(in other words, the population of families that pay for coverage).
It may do so in the public interest, but it may also do so to save
money. Motivations may not matter; people can do the right thing
for the wrong reasons. When private sector interests are in line
with public health goals, then alliances become possible to achieve
these goals. This has happened on issues ranging from infection
control, to quality of preventive services, to problem-solving
around migrant health and teen pregnancy prevention (Leviton,
Needleman, & Shapiro, 1997).

These overlaps are often confusing to the public and to policymakers, however. The key to understanding public health is that
no single organization or governmental agency has complete
responsibility for public health goals in this country. Medicine,
government, insurance companies, employers, schools, and many

other organizations and individuals adopt the public health role when they focus on prevention and on the health of populations, in the public interest.

## GOVERNMENTAL AUTHORITY FOR PUBLIC HEALTH

### Federal Authority and Infrastructure

Although the states have constitutional authority to implement public health, a wide variety of federal programs and laws assist the states. In **TABLE 4.2** we list the federal agencies that have primary responsibility for public health, along with their abbreviations, Web sites, headquarters location, and year established. The Web sites often list the many laws authorizing and appropriating funds for these public health activities. Most of these agencies conduct other activities besides public health, so we focus on their relevance to prevention and to population health. (For further information see Sparer in the next chapter.)

**USDHHS**, also called *HHS*, is the principal federal agency for assuring health and providing essential human services. All of its agencies have some responsibility for prevention. Through its 10 regional offices, HHS coordinates closely with state and local government agencies, and many HHS-funded services are provided by these agencies as well as by private sector and nonprofit organizations.

In the *Office of the Secretary, HHS*, are two units important to public health: the Office of the Surgeon General of the United States and the Office of Disease Prevention and Health Promotion (ODPHP). ODPHP has an analysis and leadership role for health promotion and disease prevention. ODPHP produced *Healthy People 2010*, the latest in a series of reports on health objectives for the nation that have a broad consensus and a science-based rationale (2000a).

The Surgeon General is appointed by the President and has the primary duty to provide leadership and authoritative, science-based recommendations about the public's health. For example, the Surgeon General's 1964 report that smoking causes cancer stimulated most of the work leading to the dramatic decline in smoking in the U.S. (USDHHS, 2000a). Recent Surgeon General Reports on obesity and oral health are referenced in this chapter (USDHHS, 2000b, 2001). The Surgeon General has titular responsibility for the

6,000 commissioned officers of the Public Health Service, who have positions throughout HHS and may also be assigned to universities, state, and local health departments. The eight health agencies of HHS are organized under the Public Health Service, or *PHS*, as follows.

### TABLE 4.2

#### Federal Agencies with Responsibility for Public Health

| ACRONYM | AGENCY | WEBSITE | HEADQUARTERS | ESTABLISHED* |
|---|---|---|---|---|
| USDHHS (or HHS) | U.S. Department of Health and Human Services | http://www.hhs.gov/ | Washington, DC | 1953/1979 |
| PHS | Public Health Service | http://www.hhs.gov/ | Washington, DC | 1798 |
| — | Office of the Surgeon General | http://www.surgeongeneral.gov/ | Washington, DC | 1871 |
| ODPHP | Office of Disease Prevention and Health Promotion | http://odphp.osophs.dhhs.gov/ | Washington, DC | 1976 |
| CDC | Centers for Disease Control and Prevention | http://www.cdc.gov/ | Atlanta, GA | 1946 |
| ATSDR | Agency for Toxic Substances Disease Registry | http://www.atsdr.cdc.gov | Atlanta, GA | 1980 |
| NIH | National Institutes of Health | http://www.nih.gov/ | Bethesda, MD | 1887 |
| FDA | Food and Drug Administration | http://www.fda.gov/ | Rockville, MD | 1906 |
| HRSA | Health Resources and Services Administration | http://www.hrsa.gov | Rockville, MD | 1982 |
| SAMHSA | Substance Abuse and Mental Health Services Administration | http://www.samhsa.gov | Rockville, MD | 1974/1992 |
| AHRQ | Agency for Health-care Research and Quality | http://www.ahrq.gov/ | Rockville, MD | 1968/1989 |
| IHS | Indian Health Service | http://www.ihs.gov/ | Rockville, MD | 1921 |
| CMS | Centers for Medicare & Medicaid Services | http://www.cms.hhs.gov/ | Baltimore, MD | 1977 |
| ACF | Administration for Children and Families | http://www.acf.hhs.gov/ | Washington, DC | 1912/1991 |

**(Continued)**

## TABLE 4.2 (Continued)

**Federal Agencies with Responsibility for Public Health**

OTHER AGENCIES

| ACRONYM | AGENCY | WEBSITE | HEADQUARTERS | ESTABLISHED* |
|---|---|---|---|---|
| AoA | Administration on Aging | http://www.aoa.gov/ | Washington, DC | 1965 |
| VA | U.S. Department of Veterans Affairs | http://www.va.gov/ | Washington, DC | 1930/1989 |
| USDA | U.S. Department of Agriculture | http://www.usda.gov/ | Washington, DC | 1862 |
| EPA | Environmental Protection Agency | http://www.epa.gov/ | Washington, DC | 1970 |
| NHTSA | National Highway Traffic Safety Administration | http://www.nhtsa.dot.gov/ | Washington, DC | 1966/1970 |
| OSHA | Occupational Safety and Health Administration | http://www.osha.gov/ | Washington, DC | 1970 |

NOTE: Many agencies were reorganized and renamed over time. Where possible, the entire set of dates is listed.

The CDC is the lead federal agency that develops and implements disease prevention and control, environmental health, and health promotion/health education activities. CDC serves as an authoritative source of information and guidance for state and local health departments. A hallmark of the approach used by the CDC is the promotion of health through strong community partnerships in the U.S. and abroad. Working with states and other partners, CDC provides a system of health surveillance to monitor and prevent disease outbreaks (including bioterrorism), implement strategies for both infectious and chronic disease prevention, and maintain national health statistics. Working with the WHO, the CDC also guards against international disease transmission, with U.S. personnel stationed in more than 25 foreign countries.

The CDC director is also administrator of the ATSDR, which helps prevent exposure to hazardous substances from waste sites on the U.S. Environmental Protection Agency's National Priorities List. It also creates toxicological profiles of chemicals at these sites. The CDC has recently undergone a reorganization of its many centers and offices.

The *NIH* is the world's premier medical research organization, comprised of more than 27 institutes and centers. The NIH supports over 35,000 research projects on diseases such as cancer, Alzheimer's disease, mental illness, arthritis, and HIV/AIDS. Much of the basic science and clinical research supported by the NIH is directly or indirectly relevant to prevention, and epidemiological (population-level) studies into the causes and risk factors for disease are often generously funded. The NIH also conducts some population-level prevention programs and demonstrations, but the agency faces a challenge when it comes to translating its research into practical services for widespread use (see chapter 10 this volume; Leviton & Guinan, 2003).

The *FDA* assures the safety of all food except for meat and poultry; all prescription and nonprescription drugs; all blood products, vaccines, and tissues for transplantation; all medical equipment and all devices that emit radiation, including microwave ovens; all animal drugs and feed; and even cosmetics. New products that are designed to treat human conditions or diseases are evaluated by the FDA reviewers for safety and effectiveness before being made available to consumers. Products can be as simple as a toothbrush or a nonprescription analgesic and as complex as a state-of-the-art excimer laser or the latest drug to treat HIV. To be approved, these products must meet the FDA's rigorous standards, and they must continue meeting them while on the market.

The *HRSA* helps build the health care workforce through many training and education programs. It also helps prepare the nation's health care system and providers to respond to bioterrorism and other public health emergencies. Through the Bureau of Maternal and Child Health the HRSA administers a variety of programs to improve the health of mothers and children. Working with the CDC, it coordinates HIV prevention and treatment for persons living with HIV/AIDS.

The *SAMHSA* works to improve the quality and availability of substance abuse prevention, addiction treatment, and mental health services. The SAMHSA provides funding through block grants to states to support substance abuse and mental health services and helps to improve substance abuse prevention and treatment services through the identification and dissemination of best practices. The SAMHSA also monitors prevalence and incidence of substance abuse.

The *AHRQ* supports research on health care systems and quality, including ways to introduce more preventive services into primary care. It also houses the U.S. Preventive Services Task Force, an independent panel that reviews evidence of the effectiveness of clinical preventive services and develops recommendations for primary care and preventive practice.

The IHS provides health services to federally-recognized American Indian and Alaskan native tribes. The IHS is the principal federal health care provider and health advocate for Indian people, and its goal is to raise their health status to the highest possible level.

### CMS

Readers may find it very odd to see the CMS on a list of public health agencies. However, the CMS has a vital role in primary, secondary, and tertiary prevention through the reimbursement of medical care services and its influence on state Medicaid and SCHIP programs. Through its policies on reimbursement for preventive services, the CMS can determine whether doctors get paid to provide routine mammograms and adequate prenatal care. By paying for quality, the CMS can require that the most effective and cost-effective prevention practices get widespread use.

### ACF

The Administration for Children and Families is not a health agency, but it is responsible for approximately 60 programs that promote the economic and social well-being of children, families, and communities. Many of these programs are strongly linked to prevention and to population health. The ACF administers the state-federal public assistance program, Temporary Assistance for Needy Families, the national child support enforcement system, and the Head Start Program. The ACF provides funds to assist low-income families in paying for child care; supports state foster care and adoption assistance programs; and funds programs to prevent child abuse and domestic violence.

### AoA

The AoA's mission is to promote the dignity and independence of older people, and to help society prepare for an aging population. The AoA is not a health agency but it is part of a federal, state, tribal, and local partnership called the National Network on Aging. This network consists of 56 State Units on Aging; 655 Area Agencies on Aging; 233 tribal and native organizations; and 2 organizations that serve Native Hawaiians. Ranging from primary prevention activities in senior centers to tertiary prevention through Adult Day Care Centers, AoA serves health by promoting successful aging.

**Other federal agencies:** The **VA** is the second largest cabinet level agency, serving the needs of veterans. As a major provider of health care, the VA system, like CMS, provides preventive services.

**USDA:** Although the USDA was created to help America's farmers and ranchers, today it also focuses on prevention and the health of populations. It is responsible for the safety of all meat, poultry, and egg products. Through the Food and Nutrition Service (FNS), the USDA also leads the federal anti-hunger effort and promotes good nutrition through the Food Stamp, School Lunch, School Breakfast, and the Women, Infant and Children (WIC) programs. It sets nutrition guidelines and publicizes its food pyramid. It is a research leader in everything from human nutrition to new crop technologies that allow increased food and fiber productivity using less water and fewer pesticides. It works with state agriculture extension services in both urban and rural areas to educate the public on nutrition, sanitation, health education, and family life (e.g., parenting skills). The USDA brings housing, modern telecommunications, and safe drinking water to rural U.S communities. Finally, the USDA also plays a role in environmental health through the Forest Service (Forest Service, www.fs.fed.us/aboutus/) as the steward of the national forests and rangelands. It is the country's largest conservation agency, encouraging efforts to protect soil, water, and wildlife on the 70% of America's lands that are in private hands.

The **EPA** is an independent agency that develops and enforces environmental regulations for clean air and water; keeping food free of pesticide contamination; preventing pollution and reducing risks to communities, homes, workplaces, and ecosystems; improving waste management; cleaning up already contaminated sites; handling hazardous materials and emergency responses to problems posed by these materials; and providing credible deterrents to pollution and compliance with the law. The EPA delegates monitoring and enforcement to states and tribes. About 50% of the EPA's budget supports state environmental programs. Where national standards are not met the EPA has legal authority to enforce the standards and penalize noncompliance. It also supports research and assessment to improve decision-making about environmental issues. It educates the general public about the environment. It also fosters and partners with a wide variety of private, nonprofit, state, and local organizations on voluntary programs and research.

The **NHTSA**, an agency of the U.S. Department of Transportation, is responsible for preventing death, injury, and economic loss due to motor vehicle crashes. This is accomplished by setting and enforcing safety performance standards for motor vehicles. Grants to state and local governments support local highway safety programs. These include reducing the threat of drunk drivers and promoting the use of seat belts, child safety seats, and air bags.

**OSHA**, an agency of the U.S. Department of Labor, sets standards for the safety and health of workers, enforces those standards, encourages continual improvement, partners with state health and safety organizations, business, and labor to achieve improvements, and provides training, outreach and education on health and safety.

**Other federal agencies.** Several other federal agencies are relevant to public health, for example, the Department of Housing and Urban Development (to provide clean and safe places to live) and even the Department of Homeland Security (to prevent, and to coordinate the response to, terrorist attacks). In fact, the list could go on. For example, assurance of pure foods goes far beyond the FDA, USDA, and EPA, to include the Consumer Product Safety Commission (enforcing the Poison Prevention Packaging Act), the FBI (enforcing the Federal Anti-Tampering Act), the Department of Transportation (enforcing the Sanitary Food Transportation Act), and the U.S. Postal Service (enforcing laws against mail fraud; FDA, 1998).

## State and Local Authority and Infrastructure

**State and federal relations.** Under the Tenth Amendment to the U.S. Constitution, states have primary responsibility for public health. State responsibilities for public health include: disease and injury prevention, sanitation, water and air pollution, vaccination, isolation and quarantine, inspection of commercial and residential premises, food and drinking water standards, extermination of vermin, fluoridation of municipal water supplies, and licensure of physicians and other health care professionals.

However, states vary greatly on how they define and delegate authority and responsibility. The lack of uniformity is due in part to the power struggle between the states and the federal government. Both levels of government have strengths and resources to respond to the concerns of the country's citizens. States and localities are closer to the communities that they serve and thus understand health threats and potential solutions that combine local insight into the root causes and can allocate locally-identified assets. However, the state legislatures and governors give different priorities to public health in terms of budget and authority. Sometimes state and local standards and services for public health exceed those that are required or recommended, and sometimes they do not or cannot meet these standards and recommendations.

On the other hand, the federal government generally has greater resources and scientific expertise necessary to tackle complex health threats. The CDC, for example, leads the investigation of certain disease outbreaks such as SARS. The federal government also steps in when states cannot meet regulated standards, as in the case of EPA pollution standards. When states cannot meet recommended guidelines for service, the federal government can provide some technical assistance, as in the case of public health performance standards and competencies (Institute of Medicine, 2003b,c). The federal government also provides financial support, such as block grants to the states for maternal and child health, preventive services, various child welfare services, and substance abuse and mental health. Finally, the federal government also gets involved when health threats such as SARS cross state borders; however, such actions can add to the already fragmented provision of public health services within states and local communities.

**Power and position of state public health agencies.** The state health officer (SHO) directs the department of health. The SHO may report directly to the governor, or to an officer in the governor's cabinet. The SHO's position affects the quality, influence, and coordination of state health departments. For example, a state's Medicaid program, its human services and welfare programs, and its environmental programs can all be free-standing, combined with the health department or with each other, or coordinated under a cabinet level officer. Medicaid and public assistance programs may take most of the governor's attention in any case, but the influence of the SHO can be impaired by the chain of command.

The organization of these functions also matters for coordination of public health activities. For example, environmental protection is often located outside the health department, in which case conservation, wilderness preservation, or legal responses to toxic spills may take center stage. When an independent agency deals with environmental protection, the health department coordinates activity to monitor potential health consequences of environmental exposures.

**Organization of state and local public health agencies.** Several designs are common for state-level public health provision and management, with varying administrative models, scope of authority and responsibility, and associated challenges.

Some states centralize their public health powers within a few state agencies. These agencies are responsible for the administration of public health care, the control of communicable diseases, population-focused health promotion, and environmental health. Both general and specific public health responsibilities are legislatively assigned to a comprehensive department of health. Even within the centralized model, however, other agencies have a role in the implementation of public health. For example, the South Carolina Department of Health and Environmental Control (SCDHEC) is the central agency charged to "promote and protect the health of the public and the environment." However, the SCDHEC is not the only state-level agency contributing to public health. Examples of other agencies include: the South Carolina Department of Alcohol and Other Drug Abuse Services, which is charged with preventing and treating substance use, the South Carolina Board of Barber Examiners, which licenses barbershops, and the South Carolina Department of Disabilities and Special Needs, which serves persons with mental retardation or other disabilities.

In the decentralized approach, by contrast, the state public health agency does not directly perform public health services, and minimally regulates local and municipal services. A decentralized approach confers local-level autonomy to meet local needs. Local communities are often the first to be affected by public health challenges. Citizens expect both formal and informal community leaders to offer solutions and provide services. Thus, in the decentralized approach, the state delegates public health authority and direct responsibility to local communities.

Most states take a hybrid approach to the distribution of public health powers. These states share the public health functions between the state and local governments. For example, the state legislature may assign primary responsibility for certain functions to the state department of health while simultaneously delegating specific functions to local governments. These local public health authorities enjoy independence from state control over their assigned responsibilities, but they must defer to the state department of health on other matters.

The National Association of County and City Health Officials (NACCHO) website (www.naccho.org) offers further detail on the range of organizational arrangements, responsibilities, and authority of local health departments. One reason that local health departments have such a varied relationship with state health departments is the cycle of growth. The first public health agencies were formed in the early 1800s and were primarily city based. The next wave occurred later in the nineteenth century when state health agencies began to form. Finally, the early 1900s saw the development of county based health departments. Their development continued throughout the twentieth century (Institute of Medicine, 2003b).

**State public health codes.** State law was created over time to respond to specific diseases or health threats. For that reason, as of 2004 many codes are in need of revision (Gostin, 2000). For example, some state laws have separate sections for specific communicable diseases instead of standard approaches to address infectious disease. Where state laws deal separately with communicable diseases such as smallpox, tuberculosis, and HIV/AIDS, the state has no standard to address new infectious diseases such as SARS or the West Nile virus.

Some state public health laws do not reflect advances in public practice and constitutional law, neglecting important safeguards for privacy and against discrimination. For example, in many states, statutes give broad discretionary power to health departments and boards of health without due process. Some state laws authorize health departments to quarantine individuals whenever officials determine it is necessary, providing little guidance on the factors necessary. Public health laws are also inconsistent within and among states. This inconsistency creates problems when diseases or public health challenges cross state lines. All these flaws could be a serious problem in the event of bioterrorism or other emergencies.

Many public health laws at the federal, state and local levels are antiquated and internally inconsistent, and thus insufficient and ineffective. The Institute of Medicine (1988, 2003b, c) has recommended that states review and revise their public health statues in order to (a) clearly delineate the basic authority and responsibility entrusted to public health entities and (b) develop and support a set of modern disease control measures, adapted to contemporary health problems and threats. To that end, a Model State Public Health Act has recently been developed. This Act provides a systematic approach to public health authority and implementation of public health responsibilities. Divided into nine articles to address current and future health threats, a public health law should include: modern surveillance techniques including reporting practices; epidemiologic investigations in response to specific outbreaks or high rates of diseases or conditions among subpopulations; testing and screening for existing and emerging conditions; vaccination for vulnerable populations, including children and others at risk of disease transmission; and responsible and respectful use of quarantine and isolation, where warranted, in cases of communicable conditions.

**Essential public health services.** In the face of tremendous

---

### EXHIBIT 4.2

**Essential Public Health Services**

**Assessment**
1. Monitor health status to identify community health problems
2. Diagnose and investigate health problems and health hazards in the community

**Policy Development**
3. Inform, educate, and empower people about health issues
4. Mobilize community partnerships to identify and solve health problems
5. Develop policies and plans that support individual and community health efforts

**Assurance**
6. Enforce laws and regulations that protect health and ensure safety
7. Link people to needed personal health services and assure the provision of health care when otherwise unavailable
8. Assure a competent public health and personal health care workforce
9. Evaluate effectiveness, accessibility, and quality of personal and population-based health services

**Serving All Functions**
10. Research for new insights and innovative solutions to health problems

SOURCE: Institute of Medicine, 2003c.

variation in services and functions, public health professionals agree that all health departments should provide 10 essential services. They are listed in EXHIBIT 4.2. However, health departments' abilities in these areas are often in question. Most of them are seriously understaffed. Local health departments have serious needs to upgrade the skills of their employees. In fact, the qualifications of the workforce have been eroding over time, and experienced professionals are not being replaced. Effective partnerships with other organizations are a problem when public health has become marginal. In many locales, this was a problem in the case of emergency response to terrorism. The erosion of resources, workforce competencies, and leadership are all issues that public health needs to address. The way they are doing so is the subject of the final section of this chapter.

## CHALLENGES AND OPPORTUNITIES

Public health has set a daunting task for itself. In order to maintain public protections and make further progress, public health must overcome three major challenges. It must find ways to improve the infrastructure. It must better communicate its value to the public, and it must restore both leadership and effective advocacy.

### Improving the Infrastructure

Throughout this chapter we have illustrated how the public health infrastructure is in trouble. This can lead to absurd situations. We know an infectious disease physician who was bitten by a bat but her local health department could not get a quick lab test for rabies. A colleague dialed the state health department hotline one evening during the anthrax crisis, and the state epidemiologist answered the phone—no one else was available. These represent serious flaws in the infrastructure. However, there are several recent developments that provide hope for improving the infrastructure.

**Public health competencies and performance standards.** Working with national public health organizations such as NACCHO and the Association of State and Territorial Health Officials (ASTHO), the CDC has developed the National Public Health Performance Standards Program (CDC, 2004). This program provides guidance on specific competencies for public health workers in areas such as laboratory, informatics, and environmental health technology (Institute of Medicine, 2003). The performance standards may eventually become requirements, but in 2004 they help to clarify what is expected of public health workers providing state and local services. The standards may also help to motivate improvements, by identifying and publicizing gaps in the infrastructure of states and localities.

Some public health competencies are less technological and more administrative or developmental. For example, culturally competent public health services will become increasingly important as our nation becomes ever more diverse (Institute of Medicine, 2003). Creating coalitions, gaining allies to address public health problems, and managing the process requires a skill set for interpersonal relations, not technical excellence (Nelson & Essien, 2002).

Schools of public health are vital to many of the country's public health functions. However, a relatively small percentage of health department employees have an advanced public health degree. New opportunities to develop the existing workforce include continuing education, management academies, and certificate programs. The curriculum in schools of public health is moving toward more of a focus on community problems and greater relevance to the needs of the public health infrastructure (Institute of Medicine, 2003c).

**Other national developments.** The terrorist attacks of 2001 led both the public and policymakers to pay renewed attention to public health. The anthrax attacks in particular, highlighted these problems, and facing the possibility of biological attack, Congress appropriated much more funding to the CDC and to state health departments. This influx has permitted some improvements by making it possible to hire new staff, upgrade the Health Alert Network, and improve computer-based informatics. ASTHO's experience, in particular, is that this additional funding has strengthened the overall public health infrastructure, at the same time that it helps to prepare the country for defense against terrorism (Steib, 2004).

Another positive national development is the emergence of state-level Public Health Institutes (PHIs). These institutes are outside the state government, which offers several advantages. First, state employees are restricted as to what they can say in terms of advocacy for public health programs and funding. PHIs are not. Second, PHIs are fast and flexible where state bureaucracies are not, to address emerging problems, hire new staff, conduct timely research, or mount new programs. Third, PHIs can sometimes offer a credible, neutral third party approach on issues where the health department cannot serve this function. They can convene all the interested parties to address a health problem and can implement a multi-sector approach that is sometimes just not possible for health departments, given their categorical funding and staffing process. This ability to partner effectively is important, since so many different sectors and organizations have an influence on public health. We have said that partnerships are effective when there is a cross-sectoral interest in public health, and that people can do the right thing even for the wrong reasons. PHIs are a good vehicle to make this happen. In general, health departments are quite positive about the PHIs and see their value (Institute of Medicine, 2003c).

The Turning Point Initiative is an effort to transform the U.S. public health system into a more effective, more community-based, more collaborative, and more responsive system. Initiated in 1997, Turning Point operated through state and local partnerships within selected states, and through several collaboratives. A Public Health Law collaborative working group guided states through a comprehensive analysis of the structure and appropriateness of current state public health statutes, including an examination of how statutes prescribe financing for public health programs and services. A performance measurement collaborative worked to assess and monitor agency performance using the standards set forth by the CDC. Several other positive consequences came out of Turning Point (see the NACCHO website for an overview, at http://www.naccho.org/project30.cfm).

## Public Relations for Public Health

### The Challenge of Communication

The Institute of Medicine (2003b,c) asserts that effective communication about public health issues is a key competency that needs much more attention. The general public does not understand what public health is. People often view public health as programs for the poor, nor do other terms such as disease prevention or health protection do much better in conveying what public health is all about.

Public health has difficulty conveying the importance of its work and the issues it addresses. For example, when public health professionals talk about "infrastructure," they too often assume that outsiders know what it means concretely, and why it is so important. People are more likely to respond to crisis, as seen in the reaction to our limited public health capability to deal with anthrax deaths in 2001.

## Public Health Flashpoints

Public health goals can sometimes conflict with other social or political agendas. The most prominent example in recent years has been the prevention of AIDS. Because men who had sex with men were the first group known to contract AIDS, policy support for its prevention was slow in coming, and many social conservatives expressed the belief that gays deserved AIDS (Shilts, 1987). These views certainly did not change when injection drug users started to contract AIDS, and opposition to dealing with AIDS remained high, even when HIV began to move into the larger population, infecting women and infants. Such world views are surprisingly common for a range of public health issues. Throughout history people have blamed outsiders for epidemics of infectious disease, and believed that personal character flaws caused illnesses such as tuberculosis (Fee & Fox, 1988). The very methods of public health can also conflict with other definitions of the public interest. For example, although condom use is one of the few effective ways to prevent HIV/AIDS, social conservatives are unwilling to promote condom use because it appears to sanction sex outside of marriage.

The best of intentions can lead to such conflicts. Public health workers can walk into these problems, completely unaware of the flashpoints, unless they have careful preparation. We once saw a toxicologist tell an audience of air pollution activists that opening a factory near their community would not harm their health. Although he was world-famous in his field, the audience almost physically attacked him. Speaking the truth is not enough—truth deserves effective communication.

Fluoridation offers another case in point with a surprising political twist. Originally, opposition to its use came from groups that were fearful of sabotage by the Communists. Today, new opposition comes from small segments of anti-government, alternative medicine, and environmental movements. Over one third of the population does not have fluoridated water. Yet fluoridation is the single most cost-effective way to achieve oral health and one with decades of demonstrated safety (USDHHS, 2000b).

### What Is Being Done

Public health professionals are addressing the challenges of public relations in a variety of creative ways. To improve communication about specific health risks and strategies, the CDC has developed *CDCynergy*, a computer based tool. Materials for improved communication are updated constantly at the CDC website (http://www.cdc.gov/communication/cdcyenergy.htm). The problem of risk communication has also received substantial attention (National Research Council, 1989). People do not understand risk very well. At least as important, communication about risks has to address people's interests and fears, as well as convey information. The early experience of the Environmental Protection Agency, the AIDS epidemic, and revelations about radiation at nuclear defense sites all make this abundantly clear (Leviton, Needleman, & Shapiro, 1997). If our toxicologist expert had been trained in risk communication, he would have prepared his remarks and framed them differently—or perhaps chosen a more effective spokesperson.

A second trend to improve public relations is the reemergence of community and cross-agency partnerships. Local public health departments have always connected to grassroots leadership and other public services, which is the way to solve collective problems at a local level. However, public health can sometimes tend to be authoritarian and paternalistic, especially if it prizes science and technology while ignoring collaboration and democratic process. This tendency weakens the connections to grassroots and local leadership. In some cases, it can actively undermine the public trust.

Several events spurred a renewed focus on regaining public trust. The most difficult lesson for public health came from the Tuskegee Syphilis Study (Jones, 1993). In 1932, 600 poor African-American men in Macon County, Alabama, became syphilis research subjects without their knowledge, when the PHS and the Tuskegee Institute began a study of the natural course of syphilis, offering the men free medical care. Of 600 subjects, 339 had syphilis but were denied treatment for up to 40 years, even though a penicillin cure became available in 1947. As many as 100 died of syphilis before a public outcry and a federal advisory panel's recommendations halted the study in 1972. Along with the Nuremberg Code on medical experiments, the misfortune of the Tuskegee Study led Congress to require a wide variety of new protections for human subjects in research. In 1997 President Bill Clinton offered an official public apology to the eight survivors and families of the Tuskegee Study. However, African Americans never fully regained a trust in public health.

The environmental movement produced a new recognition of the need to partner with other organizations and to communicate with people on their own terms. Bureaucratic ways of doing business were simply less effective than community engagement to solve problems (Leviton, Needleman, & Shapiro, 1997). The AIDS epidemic also led to a renewed focus on community engagement: the populations at highest risk did not trust authority figures, and might not be seen in health care systems until it was too late (Leviton & Guinan, 2003).

The Turning Point initiative has helped to reinvigorate community partnerships. Turning Point helped public health workers to share experiences about how to create these partnerships, in what has come to be known as "collaborative leadership." At least as important, Turning Point helped to legitimize coalition building as a vital public health activity, at both state and local levels. Finally, Turning Point crystallized for many professionals, the importance of community partnerships for reestablishing effective leadership and advocacy, the third and final challenge.

## Restoring Leadership and Advocacy

### An Effective Policy Voice

Like the public, policymakers have difficulty understanding public health, or paying much attention to it except in a crisis. One reason may be that formally recognized public health programs have such small federal budgets compared to entitlement programs such as Medicare and Medicaid. For the most part, the NIH draws a constituency from basic and clinical researchers, not from prevention in general. The general public tends to rally around prevention and treatment of specific diseases, not prevention infrastructure. Therefore, can public health develop an effective public constituency?

### What Is Being Done

Professional organizations such as the American Public Health Association attempt to convey the importance of the mission and to advocate for needed change. ASTHO and NACCHO offer important tools to their membership to increase effectiveness in state and local policy and politics. The Trust for America's Health at http://healthyamericans.org/ is emerging as a vigorous and articulate champion.

Beyond such advocacy efforts, public health has a renewed recognition that coalition building and convening are central strategies for public health problem-solving. Throughout this chapter, we have attempted to show the many ways in which a wide variety of organizations take on the public health role when they focus on populations. This approach means that other interests can be aligned with the public health mission. For example, if neighborhoods have sidewalks, they allow people to be more physically active. At the same time, neighborhoods with sidewalks are more desirable and appreciate in value. Across the nation, public health professionals are now working with city planners, the police, developers, and others, reframing "suburban sprawl" as a health issue.

In the same way, public health organizations are now participating more effectively in combating terrorist attack, because they can show where the public health interest is aligned with national defense and emergency preparedness. In the process, they have

## CASE STUDY

You are an analyst for a federal agency. Congress has ordered your agency to come up with policy options to find a cure for birth defects. You recognize that (a) birth defects have many causes, (b) some can be treated, (c) some can also be prevented, but (d) not all of them can be "cured." You analyze this issue using the core functions of public health and the problem-solving process outlined under Core Functions of Public Health.

Based on the information about spina bifida later in that section, you decide it should be the focus for policy making on birth defects. You decide to propose three options to Congress: more research on treatment of spina bifida, more health education for women about folic acid, and new regulations to increase the amount of folic acid in grain products. You may also see other options, so be sure to discuss them! For each option, what would you need to know to determine effectiveness? Cost-effectiveness? What are the tradeoffs in each course of action? Who would support this option, who would be opposed, and does it matter? Is there a single best option? Why?

been able to show the relevance of public health preparedness to a wide range of public interest problems. Through this type of coalition building, at all levels, public health can leave the sidelines. It will require knowing when to lead and when to follow, but coalition building offers an exciting future for the field.

## DISCUSSION QUESTIONS

1. What is the difference between individual- and population-based prevention efforts? For population-based prevention, what is the difference between universal and targeted strategies?
2. What does a population focus take, in terms of planning, consensus building, and resources for implementation? In the case of safety belts? Heart attack prevention?
3. Why can't public health do more to achieve its goals? Name some of the political, legal, logistic, and resource problems.
4. What should be left to the public sector to do, to achieve public health goals? Where could other health care delivery systems do more to help? Why?
5. Give some examples of the constituencies that public health will have to reach in order to implement its goals. In the case of environmental health. In the case of HIV/AIDS.
6. Why do some public health problems pose "flashpoints" for conflict? What could be done about them? Give examples in the cases of STD, HIV, and fluoridation.
7. How would you personally balance individual liberty, the common good, and social justice in public health? What would have to change to achieve this balance? Give specific examples in the area of public health that you are best acquainted with.

## REFERENCES

Centers for Disease Control and Prevention. (1999). Achievements in public health, 1900–1999: Decline in deaths from heart disease and stroke—United States, 1900–1999. *Morbidity and Mortality Weekly Report, 48,* 649–656.

Centers for Disease Control and Prevention. (2004). *The National Public Health Performance Standards Program.* Atlanta, GA: Author. Retrieved July 30, 2004, from http://www.cdc.gov/programs/partnr07.htm

de Tocqueville, A. (2001). *Democracy in America.* New York: Signet.

Duffy, J. (1992). *The sanitarians: A history of American public health* (Reprinted ed.). Urbana, IL: University of Illinois Press.

Eng, T. R., & Butler, W. T. (Eds.). (1997). *The hidden epidemic: Confronting sexually transmitted diseases.* Washington, DC: National Academy Press.

Fee, E., & Fox, D. M. (1988). *AIDS: The burdens of history.* Berkeley, CA: University of California Press.

Food and Drug Administration. (1998). *Food safety: A team approach.* Washington, DC: USDHHS, FDA.

Gostin, L. (2000). *Public health law: Power, duty, restraint.* Berkeley, CA: University of California Press.

Green, L. W., & Kreuter, M. (1999). *Health promotion planning: An educational and ecological approach.* New York: McGraw Hill.

Haddix, A. C., Teutsch, S. M., & Shaffer, P. (1996). *Prevention effectiveness: A guide to decision analysis and economic evaluation.* Oxford, UK: Oxford University Press.

Hooker, T., & Speisseger, L. (2002). *Public health: A legislator's guide.* Denver, CO: National Conference of State Legislators at http://www.ncsl.org/programs/health/publichealth.htm

Institute of Medicine. (1988). *The future of public health.* Washington, DC: National Academy Press.

Institute of Medicine. (2003a). *Scientific criteria to ensure safe food.* Washington, DC: National Academy Press.

Institute of Medicine. (2003b). *The future of the public's health in the 21st century.* Washington, DC: National Academy Press.

Institute of Medicine. (2003c). *Who will keep the public healthy? Educating public health professionals for the 21st Century.* Washington, DC: National Academy Press.

Janssen, R. S., Holtgrave, D. R., Valdiserri, R. O., Shepherd, M., & Gayle, H. D. (2001). The serostatus approach to fighting the HIV epidemic: Prevention strategies for infected individuals. *American Journal of Public Health, 91,* 1019–1024.

Jones, J. H. (1993). *Bad blood: The Tuskegee syphilis experiment.* New York: Free Press (New and expanded ed.).

Kreuter, M., & Lezin, N. (2001). *Improving everyone's quality of life: A primer on population health.* Seattle: Group Health Community Foundation.

Leviton, L. C., & Guinan, M. E. (2003). HIV prevention and the evaluation of public health programs. In R. O. Valdiserri (Ed.), *Dawning answers: How the HIV/AIDS epidemic has helped to strengthen public health.* Oxford, UK: Oxford University Press.

Leviton, L. C., Needleman, C. E., & Shapiro, M. (1997). *Confronting public health risks: A decision maker's guide.* Thousand Oaks, CA: Sage.

McGinnis, J. M., & Foege, W. H. (1993). Actual causes of death in the United States. *Journal of American Medical Association, 270,* 2207–2212.

McGinnis, Williams-Russo, P., & Knickman, J. R. (2002). The case for more active policy attention to health promotion. *Health Affairs, 22,* 78–93.

March of Dimes. (2004). Spina bifida. *Quick references and fact sheets.* Retrieved March 15, 2004, from http://www.marchofdimes.com/professionals/681 1224.asp

National Heart, Lung and Blood Institute. (2004). *National Heart Attack Alert Program: Program description.* Bethesda, MD: Author. Retrieved July 29, 2004, from http://www.nhlbi.nih.gov/about/nhaap/nhaap_pd.htm

National Highway Traffic Safety Administration. (1997). *Compendium of traffic safety research projects, 1987–1997.* Retrieved July 28, 2004, from http://www.nhtsa.dot.gov/people/injury/research/COMPEND2.HTM

National Institute of Neurological Disorders and Stroke. (2003). *Understanding sleep: Brain basics.* Bethesda, MD: National Institutes of Health.

National Research Council. (1989). *Improving risk communication.* Washington, DC: National Academy Press.

Nelson, J. C., & Essien, J. D. K. (2002). *The public health competency handbook: Optimizing individual and organizational performance for the public's health.* Atlanta, GA: Emory University. Online at www.naccho.org/GENERAL810.cfm-7k

Rosen, G. (1993). *A history of public health* (Expanded ed.). Baltimore: Johns Hopkins University Press.

Shilts, R. (1987). *And the band played on: Politics, people and the AIDS epidemic.* New York: St. Martin's Press.

South Carolina Department of Health and Environmental Control. (2004). *About DHEC.* Available: www.scdhec.net/board.htm

Steib, P. A. (2004). Federal funding key to public health preparedness. *ASTHO Report, 12*(2), 1, 5.

U.S. Department of Health and Human Services. (2000a). *Healthy People 2010: Understanding and improving health* (2nd ed.). Washington, DC: U.S. Government Printing Office, November 2000. Stock Number 017–001–001–00–550–9.

U.S. Department of Health and Human Services. (2000b). *Oral health in America: A report of the Surgeon General.* Rockville, MD: USDHHS.

U.S. Department of Health and Human Services. (2001). *The Surgeon General's call to action to prevent and decrease overweight and obesity.* Rockville, MD: Author.

U.S. Environmental Protection Agency. (2003). *Water on tap: What you need to know.* Washington, DC: EPA (EPA 816-K-03-007).

U.S. Preventive Services Task Force. (1996). *Guide to clinical preventive services* (2nd ed.). Washington, DC: USDHHS.

Warner, K. E. (1983). Bags, buckles, and belts: The debate over mandatory passive restraints in automobiles. *Journal of Health Politics, Policy and Law, 8*, 44–75.

World Health Organization. (1978). Declaration of Alma-Ata International Conference on Primary Health Care. Alma-Ata, USSR, 6–12 September 1978. www.who.int/hpr/NPH/docs/declaration_almaata.pdf

# 5

# THE ROLE OF GOVERNMENT IN U.S. HEALTH CARE

Michael S. Sparer

**LEARNING OBJECTIVES**

- Review the evolution of government's role during the course of American history
- Describe the roles of the federal, state, and local governments in the U.S. health care system.
- Examine the key issues and options on the current health policy agenda.

**TOPICAL OUTLINE**

- The government as payer: The health insurance safety net
- The government as regulator
- The government as health care provider
- Key issues on the health care agenda

**KEY WORDS**

Government, regulation, Medicare, Medicaid, Child Health Insurance Program, Employee Retirement and Income Security Act (ERISA), public hospitals, the uninsured

GOVERNMENT IS DEEPLY entrenched in every aspect of the American health care system. The federal government provides tax incentives to encourage employers to offer health insurance to their employees, provides health insurance to the poor, the aged, and the disabled, and operates health care facilities for veterans. State governments administer and help pay for Medicaid, regulate private health insurance and medical schools, license health care providers, and operate facilities for the mentally ill and developmentally disabled. Local governments own and operate public hospitals and public health clinics, and develop and enforce public health codes.

Even with this extensive agenda, government officials seem certain to add new tasks and new programs. The nation is engaged in an ongoing debate over whether government should guarantee health insurance to the 45 million people who are currently uninsured. Federal and state officials are engaged in an equally controversial debate over the rise of managed care and the extent to which government should regulate the managed care industry. And the aging of the baby boom generation prompts many to suggest that the nation needs to do more to develop an adequate and affordable system of long-term care.

The goal of this chapter is to provide an overview of government's role in the health care system. The chapter is divided into three sections. First is a discussion of government as a payer for health care services. The theme is that government provides health insurance to many of those who are not covered by the employer-sponsored private health insurance system. The section describes the evolution of the private system, the gaps in that system, and the government efforts to aid those outside of the private system. Second is a summary of government as regulator of the health care system. The focus is on state and federal efforts to enact patient protection legislation. Third is a discussion of government as a provider of health care. The section reviews the health systems operated by the three levels of government: the Veteran's Administration facilities run by the federal government, the institutions for the mentally ill operated by the states, and the public hospitals and public health clinics owned and administered by local governments.

## THE GOVERNMENT AS PAYER: THE HEALTH INSURANCE SAFETY NET

For much of U.S. history, the national government and the states were minor players in the nation's health and welfare system. The nation's social welfare system was shaped instead by the principles that governed the English poor law system. Social welfare programs were a local responsibility, and assistance was to be provided only to those who were outside of the labor force through no fault of their own (the so-called deserving poor). National welfare programs were considered unwise and perhaps even unconstitutional. The main exception was the Civil War pension program, which provided federal funds to Union veterans, but even this initiative was administered and implemented at the local level.

Lacking federal or state leadership (and dollars), local governments tried to provide a social and medical safety net. The most common approach was to establish almshouses (or shelters) for the indigent aged and disabled. There was often also a medical clinic that provided health care to almshouse residents. These clinics eventually evolved into public hospitals, offering services without charge to the poor. Generally speaking, however, the clinics (and hospitals) provided poor quality care and were avoided by those that had any alternative. Similarly, the few private hospitals then in operation were charitable facilities that served only the poor and the disabled. These hospitals, like their public counterparts, represented only a small (and rather disreputable) portion of the American health care system.

Most 19th century Americans instead received health care in their homes, often from family members who relied on traditional healing techniques. At the same time, an assortment of health care providers (including physicians, midwives, medicine salesmen, herbalists, homeopaths, and faith healers) offered their services as well. Generally speaking, these providers charged low fees and people paid out of pocket, much as they would for other commodities.

As the nineteenth century drew to a close, however, two developments fundamentally changed the nation's health care marketplace. First, the physician community began to dominate the competition between the various individual providers. Americans increasingly believed that medicine was a science and that physicians were best able to deliver high quality health care. The status and prestige accorded to physicians grew while the role of alternative medicine providers declined.

The emergence of a physician-dominated health care system was accompanied by dramatic growth in the size and the status of the hospital industry. Indeed, the nation's stock of hospitals grew from fewer than 200 in 1873 to 4,000 (with 35,500 beds) in 1900, to nearly 7,000 (with 922,000 beds) by 1930 (Rosenblatt, Law, & Rosenbaum, 1992). This growth was prompted by several factors. First, advances in medical technology (antiseptics, anesthesia, x-rays) encouraged wealthier persons to use hospitals, thereby eliminating much of their prior social stigma. Second, the number of nurses expanded dramatically (as nurses evolved from domestics to trained professionals), and hospital-based nurses worked hard to improve hygienic conditions. Third, the growing urbanization and industrialization of American life produced an increasingly rootless society, that in turn lessened the ability of families to care for their sick at home. Fourth, the medical education system begin to require internships and residencies in hospitals as part of the training of the physician.

As the hospital industry grew, so too did the cost of care. By the mid-1920s, there was growing recognition that middle-income folks needed help in financing the rising costs of hospital-based and increasingly high-tech medicine. The onset of the Depression only made the situation more problematic. In response to the emerging crisis, various hospital associations formed health insurance companies to cover the high cost of hospital care (Blue Cross plans). At the same time, medical associations formed health insurance companies to cover the cost of physician care (Blue Shield plans). More and more Americans began to rely on private health insurance.

During the 1940s and 1950s, the federal government for the first time became a key player in the U.S. health care system, taking several actions that accelerated the trend toward a hospital-dominated delivery system and an employer-sponsored health insurance system. The federal activity was spurred in large part by the era of American optimism that arrived with the end of World War II. Advances in medical technology had prompted confidence that the medical system would in time conquer nearly all forms of disease. This perception prompted the federal government (through the National Institutes of Health) to funnel billions of dollars to academic medical researchers. And with federal dollars so readily available, medical schools soon emphasized research and medical students increasingly chose research careers. Around the same time, Congress enacted the Hill-Burton Program, which provided federal funds to stimulate hospital construction and modernization. The policy assumption was that all Americans should have access to the increasingly sophisticated medical care rendered in state-of-the-art hospital facilities.

The congressional decision to exempt fringe benefits, such as health insurance, from the wage and price freeze enacted during the 1940s, also had a profound effect on the health care system, encouraging employers to provide health insurance in lieu of wage increases. The growth of employer-sponsored health insurance accelerated even more following the decision by the Internal Revenue Service that employers could take a tax deduction for the cost of health insurance provided to employees. Over the next several decades, the employer-based health insurance system became increasingly entrenched. By the end of 2002, more than 64% of Americans received health insurance through their employer (Glied & Borzi, 2004).

As the employer-sponsored health insurance system grew, so too did concern about those unable to access such coverage (such as the aged, the disabled, and the otherwise unemployed). For many years, liberal politicians had argued without success in favor of government-sponsored health insurance. In 1949, President Harry Truman had even proposed that health insurance was part of the "Fair Deal" that all Americans were entitled to. However, neither Truman nor his liberal predecessors ever came close to overcoming the opposition to national health insurance from doctors, businessmen, and others who viewed it as "un-American" and "socialistic."

With the growth of the employer-based insurance system, the likelihood of a government-funded program became even more remote. As a result, by 1949 the mainstream Democrats abandoned their visions of universal insurance and proposed instead that the Social Security (retirement) system be expanded to provide hospital insurance to the aged. After all, the elderly were a sympathetic and deserving group, and hospital care was the most costly sector of the health care system.

Conservatives opposed the effort to provide hospital insurance to the aged, arguing that it unfairly (and unnecessarily) offered free coverage to many that were neither poor nor particularly needy. The conservatives argued instead that government's role is to be a safety net to the deserving poor who are unable to access employer-sponsored coverage. The result was an amendment to the Social Security Act in 1950 that, for the first time, provided federal funds to states willing to pay health care providers to care for welfare recipients. Interestingly, this "welfare medicine" approach passed with bipartisan support (Sparer, 1996; Stevens & Stevens, 1974). For liberals it was an acceptable, if inadequate, first step. At least some poor persons could now receive previously unavailable medical care. Conservatives also went along both because a medical safety net for the poor would undermine arguments for a more comprehensive health insurance program, and because responsibility for the program was delegated to state officials.

In 1960, newly elected President John F. Kennedy revived the effort to enact hospital insurance for the aged. Congress responded by expanding its "welfare medicine" model, enacting the Kerr-Mills Program, which distributed federal funds to states willing to pay health care providers to care for the indigent aged. Congress later expanded the program to cover the indigent disabled. These initiatives again deflected support from the Kennedy social insurance proposal.

The political dynamic seemed to be quite different, however, in 1965. President Lyndon B. Johnson and the Democrats now in control of Congress were enacting various laws designed to turn America into a "Great Society." This seemed to be an opportune time to renew the effort to enact national health insurance. Even longtime opponents of health insurance expansions expected Congress to enact legislation far more comprehensive than that embodied by the Kerr-Mills Program. Perhaps surprisingly, however, Johnson followed the path set by Truman and Kennedy and proposed again hospital insurance for the aged. At the same time, various Republican legislators, citing the nation's oversupply of hospitals, and proposing to return to a physician-centered delivery system, recommended that Congress enact physician insurance for the aged. And the American Medical Association (AMA), hoping to deflect yet again the social insurance model, urged Congress simply to expand the Kerr-Mills Program.

As Congress debated the various proposals, congressman Wilbur Mills, then powerful chair of the House Ways and Means Committee, and an aspiring presidential candidate, convinced his colleagues to enact all three expansion initiatives. Thus, Johnson's proposal for hospital insurance for the aged became Medicare Part A. The Republican proposal for physician insurance for the aged became Medicare Part B. The AMA's effort to expand Kerr-Mills became Medicaid. And the government for the first time became the health insurance safety net for those unable to access employer-sponsored coverage (Marmor, 2000).

## Medicaid

Medicaid is not a single national program, but a collection of 50 state-administered programs, each providing health insurance to low-income state residents. Each state initiative is governed by various federal guidelines, and the federal government then contributes between 50% and 78% of the cost (the poorer the state, the larger the federal contribution). In 2002, the various Medicaid programs covered roughly 51 million persons at a cost of more than $248 billion (Kaiser Family Foundation, 2004a).

Given its decentralized structure, state officials have considerable discretion to decide who in their state receives coverage, what benefits beneficiaries receive, and how much providers are paid. One not surprising result is that states like New York have more generous eligibility criteria than do Alabama or Mississippi. Interestingly, however, there is also a stark contrast between states that can be classified as both large and liberal. New York, for example, spends more than $7,600 per enrollee while California spends only

$2,068 (Kaiser Family Foundation, 2004b). During the late 1980s, Congress (for the first time) imposed rules designed to increase state coverage. In 1988, for example, Congress required states to cover pregnant women and infants with family income below 100% of the poverty line. State coverage for these populations had previously hovered around the 50% level. The next year, Congress required states to cover pregnant women and children under seven years of age with family income below 133% of the poverty level. Then, in 1990, Congress required states to phase in coverage for all children younger than 19 with family income below 100% of the poverty level. As a result of these mandates, the number of children on Medicaid nearly doubled between 1987 and 1995, growing from 10 million to 17.5 million. The overall number of beneficiaries increased from roughly 26 million to nearly 40 million.

During this era, the Medicaid expansions were the nation's main effort to reduce the ranks of the uninsured. At the same time, however, the Medicaid price tag grew from $57.5 billion in 1988 to $157.3 billion in 1995. State officials blamed this increase on the federal mandates. Federal regulators disputed the claim and suggested that the states themselves were largely responsible for the increase in Medicaid costs. Hence, there was significant intergovernmental tension (Holahan & Liska, 1997).

During the early 1990s, President Clinton, a former state governor (and critic of Medicaid mandates) stopped using Medicaid as the linchpin in an effort to reduce the number of uninsured. Clinton proposed instead to require employers to offer health insurance to their employees, thereby replacing public dollars with private in the effort to subsidize the cost of covering the uninsured. Clinton's proposal for national health insurance failed, but the shift away from federal Medicaid mandates remained. Instead of imposing Medicaid mandates, federal officials were approving state requests for waivers from federal Medicaid laws, thereby granting states additional flexibility and autonomy.

During most of the 1990s, there were two trends that dominated Medicaid policy. First, states used their expanded discretion to encourage or require beneficiaries to enroll in managed care delivery systems. Between 1987 and 1998, the percentage of enrollees in managed care increased from less than 5% to more than 50%, from fewer than 1 million to more than 20 million. Second, the growth in the number of Medicaid beneficiaries ended, and a slow decline in enrollees began.

The most convincing explanation for the enrollment decline was federal welfare reform, enacted in 1996. Before then, beneficiaries enrolled in Aid to Families with Dependent Children (AFDC) were automatically enrolled in Medicaid. Thereafter, however, those on welfare needed to apply separately for Medicaid, as did those no longer entitled to welfare (but still eligible for Medicaid). Millions do not know they are Medicaid eligible, the administrative hurdles deter others from applying, whereas still others are dissuaded by the stigma attached to receiving public assistance. For all of these reasons, the number of adult Medicaid beneficiaries declined by 5.5% between 1995 and 1997, and the number of child beneficiaries declined by 1.4% during the same period.

During the late 1990s, however, state and federal officials undertook a major effort to increase Medicaid enrollment. One strategy was to simplify the eligibility process (shortened application forms, mail-in applications, more eligibility sites). A second strategy was to simplify eligibility rules (eliminate asset tests and ensure 12-month continuous eligibility). A third strategy was to expand outreach and education (by increasing marketing activities and by encouraging community-based institutions to educate and enroll). These efforts to increase enrollment succeeded. Beginning in mid-1998, Medicaid enrollment began to increase, a trend that has continued into 2004.

The growth in enrollment, along with higher costs for prescription drugs, the disabled and long-term care, has led to escalating Medicaid costs in the last few years. At the same time, state tax revenue declined precipitously in the early 2000s. The ensuing budget crises prompted Medicaid cost-containment efforts in every state. The most popular option was an effort to control the rising cost of pharmaceuticals, either through leveraged buying (purchasing pools) or limits on access (formularies). Other Medicaid cost-containment strategies have included freezing or cutting provider reimbursement, reducing benefits (such as dental and home care), cutting eligibility, increasing co-pays, and expanding disease management initiatives.

## Medicare

Like Medicaid, Medicare was enacted in 1965 to provide health insurance to segments of the population not generally covered by the mainstream employer-sponsored health insurance system. And like Medicaid, Medicare has become a major part of the nation's health care system, providing insurance coverage to nearly 35 million persons over the age of 65, and to roughly 6 million of the young disabled population, at a total cost of just over $259 billion (Kaiser Family Foundation, 2004c).

In other respects, however, Medicare differs significantly from its sister program. Medicare is a social insurance program, providing benefits to the aged and the disabled regardless of income, whereas Medicaid is a welfare initiative, offering coverage only to those with limited income. Medicare is administered by federal officials (and the private insurers they hire to perform particular tasks), whereas Medicaid is administered by the states (pursuant to federal guidance). Medicare is funded primarily by the federal government (and by beneficiary co-payments and deductibles), whereas Medicaid is funded by the federal government and the states (without any beneficiary contribution). Medicare has a relatively limited benefit package (that excludes much preventive care, long-term care, and, until 2003, prescription drugs outside of the hospital and the oncologist's office), whereas Medicaid offers a far more generous set of benefits.

Medicare also is comprised of two separate parts, with different funding sources and different eligibility requirements. Medicare Part A covers inpatient hospital care. It is financed by a 2.9% payroll tax (1.45% paid by the employer and 1.45% paid by the employee). All beneficiaries automatically receive Part A coverage. Medicare Part B, in contrast, is a voluntary program, providing coverage for outpatient care for beneficiaries who choose to pay a $67 monthly premium (95% of beneficiaries choose to enroll). The balance of the Part B bill is paid by general federal revenues.

Prior to 1994, the revenue contributed to the Part A Trust Fund exceeded the program's expenses and the Trust Fund built up a significant surplus. Beginning in 1994, however, expenses began to exceed revenue, the surplus was used to pay bills, and the surplus began to decline. Medicare experts predicted that the surplus would be gone by the early 2000s, that the Trust Fund would be unable to pay its bills, and that Medicare would therefore slide into bankruptcy.

In response to this crisis, Congress in 1997 enacted a broad effort to reduce Medicare costs, mainly by cutting provider reimbursement. The legislation also contained provisions designed to encourage beneficiaries to enroll in managed care. While the managed care initiative has had only mild success (roughly 11% of Medicare beneficiaries are enrolled in managed care), the effort to cut Medicare spending was remarkably successful. In 1998, for example, Medicare spending actually declined, the first decline in the program's 33-year history (Kaiser Foundation, 2001).

The rapid shift in the economics of Medicare prompted an equally rapid change in the politics of Medicare (Oberlander, 2003). No longer were politicians claiming that the program was about to go bankrupt. No longer was there talk of greedy providers overcharging and generating excess profits. No longer was there an intense effort to enroll beneficiaries in managed care. There were instead three competing views about how to respond to the changed Medicare market. One camp emphasized the need to undo some of the cuts in provider reimbursement, others focused on the importance of expanding the Medicare benefits package, and still others argued against new spending measures (whether on behalf of providers or beneficiaries). This last group, the fiscal conservatives, proposed that any surplus remain in the Trust Fund to be used in years to come.

Faced with these options, Congress chose in 1999 to undo some of the cuts in provider reimbursement. Provider organizations argued that the prior cuts in reimbursement were unnecessarily endangering the financial health of thousands of health care providers. Even supporters of the cuts conceded that the extent of the reductions was far greater than expected. As a result, the Congress reduced the impact of the cuts by $16 billion (over the following 5 years) and $27 billion (over the following 10 years). The following year, Congress passed another giveback initiative, this time delivering to providers $35 billion (over 5 years) and $85 billion (over 10 years).

Following the provider giveback legislation, newly elected President George Bush and Congress took up the issue of prescription drug coverage, eventually enacting the Medicare Prescription Drug Improvement and Modernization Act of 2003. Under this legislation, beginning in 2006, beneficiaries can receive drug coverage through a managed care plan or, if they wish to stay in, fee-for-service Medicare, through a private prescription drug plan. The monthly premium for the drug coverage will be $35 (though the premium will be waived for the low-income). There will be a $250 deductible, after which the plan will pay 75% of drug costs up to $2250 and 95% of the costs beyond $3600 (the beneficiary will pay 100% of the costs between $2250 and $3600). Moreover, to compensate for the two-year delay in implementing the new initiative, Congress agreed to offer beneficiaries a Medicare-endorsed drug discount card for the period between June 2004 and January 2006. More than 70 organizations now offer these plans, which promise discounts of 10–15% off standard prices.

The Medicare drug legislation was extraordinarily controversial and partisan. President Bush and leading Republicans note that the legislation, expected to cost $410 billion over its first 10 years, is the largest public insurance expansion since Medicare was first enacted, and that it will provide significant coverage to millions of seniors. Leading Democrats, while supporting the goals of the legislation, complain that the initiative gives too little to needy seniors and too much to HMOs, big business, and the pharmaceutical industry. Four issues illustrate the conflict. First, the legislation prohibits Medicare officials from negotiating rates with pharmaceutical companies, instead requiring that prices be set by marketplace negotiations between drug companies and health plans. Second, in order to convince big business not to scale back retiree health coverage (which now provides drug coverage to 34% of all Medicare beneficiaries), the legislation provides $71 billion in subsidies to companies that retain retiree coverage. Third, the so-called dual-eligibles (those on Medicaid and Medicare), who now receive drug coverage from Medicaid, will instead be covered by Medicare, even though the Medicare coverage is typically less comprehensive. Finally, the legislation calls for a premium support demonstration in 2010, under which beneficiaries in six cities will receive a defined contribution (essentially a voucher with which to buy insurance coverage) rather than a defined benefit (entitlement to the current Medicare benefits package regardless of cost), thus raising fears among some about the long-term viability of the traditional Medicare program.

As suggested by its provision for the premium support demonstration, Bush's proposal on prescription drugs was designed, in part, to revive the effort to encourage beneficiaries to enroll in managed care. The managed care initiative was sagging, in part, because of declining health plan interest. In 1998, for example, there were over 6 million beneficiaries enrolled in 346 health plans. By early 2004, however, there were only 4.6 million enrolled in 145 plans (Kaiser Family Foundation, 2004d). The health plans cited inadequate reimbursement as the main explanation for their exit (even though several studies suggested that federal officials were actually losing money on the managed care initiative, since Medicare capitation rates were set based on the health care experience of the average client in a particular community, while the typical enrollee was healthier and less costly than average).

In an effort to reverse the decline in health plan participation, and to advance the goals of privatization and competition, the Bush administration proposed that the new drug benefit be delivered exclusively by managed care plans. While the legislation as enacted does not go so far, it does dramatically increase health plan capitation rates in an effort to encourage greater health plan participation. In 2004, for example, average monthly capitation rates increased by 10.9%, and in some communities, rates went up by more than 40% (Kaiser Family Foundation, 2004d).

## Recent Efforts to Help the Uninsured

Over the last decade, the number of persons without health insurance has grown from roughly 35 million to approximately 45 million (or more than 15% of the nation's population). Moreover, nearly 82 million went without health insurance for some part of 2002 and 2003 (Families USA, 2004). Most of the uninsured (more than 80%) are in families with a full or part-time worker, and most of these workers are self-employed or employed by small businesses. States with a strong industrial and manufacturing base are likely to have fewer uninsured, while states with large numbers of immigrants and a service-based economy are likely to have more. In Iowa, Massachusetts, and Wisconsin, for example, less than 10% of the population is uninsured, while in California, Louisiana, and Texas the percentage hovers between 20% and 25%.

Rather remarkably, the national increase in the number of uninsured began during a time of unprecedented economic growth, low unemployment, and relatively small rises in health care costs (the mid-1990s), although it accelerated during the economic downturn of the early 2000. Much of the increase in the uninsured population also occurred during a time when the Medicaid rolls were expanding dramatically.

The best explanation for the rise in the number of uninsured is the decline in the number of Americans with employer-sponsored private health insurance. Between 1977 and 1996, the percentage of Americans under age 65 with employer-sponsored coverage dropped from 67% to 60%.

The decline in employer-sponsored coverage is due to several factors. Many employers have increased the share of the bill that the employee is required to cover, prompting some employees to abandon the coverage. Other employers are reducing dependent coverage (for spouses and children) or phasing out retiree health coverage. Still other employers are hiring more part-time workers and outside contractors, thereby avoiding the need to even offer health insurance. At the same time, much of the recent job growth is in the service sector of the economy. These jobs are relatively low paying and often do not provide health insurance.

In response to these trends, and to media and political attention to the problems of the uninsured, state and federal officials tried during the early 1990s to enact new programs for the uninsured (Brown & Sparer, 2001; Sparer, 2003). These proposals generally sought to require employers to provide health insurance to their employees (and to use public dollars as a safety net for those outside the labor market). The idea was to retain and reinvigorate the employer-sponsored health insurance system. By the mid-1990s, however, the various employer mandate proposals (including the plan proposed by Bill Clinton) had disappeared, defeated by vehement opposition from the business community. Business opponents argued that the mandate would be too costly and would force employers to eliminate jobs (rather than provide health coverage).

Following the collapse of the employer mandate strategy, policymakers (especially at the state level) enacted a host of efforts designed to make health insurance more available and more affordable in the small group and individual insurance markets. These reforms focused on three problems in the health care system. First, employers in the small business community often cannot afford to provide health insurance to their employees. These employers lack the market clout to negotiate a good deal, particularly given the high administrative costs associated with insuring a small group. Second, the self-employed and the employee in the small business community generally earn too little to purchase their own health insurance policy. Third, individuals with a high risk of catastrophic medical costs are often excluded from the individual insurance market regardless of their ability to pay.

The most common of the insurance reform initiatives seeks to ensure that health insurance is available to all. As of late 1997, for example, 47 states had enacted legislation that requires insurers in the small group market to provide insurance to all small group applicants (so-called "guarantee issue" provisions). The same number of states also limit the insurer's ability to deny coverage for medical conditions that began prior to the insurance coverage (Robert Wood Johnson Foundation, 2000). And 33 states subsidize special insurance products (known as high-risk pools) for individuals who have been denied health insurance because of their medical condition.

Far more controversial, however, are state efforts that seek to make insurance more affordable. One strategy is to encourage small businesses to join state-run or state-regulated purchasing alliances. The goal is to supply increased market clout, decreased administrative costs, and therefore less expensive insurance premiums. Twelve states have launched such initiatives. In 1982, for example, California established the Health Insurance Purchasing Cooperative (the HIPC), which now purchases insurance on behalf of approximately 7,700 small business owners and 147,000 employees. In Colorado, in contrast, the state licenses and regulates privately administered small business insurance purchasing cooperatives. In neither state, however, has the alliance model provided significant aid to the uninsured: In California, for example, nearly 80% of the businesses that participate in the HIPC had previously offered insurance to their employees (but because of the alliance can now do so at a lower cost).

A second strategy is to allow health insurers to sell no-frills insurance policies, presumably at a lower cost than the more comprehensive packages states often require. As of late 1997, for example, more than a dozen states had enacted this sort of "bare-bones" insurance program. By most accounts, bare-bones policies have also not sold well. Those that can afford health insurance prefer a more comprehensive policy, while those unable to afford the traditional policies are typically unable to afford even the scaled back insurance product.

There are also efforts in several states to prohibit insurers from relying on the health status of the insured when determining the individual or the small group premium. These initiatives challenge the underwriting that underpins the insurance industry: the practice known as experience rating, under which persons with a high risk of catastrophic medical care are charged higher premiums than are healthy young adults at low risk of incurring significant medical costs. The goal instead is to require a single rate (called a "community rate") for all insured, thereby requiring the healthy to subsidize the expected medical costs of the ill. By late 1997, several states had enacted some form of community rating, though most allowed some variation in rates based on age, gender, or location.

The various insurance reform initiatives have had a modest impact. According to one study, roughly 11% of the insured who work for small businesses owe their coverage to the various reforms. At the same time, however, the reform initiatives have themselves generated significant political controversy, especially from healthy younger workers who complain about paying higher rates to subsidize the older and the sicker, and from insurance companies threatening to exit reform-minded states rather than comply with the new rules.

By the late 1990s, state and federal policymakers had shifted their focus away from the (disappointing) insurance reforms and toward programs that expanded health insurance for children. There were several factors that explained the emerging consensus. Children are considered a deserving group: there is bipartisan agreement that youngsters should not go without health care services because their parents cannot afford to pay. Children are also a relatively low-cost population. In 1993, for example, the average child on Medicaid cost just under $1,000; in contrast the typical aged beneficiary cost over $9,200, while the disabled population averaged just under $8,000. Child health initiatives are also consistent with the political agendas of both Republicans and Democrats. Republicans (along with many moderate Democrats) support insurance expansions as a counterbalance to other social welfare cutbacks. Families that move from welfare to work would still have health insurance for their children. At the same time, liberal Democrats, still reeling from the defeat of national health insurance proposals, see health insurance for children as an incremental step on the path to universal health care coverage.

Given this bipartisan support, Congress enacted the State Child Health Insurance Program (SCHIP) as part of the 1997 Balanced Budget Act. SCHIP provides states with just over $40 billion (over a 10-year period) to expand insurance programs for youngsters. States are generally required to spend SCHIP dollars on children who are not Medicaid eligible and who are in families with incomes below 200% of the federal poverty line. The main exception is for states that already provide Medicaid coverage to children in families with income more than 150% of poverty: these states can use SCHIP dollars to raise their income levels by 50%.

States can use the SCHIP funds to liberalize their Medicaid eligibility rules, or to develop a separate state program, or to do a combination of both. The main advantage to using the funds to expand Medicaid is administrative simplicity (for both the client and the state). This is especially so for families in which some children are eligible for Medicaid and others for SCHIP. At the same time, there are several advantages to creating a separate state program. Enrollment can be suspended when the dollars are spent (unlike Medicaid, which is an entitlement program). The state has more discretion when developing the benefit package. The state can impose co-payments and premiums (that are not allowed under Medicaid). Beneficiaries (and providers) may be more likely to enroll because the new program may lack the stigma associated with Medicaid. As of late 2002, to implement SCHIP, 21 states were relying on a Medicaid expansion, 16 states had implemented a separate state program, and 19 had instituted a combination of both.

By all accounts, the early efforts to enroll children into SCHIP were disappointing. By the end of 1999, roughly 1.5 million youngsters were enrolled in the program, far fewer than predicted. The low enrollment was due to several factors. Large numbers of eligible families did not know they were eligible. Others were deterred by the administrative burden of the application process. Still others were dissuaded by the stigma associated with many government insurance programs. And the premiums and other cost-sharing requirements clearly discouraged others. As a result, by the end of 2000, 38 states had not spent their full allotment of federal SCHIP dollars: funds not expended in these states were then reallocated to the dozen other participating states.

Beginning in early 2000, however, the SCHIP enrollment numbers began to significantly rise. By the end of the year, there were roughly 3.3 million enrollees, nearly double the number from the prior year, and by 2003 there were more than 5 million enrollees. Policymakers attribute the turnaround to improved outreach and education initiatives and to simplified processes for eligibility and enrollment. Moreover, there was bipartisan support for expanding SCHIP. In early 2001, for example, federal regulators authorized several states to use SCHIP dollars to cover parents (as well as their children). SCHIP even "dodged the first budget ax" in 2002 when state budget crises forced cutbacks in numerous other programs (Howell, Hill, & Kapustka, 2002).

## THE GOVERNMENT AS REGULATOR

One of the key issues in contemporary health politics is the extent to which the states and the federal government should regulate the managed care industry. Between 1997 and 2000, for example, 35 states enacted laws designed to protect patients who are enrolled in managed care. In 1999, both the United States Senate and the House of Representatives passed their own versions of a managed care bill of rights, and the effort to resolve the differences between the two bills became a bitter partisan battle. During the 2000 presidential campaign, George Bush and Al Gore debated vigorously over the content of a good patient protection act, both claiming to be fully in favor of the concept. While the issue slid off the political agenda during the early 2000s, a Supreme Court decision in mid-2004 limiting patients' right to sue their HMO is likely to generate renewed interest in legislative action.

The focus on patient protection during the late 1990s was prompted by a consumer backlash against managed care. Interestingly, however, the proposed federal legislation, if enacted, would represent an important policy shift as there is little precedent for federal regulation of the health insurance industry. At the same time, state legislators, while more accustomed to regulating private insurers (as well as other sectors of the health care industry) complained that their efforts are undermined by a federal pension law that restricts state regulatory activity. These officials urged Congress to repeal or amend the pension law and thereby provide the states with far greater regulatory autonomy.

This tale of regulatory uncertainty begins with the general proposition that the states have traditionally played a dominant role in regulating all aspects of the nation's health care system, although the federal government has also played a role in regulating the health care system. In the late nineteenth century, for example, federal officials began regulating the nation's food supply, and since 1938, the Food and Drug Administration (FDA) has regulated the introduction and use of new drugs into the medical marketplace. Indeed, the speed (or lack thereof) of the FDA's approval of new drugs is an ongoing source of controversy. Moreover, federal officials also require providers who participate in federal health insurance programs (such as Medicare and Medicaid) to comply with a host of regulatory conditions.

Despite these federal efforts, however, there remains a longstanding bias in favor of state regulatory activity. The states supervise the nation's system of medical education, license health care professionals, and oversee the quality of care delivered by health care providers. States also administer the workers' compensation system (which provides benefits to workers injured on the job), and they govern consumer efforts to hold providers accountable (whether through medical malpractice litigation or otherwise). Beginning in the early twentieth century, the states also began to regulate the nation's private health insurance system, establishing capitalization and reserve requirements, regulating marketing and enrollment activities, and (in some states) establishing the rates paid by insurers to various providers, especially hospitals.

Prior to the 1960s, however, state insurance departments rarely exercised their regulatory power, imposing few substantive requirements on insurance companies. Liberal critics complained that the relationship between providers, insurers, and regulators was far too cozy. Providers (especially hospitals) charged high rates, insurers paid the bill with few questions asked, and regulators did little to ensure that insurance companies were adequately capitalized (and even less to guarantee that clients were treated fairly).

In response to the critics, several states imposed new administrative requirements, most of which dealt with health plan finances, benefit packages, and marketing practices. In the mid-1960s, for example, New York regulated the rates that hospitals could charge insurers. About the same time, states also imposed tougher capitalization and reserve requirements. Over the next two decades, states required insurers to cover certain medical services (from mental health to chiropractor visits) in every insurance package they issued. Indeed, there are now more than 1,000 of these benefit mandates. For example, 40 states require that insurers cover alcohol treatment services, 39 require coverage for mammography, and 29 require mental health coverage.

The states' ability to regulate health insurers was limited, however, in 1974, when Congress enacted the Employee Retiree Income and Security Act (ERISA). Ironically, the issue Congress focused on when enacting ERISA was the unfair denial of pensions to employees. The law requires that pension plans be adequately funded, that investing requirements be reasonable, and that companies provide employees with understandable information about their pension programs. But the law also contains a provision that prohibits states from regulating employee benefit programs unless the law is part of the traditional state regulation of insurance. This clause has in turn led to ongoing controversy and litigation.

Consider, for example, the convoluted legal reasoning that governs state efforts to require insurers to cover certain medical services. These laws clearly relate to employee benefit programs. The courts have ruled, however, that the validity of the laws depends on whether the coverage is provided by a traditional insurance company (like Blue Cross or Prudential) or by a company that self-insures. The policies sold by the traditional insurers must include the mandated benefits, but the policies provided by the companies that self-insure need not. Indeed, following the same reasoning, the courts have held that companies that self-insure are exempt from state capitalization and reserve requirements, state taxes imposed on insurers, and all other state regulatory requirements (such as patient protection laws).

To be sure, companies that self-insure are required to implement any federal regulatory requirements: ERISA simply exempts them from state regulation. But federal officials have generally steered clear of imposing any such requirements. As a result, self-insured companies are generally unregulated: the states cannot regulate them, and the federal government rarely does. Not surprisingly, this regulatory vacuum encourages firms to self-insure: by the mid-1990s, more than 70% of large firms offered self-insured plans to their employees (Dranove, 2000), and more than 56 million Americans were covered by self-insured health plans.

ERISA also makes it extremely difficult for subscribers to sue their health plan. Consider, for example, the situation in which an individual claims she was injured when her health plan wrongfully refused to authorize needed care. The woman seeks to sue the health plan for negligence. Prior to ERISA, she could have initiated such a lawsuit in state court and demanded damages to cover the cost of the denied services, as well as compensation for the injury and the unnecessary pain and suffering endured. She might also have won punitive damages (intended to punish the health plan for its wrongful behavior). But because of ERISA, our hypothetical victim cannot bring her case to state court (unless she is a government employee, is in a government-funded health plan, or buys health insurance in the nongroup market). She must instead proceed in federal court under a very different set of rules. Yet, in her federal action, the most the woman could win would be the cost of the wrongfully denied care; she could not win compensation for pain and suffering, nor could she win punitive damages.

The impact of the ERISA barrier is also illustrated by the case of Goodrich vs. Aetna. Mr. Goodrich was a government prosecutor in California, suffering from stomach cancer, whose request for surgical relief was wrongfully denied and delayed (even though Aetna's own doctors were in favor of the procedure). After Mr. Goodrich died, his estate brought a lawsuit in state court seeking damages for the wrongful denial of care. The jury awarded his estate $4.5 million in actual compensatory damages, and $116 million in punitive damages (Johnston, 1999). Rather remarkably, however, had Mr. Goodrich not worked for the government, his estate would have had to proceed in federal court, and could have collected a maximum of roughly $400,000 (the cost of the surgical procedure).

Until recently, ERISA was also viewed as a barrier to cases in which patients sue the health plan for the poor care delivered by an affiliated doctor. During the late 1990s, however, several states (led by Texas) enacted laws designed to overcome this barrier and to permit such cases to proceed in state court. The courts have consistently distinguished these "poor quality of care" cases from the "wrongful denial of care" cases described above, and have so far permitted the cases to proceed. Whether the health plan is then held liable for the malpractice of the provider depends on the relationship between provider and plan. Staff model HMOs, which exercise close oversight of their salaried doctors, are more likely to be liable than are independent practice associations, with their large and loosely controlled provider network.

Patients' right to sue their HMO thus depends on the source of their health insurance (The Columbia University employee generally must sue in federal court and gets limited compensation, while the civil servant can sue in state court and has no limit on damages) and the nature of the claim (Even the Columbia University employee can sue in state court alleging poor quality care). In June 2004, the Supreme Court upheld this unwieldy and unfair set of rules, ruling that only Congress could remedy the inequity and that it could do so only by amending ERISA (Aetna vs. Davila, 2004).

ERISA has also emerged as a key component in the national debate over patient protection laws. As discussed earlier, more than 35 states have enacted such laws. Most of the laws require an appeal process when care is denied. Most also have rules governing access to the hospital emergency room. Some states require that subscribers have direct access to certain medical specialists. Others restrict the ability of health plans to censor what doctors say to their patients. Still others guarantee new mothers the right to spend at least 48 hours in the hospital following the birth of their child. Because of ERISA, however, none of these state laws protect persons enrolled in self-insured health plans.

The regulatory vacuum became especially controversial during the mid-1990s as there emerged a consumer backlash against much of the managed care industry. There was increased pressure on Congress either to amend ERISA (to allow state regulation of the self-insured) or to enact federal consumer protection legislation.

The effort to amend ERISA faces significant political opposition. The sponsors of the self-insured plans (especially multistate employers and labor unions) are well-organized and influential. The lobbyists for the self-insured argue that the goal of the law is to avoid inconsistent state regulation that would undermine the effective administration of their organizations.

Congress, however, has begun to experiment with federal consumer protection legislation, and may move further in this direction. In 1996, for example, Congress enacted a law that guarantees new mothers the right to spend at least 48 hours in the hospital following the birth of their child. The next year, Congress enacted the Health Insurance Portability and Accountability Act (HIPAA), which seeks to make health insurance more available to the self-employed and to those that work in small companies.

More recently, in 1999, both the House of Representatives and the Senate enacted versions of a managed care bill of rights. There were two main differences between the House and Senate legislation. First is the scope of the bills. The House version would cover all Americans with private health insurance, while the Senate bill would cover only those who work for self-insured companies (and are thus beyond the scope of the state patient protection initiatives) The second difference is the right to sue: the House bill enables consumers to sue their health plan; the Senate bill does not.

## THE GOVERNMENT AS HEALTH CARE PROVIDER

Each of the three levels of government owns and operates large numbers of health care institutions. The federal government provides care to veterans through the massive Veterans Affairs (VA) health care system. The states care for the developmentally disabled in both large institutional facilities as well as in smaller group homes. And local governments own and operate acute care hospitals and public health clinics that provide a medical safety net for the poor and the uninsured.

## The Veterans Affairs Health Care System

The Department of Veterans Affairs (VA) is required to offer health care to veterans and their dependents. There are approximately 70 million persons now eligible for these services (25 million veterans and 45 million dependents or survivors of deceased veterans).

In order to serve this population, the VA owns and operates 163 hospitals, 134 nursing homes, more than 800 outpatient clinics, and 206 readjustment counseling centers. These facilities are divided into 22 integrated service networks. In 2000, more than 3.6 million people received care in one of these facilities, at a cost of more than $19 billion.

The VA health care system is also an integral part of the nation's system of medical education. There are 107 medical schools and 55 dental schools that use VA facilities to train students and residents. Indeed, more than 50% of the nation's physicians have received part of their education and training in the VA health care system.

In recent years, the VA system has engaged in a wide-ranging effort to improve the quality of care provided in its facilities. The focus is a system designed to reduce the number of medical errors. The VA created the National Center for Patient Safety (NCPS) to take the lead in the effort. The NCPS program is considered so innovative and important that it was recently nominated as a finalist in the Innovations in American Government Program, sponsored by the Ford Foundation and the Kennedy School of Government at Harvard University.

The issue of medical errors received national attention when the Institute of Medicine reported that an estimated that 44,000 to 98,000 persons die each year because of medical errors. Much of the effort to reduce medical error focuses on individual wrongdoing: If only Dr. Jones had operated on the right leg; if only Nurse Smith had given the right medication, if only Nurse's Aide Wilson had held the patient and prevented the fall. As a result, hospitals and other providers respond to medical error (if at all) by trying to identify and punish the "culprit," while policymakers press for a practitioner data bank that will list the providers guilty of committing medical errors.

In contrast, the NCPS focuses less on individual blame and more on finding the root cause of the error, aimed at avoiding errors. For example, if the medication error is due to inadequate labeling of drugs, then better labeling would reduce the likelihood of future error. In the NCPS system, health care staff are encouraged to report "close calls" as well as "adverse events." For example, if Patient Jones is given the wrong medication but suffers no adverse consequences, that is a close call. If the surgeon uses instruments that are not properly sterilized but the patient does not develop an infection, it is a close call. In the past, no one was likely to report or investigate the event. The nurse would be too embarrassed and the system too uninterested. The goal now is to encourage the nurse to report, promising that the report will be completely confidential; to create a 3 to 4 person team to investigate the root cause of the error; and to develop a plan of action to make it less likely that a similar error will occur in the future.

## State Facilities for the Mentally Ill

Prior to the 1860s, caring for the mentally ill was considered a local responsibility, part of the safety net provided to the so-called "deserving poor." Perhaps the most common strategy utilized by county governments was to house the indigent insane in almshouses (or shelters) for the poor. County officials also locked away many of the severely mentally ill in local jails. And, by the mid-nineteenth century, several counties had also established hospitals for the mentally ill, though there was little effort at treatment even in the best of these facilities. The goal instead was to warehouse the mentally ill and keep them separate from the rest of society.

Dorothea Dix and other reformers slowly persuaded nearly every state legislature to assume responsibility for the mentally ill, and to construct state hospitals to provide for their care. The state hospitals generally were located in rural communities: reformers believed that the patients were more likely to improve in a quiet and serene environment (and of course most communities seemed perfectly content to ship their mentally ill off to distant facilities). State mental hospitals were also extraordinarily large, some with as many as 2,000 patients. In 1920, for example, the 521 state hospitals had an average bed capacity of 567. In contrast, the nation's 4,013 general hospitals then had an average bed capacity of only 78 (Starr, 1982).

By the turn of the twentieth century, state governments had emerged as the primary providers of care for those with mental—and other behavioral—disorders. Behavioral health became the only health problem with a separately financed and managed treatment system, and state governments assumed responsibility for the entire system (Hogan, 1999). The system grew exponentially, as county governments transferred many of those still under their jurisdiction (such as the old and the senile) to the state facilities (thereby transferring the cost of their care as well). By 1959, there were roughly 559,000 patients housed in state mental hospitals across the country (Katz, 1989).

Beginning in the 1960s, however, a new generation of reformers challenged the conditions in many of the state institutions. Patients were generally warehoused rather than treated, were kept isolated from families and friends, and were often brutalized by staff or other patients. At the same time, medical researchers were developing a host of new drugs that enabled large numbers to cope (more or less) in the community, thereby avoiding the harsh and dismal conditions in the hospitals. Perhaps most importantly, the federal government provided funding (both directly and through Medicaid) for community-based mental health services, while restricting federal funding for services provided in the hospital. Medicaid, for example, prohibited coverage for inpatient care in psychiatric institutions for persons between ages 22 and 64, while providing coverage for a host of mental health services provided to those in community-based settings. Similarly, Congress provided direct funding to help establish a system of community mental health centers.

For all of these reasons, state governments began a massive effort to discharge patients from the state hospitals and to divert others from admission. As a result, by 1980, the number of persons in state mental hospitals had dropped to roughly 130,000 (from a previous high of nearly 560,000) (Katz, 1989). In Ohio, for example, the number of patients in state hospitals dropped from 30,000 in the early 1960s to 1,200 today, while the number receiving publicly funded community care grew from 20,000 to around 250,000 (Hogan, 1999).

Despite the reallocation of resources, however, experts suggest that the new balance of responsibility for the mentally ill has replaced one set of problems (overcrowded and poor quality institutions) with another: Large numbers of mentally ill are unable to find adequate housing (and often end up homeless), and many of those in need are unable to access adequate mental health services—despite the growth in community-based services. Interestingly, however, few advocate a return to large-scale institutionalization. The most popular alternative among state officials is to delegate the problems of the indigent mentally ill to managed care plans that mainly serve those with behavioral health problems. It remains to be seen whether the managed care revolution will provide solutions to the long-standing problems of the mentally ill. What is quite clear, however, is that state governments will continue to have the overall responsibility for the mentally ill.

## Local Government and the Safety Net for the Poor

Scattered throughout America are more than 1,500 publicly owned general hospitals, nearly all of which are owned and operated by local governments. More than two thirds are small (fewer than 200 beds), located in rural communities, and have low occupancy rates (generally well below 50%). Many of the urban institutions, in contrast, are quite large and have high occupancy rates. For example, the 100 largest average nearly 600 beds and have an occupancy rate of roughly 80%. Indeed, the average big city hospital is three times the size of the typical, privately owned facility, has four times as many inpatient admissions, provides five times as many outpatient clinic visits, and delivers seven times as many babies.

The urban public hospital also treats a disproportionately high percentage of the poor and uninsured. In 1991, nearly 50% of their patient population was on Medicaid, 25% was uninsured, and only 12% had private insurance. These institutions also treat a sicker and more difficult population than do most of their commercial or nonprofit counterparts. These are the providers of last resort, treating the homeless mentally ill, the babies addicted to cocaine, and the victims of violence.

Local governments also fund and administer more than 3,000 public health departments. Each of these departments makes an effort, at least some degree, to assess the public health needs of the community, to develop policies that address those needs, and to assure that primary and preventive health are provided to all.

For most of the last century, health department officials focused their efforts on assessment (such as collecting data on diseases and epidemics) and general public health activities (regulating the quality of the water supply, enforcing local health codes, conducting health education campaigns). Indeed, the focus on populations and community-based services is what has distinguished public health from the traditional medical system. Only rarely would health department doctors themselves deliver health care, and when they did, it was usually to supplement a broader health campaign (immunizing children, for example, as part of an immunization campaign).

Beginning in the mid-1970s, however, local health departments shifted their resources away from infectious disease control (and other public health initiatives) and increased their efforts to become direct providers of primary and preventive care. Health departments have become an increasingly important part of the medical safety net. By the late 1980s, for example, 92% of local health departments were immunizing children, 84% were providing other child health services, and nearly 60% were offering prenatal care services. At the same time, many health departments provide large amounts of specialty care services, especially to populations underserved by the traditional medical community. For example, most county health departments provide mental health services. Others treat sexually transmitted diseases. Still others care for persons with AIDS (Wall, 1998).

The emphasis on direct-care services was prompted by the growing number of persons without health insurance and by the growing number of communities in which the local health department was the only (or the primary) source of care for the medically indigent. At the same time, however, the growing emphasis on direct-care services meant fewer resources for population-based activities. This shift prompted concern among many public health leaders. The public health department seemed to be retreating from its core mission (population-based activities) just as the nation seemed to be experiencing an epidemic of public health problems (from sexually transmitted diseases to tuberculosis to foodborne illnesses). Indeed, in 1998, the Institute of Medicine declared the nation's public health infrastructure to be inadequate and insufficient.

The risk posed by an inadequate public health infrastructure was illustrated clearly by the terrorist attacks on September 11, 2001, and by the efforts to use the mail to distribute anthrax in the weeks thereafter. While the public health community responded courageously to these various attacks, the need for additional resources was also clear. In response, Congress enacted the Public Health Security and Bioterrorism Preparedness and Response Act of 2002, which has appropriated over $2 billion to state and local health departments throughout the country. Early reports suggest that health departments have used the additional resources to improve preparedness, both against terrorism as well as for naturally occurring emergencies (from hurricanes to outbreaks of the West Nile virus), by engaging in preparedness planning, developing improved laboratories, and improving communication capacities (Trust For America's Health, 2003). At the same time, however, there is no question that the public health workforce remains inadequate (and still without a supply of new public health workers) and that our capacity to respond effectively to a biological or chemical attack remains one of the most important unknowns of the twenty-first century.

## KEY ISSUES ON THE HEALTH CARE AGENDA

Health care policymakers are grappling with a host of difficult issues, ranging from the uninsured to the long-term care system to how best to serve those with special needs (such as mental illness or substance abuse). In this section, three such issues are identified, and the key options on the policy agenda are summarized.

### The Uninsured

There were about 45 million Americans without health insurance in 2004. Policymakers need to make a series of decisions about this population. Should government target its dollars on further expanding the various public insurance initiatives? How can government encourage those who are eligible but not enrolled in the public programs to sign up? Is it wiser to spend public dollars providing tax credits and other incentives to encourage persons to purchase their own private insurance policies? Are there other ways to help the uninsured, and if so, are they politically and financially feasible?

During the 2004 campaign, President Bush proposed four strategies for helping the uninsured: (a) offering a tax credit ($1,000 per individual and up to $3,000 per family) to enable the uninsured to buy health insurance in the individual market; (b) providing small businesses the opportunity to join "association health plans," which would pool their purchasing power and which would be immune from state regulation; (c) making tax exempt the cost of premiums for high deductible health plans purchased in tandem with health savings accounts, and (d) funding hundreds of new community health centers to provide health care to the poor and the uninsured. The Bush plan, which would rely primarily on the private marketplace to aid the uninsured, would cost roughly $90 billion over 10 years and would provide coverage to 4 to 5 million of the uninsured.

During the same campaign, U.S. Senator John Kerry argued that the federal government needs to play a key role in aiding the uninsured. Kerry proposed (a) making dramatic expansions in Medicaid eligibility (with the federal government bearing the cost of the expansions); (b) permitting individuals and businesses to join a new federal purchasing pool (the Congressional Health Plan) that would build on the Federal Employees Health Benefits Program; and (c) having the federal government reinsure employer-sponsored coverage (by paying 75% of the medical bills that exceed $50,000 per year) as long as the employer used the savings to lower premiums). The Kerry plan would cost roughly $653 billion over 10 years and would provide coverage to about 27 million of the uninsured. Kerry recommended financing the cost of the initiative by rescinding recent tax cuts for annual incomes above $200,000.

## Medicare and Prescription Drugs

Even before the enactment of the Medicare Prescription Drug, Improvement, and Modernization Act of 2003, more than 75% of Medicare beneficiaries had some coverage for the cost of prescription drugs, either from a retiree health plan, a managed care plan, a Medi-gap policy, Medicaid, or a state-financed pharmaceutical assistance program. Nonetheless, with rising drug costs, more than 10 million seniors without any drug coverage whatsoever, and health plans and large companies scaling back the scope of their drug coverage, the political pressure to produce Medicare drug coverage became irresistible.

Over the next several years, policymakers will undoubtedly revisit some of the more controversial elements of the recent drug legislation. Among the key issues sure to resurface are the provisions prohibiting Medicare officials from negotiating prices with the pharmaceutical industry; the subsidies provided to large employers to retain retiree coverage; the higher rates paid to managed care plans; the imposition of income-based premiums on persons with annual income above $80,000; the so-called "donut hole" which requires beneficiaries to pay a large percentage of their drug costs; the premium support demonstration to be implemented in 2010; and the requirement that dual eligibles receive coverage from Medicare and not Medicaid.

## Regulating the Managed Care Industry

Just as in the debate over Medicare prescription drug coverage, there is bipartisan support for the concept of a national patient protection act; but sharp differences exist between the political parties as to the best way to achieve the goal. There are two key issues that dominate the debate. First, most liberals want the national law to apply to all those with private health insurance (roughly 158 million Americans). The Republican leadership, in contrast, suggests that the bill cover only those 57 million or so who are in self-insured health plans and thus exempt from state patient protection laws.

Second, the more expansive proposal allows consumers to bring lawsuits to state court against HMOs for the denial (or delay) of needed health care treatment. In these state court proceedings, injured parties could receive compensation for pain and suffering, as well as punitive damages designed to punish especially malicious acts. The Republican leadership opposes such a broad right to sue, preferring instead to allow lawsuits only in federal court (if at all), with limited rights to compensation for pain and suffering and without any right to punitive damages.

## CASE STUDY

There are more than 7 million children without health insurance in the United States. In response to this crisis, Congress both expanded the Medicaid program and enacted the Child Health Insurance Program. Millions of uninsured children are eligible for these public programs but are not enrolled. Others are in families with income too high to qualify for eligibility. Why are so many youngsters eligible but not enrolled? What can government do to make it more likely that these youngsters will enroll? What should government do for those who are not eligible for these public programs? Respond from the viewpoint of a congressman, a state legislator, an insurance executive, a hospital manager, and a consumer advocate.

## DISCUSSION QUESTIONS

1. What is and should be the role of the various levels of government in the health care system?

2. Should Congress enact a managed care bill of rights, and if so, what should be its content?

3. Should the recent Medicare drug legislation be amended to enable Medicare officials to negotiate directly with pharmaceutical companies?

4. What should government do to aid the uninsured?

5. How should public health departments balance the following three tasks: operating clinics that provide medical care to low-income populations, engaging in population-based efforts to improve the overall health of the population, and serving as the linchpin of bioterror preparedness activities?

## REFERENCES

*Aetna Health, Inc. v. Davila.* (2004).

Brown, L. D., & Sparer, M. S. (2001, January/February). Window shopping: State health reform politics in the 1990s. *Health Affairs, 20,* 50–67.

Dranove, D. (2000). *The economic evolution of American health care.* Princeton, NJ: Princeton University Press.

Families USA. (2004). One in three: Non-elderly Americans without health insurance.

Glied, S. A., & Borzi, P. C. (2004). The current state of employer based health care. *Journal of Law, Medicine, and Ethics, 32,* 404–409.

Hogan, M. (1999, September/October). Public sector mental health care: New challenges. *Health Affairs, 18,* 106–111.

Holahan, J., & Liska, D. (1997). The slowdown in Medicaid growth: Will it continue? *Health Affairs, 16,* 157–163.

Howell, E., Hill, I., & Kapustka, H. . (2002). *SCHIP dodges the first budget ax.* The Urban Institute, Assessing the New Federalism. Policy Brief A-56.

Institute of Medicine. (1998). *The future of public health.*

Johnston, D. (1999, January 21). $116 million punitive award against Aetna. *New York Times,* C1.

Kaiser Family Foundation. (2004a). *The Medicaid program at a glance.* Washington, DC: The Kaiser Foundation.

Kaiser Family Foundation. (2004b). *State health facts.* Washington, DC: The Kaiser Foundation.

Kaiser Family Foundation. (2004c). *Medicare at a glance.* Washington, DC: The Kaiser Foundation.

Kaiser Family Foundation. (2004d). *Medicare advantage*. Washington, DC: The Kaiser Foundation.

Katz, M. (1989). *The undeserving poor*. New York: Pantheon Books.

Marmor, T. (2000). *The politics of Medicare* (2nd ed.). New York: Aldine de Gruyter.

Oberlander, J. (2003). *The political life of Medicare*. Chicago: University of Chicago Press.

Robert Wood Johnson Foundation. (2000, January). *The state of the states*. Princeton, NJ: Author.

Rosenblatt, R., Law, S., & Rosenbaum, S. (1997). *Law and the American health care system*. The Foundation Press.

Sparer, M. S. (2003). Leading the health policy orchestra: The need for an intergovernmental partnership. *Journal of Health Politics, Policy and Law, 28,* 245–270.

Sparer, M. S. (1996). *Medicaid and the limits of state health reform*. Philadelphia: Temple University Press.

Starr, P. (1982). *The social transformation of American medicine*. New York: Basic Books.

Stevens, R., & Stevens, R. (1974). *Welfare medicine in America: A case study of Medicaid*. New York: Free Press.

Trust for America's Health. (2003). Ready or not? Protecting the public's health in the age of bioterrorism.

Wall, S. (1998, May/June). Transformations in public health systems. *Health Affairs, 17,* 64–80.

# 6

# A COMPARATIVE ANALYSIS OF HEALTH SYSTEMS AMONG WEALTHY NATIONS

Victor G. Rodwin

WINDOWS CAN SOMETIMES be mirrors. A look at health systems abroad—particularly in nations at similar levels of economic development—can enable us to develop a better understanding of our own health system at home. That, at least is the presumption of this chapter.

We tend to be ethnocentric in our views of health care organization and policy. Despite differences in the organization and financing of their health care systems, however, most health policymakers in other wealthy nations share a number of common problems with their counterparts in the United States. First, how should they decide—or explicitly not decide—what proportion of gross domestic product (GDP) should be devoted to health and welfare? Second, how should they agree on appropriate criteria to allocate health and social service expenditures? Third, how can they implement established policies: through regulation, promotion of competition, budgeting, or reimbursement incentives directed at health care providers?

Although this chapter does not answer these questions, it does provide an historical context, an overview of health system models, and a broader framework within which to compare health systems.

## THE EVOLUTION OF HEALTH SYSTEMS AND POLICY IN WEALTHY NATIONS

Over the course of the twentieth century, national governments have gradually extended their role over the financing and organization of health care services. What was once largely the responsibility of the family, philanthropy, religious institutions, and local governments has largely been taken over by national and subnational governments—a trend that has accompanied the rise of the welfare state (De Kervasdoué, Kimberly, & Rodwin, 1984). This evolution has affected all wealthy, industrially advanced nations that form the majority members of the Organization for Economic Cooperation and Development (OECD).[1]

The pattern of increasing government expenditure and intervention in the health sector became more pronounced in the decades following World War II to the point where few people could claim not to have benefited from many dimensions of this government largesse. Even in the United States where conservatives have resisted this trend, who could claim not to have benefited—directly or indirectly—from hospitals that were granted tax-exempt status or other government subsidies, health professionals who were trained with government grants, medical research that was financed by the federal government, private health insurance that was tax deductible to an employer, or a whole host of public health programs, including Medicaid or Medicare?

The growth of government involvement in health care systems

---

[1] I define "wealthy nations," in this chapter, as the top two-thirds of all OECD members, measured in terms of gross domestic product (GDP) per capita, in 2002 U.S. dollars, after adjusting for the relative purchasing power of the currencies in these nations. This includes all OECD members except for Greece, Portugal, Korea, Czech Republic, Hungary, Slovak Republic, Poland, Mexico, and Turkey.

> ### TABLE 6.1
>
> #### Health System Components: Organizational Arrangements and Sources of Financing
>
> | ORGANIZATION | FINANCING | | | |
> | --- | --- | --- | --- | --- |
> | | **Government** <br> 1 | **Social security/NHI** <br> 2 | **Private insurance** <br> 3 | **Out-of pocket** <br> 4 |
> | **Public** <br> A | Veterans Administration | Medicare pays for patient in public hospital | Private insurer pays for patient in public hospital | Patients pay for their own care in a public hospital |
> | **Private nonprofit/ quasi-government** <br> B | Medicaid pays for patient in a non-profit hospital | Medicare pays for patient in a non-profit hospital | Private insurer pays for patient in non-profit hospital | Patients pay for their own care in a nonprofit hospital |
> | **Private for-profit** <br> C | Medicaid pays for patient in a for-profit hospital | Medicare pays for patient in a for-profit hospital | Private insurer pays for patient in for-profit hospital | Patients pay for their own care in a for-profit hospital |

characterized OECD nations during the great boom years of health sector growth (the 1950s and 1960s), when governments encouraged hospital construction and modernization, workforce training, and biomedical research. It has continued since the 1970s, when the goals shifted more in the direction of rationalization and cost containment (Rodwin, 1984). As we begin the twenty-first century, public and other forms of collective private financing, e.g., health insurance, have become the dominant sources for funding health care (see **TABLE 6.1**), and public expenditure on health care has become the largest category of social expenditure, as a share of GDP, after social security payments. What is more, as in the United States, governments have increasingly broadened the scope of their intervention to encompass new regulatory functions (see Sparer, chapter 5 this volume).

These trends are so powerful that they have affected the way we conceptualize health care systems. Indeed, the comparative study of health systems is dominated by attention to the role of the nation state. Thus, in this chapter, we first provide an overview of health system models across OECD nations. Next, we review some general issues raised by the comparative analysis of health systems. To provide further context for some health system models that are important for the United States—Canada, Great Britain, and France—we also review some common problems of health care organization and policy in these nations. Finally, we analyze the U.S. health system from a comparative perspective; examine the uses of comparative analysis for Americans, in learning from abroad; and present some new and promising approaches to the comparative analysis of health systems.

## OVERVIEW OF HEALTH SYSTEM MODELS

Whether one's image of a health system is private and market-based, as in the United States and Switzerland, or public and state-controlled, as in Great Britain and Scandinavian nations, or at some intermediary point along such a continuum, as in France, Canada, and Japan, it is possible to make some useful distinctions with respect to the financing and organization of health services. Table 6.1 classifies components of health systems by distinguishing the sources of health care financing (in the columns) and organizational arrangements (in the rows).

The four principle sources of financing to pay for health services are (a) *government*—general revenue funds from the fiscal tax system; (b) *social security/NHI*—funds from compulsory payroll taxes through the social security system; (c) *private insurance*—funds raised through voluntary premiums assessed by private health insurance companies; and (d) *out of pocket*—funds from individual payments. There are of course other sources of health care financing, particularly for capital expenditures, for example, direct employer contributions and philanthropic funds. But these are no longer major sources of financing for health care services.

The organizational arrangements in Table 6.1 refer to the supply of health services: public, private not-for-profit, or private for-profit. Within these categories, many distinctions may be added. For example, in the United States some publicly capitalized organizations (row 1) are national (the Veterans Administration); others are subnational (state mental hospitals); and many are local (municipal hospitals). Likewise, the not-for profit category may include a variety of quasi-public organizations, for example, hospital trusts in Britain. The for-profit form of organization, an important subcategory in the U.S., would include investor-owned hospitals and managed care organizations (MCOs). Indeed, the growth of large investor-owned MCOs distinguishes the health system of the United States from that of most other OECD nations.

In summary, Table 6.1 highlights components of the U.S. health system that are characterized by specific relationships among organizational arrangements and sources of health care financing. This matrix may be used as a framework for cross-national comparative analysis of health systems.

## National Health Service Systems

National Health Service (NHS) systems, such as those in Great Britain, Sweden, Norway, Finland, Denmark, Portugal, Spain, Italy, and Greece, are typically traced back to Lord Beveridge, the British economist who wrote the blueprint for that country's NHS immediately following World War II. Such systems are characterized by a dominant share of financing derived from taxes (column 1). Likewise, their systems of hospital provision were dominated by public sector organizational forms (row A) that are now coming to resemble quasi-public organizations in Great Britain (row B). These general characteristics do not preclude other forms of financing (columns 2, 3, and 4), nor do they preclude a significant mix of other associated organizational forms. Indeed, some of the most interesting differences among NHS systems revolve around the extent to which they combine a different mix of columns and rows. For example, the relative size of a legal private system of financing and provision (I2) is much higher in Italy and Spain than in Sweden or Denmark.

Another distinguishing characteristic of NHS systems is their tendency to rely largely on budgets to allocate government resources in the health sector. National health insurance (NHI) systems, by contrast, have had a more open-ended reimbursement system for health care providers, but this distinction is rapidly blurring as NHI systems are increasingly under pressure to operate within budget limits.

## National Health Insurance Systems

National Health Insurance (NHI) systems, such as those in France, Germany, Belgium, Luxemburg, and Japan, are typically traced back to Chancellor Otto von Bismarck who established the first NHI program for salaried industrial workers in Germany in 1883. NHIs tend to be characterized by a dominant share of financing from column 2. Canada is an exception to this pattern as the dominant share of financing is from general revenue funds. Likewise, their systems of provision are characterized by a more balanced public-private mix than in NHS systems. Once again, these general characteristics do not preclude the contributions of other forms of financing (columns 1, 3, and 4), nor do they preclude a dominant share of public hospitals in nations such as France and Germany (row A).

As with NHS systems, NHI systems are also characterized by significant variation in their financing and organizational arrangements. For example, the share of French health care expenditures financed from general tax revenues (column 1) has increased beyond 40%. Likewise, the relative share of proprietary hospital beds ranges widely across NHI systems from none in Canada to 26% in France.

## Other Health System Models

Although this chapter focuses on health systems of wealthy nations, it should be noted that Table 6.1 can be used to classify health systems around the world. Developing nations still finance most of their health care expenditures from out-of-pocket payments (column 4), although experiments are underway to develop systems of mutual aid through voluntary private health insurance (Preker, 2002). Also, with regard to contagious diseases such as HIV/AIDS that have what economists call negative externalities, there is an increasing role for external international health care financing, however insufficient. Likewise, in the independent states of the former Soviet Union (FSU)—so-called transitional economies—out-of-pocket payments usually exceed one half of all health care expenditures. The same is true in China and India. In Latin American nations, by contrast, although there are few systems of universal NHI coverage, social security financing based on payroll taxes (row B) covers an important share of health care expenditures.

## An Emerging Paradigm

In all the columns and rows of Table 6.1, it is hard to locate any existing health system within any one category. The enormous pluralism of the U.S exhibits components of its health system within each category. Among most OECD nations, which include Japan and the United States, there is increasing recognition that no existing systems actually correspond to the pure NHI and NHS models. In fact, most health systems in wealthy nations have converged along the lines of what the OECD (1994) has called the "contractual model." This model indicates that there is an important dimension

missing in Table 6.1—the relationships between health care purchasers and health care providers. Chernichovsky (1995, 2002) analyzes this emerging paradigm in relation to what he calls the
"organization and management of care consumption (OMCC)."

The contractual model and the functions of OMCC suggest that
what is important in the comparative analysis of OECD health systems—beyond the question of how to finance health services or
how to achieve the right balance between public and private organizational arrangements—is how to allocate available resources to
achieve the best results. This challenge raises issues of health system performance, governance, accountability, consumer control,
management of care, and overall integration of health services
across the full continuum of care.

## COMPARATIVE ANALYSIS OF HEALTH SYSTEMS

Comparative analysis of health systems in wealthy OECD nations
has resulted in a large and growing literature that provides profiles and improves our understanding of health care systems
abroad. Three stages may be distinguished in the evolution of such
research (Dumbaugh & Neuhauser, 1979), all of which are apparent
in contemporary studies of health systems abroad. The first stage
dominated the field until the mid-1960s and continues today in the
form of "travelogues" written by physicians returning from overseas tours. During the second stage, researchers described health
systems from a variety of perspectives—often with hopes of promoting health care reform. During the third stage, there has been
an attempt to make the comparative analysis of health systems into
a kind of social science. This kind of research focuses largely on
explaining variation across health systems on the basis of received
theories within such disciplines as anthropology, sociology, political science, and economics.

The social science approach to the comparative analysis of
health systems has some of the defects of its virtues. To achieve a
rigorous study design, it classifies data on health systems, formu-
lates hypotheses, and tests them against available evidence. Economists, for example, focus on cross-sectional comparisons of health
services utilization and expenditures, thus narrowing the scope of
research questions and eroding the ideals shared by stage 2 scholars, who were more motivated by the pragmatic concerns of
improving the health care delivery in their countries.

Social scientists tend to display more interest in the theoretical concerns of their disciplines than in social change. Nevertheless, some excellent studies have been produced, which have raised some conceptual and methodological issues that remain at the center of health systems research.

## Conceptual Issues

The concept of a "health system" is critical in efforts to compare health systems across nations. There is yet no fully satisfactory definition of this concept, for it is difficult to agree on both the boundaries of the system and on a definition of health. Blum (1981) provided a graphic model of health, which suggests that health care services are merely one input to health among three others—heredity, behavior, and environment (see FIGURE 6.1). McGinnis and Foege (1993) have since estimated that behavioral factors account for roughly half of all deaths in the United States.

Viewing the concept of a health system at a macrosociological

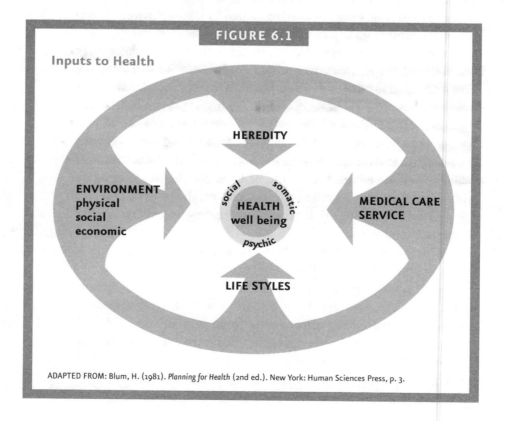

FIGURE 6.1

Inputs to Health

HEREDITY

ENVIRONMENT
physical
social
economic

social somatic

HEALTH
well being

psychic

MEDICAL CARE
SERVICE

LIFE STYLES

ADAPTED FROM: Blum, H. (1981). *Planning for Health* (2nd ed.). New York: Human Sciences Press, p. 3.

level, Field (1973) proposed the following formal definition: A health system is "that societal mechanism that transforms generalized resources . . . into specialized outputs in the form of health services." He added that "the 'health system' of any society is that social mechanism that has arisen or been devised to deal with the incapacitating aspects of illness, trauma, and (to some degree) premature mortality . . . the five D's: death, disease, disability, discomfort, and dissatisfaction" (pp. 768, 772). Anderson (1972) outlined more concretely the "boundaries of a relatively easily defined system with entry and exit points, hierarchies of personnel, types of patients"—in short what he calls "the officially and professionally recognized 'helping' services regarding disease, disability and death" (p. 22).

Another approach to the concept of a health system is to define it implicitly by postulating a causal model of it. Thus, De Miguel (1975) outlined four subsystem levels that influence health status: individual, institutional, societal, and environmental. Such an approach allows one to analyze a health system by investigating the effects of a hierarchy of independent variables on the dependent variable, health status. It also raises questions about the most effective levels at which to effect system change.

## Methodological Issues

A key methodological issue in comparative health systems research involves the selection of two or more health systems that allow the analyst to hold some variables constant while manipulating experimental ones. With respect to the performance of a health system, for example, how does one evaluate health system outcomes among different systems characterized by different patterns of financing, organization, and access? Quasi-experimental research designs suggest matching two health systems on all but a few policy-related factors. But "matching," let alone a real experiment, is rarely feasible in policy research.

One response to this difficulty has been to match health systems on at least some criteria (e.g., levels of economic development and health resources) and then to call for "in-depth studies of contrasting cases" (Elling & Kerr, 1975). Another response has been to use the language of natural experiment and view "most similar systems" as laboratories in which to assess the effects of alternative policy options at home (Marmor, Bridges, & Hoffman, 1978). A more recent response has been to adopt a "modular approach" that examines, systematically and sequentially, diverse components of health systems, e.g., needs, inputs, the delivery process, and health system outcomes (Ellencweig, 1992).

A second methodological issue in the social science approach to comparative health systems research is whether the descriptive studies and data collected during stages 1 and 2 (previously described) are actually comparable. If they are not, this casts great doubt on the utility of making international comparisons. If they are, qualifications must usually be given.

The most difficult issues in evaluating health system performance involve specifying the relationship between the elements of a health system (inputs and outputs) and their impact on health status (outcomes). But how does one differentiate the effects of health services on health from the effects of improvements in social services, income security, education, and transportation, not to mention individual behaviors, as well as on the social and physical environments? This question raises the problem of devising indicators of health status. It also explains why, in his comparative study of the United States, Sweden, and England, Anderson (1972) found it impossible to attribute differences in the usual health indices of morbidity and mortality to patterns of medical care organization in these countries.

Nonetheless, there has been some progress on this score over the past 32 years. To evaluate health systems, however, it is necessary to agree on consistent definitions of health system inputs and outputs, and to devise health status indicators to measure outcomes. The World Health Organization (WHO) recently published a study of health system performance in which member health systems were ranked on the basis of eight measures (WHO, 2000). OECD (2003) has embarked on a more compelling "disease-based comparison of health systems" (see later section on New Approaches). The results of the WHO study, however, are controversial and suffer from grave methodological problems (Coyne & Hilsenrath, 2002; Navarro, 2002). Likewise, the OECD approach suffers from lack of available data. Thus, both of these efforts will no doubt be followed by many more.

## Learning from Abroad

Comparative studies of health policy are sparse. Most often, they describe an experience in a range of policy areas; only rarely have they interpreted, let alone evaluated, this experience. Exceptions to this general rule are of interest because they have contributed at least three ideas with implications for how we might learn from health systems abroad.

First, is the idea of evolutionary progress in health systems. Roemer (1977) described the evolution of health systems as a march toward a health ideal characterized by increasing shares of public expenditure on health services and increasing government control over the health care sector. Medical sociologists Field (1973) and Mechanic (1976) argued that health systems in Western industrialized nations evolve in similar directions. Unlike Roemer, however, Field and Mechanic were not convinced that such change necessarily implies "progress."

The second idea, the notion of public policy learning, is methodological in nature. For example, the "most similar systems approach" (Marmor, Bridges, & Hoffman, 1978) views health systems as laboratories in which to assess the effects of alternative policy options at home. Examples of this approach include Evans' (1984) book on health economics in Canada, as well as Marmor's (1994) analyses of the Canadian experience. The "most similar systems approach" is also highlighted in Glaser's (1970, 1978, 1987, 1991) studies of health policy in Western Europe and Canada. These studies are distinctive, however, in that they begin with the presumption that the U.S. health care system has many problems and that the policies and experiences of Western Europe and Canada can shed light on and provide a useful range of solutions for the United States.

The third idea focuses on understanding either determinants of health policies or at least their effects. Leichter (1979), for example, analyzed the determinants of health policies in Britain, Germany, Japan, and the former Soviet Union. Similarly, Altenstetter (1974), Stone (1980), Hollingsworth (1986), Immergut (1992), and Tuohy (1999) have attempted to relate differences in structure, performance, and policy among such nations as the United States, France, Germany, Britain, and Canada. This approach views "most similar systems" (Marmor, Bridges, & Hoffman, 1978) as laboratories in which to assess the effects of alternative policy options at home (Teune, 1978), which is exemplified by Evans (1984) in his book on health economics and Canada.

The idea of evolutionary progress in the development of health systems suggests that the United States can learn about and determine future policy issues by studying nations whose systems are more advanced, i.e., to bring foreign solutions to bear on American problems. Finally, the idea of using comparative analysis to understand the determinants and effects of health policies abroad can assist us in evaluating alternative policy options at home.

There is, however, an important caveat to these views. The ideas briefly discussed above—indeed most of the literature in comparative health policy—often minimize or overlook the substantial problems of health systems abroad. An alternative, problem-oriented approach reverses this emphasis. For example, another way to think about learning from health systems abroad is to begin with the recognition that most countries, irrespective of their particular health system, face common, serious problems with regard to the efficient and equitable allocation of scarce health care resources. OECD and the World Bank have published important comparative studies that reflect this approach (see Suggested Readings at the end of this chapter). Within this problem-oriented approach, there are at least three ways of viewing the problems.

Economists, for example, emphasize the problem of inefficiency in the allocation of health care resources. They point out that cost containment should not be confused with allocative efficiency in the use of health care resources, and they study the possibilities for obtaining more value for the money spent on health care. This applies not only with regard to improving health status but also with respect to altering input mixes in the provision of health services that take advantage of cost-effective treatment settings (e.g., ambulatory surgery) and personnel (e.g., nurse practitioners).

Public health and medical care analysts criticize the lack of integration among primary, secondary, and tertiary levels of care. They have called for redistributing resources away from hospitals to community-based ambulatory care services and public health programs. Despite these views, the allocation of resources within health regions has been notoriously biased in favor of more costly technology-based medical care at the apex of the regional hierarchy (Fox, 1986; Rodwin, 1984). The consequence of this allocational pattern has been to weaken institutional capability for delivering primary care services and has exacerbated the separation of primary, secondary, and tertiary levels of care, thus making it difficult for providers to assure that the right patient receives the right kind of care, in the right place, and for the right reason.

Consumers have noted the inflexibility of bureaucratic decision-making procedures and the absence of opportunities for exercising what Hirschman (1970) calls "voice" in most health care organizations. Indeed, the problem of control and how it should be shared among consumers, providers, managers, and payers is at the center of most criticisms leveled against the current structure of health systems in Western industrialized nations. In all of these systems, decisions about what medical services to provide, how and where they should be provided, by whom, and how often are separated from the responsibility for financing medical care.

## COMMON PROBLEMS OF HEALTH CARE ORGANIZATION AND POLICY IN THREE NATIONS

Drawing on the problem-oriented approach presented above, this section provides an analysis of common problems with regard to the efficient and equitable allocation of scarce health care resources in three OECD nations: France, Canada, and Britain. These nations are far smaller than the United States in terms of population size (see TABLE 6.2). They have slightly lower gross domestic product (GDP) per capita and spend less on health care as a percentage of GDP. In the aggregate, they deliver more hospital bed-days and doctors' consultations per capita. With respect to health outcomes, measured against most traditional health indicators, they appear to be better off. All of them have lower infant mortality rates, higher life expectancy at birth, and (except for the U.K.) higher life expectancy at age 65.

The health systems of all three nations deserve to become better known in the U.S., for they represent models that have been invoked time and again in U.S. efforts to achieve health care reform. France is a prototype model of a traditional European employment-based NHI system; Canada represents 12 different examples of a newer NHI system operating in a federal institutional structure that resembles more closely the United States; Britain is the model, par excellence, of a NHS operating under a highly centralized government.

### France

The French health system combines NHI with solo, office-based, fee-for-service private practice in the ambulatory care sector and a mixed hospital care sector of which two thirds of all acute beds are

## TABLE 6.2

### National Indicators, Health System Characteristics and Outcomes: U.S., Canada, France, and U.K.

| NATIONAL INDICATORS | YEAR | U.S. | CANADA | FRANCE | U.K |
|---|---|---|---|---|---|
| Total population in thousands | 2002 | 288,369 | 31,414 | 59,486 | 59,232 |
| Percent of population age 65 and over | 2002 | 12.3% | 12.7% | 16.3% | 15.9% |
| GDP $ per capita[a] | 2002 | $36,006 | $30,429 | $28,094 | $27,959 |

| HEALTH SYSTEM CHARACTERISTICS | YEAR | U.S. | CANADA | FRANCE | U.K |
|---|---|---|---|---|---|
| Health expenditure as a percent of GDP | 2002 | 14.6% | 9.6% | 9.7% | 7.7% |
| Per capita health expenditures in $US (PPP) | 2002 | $5,267 | $2,931 | $2,736 | $2,160 |
| Public expenditures on health as a % of GDP | 2002 | 6.6% | 6.7% | 7.4% | 6.4% |
| Doctors' consultations per capita | 2002 | 8.9 | 6.2[f] | 6.9[f] | 4.9[g] |
| Acute care bed-days per 1,000 population | 2002 | 700 | 1,000[f] | 1,100[f] | 1,200[f] |

| HEALTH OUTCOME CHARACTERISTICS | YEAR | U.S. | CANADA | FRANCE | U.K |
|---|---|---|---|---|---|
| Infant mortality per 1,000 live births | 2002 | 6.8f | 5.2f | 4.2 | 5.3 |
| Life expectancy (females) at age 65 | 2002 | 19.4 | 20.6 | 21.3 | 18.9[g] |
| Life expectancy at birth (males) | 2002 | 74.4f | 77.1f | 75.6 | 75.7[f] |
| Self-evaluation as "very good" or "good," pop. 15 and over[c] | 2002 | 88.8% | 88.0%[f] | 72.9% | 77.8% |
| Percent of population satisfied with their health system | 1999–2000 | 40%g | 46.0% | 65.0% | 57.0% |
| DALE (Disability-adjusted life expectancy) (total populations) at birth[h] | 1999 | 70.0 | 72.0 | 73.1 | 71.7 |
| Years of life lost (total pop.) per 100,000, years < 70 All causes | 2000 | 5,120 | 3,571 | 4,182 | 3888[i] |

[a]In purchasing power parities.
[b]Blendon, R. Kim, M., & Benson, J. (2001). The public versus the World Health Organization on health system performance. *Health Affairs*, (20)3.
[c]Percentage of population that evaluates their own health status as "very good" or "good" based on national surveys.
[d]Number of deaths caused by adverse effects from medicines as reported by WHO World Statistics Manual and complemented by national sources.
[e]Public current expenditures.
[f]2001.
[g]2000.
[h]Annex Table 5 Health attainment, level and distribution in all member states, estimates for 1997 and 1999. *The World Health Report* (2000).
[i]1999.
SOURCE: Unless otherwise indicated, data are from the Organization for Economic Cooperation and Development (OECD) Health Data (2004).

in the public sector and one third are in the private sector (Rodwin, 2003). Physicians in the ambulatory sector and in private hospitals are reimbursed on the basis of a negotiated fee schedule. Roughly 30% of all physicians selected the option to extra-bill beyond the negotiated fees that represent payment in full for the remaining 70% of physicians (Rodwin & Sandier, 1993). They may do so as long as their charges are presented with "tact and measure," a standard that has never been legally defined but which has been found, empirically, to represent a 50 to 100% increase in the negotiated fees. Physicians based in public hospitals are reimbursed on a part-time or full-time salaried basis. Private hospitals used to be reimbursed on the basis of a negotiated per diem fee, but in the late 1990s, they gradually moved to a case-mix reimbursement system. Before 1984, public hospitals were reimbursed on the basis of a retrospective, cost-based, per diem fee; since then they have received prospectively set "global" budgets adjusted for patient case mix.

Although the French NHI was rated No. 1 on the basis of its overall efficiency and fairness, by the 2000 WHO study of health system performance, there are still several problems with the French system. From a public health point of view, there is inadequate communication between full-time salaried physicians in public hospitals and solo-based private practice physicians working in the community. Although general practitioners in the fee-for-service sector (roughly one half of French physicians) have informal referral networks to specialists and public hospitals, there are no formal institutional relationships that assure continuity of medical care, disease prevention and health promotion services, posthospital follow-up care, and, more generally, systematic linkages and referral patterns between primary-, secondary-, and tertiary-level services.

From an economic perspective, there still remain problems of economic efficiency. On the demand side, two factors encourage consumers to increase their use of medical care services: the uncertainty about the results of treatment and the availability of universal and comprehensive insurance coverage. To reduce the risk of misdiagnosis or improper therapy, physicians are always tempted to order more diagnostic tests. Since NHI covers most of the cost, there is no incentive—for either the physician or for the patient—to balance marginal changes in risk with marginal increases in costs. This results in excessive (and often inappropriate) use of services.

On the supply side, fee-for-service reimbursement of physicians provides incentives for them to increase their volume of services so as to raise their income. Likewise, case-based reimbursement of private hospitals provides incentives to increase patient admissions as long as revenues exceed costs. The imposition of global budgets in 1984 eliminated this problem for the French public hospitals. The move toward using indicators of case mix for setting public hospital budgets and negotiating per diem fees for private hospitals has also weakened the incentives to increase hospital services. However, the budgets for public hospitals represent a blunt policy tool—one that tends to support the existing allocation of resources within the hospital sector and possibly to jeopardize the quality of public hospital services. It is relatively easy for a hospital to receive an annual budget to maintain its ongoing activities but extremely difficult to receive additional compensation for higher service levels, institutional innovation, or improvements in the quality of care. Since 1996, even with prospectively set budgets for public as well as private hospitals, these institutions naturally have sought to maximize the level of their annual allocations and to resist budget cutbacks.

In summary, under French NHI, providers have no financial incentives to achieve savings while holding quality constant or even improving it, nor are there incentives—in public hospitals, for example—to increase service activity in exchange for more revenues. Therefore, consumers have few incentives, other than minimal copayments, to be economical in their use of medical care. Also, there are no incentives to move the French system away from hospital-centered services toward new organizational forms that encourage teamwork between general practitioners, specialists, and hospitals and greater responsiveness to emerging market demands (Rodwin, 1997).

In 1996, as part of a broader reform of the social security system, Prime Minister Alain Juppé attempted the most far-reaching reform of the French health sector since 1958 (Le Pen & Rodwin, 1996). The central state's supervisory role over the NHI system was reinforced. In addition, the French Parliament was made accountable for health expenditures. It was required to set a global expenditure target for total health care expenditures reimbursed by French NHI and to set targets for each of France's 21 regions. To advise Parliament in this new responsibility and assist the Ministry of Health in overseeing the health system, a number of new institutions were created: the National Committee on Public Health, a National Agency for Hospital Accreditation, and Quality and Regional Agencies for hospital planning and control.

Although President Jacques Chirac dissolved Parliament shortly after the national strikes in protest of the social security reforms, almost all of the health care reforms were maintained by the socialist government of Prime Minister Lionel Jospin. Perhaps most noteworthy has been the increased role of the National Agency on Health Accreditation and Evaluation in setting standards for the quality of hospital care and developing national medical guidelines for physicians in private practice, which the NHI Administration is trying to enforce. The problems identified earlier are still not resolved; the reforms were not successfully implemented by either the Jospin government or by his successor, Prime Minister Jean-Pierre Raffarin. But the French central government is increasingly intervening to modernize and rationalize their health care system.

## Canada

Under Canadian NHI, although coverage for prescription drugs is far less generous than in France (only two provinces have a program to cover prescription drugs), most provinces have no copayments for any covered hospital and medical services (Deber, 2003). This means that patients are not required to pay a portion of their medical bills; there is a "first-dollar" coverage for a comprehensive "package" of hospital and medical services. Physicians in ambulatory care are paid predominantly on a fee-for-service basis, according to fee schedules negotiated between physicians' associations and provincial governments. All physicians must accept these fees as payment in full. In contrast to France, where physicians in public hospitals are largely paid on a salary basis, most physicians in Canadian hospitals are paid on a fee-for-service basis, as in the United States.

There are few private, for-profit hospitals in Canada, as in France and the U.S. Most acute-care hospitals in Canada are private, nonprofit institutions. But their operating expenditures are financed through the NHI system, and most of their capital expenditures are financed by the provincial governments. In the United States, among advocates of NHI, Canada's health system has often been depicted as a model that could save almost $300 billion in U.S.

administrative costs and to extend coverage for Americans (Wool-handler, Campbell, & Himmelstein, 2003; Himmelstein, Woolhandler, et al., 1989). Its financing—through a complex shared federal and provincial tax revenue formula—is more progressive than the European NHI systems financed on the basis of payroll taxes. As well, Canada's levels of health status are high by international standards. In comparison to the United States, it has achieved notable success in controlling the growth of health care costs. What then are the problems in this system?

From the point of view of health care providers, Canada's successful cost-containment program is perceived as a crisis of "under financing." Physicians complain about low fee levels. Hospital administrators complain about draconian control of their budgets. And other health care professionals note that the combination of a physician "surplus" and excessive reliance on physicians prevents an expansion of their roles.

Although Evans (1992) contends that Canadian cost-control policies cannot be shown to have jeopardized the quality of care, providers and administrators alike claim that there has been deterioration since the imposition of restrictive prospective budgets. Leaving aside the issue of quality, the same issues discussed in the context of France are present in Canada with respect to economic efficiency. There is no incentive for the hospital, the physician, or the patient to be economical in the use of health care resources. On the demand side, because patients benefit from what is perceived as "free" tax-financed, first-dollar coverage, they have no incentive to choose cost-effective forms of care. For example, in the case of a demand for urgent care, there is no incentive for a patient to use community health centers rather than rush directly to the emergency room.

On the supply side, physicians lack incentives to make efficient use of hospitals, which are essentially a free service at their disposal. There are no incentives for altering input mixes to affect practice style, nor are there incentives for providers to evaluate service levels and the kinds of therapy performed in relation to improving health status. It could be argued that these problems are common to all health systems, but they are especially acute in a system characterized by concentrated political interests—health care providers, on the one hand, and a "single payer," on the other—that tend to support the status quo. On the one hand, providers organized in strong associations have strong monopoly power, which they use to defend their legitimate interests; on the other, the monopoly power of sole-source financing (NHI) keeps provider interests in check at the cost of not intervening in the organizational practice of medicine.

Stoddard (1984) characterized the problems of the Canadian health system as "financing without organization," and this is still a fundamental problem in the Canadian system. In his view, Canadian provinces "adopted a 'pay the bills' philosophy, in which decisions about service provision—which services, in what amounts, produced how, by whom and where—were viewed as the legitimate domain of physicians and hospital administrators" (p. 3). The reason for this policy is that provincial governments were concerned about maintaining a good relationship with providers, though this concern has not avoided tough negotiations and periodic confrontations. But there have been only limited efforts to devise new forms of medical care practice—for example, health maintenance organizations (HMOs) or new institutions to handle long-term care for the elderly. The side effect of Canadian NHI has been to support the separation of hospital and ambulatory care and to reinforce traditional organizational structures.

As in France, there are, in essence, two strategies for managing the Canadian health system and making needed adjustments. The first involves greater regulation on the supply side: even stronger controls on hospital spending, more rationing of medical technology, and more hospital mergers and eventually closures. The second involves increased reliance on market forces on the demand side: various forms of user charges such as copayments and deductibles now advocated as a form of privatization. Neither strategy is likely to succeed on its own. The former will control health care expenditures in the short run, but it fails to affect practice styles. Its effectiveness runs the risk of exacerbating confrontations between providers and the state, and jeopardizing health care needs. The latter deals with only part of the problem—the demand side—and neglects the issue of supply-side inefficiency. It provides no mechanism by which consumer decisions can generate signals to providers to adopt efficient practice styles. Moreover, to the extent that it has been used, it has raised the level of private expenditures.

Between these two strategies, there is increasing recognition among Canadian policymakers that the health sector requires significant reorganization. In Ontario, in 1996, the Health Services Restructuring Commission (HSRC) was formed; in Quebec, the Federation of general practitioners (GPs) formed a task force on the reorganization of primary care. Both of these efforts reinforced a trend toward "integrated health systems" and the use of gatekeepers in primary care. In Ontario, the main accomplishment of HSRC was to devise a seven-point plan to restructure the balance of resources among hospitals and community health services. In Quebec, the main accomplishment of the task force was also limited to planning for needed reforms. The Canadian system has been remarkably resistant to organizational reform, in practice.

Throughout the 1990s, the major health policy battles in Canada were fought over the problem of funding health services. Hospital budget cuts held per-capita public spending on health care roughly constant from 1992 to 1997, but total health care spending, as a percent of GDP, fell by a full percentage point (Naylor, 1999). The combination of escalating drug costs and hospital cuts has eroded public confidence in the system (Evans, 2000). But in the spring of 2000, contentious meetings between provincial health ministers and federal officials resulted in a deal to restore federal cash payments for health care and other social welfare services.

From 2000 to 2004, the federal government agreed to provide 1 billion Canadian dollars to purchase medical equipment in hospitals and 800 million Canadian dollars to support projects that reform the delivery of primary care services (Kondro, 2000). The strings attached to this deal commit the provinces to develop a formulary service for prescription drugs and to produce annual "report cards" on the performance of their respective systems. Thus, the pressure is still on to produce some organizational reform and hold the supply side more accountable to those paying the bill.

## Britain

There are many models of an NHS in Europe, ranging from decentralized systems in Sweden, Norway, Finland, and Denmark to more centralized systems in Spain, Greece, Portugal, and Italy. Because the British NHS is one of the oldest and most thoroughly studied models (Klein, 1995), it stands as an exemplar. It is financed almost entirely through general revenue taxation and is accountable directly to the central government's Department of Health and

Social Security (DHSS) and Parliament. Access to health services is free of charge to all British subjects and to all legal residents. But despite the universal entitlement, health expenditures in the U.K. represent only 7.7% of the gross domestic product (GDP)—nearly half that in the United States (see Table 6.2).

Although the NHS is cherished by most Britons, there are, nevertheless, some serious problems concerning both the equity and efficiency of resource allocation in the health sector. With regard to equity (defined as "equal care for those at equal risk"), in 1976, the Resource Allocation Working Party (RAWP) developed a formula for narrowing inequities in the allocation of NHS funds among regions (Townsend & Davidson, 1982). The formula (DHSS, 1976) represents one of the most far-reaching attempts to allocate health care funds because it incorporated regional differences in health status based on standardized mortality ratios. Some progress was made in redistributing the aggregate NHS budget along the lines of the RAWP formula in the 1980s, but it was eventually eliminated in the 1990s. Yet substantial inequities still remain, from the point of view of both spatial distribution and social class.

With regard to efficiency, the problems are even more severe because NHS resources are extremely scarce by OECD standards. Perhaps because there are fewer health care resources in Britain than in the rest of Western Europe or the United States, the British have been more aggressive in weeding out inefficiency than have wealthier countries. And because the NHS faces the same demands as other systems to make available technology and to care for an increasingly aged population, British policymakers recognize that they must pursue innovations that improve efficiency. But there have been numerous obstacles: opposition by professional bodies, difficulties in firing and redeploying health care personnel, and the institutional separation between hospitals, general practitioners, and community health programs.

The tripartite structure of the NHS has, since its establishment in 1948, been a source of inefficiency:

1. Regional Health Authorities (RHAs) had been responsible (until the mid-1990s) for allocating budgets to districts and hospitals. Hospital-based physicians, known as "consultants," are paid on a salaried basis, from these budgets, with distinguished clinicians

receiving "merit awards"; and all consultants have the right to see a limited number of private, fee-paying patients in so-called pay beds within their service units.

2. Outside the RHA budget (until the mid-1990s) were the Family Practitioner Committees (FPCs) responsible for paying general practitioners (GPs), ophthalmologists, dentists, and pharmacists. These are now called Primary Care Trusts from which GPs are reimbursed on a capitation basis, with additional remuneration coming from special "practice allowances" and fee-for-service payment for specific services (e.g., night visits and immunizations).

3. Separate from both the RHAs and the FPCs are the local authorities (LAs), which are responsible for the provision of social services, public health services, and certain community nursing services.

This institutional framework has created perverse incentives—for example, to shift borderline patients from GPs to hospital consultants, to the community, and back to the hospital. Until the reforms introduced by the Thatcher government in 1991, GPs had no incentive to minimize costs and could even impose costs on RHAs by referring patients to hospital consultants or for diagnostic services. NHS managers could shift costs from the NHS to social security by sending elderly hospitalized patients to private nursing homes. And consultants could shift costs back onto the patient by keeping long waiting lists, thereby increasing demand for their private services. As in France and Canada, neither the patient nor the physician in Britain bears the cost of the decisions they make; it is the taxpayers who pay the bill.

Four strategies—all of them inadequate—have attempted to deal with this problem. The first came promptly with the arrival of the first Thatcher government in 1981. After cautious attempts to denationalize the NHS by promoting a shift toward NHI and privatization, the conservative government backed off when they realized that such an approach would not merely provoke strong political opposition but would also increase public expenditure and therefore conflict with their budgetary objectives. Instead, the strategy was narrowed in favor of encouraging competition and market incentives in limited areas. To begin with, the government allowed a slight increase in private pay beds within NHS hospitals. In addition, it introduced tax incentives to encourage the purchase of private health insurance and the growth of charitable contributions. Also, the government encouraged local authorities to raise money through the sale of surplus property and to contract out to the private sector such services as laundry, cleaning, and catering.

The second response was the Griffiths Report (1983), which resulted in yet another reorganization in the long history of administrative reform within the NHS. Roy Griffiths, the former director of a large British department store chain, introduced the concept of a general manager at the department (DHSS), regional, district, and unit levels. This manager was presumably responsible for the efficient use of the budget at each level of the NHS. In summary, the report observed, in a sentence that has since become well known, "If Florence Nightingale were carrying her lamp through the corridors of the NHS today, she would almost certainly be searching for the people in charge" (Griffiths, 1983, p. 12). The problem is, however, that, following the Griffiths Report, the tripartite structure of the system remained largely unchanged, and the general managers had very little information about least-cost strategies (across the tripartite structure) for generating improvements in health status.

The third response to the problem of improving efficiency was to reduce the drug bill (Maynard, 1986). In April 1985, the government limited the list of reimbursable drugs and reduced the pharmaceutical industry's rate of return. These measures helped contain the costs of the formerly open-ended drug budget within the NHS, but there is no evidence that they had any impact on the efficiency of health care expenditures.

Finally, the fourth and most significant reform for improving efficiency in the NHS was announced in a government white paper, *Working for Patients* (1989): The National Health Service and Community Care Act was passed in 1990 and implemented on April 1, 1991. The white paper proposed a range of significant changes, all of which attempt to create "internal markets" within the public sector, by giving providers incentives to treat more patients and having "money follow patients." On the demand side, the government proposed that, instead of operating as monopoly suppliers of services, district health authorities be required to purchase services for the patients they serve. On the supply side, the government proposed that NHS hospitals be given the option to convert from purely "public" status to that of independent, self-governing "trusts." Also, the government proposed that GPs be given the option to serve as "fundholders" for their enrolled patients and thereby serve as purchasers on their behalf for basic specialty and hospital services.

In July 1990, RHAs were streamlined and FPCs were transformed into newly named Family Health Service Authorities (FHSAs), with stronger management over primary care. In 1996, the districts were merged with the FHSAs into roughly 80 Health Authorities (HAs) and placed under a new National Health Service Executive (NHSE) with eight regional offices. The HAs were supposed to function as integrated purchasing coalitions, thereby strengthening the role of internal markets in the allocation of health resources. There have been some preliminary evaluations of these reforms, but they are still too recent to permit one to conclude very much about the effects of internal markets on efficiency of resource allocation, continuity of care, and responsiveness to patient demands. There is, however, general agreement that the reforms shifted the balance of power between GPs and hospital specialists, encouraged innovation in primary care, encouraged greater cost consciousness, and raised administrative costs (Smee, 2000).

Following Tony Blair's election as Prime Minister in 1994, the New Labour party's "third way" reforms focused more on collaboration and less on competition, but the government's white paper retained the major elements of the Thatcher reforms (1997). The purchaser/provider split was retained albeit with more emphasis on cooperation. All GPs have been brought into primary care trusts (PCTs), thus bringing important elements of managed care to the NHS. Fundholders have now been largely absorbed by PCTs, and the HAs are losing their former purchasing role as they become increasingly responsible for providing a framework for PCG accountability (Dobson, 1999). Finally, as in France and Canada, there have been efforts to improve quality and standards in the British NHS. The National Institute for Clinical Effectiveness (NICE) is setting standards, and the Council for Health Improvement (CHIMP) will enforce them (Le Grand, 1999).

In retrospect, it is no exaggeration to suggest that the history of the British NHS is largely a story of successive organizational reforms to improve the efficiency and equity of resource allocation within the health care sector. An additional and more recent goal has been to increase responsiveness of health care providers to consumers. Nonetheless, most astute observers of the NHS concur that even the most radical reforms under Prime Ministers Margaret Thatcher and Blair have had limited effects on the basic structure and problems of the system (Kein, 1998; Le Grand, 1999). The fundamental tension between the push to introduce market mechanisms and the need for central control to preserve political accountability has remained intact. Moreover, the institutional power of central control appears to have the upper edge.

## THE U.S. HEALTH SYSTEM IN COMPARATIVE PERSPECTIVE

How does the U.S. health care system measure up in comparison to the health systems in France, Canada, and Great Britain? To answer this question, we review the ways in which the U.S. health system differs from and resembles that of other OECD nations. We examine this issue from the perspectives of two characteristics that typically distinguish the United States from Western Europe and Canada: (a) the structure of health care financing and organization (see Table 6.1) and (b) values and popular opinion.

### The Structure of Health Care Financing and Organization

The prevailing image of the American health care system is one of a privately financed, privately organized system with multiple payers. These characteristics derive, in large part, from the absence of a publicly mandated NHI program. In comparison with other wealthy OECD nations, the United States is ranked lowest at 44.9% with respect to the public share of total health care expenditures (see TABLE 6.3). Although the United States has the highest per capita health care expenditures—public and private combined (see TABLE 6.4)—its share of public expenditure as a percentage (6.5%) of total health expenditures (Table 6.4) is relatively high.

Organizational arrangements for health care in the United States are noted for being on the private end of the public-private spectrum (see Table 6.1). In comparison with Western Europe, the United States has one of the smallest public hospital sectors. In the organization of ambulatory care, American private fee-for-service practice corresponds to the norm, at least in comparison with NHI systems. However, the absence of an NHI program in the United States

## TABLE 6.3

GDP Per Capita and Sources of Finance for Health Care Expenditure: The Relative Share of Public and Private Spending (2002)

| COUNTRY | GDP PER CAPITA[d] | PUBLIC | PRIVATE |
| --- | --- | --- | --- |
| Luxembourg | $49,207 | 85.4 | 14.6 |
| United States | $36,006 | 44.9 | 55.1 |
| Norway | $35,531 | 85.3 | 14.7 |
| Ireland | $32,571 | 75.2 | 24.8 |
| Switzerland | $30,725 | 57.9 | 42.1 |
| Canada | $30,429 | 69.9 | 30.1 |
| Denmark | $29,228 | 83.1 | 16.9 |
| Netherlands | $28,983 | 67.8[a] | 32.2 |
| Austria | $28,842 | 69.9 | 30.1 |
| Iceland | $28,404 | 84.0 | 16.0 |
| Australia | $28,168 | 68.2[b] | 31.8 |
| France | $28,094 | 76.0 | 24.0 |
| United Kingdom | $27,959 | 83.4 | 16.6 |
| Belgium | $27,652 | 71.2 | 28.8 |
| Sweden | $27,255 | 85.3 | 14.7 |
| Japan | $26,860 | 81.7[b] | 18.3 |
| Finland | $26,616 | 75.7 | 24.3 |
| Germany | $25,843 | 78.5 | 21.5 |
| Italy | $25,569 | 75.3[c] | 24.7 |
| New Zealand | $21,943 | 77.9 | 22.1 |
| Spain | $21,592 | 71.4 | 28.6 |

[a]1997  [c]2003
[b]2001  [d]in purchasing power parities
SOURCE: OECD Health Data (2004).

has resulted in a system of multiple payers and has encouraged a more pluralistic pattern of medical care organization and more innovative forms of medical practice—for example, multispecialty group practices, HMOs, ambulatory surgery centers, and Preferred Provider Organizations (PPOs) (see chapter 3 in this volume).

## TABLE 6.4

Total Expenditures on Health Care as a Percentage of GDP: 2002

| COUNTRY | PUBLIC EXPENDITURE ON HEALTH IN GDP (%) | TOTAL EXPENDITURE ON HEALTH IN GDP (%) | PER CAPITA HEALTH CARE EXPENDITURES IN $US (PPP) | OUT-OF-POCKET PAYMENT AS % IN P TOTAL HEALTH |
|---|---|---|---|---|
| Luxembourg | 5.3 | 6.2 | 3 065 | 11.9 |
| United States | 6.6 | 14.6 | 5 267 | 14.0 |
| Norway | 7.4 | 8.7 | 3 083 | 14.2 |
| Ireland | 5.5 | 7.3 | 2 367 | 13.2 |
| Switzerland | 6.5 | 11.2 | 3 445 | 31.5 |
| Canada | 6.7 | 9.6 | 2 931 | 15.2 |
| Denmark | 7.3 | 8.8 | 2 580 | 15.3 |
| Netherlands | 5.5[b] | 9.1 | 2 643 | 10.1 |
| Austria | 5.4 | 7.7 | 2 220 | 17.5 |
| Iceland | 8.3 | 9.9 | 2 807 | 16.0 |
| Australia[a] | 6.2 | 9.1 | 2 504 | 19.3 |
| France | 7.4 | 9.7 | 2 736 | 9.8 |
| United Kingdom | 6.4 | 7.7 | 2 160 | 11.0[c] |
| Belgium | 6.5 | 9.1 | 2 515 | N/A |
| Sweden | 7.9 | 9.2 | 2 517 | N/A |
| Japan | 6.4 | 7.8 | 2 077 | 16.5 |
| Finland | 5.5 | 7.3 | 1 943 | 20.0 |
| Germany | 8.6 | 10.9 | 2 817 | 10.4 |
| Italy | 6.4[f] | 8.5[f] | 2 166 | 20.6[f] |
| New Zealand | 6.6 | 8.5 | 1 857 | 16.1 |
| Spain | 5.4 | 7.6 | 1 646 | 23.6 |

[a]2001. [d]1990.
[b]1997. [e]2000.
[c]1996. [f]2003.
SOURCE: OECD Health Data (2004).

The United States is also different, in comparison with wealthy OECD nations, with regard to the ways in which health resources are used. For example, the United States is among the OECD countries with the lowest number of acute care hospital beds per 1,000 population (see **TABLE 6.5**). These data should not necessarily lead

## TABLE 6.5

### Acute Care Hospital Beds and Use of Inpatient Care, 2002

| COUNTRY | NO. OF BEDS PER 1,000 POPULATION | BED DAYS PER 1,000 POPULATION |
|---|---|---|
| Luxembourg | 5.8 | 1,400 |
| United States | 2.9 | 700 |
| Norway | 3.1 | 900 |
| Ireland | 3.0 | 900 |
| Switzerland | 3.9 | 1,200 |
| Canada | 3.9[b] | 1,000[a] |
| Denmark | 3.4[a] | 1,000[c] |
| Netherlands[a] | 3.3 | 800 |
| Austria | 6.1 | 1,700 |
| Iceland[d] | 3.7 | 1,100 |
| Australia[a] | 3.7a | 1,000 |
| France[a] | 4.0 | 1,100 |
| United Kingdom | 3.9 | 1,200[a] |
| Belgium[b] | 4.6 | 1,300 |
| Sweden | 2.4[e] | 800[f] |
| Japan | N/A | N/A |
| Finland | 2.3 | 900 |
| Germany[a] | 9 | 2,600 |
| Italy[a] | 4.6 | 1,100 |
| New Zealand | 6.9[h] | 300[g] |
| Spain[g] | 2.9 | 900 |

[a]2001.  [e]2000.
[b]1997.  [f]1996.
[c]1999.  [g]1998.
[d]1995.  [h]1991.

SOURCE: OECD Health Data (2004).

one to the conclusion that the United States is less prone to institutionalize patients than other nations. They probably reflect the
size of the American private nursing home industry, which has no
equivalent in Western Europe or Canada, where a portion of long-
term care for the elderly is still provided in hospitals. In addition

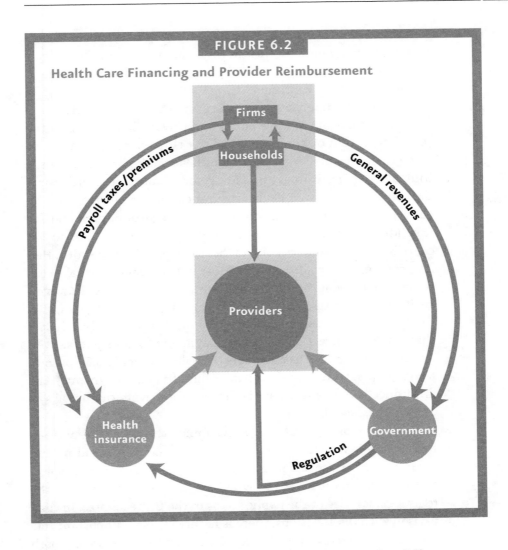

**FIGURE 6.2**

Health Care Financing and Provider Reimbursement

to the low number of acute care beds, the United States also differs from other OECD nations in having the lowest number of bed days per 1,000 population (700). This reflects a combination of low hospital admission rates compared with short lengths of stay in acute care hospitals.

There are also noteworthy points of similarity among the United States and other OECD nations in the broad structure of health care financing and provider reimbursement (see FIGURE 6.2). From the point of view of both consumers and providers, the essential feature of modern health care systems is the central role of third-party payment, by either government or health insurers. On the financing end, all health systems are supported primarily by either general revenue taxes or by payroll deductions in the form of compulsory taxes or voluntary health insurance premiums. On the payment end, the magnitude of third-party payment dwarfs the out-of-pocket payment by consumers.

For the consumer, what matters with regard to health care financing is not the relative public and private mix but rather the relative portion of *direct versus indirect* third-party payment. To emphasize that the larger portion of health care financing in the United States is private is misleading, for the more critical factor is that public and private health insurance are both forms of third-party payment. This amount was equal to 78.3% of national health expenditures in 1999, leaving consumers with direct out-of-pocket contributions equal to 17% of total health expenditures (Smith, Heffler, & Freeland, 1999). The OECD does not routinely compare consumers' out-of-pocket payments to total expenditures. However, available data on this important indicator suggest, once again, that the United States is different (see Table 6.4). It has the highest share (14%) of direct out-of-pocket payments by consumers. Even under the French NHI, consumers contribute roughly 9.8% of total health expenditures in the form of out-of-pocket payments. The difference is not as large as the image of a private financing system would suggest.

The image of a private organizational structure in American health care is well founded. But that view, too, is misleading and incomplete. In spite of a notable but small investor-owned hospital sector, a dominant investor-owned managed care sector, and the *relatively* small size of the public sector in the United States, in comparison with OECD nations, there is nevertheless an important role for the public sector in the United States health care system—both in ambulatory services for the non-institutionalized patient and in the provision of hospital services.

With regard to ambulatory care, there is a maze of special federal programs and a network of local government services largely for the poor. The services are provided either in county or municipal hospital emergency rooms, in local health departments, or in nonprofit community health centers receiving significant public financing from the federal, state, and/or local governments. As for hospitals, almost 30% of all registered hospitals (private nonprofit, local, state, and federal institutions) are owned and operated by governments (American Hospital Association [AHA], 2000). This includes the federal Veterans Health Administration hospitals, marine and military hospitals, as well as state, county, and municipal hospitals. Although Medicare and Medicaid were intended to bring the poor into "mainstream medicine" (i.e., into the private sector), local county governments continue to finance care for the "medically indigent" uninsured, either through private vendors or directly in public hospitals. These hospitals are a major source of care not only for Medicaid beneficiaries but also for more than half of the poverty population who do not meet Medicaid eligibility levels and consequently often do not have access to private physicians or voluntary hospitals.

To sum up, there are distinctive characteristics of health care financing and organization in the United States, but there are also striking points of similarity when compared with Western Europe nations and Canada. The distinctive characteristics of the U.S. health care system include the absence of an NHI program, preferences for institutional flexibility, and innovative forms of medical care organization. The points of similarity—the coexistence of both public and private provision and third-party payment— are structural features of the American health system as well as those of most other OECD health systems.

## American Values and Popular Opinion

The prevailing image of American values and popular opinion is that of nineteenth-century liberalism, which has colored American perceptions of equity, the proper role of government, and citizenship. These perceptions represent a range of American values and popular opinions that distinguish the United States from Western Europe and Canada.

American attitudes about equity with regard to health care were formed in the nineteenth century as the country became populated by immigrants in its urban centers. During this period, the concept of "truly needy" emerged (Rosner, 1982). Many Americans assumed a sense of responsibility and came to these newcomers' aid, but there were also harsher attitudes, inspired by social Darwinist notions, that distinguished between the "truly needy" and the "undeserving" or "unworthy" poor. Whereas in Western Europe broadly based socialist parties viewed poverty as an outcome of the economic system, in the United States there was an inclination to regard poverty as an individual problem. Hence, the greater attention to *equality of opportunity* in the United States as compared with *equality of results* in the more left-leaning European social democracies.

As far as the proper role of government is concerned, in contrast to Western Europe and Canada, the United States has a history of anti-government attitudes. The suspicion about excessive governmental authority and the attachment to individual liberties is a pervasive American value.

American perceptions of citizenship also present a striking contrast to Western European perceptions. In the United States, individualistic values, on the one hand, and social and ethnic heterogeneity, on the other, have resulted in more "fractionalized understandings of citizenship" (Klass, 1985). In Western Europe and Canada, the understandings of citizenship are grounded in notions of solidarity and universal entitlements. The result is that Western Europe and Canada have largely succeeded in covering all of their citizens under some form of national health insurance (NHI); the United States has not.

There is also a general aversion among Americans to universal entitlements. As Reinhardt (1985) observed, when Americans face a trade-off between establishing tax-financed entitlements and leaving the uninsured on their own, they prefer to do the latter. It would be misleading, however, to draw any conclusions about how generous Americans are or how much social welfare they provide based only on the image of liberalism outlined above. In contrast to Western Europe and Canada, Americans prefer to promote redistribution policies through local assistance and indirect subsidies to the voluntary sector via tax exemptions.

Clearly, in comparison with Western Europe and Canada, there are important differences in the United States with regard to values and popular opinion. But how much of a difference do these differences make?

## The Uses of Comparative Analysis in Learning from Abroad

Given the ways in which the health sector in the United States resembles that of Western Europe and Canada and the ways in which it is exceptional, what inferences can be drawn about the uses of comparative analysis for purposes of learning from abroad? If the United States is truly exceptional in the health sector, then it can be argued that there is little to learn from Western Europe and Canada. Countries often rely on this "assumption of uniqueness" to reject ideas from abroad (Stone, 1981). To the extent that the United States is unexceptional, however, a case can be made for drawing lessons from comparative experience.

For example, there is a widely shared belief among American policymakers that a national program providing for universal entitlement to health care in the United States would result in runaway costs. In response to this presumption, nations that entitle all of their residents to a high level of medical care while spending less on administration and on medical care than the United States, are often held up as models. The Canadian health system is the most celebrated example. The French NHI, a prototype of Western European continental health systems, is another case in point. Britain's NHS, although typically considered a "painful prescription" for the United States (Aaron & Schwartz, 1984), nevertheless assures first-dollar coverage for basic health services to its entire population and, as we have seen, spends less than half as much money, per capita, as the United States (see Table 6.4).

All of these countries have produced some of the leading physicians and hospitals in the world. Judging by various measures of health outcome, they are in the same league as, or better than, the United States (see Table 6.2). But in 2003, 45 million people in the United States (CPS, 2004)—18% of the population under 65 years of age—remain uninsured for health care services while spending, as a percentage of GDP, surpasses that of all industrially advanced nations (see Table 6.4).

Should we therefore adopt a Western European or Canadian model of health care financing and organization? Or should we maintain our present system and recognize that it is a manifestation of American exceptionalism, that is, of the ways in which the United States is fundamentally different from most OECD nations? Both of these responses are probably inappropriate. The second response—that comparative analysis is not useful—insulates us from the experience of other nations. It smacks of ethnocentrism, makes us conservative, and thereby supports the status quo in the United States. The first response—that we should adopt a Western European or Canadian model—relies too heavily on the experience of those nations. It is misleading because, as we have seen, there are serious limitations in the Western European and Canadian health systems. Moreover, many of the present institutional arrangements of health care delivery in the United States are superior to those abroad.

The proliferation of medical technology combined with an aging population are trends common to all modern health care systems and have contributed to rising health care costs. Policymakers have responded largely by implementing systems with increasing control over expenditures on doctors' services as well as over hospital budgets. Virtually no one in Canada or Western Europe views the American system as a model to emulate. Even under the government of Prime Minister Margaret Thatcher there was no significant challenge to the principle of an NHS in Britain (*Working for Patients*, 1989). Nor is there any question about eliminating NHI in such countries as France, Canada, Germany, Belgium, or the Netherlands.

Despite these attitudes, one striking aspect about how some common problems are currently being dealt with abroad is the extent to which a number of fashionable American themes have drifted north to Canada and across the Atlantic to Western Europe. In the context of the problems we identified earlier—inefficiency in the allocation of health care resources, lack of continuity between levels of care, and the absence of consumer "voice" in most health care organizations—the concept of a managed-care organization (MCO), in combination with elements of market competition, has a certain appeal. Since an MCO is, by definition, both an insurer and a provider of health services, it establishes a link between the financing and provision of health services. Because its managers have a budget to care for an enrolled population, they have powerful incentives to provide needed services in a cost-effective manner while simultaneously maintaining quality to minimize the risk of disenrollment.

The idea of introducing MCOs or similar kinds of health care organizations into national systems that provide universal entitlement to health care, in many ways, resembles the American experience of encouraging Medicare beneficiaries to enroll in Medicare Choice (Part C). This idea involves two reforms. It spurs policymakers to combine regulatory controls with competition on the supply side; and it encourages them to design market incentives for both providers and consumers of health care.

To the extent that the insertion of MCOs into NHI or NHS systems represents an American "solution" to *foreign* problems, it may provide a way in which Canada and Western Europe could learn from the United States (Rodwin, 1989b). It may also, paradoxically, have more practical implications for the United States than simply transposing a European NHI system into the American context. For example, the insertion of MCOs into NHI or NHS systems might provide insights on how managed care and universal coverage could be combined in the United States. Alternatively, experience abroad with managed care and health care reform might highlight some of the obstacles faced in attempting to assure universal access in a system so reliant on decentralized control.

## NEW APPROACHES TO COMPARING HEALTH SYSTEMS

Beyond being mind-stretching, viewing one's own system with a reflective telescope, and speculating about possible policy lessons derived from comparative analyses, what can be gained from comparative analysis of health systems? There are two promising directions in which the field is moving: (a) comparison of disease-specific treatment patterns and outcomes across nations and (b) comparison of health systems and outcomes across cities. Both directions represent responses to important gaps in existing comparative research on health systems:

**The limits of OECD data:** As we have seen from Table 6.1, and from our analysis of OECD data on the U.S., in comparative perspective, we spend more on health care than any other nation, yet we rank nowhere near the top in measures of life expectancy, at birth, or infant mortality. Further analysis of OECD data (Anderson, Reinhardt, Hussey, & Petrosyan, 2003) indicates that the higher spending and lower aggregate use of health services in the U.S. is explained by the fact that average prices for medical goods and services are much higher in the U.S. Beyond this important conclusion, however, aggregate OECD data are insufficient to make any claims about average productivity and quality of medical treatments provided in the U.S. compared to other OECD countries. Unfortunately, OECD's extensive database on inputs, spending, and health status outcomes does not include information on the outcomes of medical treatments for common conditions.

**The limits of cross-national comparisons:** In addition to the limits of the OECD database, questions may be raised about whether the nation state is the most appropriate spatial unit for comparing the performance of health systems. As we live in a more urbanized world, there is increasing awareness that the city is a strategic unit of analysis for understanding the health sector (Vlahov & Gallea, 2002). Yet most health services research—both in the United States and among international organizations such as the United Nations, the World Health Organization (WHO) or the OECD—continues to assume that nations are the most relevant units of analysis for assessing the performance of health systems and health policy. There are many limitations to this view, however.

First, there are enormous variations in health and health system performance within nations, between urban and rural areas, large and small cities, depressed and prosperous ones, and even within cities (Wennberg, Andrulis, & Ginsberg, 1996; NYCDHMH, 2004). Second, it is exceedingly difficult to disentangle the relative importance of health systems from other determinants of health, including the sociocultural characteristics and the neighborhood context of the population whose health is measured (Ellen, Mijanovich, & Dillman, 2001). It is even more difficult to do so at a level of aggregation such as the nation state where important dimensions of health policy are made.

Third, despite the rise of the welfare state, even in the most centralized nations, many dimensions of health and social policy elude national and state levels. Some of the most challenging problems—care for vulnerable older persons, the severe mentally ill, the most economically disadvantaged and the uninsured—fall into a kind of residual category of problems that are passed down to local governments among which city governments bear a disproportionate share of responsibility (Rodwin & Gusmano, 2005a).

## Comparison of Disease-Specific Treatment Patterns and Outcomes

In response to the limits of OECD data, significant work is now underway but only for a subset of OECD nations. To overcome the limits of aggregate OECD data, all of this work has focused on specific diseases, drawing on individual level data related to specific health conditions. For example, the McKinsey Healthcare Productivity Project compared the management of diabetes mellitus, cholelithiasis (gall stones), lung cancer, and breast cancer in Germany, the United Kingdom, and the U.S. (McKinsey Global Institute, 1996; Baily & Garber, 1997). Also, the OECD, itself, has launched the Aging-Related Diseases Project in which an impressive team of economists has attempted to link treatments with outcomes by collecting comparative data on ischemic heart disease, stroke, and breast cancer (Cutler, 2003; Moise & Jacobzone, 2003).

Do such studies yield valid findings across OECD nations? Not yet! But others are in progress, as well. The Commonwealth Fund's International Working Group on Quality Indicators collected data for 21 indicators in Australia, Canada, New Zealand, England, and the U.S. (Hussey, Anderson, Osborn, et al., 2004). Their indicators included various dimensions of medical care, including five-year cancer relative survival rates, 30-day case-fatality rates after acute myocardial infarction and stroke, breast cancer screening, and asthma mortality rates. In her commentary on this study, McGlynn (2004) concluded that there is no perfect health system because each country has expertise in at least one area of care which it could teach others.

## Comparison of Health Systems and Outcomes Across Cities

In response to the limits of cross-national comparisons, a number of efforts are underway to examine health systems and outcomes across cities. One of the most well-known is the World Health Organization's Healthy Cities Project, which began as a WHO-led movement to promote population health in cities throughout the world (Aicher, 1998). Although this project aimed largely at sensitizing local authorities to the health implications of different urban policies, current efforts to evaluate diverse city programs may result in valuable data on the social and economic determinants of health, as well as on the role of health systems in affecting population health.

In Europe, the Mégapoles Project (Bardsley, 1999), which focused on the socially disadvantaged, represents an innovative attempt to combine research and practice by collecting a database on the major capital cities of Europe, their health systems, and population health status. Along with the compilation of comparative data across these cities, the project has initiated study groups of health and social service professionals to search for relevant innovations in the areas of services for older persons and youth. Although this project is surely the most well-developed attempt to compare the

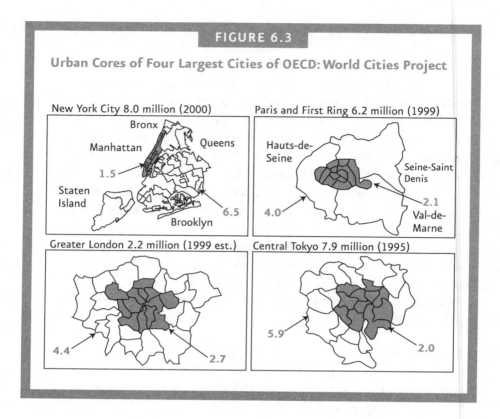

FIGURE 6.3

Urban Cores of Four Largest Cities of OECD: World Cities Project

New York City 8.0 million (2000)
Bronx
Manhattan      Queens
1.5
Staten
Island
6.5
Brooklyn

Paris and First Ring 6.2 million (1999)
Hauts-de-Seine
Seine-Saint Denis
4.0      2.1
Val-de-Marne

Greater London 2.2 million (1999 est.)
4.4      2.7

Central Tokyo 7.9 million (1995)
5.9      2.0

health of cities, it is limited by the fact that the choice of cities was driven by political criteria. European capitals, such as Vienna and Oslo, are so much smaller than London that it is questionable whether they can really learn from one another.

The World Cities Project (Rodwin & Gusmano, 2002; www.ilcusa.org/projects/research) represents a new approach to the comparison of health systems of cities because it explicitly compares the health systems and health status of the urban core of the four largest cities in the OECD nations: New York, London, Paris, and Tokyo (see FIGURE 6.3). The urban core as a unit of analysis provides a frame within which to focus cross-national comparisons on a more coherent and discernible set of health system characteristics. For example, Manhattan, Paris, and Inner Tokyo and Inner London are characterized by similar concentrations of teaching hospitals, medical schools, physicians, and acute care hospital beds (see TABLE 6.6).

> ### TABLE 6.6
>
> ### Health Care Resources: Manhattan, Inner London, Paris, and Tokyo (1995–2000)
>
> | | MANHATTAN | INNER LONDON | PARIS | INNER TOKYO |
> |---|---|---|---|---|
> | # of teaching hospitals | 19 | 13 | 25 | 9 |
> | # of medical schools | 5 | 4 | 7 | 7 |
> | Acute hospital beds per 1000 population | 8.9 (1997) | 4.1 (1990) | 9.6 (1995) | 12.8 (2000)[1] |
> | Physicians per 10,000 population | 71.2 (1995) | 36.9 (2000) | 84.6 (1997) | 70.0 (2000) |
>
> SOURCES: Manhattan: New York State Department of Health (NYSDOH), 1998; London: UK Department of Health and Health of Londoners Project; Paris: physicians- Ministère de l'Emploi et de la Solidarité, Direction de la Recherche, des Etudes, de l'Evaluation et des Statistiques (DREES) repertoire ADELI, January 1st 2002; hospitals DRESS, SAE, 2001; Tokyo: "Report on Survey of Physicians, Dentists and Pharmacists 1998", Tokyo Metropolitan Government, Bureau of Public Health, 2000.
> 1 This figure is an estimate derived by reducing the number of general hospital beds by 30% so as not to include beds in which length of stay is over 30 days.

Beyond the selection of the urban cores of New York, London, Paris, and Tokyo, the WCP illustrates how a comparative analysis, structured by comparable units of analysis, can serve to highlight some striking similarities and differences for further investigation. All four urban cores have economies based on services and information, which are closely tied to national and international transactions. They are also centers of culture, media, government, and international organizations. And their resident populations include some of the wealthiest and poorest members of their respective nations.

A major focus of this on-going project is to explore the impact of world cities—their health systems and neighborhood characteristics—on two outcomes: the use of health services and health status (Rodwin & Gusmano, 2005a). So far, this project has resulted in comparative analysis of several specific issues across these four world cities—aging and long-term care (Rodwin & Gusmano, 2005b), patterns of infant mortality (Neuberg & Rodwin, 2002; Rodwin & Neuberg, 2005), patterns of coronary artery disease (Gusmano, Rodwin, & Weisz, 2004; Weisz, Gusmano, & Rodwin, 2004), and patterns of avoidable hospital conditions. By comparing these issues in cities that share many characteristics in common (size, density, share of foreign-born, income disparities) but differ in the financing and organization of their health systems and degree of income inequalities and neighborhood segregation, it is possible to generate and begin testing hypotheses on why these cities differ from one another along a range of indicators.

## CONCLUDING OBSERVATIONS

The new approaches to comparing health systems noted above have not yet yielded important lessons for the U.S. or local units within it. At this stage, these approaches are presented to provide a sense of new direction in the field. Whether they will result in valuable lessons—indeed, just how policy learning occurs as a result of studying health care systems abroad—is not thoroughly under-

## CASE STUDY

You have just been hired by Health Care Associates (HCA), a large U.S. consulting firm specializing in health care management and policy analysis. HCA's clients range from government agencies to large health care providers, insurers, and purveyors of information-based administrative technologies. The firm has grown rapidly over the past decade and thrives on its stellar reputation for quality work and advice that has helped many clients achieve their goals.

Because many of HCA's private clients are entering the global marketplace, the CEO calls you one day and asks you to prepare a memorandum on the market opportunities for techniques of managed care in health care systems abroad. What would you advise her to do? Include in your answer a discussion of the possibilities in national health insurance systems (e.g., France and Canada), as well as national health services systems (e.g., Britain). Also, based on your understanding of the financing and organization of their respective health care systems, provide some advice on potential clients for introducing elements of managed care within each system. Finally, as an optional exercise, write a memorandum to HCA's CEO in which you explain what U.S. policymakers could learn from the experience of France, Canada, and Britain; or from new approaches to the comparative analysis of health systems in wealthy nations.

stood (Rodwin & Brecher, 1992; Freeman, 2003). But there is little doubt that comparative research on health systems in wealthy nations (and cities) could be helpful to health policymakers and managers in the U.S., who seek to draw lessons from experience abroad.

## DISCUSSION QUESTIONS

1. What are the strengths and weaknesses of the social science approach to comparative health systems?
2. How can the analysis of health systems abroad be used to promote policy learning?
3. What are three common problems in health policy development found in different countries?
4. How does the French NHI system differ from the Canadian NHI system in its financing?
5. Compare the organization and financing of the British and U.S. health systems.
6. Is there evidence of policy convergence in the evolutions of the French, Canadian, and British health systems?
7. What can be learned from new approaches to the comparative analysis of health systems in wealthy nations?

## ACKNOWLEDGMENT

I wish to thank Michael Gusmano for his comments on this chapter and Jin Liu for assistance including updating the OECD data and preparing the tables for this chapter.

## REFERENCES

Aaron, H., & Schwartz, W. (1984). *The painful prescription: Rationing hospital care.* Washington, DC: Brookings Institution.

Abelson, J., Mendelsohn, M., Lavis, J., Morgan, S., Forest, P., & Swinton, M.. (2004). Canadians confront health care reform. *Health Affairs,* 23(3), 186–193.

Aicher, J. (1998). *Designing healthy cities.* Krieger.

Altenstetter, C. (1974). *Health policy-making and administration in West Germany and the United States.* Beverly Hills, CA: Sage.

American Hospital Administration. (2000). *Hospital statistics.* Chicago: Author.

Anderson, G., Reinhardt, U., Hussey, P., & Petrosyan, V. (2003). It's the prices, stupid: Why is U.S. spending so much higher? *Health Affairs,* 22(3), 89–105.

Anderson, O. (1972). *Health care: Can there be equity? The United States, Sweden, and England.* New York: Wiley.

Andrulis, D., & Shaw-Taylor, Y. (1996). The social and health characteristics of California cities. *Health Affairs, 15,* 131–142.

Baily, M., & Garber, A. (1997). Health care productivity. *Brookings Papers on Economic Activity: Microeconomics.* 143–2002.

Bardsley, M. (1999). *Health in Europe's capitals.* Project Megapoles. London: Directorate of Public Health, East London & the City Health Authority.

Blendon, R., Leitman, R., Morrison, K., & Donelan, K. (1990). Satisfaction with health systems in ten nations. *Health Affairs, 9(2),* 185–192.

Blum, H. (1981). *Planning for health.* New York: Human Sciences.

Brown, L. (2003). Comparing health systems in four countries: lessons for the United States. *American Journal of Public Health, 93(1),* 52–56.

Brown, L. (1998). Exceptionalism as the rule? U.S. health policy innovation and comparative learning. *Journal of Health Politics, Policy and Law, 23(1),* 35–51.

Chen, L., Evans, T., & Cash, R. (2000). Health as a global public good. In Kaul,I., Grunberg, I., & Stern. M. (Eds.), *Global public goods* (pp. 284–305). New York: Oxford University Press.

Chernichovsky, D. (1995). Health system reforms in industrialized economies: An emerging paradigm. *Milbank Quarterly, 73,* 339–372.

Chernichovsky, D. (2002). Pluralism, choice, and the state in the emerging paradigm in health systems. The Milbank Quarterly, 80, 5–40.

Coyne, J., & Hilsenrath, P. (2002). The world health report 2000. *American Journal of Public Health, 92,* 30–33.

Current Population Survey. (2004, March). U.S. Bureau of the Census. Health insurance coverage status and type of coverage by selected characteristics: 2003 (Suppl.). Available: http://ferret.bls.census.gov/macro/032004/health/h01_001.htm

Cutler, D. (2003). A framework for evaluating medical care systems. In OECD 2003. *A disease-based comparison of health systems: What is best at what cost?* Paris: OECD.

Deber, R. (2003). Health care reform: Lessons from Canada. *American Journal of Public Health, 93,* 20–24.

De Kervasdoué, J., Kimberly, J., & Rodwin, V. (Eds.). (1984). *The end of an illusion: The future of health policy in Western industrialized nations.* Berkeley, CA: University of California Press.

De Miguel, S. (1975). A framework for the study of national health systems, *Inquiry, 12,* 10.

DHHS. (1976). *Sharing resources for health in England: Report of the Resource Allocation Working Party.* London: Her Majesty's Stationery Office.

Dobson, F. (1999). Modernizing Britain's national health service. *Health Affairs, 18*(3), 40–41.

Dumbaugh, K., & Neuhauser, D. (1979). International comparisons of health services: Where are we? *Social Science and Medicine, 221,* 13B.

Ellen, I., Mijanovich, T., & Dillman, K. (2001). Neighborhood effects on health: Exploring the links and assessing the evidence. *Journal of Urban Affairs, 23,* 391–408.

Ellencweig, A. (1992). *Analyzing health systems: A modular approach.* New York: Oxford University Press.

Elling, R., & Kerr, H. (1975). Selection of contrasting national health systems for in-depth study. *Inquiry (Suppl. 12), 2.*

Evans, R. (1984). *Strained mercy: The economics of Canadian health care.* Toronto: Butterworths.

Evans, R. (1992). Canada: The real issues. *Journal of Health Policy, Politics and Law, 17*(4), 739–763.

Evans, R. G. (2000). Canada. *Journal of Health Politics, Policy and Law, 25,* 890–897.

Field, M. (1973). The concept of "health system" at the macrosociological level. *Social Science and Medicine, 7,* 763–785.

Fox, D. (1986). *Health policies, health politics.* Princeton, NJ: Princeton University Press.

Freeman, R. (2005). Learning in public policy. In M. Moran, M. Rein, & R. Goodin (Eds.), *Oxford handbook of public policy.* Oxford: Oxford University Press.

Garber, A. (2003). Comparing health care systems from the disease-specific perspective. *A disease-based comparison of health systems: What is best at what cost?* Paris: OECD.

Ginsberg P. (1996). The RWJF community snapshots study: Introduction and overview. *Health Affairs, 15,* 7–15.

Glaser, W. (1970). *Paying the doctor: Systems of remuneration and their effects.* Baltimore, MD: Johns Hopkins University Press.

Glaser, W. (1978). *Health insurance bargaining: Foreign lessons for Americans.* New York: Gardner Press.

Glaser, W. (1987). *Paying the hospital,* San Francisco: Jossey Bass.

Glaser, W. (1991). *Health insurance in practice: International variations in financing, benefits, and problems.* San Francisco: Jossey-Bass.

Glouberman, S. (1996). *Beyond restructuring.* London: King's Fund.

Griffiths, R. (1983). *NHS management inquiry.* London: DHSS.

Gusmano, M. K., Rodwin, V. G., & Weisz, D. (2004). *L'affaire du coeur in the United States and France: The prevalence and treatment of ischemic heart disease in two Nations and their world cities.* Robert Wood Johnson Foundation Scholars in Health Policy Working Paper. Princeton: Robert Wood Johnson Foundation.

Hirschman, A. (1970). *Exit, voice and loyalty*. Cambridge, MA: Harvard University Press.

Holliday, I. (1992). *The NHS transformed*. Manchester, UK: Baseline Books.

Hollingsworth, J. (1986). *A political economy of medicine: Great Britain and the United States*. Baltimore, MD: Johns Hopkins University Press.

Hussey, P., Anderson, G., Osborne, R., Feek, C., McLaughlin, V., Miller J., & Epstein, A. (2004). How does the quality of care compare in five countries? *Health Affairs, 23*(3), 89–99.

Illsley, R. (1999). Reducing health inequalities: Britain's latest attempt. *Health Affairs, 18*(3), 45–46.

Immergut, E. (1992). *Health politics: Interests and institutions in Western Europe*. New York: Cambridge University Press.

Klass, O. (1985). Explaining America and the welfare state: An alternative theory. *British Journal of Political Science, 15*, 427–450.

Klein, R. (2001). What's happening to Britain's National Health Service? *New England Journal of Medicine, 345*, 305–308.

Klein, R. (2000). *The new politics of the NHS* (4th ed.). Harlow, UK: Prentice-Hall.

Klein, R. (1998). Why Britain is reorganizing its National Health Service—Yet again? *Health Affairs, 17*(4), 111–125.

Klein, R. (1991). Risks and benefits of comparative studies: Notes from another shore. *Milbank Quarterly, 69*, 275–291.

Kondro, W. (2000). Canada's ministers agree on health package. *Lancet, 356*, 1011.

Le Pen, C., & Rodwin, V. (1996). Le plan Juppé: Vers un nouveau mode de régulation des soins [The Juppé Plan: Toward a new form of health care regulation]. *Droit Social, 9*(10), 859–862.

Le Grand, J. (1999). Competition, cooperation, or control? Tales from the British National Health Service. *Health Affairs, 18*(3), 27–39.

Leichter, H. (1979). *A comparative approach to policy analysis: Health care policy in four nations*. Cambridge. Cambridge University Press.

Levit, K., Smith, C., Cowan, C., Sensenig, C., Catlin, A., et al. Health spending rebound continues in 2002. *Health Affairs, 23*(1), 147–159.

Marmor, T., Bridges, A., & Hoffman, W. (1978). Comparative politics and health policies: Notes on benefits, costs, limits. In D. Ashford (Ed.), *Comparing public policies*. Beverly Hills, CA: Sage.

Marmot, M. (1999). Acting on evidence to reduce inequalities in health. *Health Affairs, 18*(3), 45–46.

Maynard, A. (1986). *Annual report on the National Health Service*. New York: Center for Health Economics.

McGinnis, M., & Foege, W. H. (1993). Actual causes of death in the United States. *Journal of the American Medical Association, 270*, 2207–2212.

McGlynn, E. (2004).There is no perfect health system. *Health Affairs, 23*(3), 100–102.

Mechanic, D. (1976). The comparative study of health care delivery systems. In D. Mechanic. (Ed.), *The growth of bureaucratic medicine: An inquiry into the dynamics of patient behavior and the organization of medical care* (pp. 23–48). New York: Wiley.

McKinsey Global Institute. (1996). *Health care productivity.* Washington, DC: McKinsey Consulting.

Moise, P., & Jacobzone, S. (2003). *Population ageing, health expenditure and treatment: An ARD perspective. In OECD 2003. A disease-based comparison of health systems: What is best at what cost?* Paris: OECD.

Navarro, V. (2002). Can health care systems be compared using a single measure of performance? *American Journal of Public Health, 92*(1), 31–34.

Naylor, C. D. (1999). Health care in Canada: Incrementalism under fiscal duress. *Health Affairs, 18*(3), 9–26.

Neuberg, L., & Rodwin, V. (2002). Infant mortality in four world cities: New York, London, Paris and Tokyo. *Indicators—The Journal of Social Health, 2*(1), 86–90.

New York City Department of Health and Mental Hygiene. (2004). *Take care New York.* Available: www.nycdoh.gov

Preker, A., & Dror, D. (2002). *Social reinsurance: A new approach to sustainable community health financing.* Geneva: IL/World Bank.

Reinhardt, U. (1985). Hard choices in health care: A matter of ethics. In L. Etheredge, (Ed.), *Health care: How to improve it and pay for it.* Washington, DC: Center for National Policy.

Robinson, R., & Le Grand, J. (1994). *Evaluating the NHS reforms.* London: King's Fund Institute.

Rodwin, M. (2000). Exit and voice in American health care. *University of Michigan Journal of Law Reform, 32,* 1041–1066.

Rodwin, V. (1984). *The health planning predicament: France, Quebec, England and the United States.* Berkeley, CA: University of California Press.

Rodwin, V. (1989). New ideas for health policy in France, Canada, and Britain. In M. Field (Ed.), *Success and crisis in national health systems: A comparative approach.* New York: Routledge.

Rodwin, V. (1997). The rise of managed care in the United States: Lessons for French health policy. In C. Altenstetter & J. Bjorkman (Eds.), *Health policy reform, national variations and globalization.* New York: St. Martin's Press.

Rodwin, V. (2003). The health care system under French National Health Insurance: Lessons for health reform in the United States. *American Journal of Public Health, 93*(1), 31–37.

Rodwin, V., & Brecher, C. (1992). Comparative analysis and mutual learning. In V. Rodwin, C. Brecher, D. Jolly, & R. Baxter (Eds.), *Public hos-*

*pital systems in New York and Paris.* New York: New York University Press.

Rodwin, V., & Gusmano, M. (2002). The world cities project: Rationale, organization, and design for comparison of megacity health systems. *Journal of Urban Health, 79*(4).

Rodwin, V., & Gusmano, M. (2005a). Health services research and the city. In Vlahov D. & Gallea, S. *Handbook of Urban Health.*

Rodwin, V., & Gusmano, M. (Eds.). (2005b). *Growing older in world cities: New York, London, Paris and Tokyo.* Vanderbilt University Press.

Rodwin, V., & Neuberg, L. (2005). Infant mortality and income in four world cities: New York, London, Paris and Tokyo. *American Journal of Public Health, 95*(1), 86–90.

Rodwin, V., & Sandier, S. (1993). Health care under French National Health Insurance: A public-private mix, low prices, high volumes. *Health Affairs, 12*(3), 113–131.

Roemer, M. (1977). *Comparative national policies for health care.* New York: Marcel Dekker.

Rosner, D. (1982). Health care for the "truly needy": Nineteenth-century origins of the concept. *Milbank Memorial Fund Quarterly: Health and Society, 60,* 355.

Smee, C. (2000). United Kingdom. *Journal of Health Politics, Policy and Law, 25,* 945–951.

Smith, S., Heffler, S., & Freeland, M. (1999). The next decade of health spending. *Health Affairs, 18*(4), 86–95.

Stoddard, D. (1984, May). *Rationalizing the health care system.* Paper presented at the Ontario Council Conference, Toronto.

Stone, D. (1981). Drawing lessons from comparative health research. In R. A. Straetz, M. Lieberman, & A. Sardell (Eds.), *Critical issues in health policy* (pp. 135–148). Lexington, MA: D.C. Heath.

Teune, H. (1978). The logic of comparative policy analysis. In D. Ashford (Ed.), *Comparing public policies.* Beverly Hills, CA: Sage.

Tuohy, C. (1999). *Accidental logics: The dynamics of change in the health care arena in the United States, Britain, and Canada.* New York: Oxford University Press.

Townsend, P., & Davidson, N. (Eds.). (1982). *Inequalities in health: The Black report.* London: Penguin.

Vlahov, D., & Gallea, S. (2002). Urbanization, urbanicity, and health. *Journal of Urban Health, 79*(Suppl. 1), S1–S11.

Wennberg, J. E., & Gittlesohn, A. (1973). Small area variations in health care delivery. *Science, 182,* 1102–1108.

Wennberg, J. E., Freeman, J. L., & Culp, W. J. (1987). Are hospital services rationed in New Haven or over-utilised in Boston? *Lancet, 1,* 1185–1189.

Weisz, D., Gusmano, M., & Rodwin, V. (2004). Gender and the treatment of heart disease among older persons in the U.S., England and France: A comparative, population-based view of a clinical phenomenon. *Gender Medicine, 1*(1), 29–40.

Weisz, D., Gusmano, M., & Rodwin, V. (2004). *Avoidable hospital conditions in New York and Paris.* New York: International Longevity Center-USA, Working Paper.

Woolhandler, S., Himmelstein, D., Angell, M., & Young, Q. (2003). Proposal of the physicians' working group for single payer national health insurance. *Journal of the American Medical Association, 290,* 798–805.

Woolhandler, S., Campbell, T., & Himmelstein, D. (2003). Costs of health care administration in the United States and Canada. *New England Journal of Medicine, 349*(8), 768–775.

*Working for patients.* (1989). London: Her Majesty's Stationery Office.

WHO. (2000). *The World Health Report 2000. Health systems: Improving performance.* Geneva: Available: www.who.int/whr/2000

# PART II
## PROVIDING HEALTH CARE

# 7

# ACUTE CARE

Marc N. Gourevitch,
Carol A. Caronna, and
Gary Kalkut

- Provide an overview of acute care sites and practitioners.
- Describe the historical development of acute care in the U.S.
- Differentiate between ambulatory and primary care.
- Describe the role of emergency services in the spectrum of acute care.
- Describe types of hospitals and health systems involved in acute care.
- Discuss changes and challenges facing acute care providers.

TOPICAL OUTLINE

- History of acute care
- Kinds of acute care: ambulatory, primary, emergency, specialty
- Hospitals in the U.S., kinds of acute care hospitals, and hospital systems
- Current issues in acute care

KEY WORDS

Acute care, ambulatory care, primary care, primary care provider, emergency care, specialty ambulatory care, hospitals, scope of services, public hospitals, rural hospitals, teaching hospitals, hospital systems, integrated health care systems

---

THE TERM "ACUTE CARE" refers to medical services for persons with or at risk for acute or active medical conditions in a variety of ambulatory and inpatient settings. One might define acute care, as discussed in this chapter, as "medical care other than chronic care." Thus, acute care excludes care delivered in chronic care facilities such as nursing homes, but includes services provided in a complex range of settings including physicians' offices, community health centers, outpatient clinics, urgent care centers, hospital outpatient departments, emergency departments, free-standing surgery centers, and hospital inpatient units. The last few decades have witnessed many changes in acute care delivery, including the increased provision of acute care on an outpatient basis. This trend has influenced many aspects of acute care, including the roles of medical practitioners and the structures and strategies of acute care hospitals. This chapter explores the current spectrum of acute care and the challenges facing its delivery in the United States in light of these recent changes.

## THE HISTORY OF ACUTE CARE

The history of acute care can be divided into several stages of development. Prior to the mid to late 1870s, "the family, as the center of social and economic life in early American society, was the natural locus of most care for the sick" (Starr, 1982, p. 32). Family members, usually women, were responsible for treating illnesses using medicinal herbs, medical almanacs, and knowledge from oral tradition. Physicians and lay healers treated paying patients in their homes, even for surgery. Hospitals were used to care for, but not cure, the more seriously ill and the poor. Of the approximately 180 hospitals in the U.S. in the 1870s, most were simply known as poorhouses, staffed by untrained nurses, and often serving people of a certain religion, age, or ethnic group.

Advancements in biomedical science and technology in the late 1800s led to more effective medical means of cure and intervention. In the early 1900s, hospitals evolved into the medical facilities we are familiar with today, where doctors treat patients for specific illnesses and diseases. Improvements in hygiene and techniques for asepsis and surgical anesthesia prompted surgery to move from the home to the hospital. As demands for admission increased, hospitals limited their patients to those with acute care needs and sought physician contacts to fill their beds with acute care patients. More sophisticated equipment needs and consultations with other doctors also encouraged the move of acute care from the home to medical offices and hospitals. By 1909, there were more than 4,300 hospitals in the U.S. (Stevens, 1971). By the 1920s, most home care was limited to first aid and everyday hygiene (Starr, 1982).

In the 1920s and 1930s, most doctors were solo practitioners, treating patients in offices and hospitals. Some doctors practiced in clinics, whether in rural and poor areas that lacked hospitals, or in private group practices in urban areas, such as the Mayo Clinic in Minnesota and the Palo Alto Medical Clinic in northern California (Starr, 1982). Industrial workers at remote sites often received acute care at hospitals and clinics owned and staffed by their employers, such as railroads, shipyards, and construction firms. Although they were unusual at the time, many of these early clinics and industrial health plans served as models for managed care organizations and integrated health care systems formed in the latter part of the twentieth century.

The World War II era brought significant changes to the world of acute care. New developments, such as the introduction of widespread antibiotic use in 1943, markedly enhanced treatment outcomes for certain conditions. Health insurance also became more widespread after presidential action during the war froze wages but not fringe benefits. The negotiation of benefits brought health insurance to many workers as well as fostered the expectation that Americans should procure health insurance through employment. The health insurance industry developed rapidly after World War II. The Hill-Burton Act (Starr, 1982) originally passed in 1946, provided federal funds for hospital construction and brought hospitals to underserved areas. In the 1960s, the introduction of Medicare and Medicaid provided federally funded health insurance for Americans who lacked an employment relationship— namely, the elderly and the poor. Concerns about enough health care providers led to increased funding for medical training and the establishment of new health care occupations, including nurse practitioners and physician assistants.

In the 1970s more and more Americans had access to health care and insurance, and insurers reimbursed doctors on a fee-for-service basis. These factors led to an escalation of medical costs, which was of particular concern to the federal government. In the early 1980s, federal legislation created a prospective payment system for Medicare. Instead of fee-for-service reimbursement, practitioners were allowed a set payment per treatment, depending on the illness or injury. The private insurance industry also adopted strategies for cost containment, such as capitation and discounted contracts with preferred providers. Because early models of managed care saved money by reducing hospital admissions and lengths of stay, government programs and insurance companies encouraged and/or constrained physicians to limit hospitalization. As a consequence, the delivery of acute care became more and more likely to be provided on an outpatient basis.

## KINDS OF ACUTE CARE TODAY

In today's environment of financial constraints and managed care, acute care is still provided in familiar settings, but patients are likely to see nurse practitioners and physician assistants in addition to primary care physicians. Rather than practice by themselves, doctors are more likely to have formal, legally grounded linkages with other doctors, hospitals, and integrated health care systems. Patients today may see a health care provider at a clinic, doctor's office, outpatient facility owned by a hospital or group of doctors, or at a hospital, or communicate with a provider over the telephone or Internet. Decisions about where to provide acute care are made based on how it can be delivered most efficiently and cost effectively. Hospital stays are minimized and patients may be prepared for surgery, undergo rehabilitative therapy, and receive follow-up care in outpatient settings or even their homes. We describe this diverse world of acute care in the following sections.

## Ambulatory Care

Ambulatory care is health care provided to individuals who are neither inpatients in a hospital or another chronic care facility nor bed bound at home. It is provided by a variety of categories of health care providers in a broad range of settings and includes primary care, emergency care, and ambulatory subspecialty care (including ambulatory surgery). Several themes shape the face of ambulatory care today, reflecting the intense pressures of cost containment in the health care industry. As care is generally more expensive to provide in inpatient than in outpatient settings, recent trends in ambulatory care reflect efforts to prevent hospitalization. When patients are hospitalized, efforts are made to reduce the length of their stay and hasten their transition from the inpatient to the ambulatory care setting. To reduce acute care utilization, initiatives in disease management and delivery system integration are defining new paradigms for the outpatient management of patients with chronic diseases. All of these trends have contributed to the growth of outpatient care relative to inpatient care. Efforts to decrease hospital length of stay and to shift many surgical procedures to the ambulatory setting have caused a relative increase in the acuity of patients seen in some ambulatory settings. In the section that follows, we provide an overview of ambulatory care in the United States, examine the forces shaping its evolution, and discuss some of the resulting tensions and challenges faced by this vast system of care.

### Ambulatory Care Statistics

In the United States, slightly over 1 billion ambulatory care visits were made in 2000 to physicians' offices, hospital outpatient

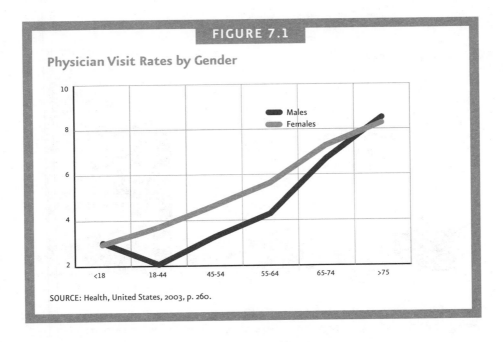

**FIGURE 7.1**

Physician Visit Rates by Gender

SOURCE: Health, United States, 2003, p. 260.

departments, and hospital emergency departments, with a mean
of 3.7 such visits per person (USDHHS, 2003, p. 260). Of these ambulatory care visits, 81% were to physicians' offices, 8% to hospital outpatient departments, and 11% to hospital emergency departments.
The frequency of physician office visits varies by age, gender, race,
and socioeconomic status (see **FIGURE 7.1**). Rates for females were
higher than for males (3.5 visits versus 2.6 visits/year), primarily
reflecting a marked difference in the 18 to 44 year-old category (3.0
for females vs. 1.5 for males, respectively). Physician office visit
rates increased with age, with highest rates (6.5/year) among those
75 years and older. Sharp differences in the pattern of ambulatory
care utilization between whites and blacks were evident (see **FIG-
URE 7.2**). Whites visited physicians' offices more often than blacks
(3.2 versus 2.4 visits/year), yet blacks used emergency department
services at nearly double the rate of whites (0.62 versus 0.37 vis-
its/year, respectively). Stated differently, emergency department
visits comprised 18% of total ambulatory care visits for blacks, compared with 10% for whites. Differences in utilization rates between
rich and poor persist, though they have diminished in recent years.
In 1964, 59% of poor and 74% of nonpoor families reported seeing a
physician within the last year, compared to rates in 1998 of 80% and
86%, respectively (USDHHS, 1995, Table 77; USDHHS, 2000, Table 71).

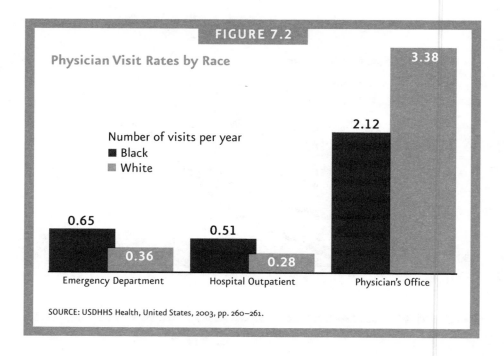

FIGURE 7.2

Physician Visit Rates by Race

Number of visits per year
■ Black
■ White

| | | |
| 0.65 | 0.51 | 2.12 |
| 0.36 | 0.28 | 3.38 |
| Emergency Department | Hospital Outpatient | Physician's Office |

SOURCE: USDHHS Health, United States, 2003, pp. 260–261.

The enactment of Medicaid and Medicare in 1965 is believed to have greatly facilitated access to medical care for low-income and elderly persons in the United States.

Utilization of ambulatory care appears to be more strongly determined by insurance status than by income bracket, however. Among uninsured persons in 1998, 37% of the poor, 36% of the near poor, and 29% of the nonpoor made no visits to a doctor's office or to a hospital emergency department. In contrast, among those with health insurance, 14% of the poor, 16% of the near poor, and 13% of the nonpoor had no such visits (U.S. Department of Health and Human Services [USDHHS], 2000, Table 71). Lack of health insurance for children less than 6 years of age, the group most in need of immunizations and psychosocial, neurological, and behavioral assessments, was associated with similar disparities in access to care.

Utilization of ambulatory care services has increased steadily in recent years, from an age-adjusted mean of 3.34 visits/person in 1995 to 3.85 visits/person in 2001 (USDHHS, 2003, p. 260). At the same time, the average length of hospital admissions has decreased, from 7.1 days in 1992 to 5.7 days in 2002 (American Hospital Association [AHA], 2002). These shifts reflect the increased emphasis on delivering care in outpatient settings whenever possible. A natural consequence of this trend is a greater likelihood that more acute patients will be seen in outpatient settings, and that only the most acute patients will be seen in many inpatient settings.

## Organization of Ambulatory Care Services

There are two major categories of ambulatory care. The greater volume of this kind of care is delivered by individual physicians either in solo practice or who have organized themselves into partnerships or private group practices. The second category, often referred to as hospital-based ambulatory services, may be thought of as care organized and delivered under the auspices of institutions. This category includes ambulatory care provided in outpatient clinics, walk-in centers, and emergency departments; hospital-sponsored group practices and health promotion centers; freestanding "surgi-centers" and "urgi"- or "emergi-centers"; health department clinics; neighborhood and community health centers (NHCs and CHCs); organized home care; community mental health centers; school and workplace health services; and prison health services. The average annual number of visits to physicians' offices increased from 2.71 per person in 1995 to 3.04 per person in 2000, while emergency department visit volume remained relatively unchanged (from 0.37 visits per person in 1995 to 0.40 visits per person in 2000) (USDHHS, Table 82).

## Primary Care

It is important to understand the distinction between primary care and ambulatory care. Primary care signifies a relationship between a patient and clinician that is longitudinal and that both patient and clinician view as the patient's principal source of general outpatient medical care. The Institute of Medicine defines primary care "the provision of integrated, accessible care services by clinicians who are accountable for addressing a large majority of the personal health care needs, developing a sustained partnership with patients, and practicing in the context of family and community" (Institute of Medicine, 1996, p. 1). Embedded within this definition are the concepts of longitudinal care characterized by continuity with a single provider and by its comprehensive approach to patients' multiple medical needs. Also implicit in this definition is the notion of primary care provider as coordinator of patients' care, ranging from subspecialist referrals to social service assistance. Primary care is thus one type of ambulatory care a patient may receive. A person seeking medical care directly from various subspecialists as the need may arise but who has no principal ongoing relationship with any of them would be using ambulatory care but not primary care.

### Primary Care Providers

Primary care is provided by four principal categories of professionals: physicians, nurse practitioners (NPs), physician assistants (PAs), and midwives. Physicians typically considered providers of primary care include those in general internal medicine, family practice, pediatrics, and geriatrics. Obstetrician/gynecologists serve as the primary care provider for many women as well. Other specialist and subspecialist physicians can provide primary care. For example, a cardiologist who sees a patient in her office following hospitalization for a first heart attack may become the patient's primary care physician. In this case, the cardiologist might care for the patient's various medical problems over time, or at least maintain awareness of the care the patient is receiving from other physicians with a view towards ensuring that the patient's overall care is comprehensive and coordinated. Over the last two decades, the percentage of primary care visits provided by generalists (general internists, family practitioners, and pediatricians) has declined (from 57% in 1980 to 51% in 2000), relative to that provided by specialists (43% in 1980 and 49% in 2000) (USDHHS, 2003, Table 84).

Nonphysicians (nurse practitioners, physician assistants, and midwives) are also gaining in importance as primary care providers. Although each follows a unique educational path, there is substantial overlap in their capabilities in many ambulatory primary care settings. It is estimated that NPs and PAs typically have the skills to perform 75% of the services that physicians provide in adult practices and 90% of those in pediatric practices (Scheffler, 1996). While physicians continue to provide the great majority of ambulatory care visits, ambulatory care encounters with nonphysician providers are on the rise. Training programs are responding to this demand for nonphysician practitioners by significantly increasing capacity. The number of PAs in practice, for example, has more than doubled in the last decade alone (American Academy of Physician Assistants, 2004).

### Sites for the Provision of Primary Care Services

Primary care in the United States is provided in a number of settings, with private physician offices continuing to be the most visited sites even as managed care organizations continue to capture market share. In recent years, community-based and hospital-based primary care clinics have expanded their primary care capabilities in response to increased numbers of persons eligible for subsidized health insurance through Medicaid managed care and the State Children's Health Insurance Plan (SCHIP) (Forrest & Whalen, 2000). Academic medical centers (teaching hospitals closely aligned with medical schools) have also been aggressive in expanding primary care operations into surrounding communities in order to maintain their traditional patient base, to invigorate education of medical students and physicians in training, and to support clinical research.

## Emergency Care

The United States has developed a complex and comprehensive system of emergency care, ranging from the national 911 emergency response system to hospital-based emergency services, which has been bolstered by the emergence of emergency medicine as a formally recognized medical specialty. Most U.S. hospitals, including over 92% of community hospitals, provide emergency department services (AHA, 2000, Table 7, p. 154). Though designed to care for the acutely ill or injured patient, emergency departments also serve as a major source of walk-in services for less sick patients. Many physicians in practice who are affiliated with a specific hospital will use its emergency department (ED) as a resource-rich setting in which to assess patients with serious problems that may lead to inpatient admission or whose evaluation requires equipment or diagnostic imaging facilities not available in the physician's office. Similarly, extended care facilities such as nursing homes and chronic disease hospitals may use the emergency services of a nearby acute care facility to evaluate a patient with a sudden change in medical status.

Emergency services are a major source of admissions to hospitals. In 1997, emergency department visits resulted in approximately 42% of the nearly 31 million admissions to acute care hospitals. Of the nearly 95 million ED visits in 1997, approximately one in seven resulted in hospital admission (Nourjah, 1999, p. 11; AHA, 2000, Table 3, p. 9). In this and other ways, the emergency department serves as an interface between the worlds of ambulatory and inpatient medicine.

Patients often err in over- or under-interpreting the gravity of symptoms they are experiencing. Most patients reporting to an emergency service believe they need immediate attention. Others know they do not have an urgent or emergent problem, but simply use the emergency service because it is the most convenient source of care available. Although emergency department visits are not particularly costly, there is broad consensus that it is a poor choice of location for receipt of general primary care, as many important elements of care (e.g., continuity of care with a single provider, preventive health screenings and immunizations) receive little or no attention in the ED. On the other hand, emergency department visits can serve as a bellwether for opportunities missed in primary care settings to prevent exacerbations of chronic medical conditions like asthma, congestive heart failure, diabetes, and vaccine-preventable, acute infections such as influenza and certain common types of pneumonia.

In fact, many hospitals have developed walk-in care centers to relieve emergency departments of having to assess and treat patients with conditions that do not demand immediate attention. Business motives in developing such centers include concentrating the attention of more costly emergency department staff and equipment on cases more likely to result in hospital admissions (the financial lifeblood of most hospitals), and competing with freestanding walk-in services or urgi-centers for ambulatory care volume. To maximize the relief such centers are able to provide, they are often open during evening and weekend hours, and patients in other hospital-affiliated outpatient settings are urged to make use of after-hours telephone access instead of visiting the emergency department. Despite attempts to conserve their services for urgent and emergency care, however, the fact remains that EDs remain a common point of contact with the health care system for a large number of persons not receiving regular or longitudinal health care. Recognizing this, some EDs have developed programs to provide brief public health-oriented preventive health interventions, such as HIV testing with risk reduction counseling and childhood immunizations (Szilagyi, 1997). Such innovative programs embody the tension between a public health outreach paradigm and the need to optimize the efficiency and fiscal viability of resource intense hospital based settings.

## Specialty Care

Subspecialty care, as distinct from general primary care, is defined as care given by physicians who have received additional training in a specific area of expertise (e.g., endocrinology, pediatric cardiology). Specialty care is practiced and delivered by physicians in a broad array of disciplines and delivered in diverse settings.

Patients are referred to specialists by their primary care providers for evaluation or treatment of conditions that require particular expertise. Thus, while most primary care clinicians are comfortable treating patients with disorders of the thyroid gland, many would refer such a patient to an endocrinologist for initial evaluation and for additional consultation when changes in the treatment regimen appeared indicated. Patients often choose to bypass generalist physicians and go directly to a specialist. This route has become less common, however, because of financial penalties associated with self-referral to specialists imposed by managed care health insurance plans.

Surgical ambulatory care consists of surgical procedures performed on patients who are not, at the time of surgery, hospital inpatients. From 1994 to 1998, ambulatory surgeries rose from 50.5 to 57.7 per 1000 persons, while the rate of inpatient surgeries fell from 47.8 to 36.0 per 1000 persons (AHA, 2000, Table 3, p. 9). This reflects a marked change from 1980, when only 16.4% of surgery was performed on an outpatient basis (USDHHS, 1995, Table 90), and demonstrates the growth of acute care provision in outpatient settings. This shift can be attributed to improved technology, economic pressures, and the demands of both patients and third-party payers.

Imaging procedures (e.g., traditional x-rays, ultrasound, CT and MRI) can be performed in a variety of settings, including ambulatory imaging facilities located in hospitals or community health centers, large multi-specialty group practice, or freestanding facilities. Some primary care physicians and a greater number of subspecialist physicians, including gastroenterologists, urologists, orthopedists, and cardiologists, perform imaging procedures in their offices. The resulting competition for these imaging procedures, which are typically well reimbursed, has mixed effects. While competition may keep costs down in other markets, this is not always the case with health care, where reimbursement rates are often only loosely tied to the cost of delivering specific services. Imaging facilities must purchase and maintain expensive equipment, and they rely on referrals from other physicians to succeed. Ethical, legal, and financial tensions may emerge, particularly when a referring physician has a financial interest in the success of an imaging center. On the other hand, this competitive market may increase convenience for patients by expanding the hours of operation and facilitating communication of test results with referring physicians.

## HOSPITALS IN THE U.S.

Although the majority of acute care visits take place in doctors' offices, hospitals play an important role in delivering acute care, in both inpatient and outpatient settings. This section gives an overview of acute care hospital types, services, and structures, with an emphasis on the ways hospitals have adjusted to the changing environment of acute care.

In 2002, there were 4,927 hospitals in the United States, with a total of 821,000 beds (AHA, 2003b). Of the $1.4 trillion spent on health care in 2001, hospital costs totaled $415 billion, or 32%. The majority of hospitals in the U.S. are nonprofit or owned by local, state, or federal governments (see TABLE 7.1). As the total number of hospitals decreased in the last 20 years, over 600 state and local government hospitals and over 300 nonprofit hospitals have closed, while the number of investor-owned hospitals has increased slightly. Hospitals of different ownership types exhibit variance with regard to several characteristics. As TABLE 7.2 illustrates, in 2000 the majority of patient admissions, births, and outpatient visits took place at nonprofit hospitals. The average length of stay at state and local government hospitals was higher than average for the whole population of acute care hospitals, while the average length of stay for investor-owned hospitals was lower than average. State and local government hospitals had almost double the number of outpatient visits compared to investor-owned hospitals, but similar numbers of patient admissions. State and local government and investor-owned hospitals also had similar expenses adjusted per inpatient day, whereas expenses at nonprofit hospitals were $100 higher on average.

There have been several significant changes in hospital utiliza-

| TABLE 7.1 | | | |
|---|---|---|---|
| **Community Hospital Ownership** | | | |
| OWNERSHIP | 1982 | 1992 | 2002 |
| Nonprofit | 3,338 | 3,173 | 3,025 |
| State and local government | 1,715 | 1,396 | 1,136 |
| Investor owned | 748 | 723 | 766 |
| Total | 5,801 | 5,292 | 4,927 |

SOURCE: AHA, Hospital Statistics, 2004. (Community hospitals are defined by the AHA as all nonfederal short-term general and special hospitals whose facilities and services are available to the public.)

tion in the last 20 years (see **TABLE 7.3**). New hospital construction increased in 2002 by 20%, accompanied by an increase in hospital bed capacity, reversing a 20-year trend of bed closures due to excess

| TABLE 7.2 | | | |
|---|---|---|---|
| **Acute Care Hospital Data by Ownership Type, for Year 2002** | | | |
| | NONPROFIT | STATE/ LOCAL GOVT | INVESTOR OWNED |
| Number of hospitals | 3,025 | 1,136 | 766 |
| Beds (thousands) | 582 | 130 | 130 |
| Patient admissions (thousands) | 25,425 | 4,688 | 4,365 |
| Births (thousands) | 2,820 | 553 | 497 |
| Outpatient visits (thousands) | 416,910 | 94,280 | 45,215 |
| Ave. length of stay (days) | 5.6 | 6.6 | 5.3 |
| Ave. daily census (thousands) | 391 | 84 | 64 |
| Full-time employees (thousands) | 3,039 | 651 | 379 |
| Expenses (adjusted per inpatient day) | $1,328.81 | $1,188.12 | $1,180.83 |

SOURCE: AHA, Hospital Statistics, 2004. (Acute care hospitals are called "community hospitals" by the AHA.)

| TABLE 7.3 | | | |
|---|---|---|---|
| **Community Hospital Data by Decade** | | | |
| | 1982 | 1992 | 2002 |
| Number of hospitals | 5,801 | 5,292 | 4,927 |
| Beds (thousands) | 1,012 | 921 | 821 |
| Patient admissions (thousands) | 36,379 | 31,034 | 34,478 |
| Births (thousands) | 3,514 | 3,925 | 3,870 |
| Outpatient visits (thousands) | 248,124 | 348,522 | 556,404 |
| Ave. length of stay (days) | 7.6 | 7.1 | 5.7 |
| Ave. daily census (thousands) | 762 | 604 | 540 |
| Full-time employees (thousands) | 3,103 | 3,620 | 4,069 |
| Expenses (adjusted per inpatient day) | $327.37 | $819.63 | $1,289.87 |
| Gross outpatient revenues (percentage of all revenues) | 13% | 25% | 35% (2001) |

SOURCE: AHA, Hospital Statistics, 2004. (Community hospitals are defined by the AHA as all nonfederal short-term general and special hospitals whose facilities and services are available to the public.)

inpatient supply. The increased demand for inpatient care is reflected in the recent trend of rising admissions. In 2002, there were 33 million hospital admissions, a 3.5% increase over 1998, after nearly two decades of declining inpatient utilization (AHA, 2002). The aging of the population is accepted as the major driver of increased demand for hospital services, although lack of access to timely ambulatory care also plays a role. A consequence of the relatively abrupt increase in inpatient demand nationally has been greater hospital crowding with longer waits for services, including emergency department care and ancillary testing. The growth in demand for hospital services is likely to continue in the short term with a 1.6 to 6.0% annual increase projected through 2006 (Health Care Advisory Board, 2002).

There have also been changes in demand for hospital outpatient services. In 1982, there were 248,124,000 outpatient visits to acute care hospitals; by 2002, this number had increased to 556,404,000. These outpatient visits contributed to a greater percentage of gross revenues for acute care hospitals, from 13% in 1982 to 25% in 1992 to 35% in 2001. As noted in the Ambulatory Care section, the average length of a hospital stay has decreased over time, from 7.6 days in 1982 to 5.7 days in 2002. The average daily hospital census has decreased over time as well, although the number of births and patient admissions has fluctuated over the last 20 years. Both the average number of full-time employees working for acute care hospitals and the expenses per inpatient day have increased. In 2002, the average expense per inpatient day was $1289.87, compared to only $327.37 in 1982.

## Types of Acute Care Hospitals

There are several types of acute hospitals under different ownership as previously described. Additionally, many hospitals in the U.S. are now part of multi-hospital and integrated health care systems. The sections that follow describe these hospitals and hospital systems.

### Teaching Hospitals

There are 400 hospitals or health systems in the U.S. that are members of the Council of Teaching Hospitals and Health Systems (COTH). To qualify as a member, a hospital must have an affiliation agreement with a medical school and demonstrate a commitment to graduate medical education by participating in at least four residency training programs. According to the Association of American Medical Colleges, "teaching hospitals are providers of primary care and routine patient services, as well as centers for experimental, innovative and technically sophisticated services. Many of the advances started in the research laboratories of medical schools are incorporated into patient care through clinical research programs at teaching hospitals" (Association of American Medical Colleges [AAMC], 2004). Teaching hospitals are among the largest facilities in the country, may be private or government supported, and provide a disproportionate share of uncompensated care compared to other hospitals. Teaching hospitals are often in large urban centers and may be part of an academic medical center, with close ties to a medical school, including physicians on staff who hold an academic appointment and teach medical students or residents in training.

Montefiore Medical Center (MMC) is an example of a teaching hospital that is part of an academic medical center. The medical center is comprised of two acute care adult hospitals and a children's hospital, all in the Bronx, the poorest of New York City's five boroughs. It is the principal training venue for medical students at the Albert Einstein College of Medicine, and sponsors residency programs in 63 medical specialties with over 865 trainees, making it one of the largest medical training programs in the country. Including patient visits in its emergency departments, MMC had nearly 2 million ambulatory visits in 2003. Inpatient volume reached 58,000 discharges in 2003, with total clinical activity that has grown by approximately 33% in the past decade. In 2003, MMC had a surplus of just over 1% on total revenues of $1.6 billion.

In a market characterized by an unfavorable payer mix dominated by government insurance, rising costs, and declining payments, MMC's strategy has been based on expanding its primary care network with over 20 community ambulatory practices throughout its service area staffed by MMC-employed physicians. MMC also has invested over $100 million in its business and clinical information systems since 1995 in order to integrate provider information across its extensive delivery system and to catalogue clinical data for quality improvement initiatives. MMC has demonstrated that medication errors have decreased by 70% because of the introduction of computerized physician orders and a pharmacy information system (B. Currie, MD, personal communication 2002).

MMC can be considered both a teaching hospital in a large academic medical center and a community hospital that has made health care delivery to the Bronx a component of its business strategy and a central element of its mission. Many urban teaching hospitals replicate this hybrid status, serving as primary care community providers while offering tertiary care and clinical research to a broad regional or national patient base.

### Public Hospitals

Public hospitals are characterized by their receipt of financial support from the local, state, or federal government, beyond the patient care reimbursement they receive from Medicaid and Medicare. The National Association of Public Hospitals and Health Systems (NAPHHS) has more than 100 member hospitals in 30 states and includes public hospitals in our largest cities, such as Bellevue in New York, Cook County in Chicago, and LA County in Los Angeles. NAPHHS categorizes its members into three models of governance: direct operation by local or state governments, operation by a separate public entity such as the Health and Hospitals Corporation in New York City, or ownership and operation by a not-for-profit corporation, usually with a contractual relationship with the local government (National Association of Public Hospitals and Health Systems [NAPHHS], 2003).

Public hospitals are larger on average than other hospitals in their market place and have about twice the number of discharges as their local counterparts (NAPHHS, 2003). All have busy emergency departments and ambulatory clinics; the average ambulatory volume for an NAPHHS member in 2001 was 346,000, a 26% increase over 1993 visits. Public hospitals have been referred to as "safety net hospitals" because they provide significant services to uninsured, underinsured, or other vulnerable populations, and offer services to all—regardless of ability to pay—as part of the hospital's mission or legal mandate (Institute of Medicine, 2000). The 100 NAPH hospitals provided $5.4 billion in uncompensated care in the U.S. in 2001, or one quarter of all uncompensated care nationally (NAPHHS, 2003). State and local subsidies contributed nearly 40% of NAPHHS hospitals' support in 2001.

Public hospitals have unique roles in the neighborhoods they serve. Given their role in serving vulnerable populations, they often offer community outreach and health education programs directed at minority communities. Their emergency departments are busy, often serving as municipal trauma centers and as home bases for local 911 systems. They have become an invaluable component of local disaster preparedness working with public health departments. Public hospitals are also training facilities, turning out over 15% of American medical and dental residents in 2001 (NAPHHS, 2003).

The hospitals of the Bureau of Health Services in Cook County, Illinois, exemplify the role of the public hospital. The mission of the Cook County Bureau of Health Services is "to provide a comprehensive program of quality health care with respect and dignity, to the residents of Cook County, regardless of their ability to pay." The Bureau of Health is comprised of two acute care hospitals, a chronic care and rehabilitation facility, 30 community and school-based ambulatory care sites, and a correctional health service. Its emergency departments are among the busiest in the country; they provide tertiary care clinical service in many specialties, including state of the art imaging technology. The Bureau of Health Services has developed centers of excellence that address inner city health issues across its care continuum, including asthma, violence prevention, lead poisoning, maternal health, and cancer treatment and prevention.

The hub of the municipal health system serving the 5 million people who live in and around Chicago is the John H. Stroger, Jr., Hospital of Cook County. Cook County Hospital was established in 1866 to provide care to indigent residents of Chicago after the city's Board of Commissioners recognized that the medical care provided at its "poorhouse" was inadequate. Cook County Hospital grew to 3,400 beds, established a school of nursing and became an important academic medical center that trained generations of physicians. In December 2002, a new $600 million hospital, named for the current president of the Cook County Board of Commissioners, John H. Stroger, Jr., replaced the facility built in 1914. The new Cook County Hospital has 464 beds, including 80 intensive care (ICU) beds, 58 neonatal ICU beds, and an 18-bed burn unit. Reflecting the growing importance of ambulatory care, 40% of this 1.2 million-square-foot hospital building is devoted to ambulatory care services. For fiscal 2004, the Cook County Bureau of Health Services appropriated $460 million for the Stroger Hospital and projects $390 million in revenue from its operation. Eighty-seven percent of the hospital's revenues come from state and federal programs (Cook County Executive Budget Recommendations, 2004).

## Rural Hospitals

A rural hospital is located outside of a metropolitan statistical area (MSA), a geographical designation by the Federal Office of Management and Budget (AHA, 2003, 2004). To qualify as an MSA, a location must contain a city of more than 50,000 or have a total metropolitan population of more than 100,000. Metropolitan statistical areas can include multiple counties if there are substantial social and economic ties to a metropolitan hub. Of the 4,927 U.S. hospitals in 2002, there were 2,178 classified as rural (44%). The number of rural hospitals has declined by less than 1% since 1998, a closure rate identical to metropolitan area hospitals. Despite the slight decline in the number of rural hospitals, admissions have risen 5.5% since 1998 (AHA, 2004). The average rural hospital has 79 beds compared to 236 for hospitals in MSAs; 74% of rural facilities have fewer than 100 beds (AHA, 2003, 2004).

Rural hospitals are under significant clinical, financial, and regulatory pressures to meet current standards of medical practice. The demographics of rural America are changing with a loss of population in many areas, increased poverty, aging of the remaining population, and a sharp increase in the population of immigrants, particularly Hispanics, in many counties. The increasing dependence of clinical medicine on expensive technologies can magnify the disparity in services offered by smaller hospitals and add to the difficulties rural hospitals have in attracting and retaining skilled providers. However, telemedicine (audio and video communication with larger medical centers for patient consultation) offers access to specialists without the need for travel. A recent study at the University of Washington showed that telemedicine resulted in better care, according to referring and consulting physicians, compared to phone consultation; resulted in a change in management in 64% of cases, and was satisfying to patients who avoided travel to a nonlocal provider (Norris, Hart, Larson, Tarczy-Hornoch, Masuda, et al., 2001). More widespread availability of broadband internet access to rural communities is critical to expanding the utility of telemedicine.

An example of a rural hospital with telemedicine capabilities is the Haxtun Hospital in Haxtun, Colorado. Founded in the 1960s, the Haxtun Hospital District serves a 300-square-mile area of western Philips County with a population of roughly 2,500 residents. The 15-bed, critical access hospital has a Colorado level 4 trauma classification with staff trained in trauma life support and trauma nursing (Philips County Economic Development Corporation, 2004). Its services include emergency medicine, surgery, obstetrics, and imaging. CAT scan and MRI services are provided by a mobile unit (Haxtun Hospital, 2004). In 1989, the Haxtun Hospital District became a member of the High Plains Rural Health Network, which connects 18 rural hospitals, 2 urban hospitals, and 1 secondary referral center in Colorado, Kansas, Nebraska, and Wyoming. In 1995, the network received a grant from the Office of Rural Health Policy to develop a telemedicine network (High Plains Rural Health Network, 2004). In 2001, the network received an additional grant from the U.S. Department of Agriculture Rural Utilities Service, Distance Learning and Telemedicine Program (U.S. Department of Agriculture [USDA], 2004). These grants allowed the network to create direct video and radio links between emergency room staff and board-certified emergency room specialists at two urban facilities with hospitals in seven rural communities. In teleconferencing with urban providers, rural providers are able to make decisions about providing local treatment to emergency room patients or have them transported to urban hospitals. Haxtun District Hospital also provides online services, providing contact with its two affiliated family practice physicians, access to a medical dictionary and a drug encyclopedia.

The Balanced Budget Act (BBA) of 1997 reduced Medicare payments to all hospitals by $119 billion (11.4%) from 1998 to 2004, including a $15 billion reduction for rural hospitals. The Balanced Budget Refinement Act (BBA) of 1999 restored about 13% of these cuts for rural hospitals. Part of the BBA, the Medicare Rural Flexibility Program, allowed Medicare to certify some rural hospitals as Critical Access Hospitals (CAH), if the facility was the sole source of inpatient care in a community (Critical Access Hospitals and the Medicare Rural Hospital Flexibility Grant Program, 2002). Critical Access Hospitals (CAHs) are reimbursed on a cost–based schedule instead of a standard case rate, a much more generous payment method. Additionally, the Medicare Reform Act of 2003 increased reimbursement to rural health facilities by $25 billion, including a premium for telemedicine, and expanded ambulance services in rural counties. Despite these enrichments, however, the financial pressures on all hospitals, including the rural, are daunting. Rural hospitals will likely require additional federal subsidies to make technology investments and to cover operating costs in order to maintain financial viability in the short term.

## Multi-Hospital and Integrated Health Care Systems

Most hospitals are integrated into their communities through ties with area physicians and other health care providers, clinics and outpatient facilities, and other practitioners. Almost half of the nation's hospitals also are tied to larger organizational entities:

multi-hospital and integrated health care systems, networks, and alliances. A network is a group of hospitals, physicians, other providers, insurers, and/or community agencies that work together to deliver health services (AHA, 2003–2004). In 2002, there were 1,343 acute care hospitals (27% of the total) in networks (AHA, 2003–2004). Multi-hospital systems include two or more hospitals owned, leased, sponsored, or contract managed by a central organization. In 1985, 27.5% of hospitals were system members, which rose to 46% by 2002 (AHA, 2003–2004). An alliance is defined as a formal organization, usually owned by shareholders/members, that works on behalf of its individual members in the provision of services and products and in the promotion of activities and ventures (AHA, 1999). In 2000, there were 3,344 hospitals in group purchasing organizations (the dominant kind of alliance). The same hospitals can be registered in more than one category (AHA, 2000).

In 2002, there were 321 multi-hospital or integrated health care systems in the U.S. The majority were not-for-profit, including religious (56) and secular (209) systems. Fifty-one systems were investor owned, and five were operated by the federal government (Departments of the U.S. Navy, U.S. Air Force, U.S. Army, Veterans' Administration, and the Bureau of Indian Affairs). Investor-owned systems tend to have more, but smaller, hospitals than nonprofit systems and to own or manage hospitals in more parts of the nation. Many of the large for-profit systems have headquarters in the South, particularly in Tennessee and Texas. HCA, formerly Columbia-HCA, owns or manages 184 hospitals in 22 states, with 41 in Florida and 40 in Texas. Quorum Health Resources operates 160 hospitals in 40 states, and Tenet Healthcare Corporation owns or manages 116 hospitals in 16 states, with the majority in California, Florida, and Texas.

Secular nonprofit systems tend to be smaller and more regional. Examples include the Great Plains Health Alliance, with 24 hospitals in 2 states (Kansas and Nebraska); the Carolinas Healthcare System, with 15 hospitals in 2 states (North Carolina and South Carolina); and Appalachian Regional Healthcare, with 9 hospitals in Kentucky and West Virginia. There are several large Catholic health care systems in the U.S., such as Ascension Health which owns 68 hospitals in 18 states, and Catholic Health Initiatives (CHI), which owns 58 hospitals in 18 states. Ascension Health has headquarters in St. Louis, Missouri, and CHI has headquarters in Denver, Colorado.

Kaiser Permanente is an example of an integrated health care system. As one of the nation's first health maintenance organizations (HMOs), Kaiser Permanente operates under the principles of prepaid insurance, physician group practice, preventive medicine, and the organized delivery of services—"putting as many services as possible under one roof" (Kaiser Permanente, 2004). The Kaiser Permanente Medical Center in Oakland, California typifies the system's integration of medical care. Several large doctors office buildings are situated in the same complex as an acute care hospital, several laboratories, and several pharmacies. Members in the Oakland area receive all of their medical care at the same medical center, which employs a full range of practitioners, including both generalists and specialist physicians. If a patient's doctor orders a medical test, the patient walks to the appropriate testing center located within the complex. The logistics of hospitalizing patients or using sophisticated medical equipment are simple and routine. Referrals to specialists are handled within the system. In addition, the complex is served by public buses and a free shuttle to and from the nearest subway station. A Kaiser health plan member conceivably could be treated for all health care needs at the Oakland medical center, from birth to death.

Kaiser Permanente serves members in seven regions: California, Oregon/Washington, Hawaii, Colorado, Georgia, Ohio, and the District of Columbia metropolitan area. The integrated system consists of three separate entities: The Kaiser Foundation Health Plan, Inc., which provides insurance; Kaiser Foundation Hospitals and Subsidiaries, which manages 30 hospitals and 431 medical office buildings, and The Permanente Medical Groups. The Health Plan and Hospitals organizations contract exclusively with each region's Permanente Medical Group to provide medical care for its members. Nationwide, Kaiser Permanente had 8.2 million members, 136,511 nonphysician employees, approximately 11,000 doctors, and operating revenues of $22.5 billion in 2002 (Kaiser Permanente, 2004).

Another example of an integrated health care system is the Department of Veterans Affairs. The hospitals and ambulatory programs of the federal Department of Veterans Affairs (VA) make it the largest health care delivery system in the country (Haugh, 2003). There are 25 million veterans currently alive in our country who are potentially eligible for health care benefits; family members of disabled veterans and survivors of veterans are also eligible. In 2002, the VA treated 4.5 million people in its 163 hospitals and ambulatory clinics (Haugh, 2003). VA care is not free to beneficiaries, but costs are usually limited to co-payments. The extent of coverage depends on Congressional appropriations with a priority list of covered beneficiaries that target fully or partially disabled veterans. Eligibility can change annually, depending on the level of funding (U.S. Department of Veterans Affairs, 2004).

VA hospitals have been referred to as an unrecognized component of the national health care safety net (Wilson, 1997). Sixty percent of the veterans who received VA medical care in 1992 had no private insurance and would potentially otherwise use public safety net hospitals and clinics (Wilson, 1997). Additionally, the veterans using the VA health care system have a high burden of chronic disease, psychiatric illness, substance abuse, and physical disability related to their military service. VA hospitals have been reorganized over the past decade and now enjoy a reputation for higher quality care that takes advantage of a sophisticated national hospital information system.

## Services and Structures of Acute Care Hospitals

Hospitals are diverse in their governance, organization, mission, and relationships to their communities. They also vary by organizational structure and the scope of services delivered. All hospitals, however, must adhere to the standards of the Joint Commission on the Accreditation of Healthcare Organizations (JCAHO) to be accredited (see Kovner, chapter 14, this volume). The medical care delivered in hospitals ranges from well patient health maintenance to organ transplantation. A majority of hospitals provide emergency care (92%), outpatient surgery (92%), CT scanning (86.6%), outpatient hospital services (73.8%), and volunteer services (78.3%) (AHA, 2003–2004). Just over half of acute care hospitals have MRI capabilities (53.7%) and provide oncology services (59.8%). A minority of hospitals provides primary care (35.6%), HIV/AIDS services (32.5%), angioplasty (25.5%), hospice care (24.4%), open heart surgery (21.7%), infertility services (18%), alcohol and drug dependency treatment (10.3%), and organ transplantation (9.3%) (AHA, 2003–2004). As the practice of medicine has grown increasingly dependent on sophisticated technology for routine diagnosis and treatment, even smaller acute care hospitals must own or have access to expensive equipment and services. At the same time, biomedical progress has driven large, tertiary care facilities, particularly university-affiliated ones, to offer cutting edge treatments and research protocols only available in select centers across the country.

Certain principles characterize all hospitals. Physicians determine who is admitted to hospitals and direct their care during the hospital stay. Other licensed health professionals, particularly nurses, but also respiratory therapists, physical therapists, social workers, pastoral caregivers, and technicians provide service components that are critical to patients' recovery. Physicians are primarily organized along the lines of the medical specialties. The larger the hospital and hospital network, and the more specialized the medical services, the greater the number of separate medical departments. Departments found in most hospitals include internal medicine, surgery, pediatrics, obstetrics/gynecology, psychiatry/neurology, radiology/diagnostic imaging, pathology, anesthesiology, family medicine, and emergency medicine. Other more specialized medical departments tend to be organized around organs and organ systems, for example, ophthalmology (eye); otolaryngology (ear, nose, and throat); urology (male sexual/reproductive system and the urinary tract of males and females); orthopedics (bones and joints); and so on.

Hospital diagnostic and therapeutic services, which may or may not be attached to one of the medical departments, include laboratory services (usually directed by the department of pathology); electrocardiography (directed by cardiology); electroencephalography (neurology); radiography (radiology); pharmacy; clinical psychology; social service; inhalation therapy (anesthesiology); nutrition as therapy; physical, occupational, and speech therapy (rehabilitation medicine, if present); home care; and medical records, among others. Nonclinical services include finance, facilities and equipment, human resources, and management.

Physicians relate to hospitals in different ways. Attending physicians on the hospital staff, who are not salaried, often conduct much of their business in private offices they own or rent. These physicians may admit patients to more than one hospital and may compete with the hospital for patients or customers. Other physicians may be salaried or paid by the hospital, according to the amount of hospital work they do. These physicians often see patients or provide diagnostic services in offices that are provided for them by the hospital. Some hospitals employ physicians to provide primary care in competition with other physicians who are attending or with local nonhospital-affiliated practitioners. Other hospitals contract with physician groups to provide emergency care or subspecialty services on hospital premises or in satellite centers. Some physicians maintain their own practices distinct from the hospital but also receive a part-time salary from the hospital for administrative work.

Shortell (1985) has conceptualized four different models of organization among physicians and hospitals: traditional (departmental), divisional, independent-corporate, and parallel. Under the *traditional* model, while each department retains relevant medical specialists, it does not provide the support services required by the physician to provide care, such as nursing, housekeeping, dietary, and clerical staff. Physicians are not a part of the hospital chain of command, as are nurses or assistant administrators. In hospitals this is referred to as a *dual authority structure* (Smith, 1955). Most physicians are not hospital employees. Many physicians do not see themselves as primarily responsible to hospital administration but function rather as independent medical practitioners who must practice according to medical staff bylaws, rules, and regulations. The *divisional* model is characterized by the placement of functional support services within medical divisions, which are organized along departmental lines. Each division, such as medicine or physical medicine, includes many of the support services, such as nursing and clerical (and sometimes dietary and medical records and other services) it needs to do its tasks. Each medical division leader is responsible for management, including financial management, of both medical and support services.

Under the *independent-corporate* model, the medical staff becomes a separate legal entity that negotiates with the hospital for its services in return for receiving support services. An independent group of physicians provides medical services to the hospital, under contract. The *parallel* model involves the creation of a separate organization in order to conduct certain activities that are not handled well by the formal hospital organization. Certain physicians are selected to participate in a parallel organization for a certain percentage of their time, to work on important problems, and to report back to the formal structure. Some of these physicians would have positions in the formal structure as well.

Physicians and other clinicians practicing in hospitals have their own staff organization, with bylaws, rules and regulations that must be approved by the hospital's governing board. Medical staff bylaws specify procedures for election of medical staff officers by membership. The officers are given authority under the bylaws to enforce rules and regulations. The officers delineate privileges and recommend disciplinary action when necessary, through the committee structure. They enforce the bylaws and must oversee the committee structure and submit reports of medical staff activities to the governing board.

There are numerous medical staff committees in the hospital, some of which may include nonphysicians, particularly nurses, as members. The executive committee, if there is one, coordinates all activity, sets general policies for the medical staff, and accepts and acts upon recommendations from the other medical staff committees. The joint conference committee, if present, acts as a liaison between the medical staff and the governing board in deliberations over matters involving medical and nonmedical considerations. The credentials committee reviews application by physicians to join the medical staff and considers the qualifications of education, experience, and interests before making recommendations for appointment to the executive committee, which will then make recommendations for appointment to the governing board. In some hospitals the joint conference committee is also involved in this process.

Through the initiative of the JCAHO, the medical staff (and the board) is increasingly structured to place higher priority on clinical quality improvement and patient care outcomes. Medical staff committees can be structured in various ways to accomplish this purpose. Commonly, there is an overall medical staff committee concerned with clinical quality improvement, as well as various subcommittees such as infection control and quality improvement. In some cases what were formerly medical staff committees have become hospital-wide committees, as physicians and others have realized that improvement of clinical performance rests increasingly on the teamwork of physicians and other clinicians and support staff, and not on physicians alone.

Many hospitals have hired salaried medical directors and quality improvement review teams. When physicians admit patients to the hospital, in most instances they are free to order whatever tests or treatments they deem necessary. Thus, a physician basically determines the amount of services used and the consequent costs of patient care. Physicians have every reason to want the best possible hospital setting in which to practice medicine, especially when it is provided at little personal cost to them.

Although the physician is technically a guest in the hospital, the hospital is responsible for the care its staff renders to patients on a physician's orders. In the past, hospitals could not be held liable for the wrongful conduct of a physician, but this principle has changed as a result of a series of judicial decisions (Southwick 1978). Legal changes regarding negligence and corporate liability of hospitals have established that hospitals are legally responsible and, to the extent that hospital negligence is involved, financially responsible for the care provided by their entire professional staff, including physicians (Showalter, 1999). Therefore, many hospitals require physicians to have malpractice insurance as a condition of staff membership (Hollowell, 1978).

For most hospitals, government reimbursement through Medicare and Medicaid is a key payer, thus requiring compliance with access and quality standards set by federal and local governments. Hospitals are highly regulated by all levels of government, and by independent organizations such as the JCAHO, and are held increasingly accountable for their performance by consumers of their services.

Since the 1999 publication of a landmark Institute of Medicine report on patient safety, *To Err is Human* (Kohn, Carrigan, & Donaldson, 1999), which estimated that up to 98,000 people had been killed annually by human errors made in American hospitals, there has been a greatly increased national focus on reducing medical errors. Hospitals have responded by using information technology, such as computerized medication order entry, bar coding of patient identification, provider education, and other techniques to standardize practices.

## CURRENT ISSUES IN ACUTE CARE

Acute care involves numerous issues, some challenging, in the changing and growing health care delivery system. This section addresses such elements of today's acute care as team-based care, hospitalists, physician training, access to care, cost containment, as well as future challenges for acute care.

### Team-Based Care

The nature of primary care delivery is likely to undergo several significant changes in the coming years. In some settings, team-based care will evolve as an important model. Pressures on providers to maximize visit volume are often at odds with pressures to provide comprehensive services to patients with complex needs. Apportioning tasks between members of a primary care team is one solution to this tension. For example, a diabetic might need to meet with the doctor to review his dose of insulin in the context of morning headaches, and, based on recent laboratory results, might be in need of dietary counseling as well. The physician might meet with the patient for 10 minutes and then refer him to a nutritionist in the practice for a 20-minute assessment and brief intervention regarding late night snacking. Such an arrangement plays to the strengths of each team member, meets the patients' needs, and enables the physician to maintain his productivity at a level compatible with supporting the practice. Similarly, the management of a patient with an acute medical condition (e.g., a bleeding ulcer) associated with a chronic illness such as alcohol abuse, can benefit greatly from integration of the provider team. The use of primary care provider teams may evolve to become standard in the treatment of chronic diseases in many settings. The continuing expansion of electronic medical information systems can facilitate such interdisciplinary team management by providing multiple caregivers with ready access to a single consolidated medical record.

### Hospitalists

Hospitalists are physicians, usually trained in internal medicine, whose practice is confined to hospital care. Their expertise is in the hospital-based management of acute illness, use of care pathways to manage common inpatient problems, and efficient use of hospital services to minimize the patient's length of stay and unnecessary utilization of resources. It is likely that primary care physicians will increasingly team up with hospitalists to care for their patients who require inpatient care. Communication with the patient and primary care physician are central to maintaining continuity of care and patient satisfaction. There are multiple advantages to such divisions of labor: office based primary care providers can concentrate on their ambulatory practice, save time by not having to travel to and from the hospital, and take advantage of the expertise of hospital "specialists" to manage the increasingly complex inpatient component of their patient's care. The primary disadvantage, lack of continuity between outpatient and inpatient treatment, can be mitigated by effective communication strategies, paradigms for which are steadily evolving.

## Panel-Based Standards

With increasing numbers of Americans receiving their health insurance through managed care organizations (MCOs), the responsibilities of primary care providers have also changed. In the fee-for-service model, the primary care provider is responsible only for the patients actually seen in his or her office, and a practice is viewed as being made up of individual patients. In fully capitated managed care settings, particularly when the provider is paid through a capitation system rather than by a modified fee-for-service system, the provider is responsible for providing care to a defined population of patients assigned to him or her by the MCO. The MCO may audit a provider's practice to determine whether standards of care are being met. In the capitated MCO setting, providers are often held responsible for each patient on their panels, whether or not the patient ever came to the office to be seen. Thus, if the standard of care set by the MCO for a pediatric practice requires that 90% of children have received all their immunizations by 2 years of age, the denominator used in assessing compliance with this goal is the total number of children 2 years of age and older in the provider's panel, not just those actually seen in the office. Standards of care, benchmarks against which the adequacy of care provided by the primary care practitioner is judged, exist for preventive services such as blood pressure and cholesterol screening, and breast and colorectal cancer screening, as well as for actual management of specific medical conditions. Although quality assurance measures have been required in hospital settings for a long time, it is only since 1991, with the advent of standards for accreditation of MCOs by the National Committee on Quality Assurance (NCQA), the accrediting body for MCOs, that widespread monitoring of standards of care in ambulatory settings has begun to gain acceptance.

## Changing Patient Expectations

As acute care delivery systems begin to break new ground with innovations in restructuring of medical visits, enhanced information systems and advances in patient education, patients will come to demand more of their medical providers. Easier access to care—same or next day appointments with their own team of providers—will likely become a standard feature of better systems

(Murray & Tantau, 2000). Patients will be less likely to accept long waits when arriving at the primary care office. Successful practices, serving large panels of patients, will thrive by excelling in three areas: efficient visit management (prompt appointments, accurate billing); a focus on patient satisfaction (courteous staff, easy telephone access, pleasant surroundings, extended hours); and quality of care (medical outcomes that meet or exceed benchmarks, rare medication errors, adherence to health management guidelines). To achieve these goals, practices will rely on effective teamwork, health care managers will have to be trained to function effectively in this new paradigm, and physicians will have to embrace participation in the health care team.

## Changes in Physician Training

Each year, approximately 12,000 residents complete training in generalist specialties (internal medicine, family medicine, and pediatrics) in the United States. It is this group of individuals, freshly trained in an evolving paradigm of how acute care services are best structured, that will effect lasting changes in care delivery in diverse settings. Changes in health care delivery have had a substantial impact on the thinking of leaders in medical education. In the early 1990s, the majority of medical school deans responsible for oversight of residency education were concerned about the impact of managed care on their training programs. But by 1997, at a meeting of the Group on Residency Affairs (GRA) of the Association of American Medical Colleges (AAMC), the tone of the discussion had changed. There was an emphasis on how to teach the "new medicine" to residents, not based on cost of care concerns but based on the best interests of patients. A variety of changes in the education and training of generalist physicians reflect the impact of these recent shifts in approach. New requirements for the accreditation of residency training programs provide an example. Experience in the continuity of care of panels of patients in community-based settings, as opposed to hospital-based outpatient clinics, is now required. Primary care residency programs are required to teach a formal curriculum that documents training in biomedical ethics, medical legal issues, cost management of health care, and the responsibility of health care providers for an entire population of individuals. As a result, physicians entering the workforce for the first time will therefore have some knowledge of the trends and forces shaping the world in which they will practice.

## Access to Care

Approximately 45 million Americans lack health insurance coverage, a tremendous barrier to their ability to access comprehensive medical care services. Access is limited for millions of others because of where they live, the language they speak, their inability to read, and for a host of other reasons.

The provision of care to under- or uninsured persons is a major financial strain for acute care facilities. For uninsured or underinsured individuals, inpatient costs are partially offset by Disproportionate Share Hospital (DSH) funds that cover a modest portion of unreimbursed care based on the volume of low income Medicare and Medicaid patients seen at a hospital. Organizational responses vary with respect to addressing the remaining uncovered costs of providing care to the uninsured. Some make it policy that they be responsible only for paying customers or for providing those services, such as emergency care, as required by law. Others may opt to provide medically appropriate services to all who live within the organization's catchment area, or who come for care, and rely on a mix of income streams for compensation, including sliding scale payments based on income, philanthropy, and cross-subsidization from profitable services.

Barriers to accessing health care are also experienced by many persons who have health insurance. Strategies to enhance access in this group can include community outreach, health education in schools and on the job, and enhancing cultural sensitivity and linguistic capability among front-line providers. Improved technology and better office management can result in shortened waiting times for physician appointments and ancillary testing. Considerable potential exists for the use of electronic communication between patient and provider, and among patients with the same symptoms or diseases. For internet users, access to an array of general and disease-specific health information is available online.

Solving the challenge of ensuring ready access to primary health care for all will require sophisticated understanding of the impact on medical costs and the lost productivity of not having such access—as well, in the end, as sustained political will.

## Cost Containment

The cost of both inpatient and ambulatory care has risen significantly over the past decade. Most projections forecast continued growth of health care spending as the population ages, new and expensive pharmaceuticals continue to be introduced, and ever-new technology becomes available for diagnosis and treatment. Cost containment is a central issue in health care today because of pressure from payers, led by the federal government, and from consumers paying ever more in insurance premiums and out-of-pocket expenses. Cost containment strategies have focused on reimbursement mechanisms, clinical practice, and more active oversight of resource utilization. For example, prepayment for health care (capitation) was designed to transfer financial risk to managed care companies and their providers, with the associated incentive to contain costs. Though credited with slowing the rise of health care spending in the last decade, the financial benefits of this model have not been sustained as providers and patients became dissatisfied with restrictions on choices. Complicating the equation are evolving requirements by accrediting organizations like the NCQA, demanding that HMOs adhere to screening and prevention guidelines. In turn, many HMOs have required that practitioners listed on their panels adhere to these standards. Clinical practice variability, i.e., diverse approaches by different doctors to managing similar problems, has thus come under scrutiny as a challenge to containing costs, particularly as evidence-based best practices are promoted as a central element of quality improvement. Reduction of medical errors by implementation of electronic medical record keeping is also projected to cut overall costs, though few data demonstrating actual costs saved from such approaches are yet available. Delivering procedurally oriented medical services in ambulatory settings, including surgical and imaging procedures, can save money by avoiding the high fixed costs of hospitals. Other approaches to cost containment in ambulatory care include preventive services, delivery of care by nonphysician providers (e.g., physician assistants or nurse practitioners), and more advanced disease management practices. Standardization of insurance forms and payment protocols can reduce ambulatory care billing costs, as can collecting payments up front rather than billing for care on a per-episode basis.

Much remains to be learned regarding the cost effectiveness of behavioral interventions that promote healthful behavior and healthy outcomes, such as improving literacy, fostering nutritional diet habits, increasing exercise, and stopping smoking.

## CASE STUDY

You are a health care consultant working in a large eastern U.S. city. Dr. Irving Freedom, the Chief of Staff at St. George Hospital, and Charlie Sweat, the Chair of the Board of the St. George Medical System, ask for your advice. The directors of the St. George Medical System, facing pressure to contain medical costs, need help deciding how (and where) to treat their patients in the most cost-effective and efficient manner. Managed care companies insure 20% of the city's population, 30% of the city's residents are over the age of 65, and the city's population has grown 10% in the last year. The System currently owns two hospitals (including St. George) and one outpatient clinic. Both of its emergency departments are oversubscribed. It also has contracts with three multispecialty physician group practices, including the Irving Freedom Medical Group. The System recently received a large anonymous donation and has enough funds to balance between building additional facilities, investing in new technologies, and/or increasing their provision of indigent care. Dr. Freedom and Mr. Sweat want to know if they should build additional wings for their hospitals, open more outpatient clinics, invest in technology, or find ways to better serve the poor. What would you advise them to do? What factors would you need to consider before you make your report? Include in your answer a discussion of what Dr. Freedom and Mr. Sweat could do in the short and long term to improve the effectiveness of patient distribution.

## Future Challenges

Effective, evidenced-based care of populations or panels of patients, offers the potential to improve health outcomes and lower costs. For example, administering influenza vaccine to an entire population of elderly patients should decrease the seasonal number of hospital admissions for pneumonia and other influenza-related complications, while improving the health status of vaccine recipients. Early recognition and management of slowly progressive diseases, as achieved by screening for breast, prostate, or colon cancer, or by maintaining tight control of diabetes, offers great potential to decrease the costs of caring for advanced illness, and decreases associated mortality and morbidity. Emphasis on wellness programs, aimed at decreasing the incidence of obesity, heart disease, or smoking-related illness, through education will become standard features of the care offered by primary care providers, either directly or indirectly, to their populations of patients. Early detection of conditions that currently have no, or only minimally effective treatments, such as Alzheimer's disease, will become more important as our ability to treat them improves. Integrating provider teams and information systems across ambulatory and inpatient settings will begin to make substantive progress in improving acute care delivery a realizable goal.

## DISCUSSION QUESTIONS

1. What factors are driving the delivery of health care away from emergency care and inpatient hospital stays?
2. How has the role of the primary care practitioner expanded?
3. In the context of this chapter, what is meant by the integrated delivery of health care services?
4. What are three factors that have contributed to the increase in patients learning to procure more of their own health care?

## REFERENCES

American Academy of Physician Assistants. (2004). Retrieved April 24, 2004, from http://www.aapa.org/researc/91–03trends-report.pdf

American Association of Medical Colleges. (2004). *Teaching hospitals.* Available: http://www.aamc.org/teachinghospitals.htm

American Hospital Association. (1999). *AHA Guide 1999–2000.* Chicago: Author.

American Hospital Association. (2000). *Hospital statistics.* Chicago: Health Forum LLC.

American Hospital Association. (2002). Accessed at http://www.hospital connect.com, March 2004.

American Hospital Association. (2003a). *Trendwatch Chartbook 2003: Trends affecting hospitals and health systems.* Prepared by The Lewin Group, Inc., for the American Hospital Association. Retrieved July 2003 from http://www.hospitalconnect.com/ahapolicyforum/trend watch/chartbook2003.html

American Hospital Association. (2003b). *Hospital statistics.* Chicago: Author.

American Hospital Association. (2003–2004). *Guide to the health care field.* Chicago: Author.

Cook County Executive Budget Recommendation. (2004). *Section I, Bureau of Health* (p. 84). November 4, 2003.

Critical Access Hospitals and the Medicare Rural Hospital Flexibility Grant Program. (2002). CAS increases and expands flexibility for critical access hospitals in rural areas. *Medicare News.* Available: http://www.cms.hhs.gov/media/press/release.asp

Forrest, C. B., & Whalen, E.-M. (2000). Primary care safety-net delivery sites in the United States: A comparison of community health centers, hospital outpatient departments, and physician offices. *Journal of the American Medical Association, 284,* 2077–2083.

Fried, V. M., Prager, K., MacKay, A. P., & Xia, H. (2003). *Chartbook on trends in the health of Americans. Health United States, 2003.* Hyatsville, MD: National Center for Health Statistics.

Haugh, R. (2003, December). Reinventing the VA. *Hospitals & Health Networks, 77,* 50.

Haxtun Hospital. (2004). Haxtun Hospital District. Available at: http://www.haxtunhospital.com/ Retrieved August 2, 2004.

Health, United States (2003).

Health Care Advisory Board. (2002). Available at: http://www.advisory boardcompany.com/public/hcap.asp

Hollowell, E. (1978). No insurance—no privileges. *Legal Aspects of Medical Practice, 6*(14), 16–19.

High Plains Rural Health Network. (2004). High Plains Rural Health Network. Available at: http://www.hprhn.org/

Institute of Medicine. (1996). *Primary care: America's health in a new era.* Washington, DC: National Academy Press.

Institute of Medicine. (2000). America's health care safety net: Alive but endangered.

Kaiser Permanente. (2004). About Kaiser Permanente. Retrieved from http://newsmedia.kaiserpermanente.org/kpweb/mediakit/navlink page.do?elementId=htmlapp/feature/164mediakit/nat_mediaabo utkp.html.xml&repositoryBean=/kp/repositories/ContentReposi tory

Kohn, L. T., Corrigan, J. M., & Donaldson, M. S. (Eds.). (1999). *To err is human: Building a safer health system.* Washington, DC: National Academy Press.

Murray, M., & Tantau, C. (2000). Same day appointments: Exploding the access paradigm. *Family Practice Management, 7,* 45–50.

National Association of Public Hospitals and Health Systems. (2003). *America's safety net hospitals and health systems, 2001.* Washington, DC: NAPH.

Norris, T. E., Hart, G. L., Larson, E. H., Tarczy-Hornoch, P., Masudo, D. L., Fuller, S. S., et al. (2002). Low-bandwidth, low-cost telemedicine consultations in rural family practice. *Journal of the American Board of Family Practice, 15*(2), 123–127.

Nourjah, P. (1999). National Hospital Ambulatory Medical Care survey: 1997 emergency department summary. In *Advance Data from Vital and Health Statistics* (No. 304). Hyattsville, MD: National Center for Health Statistics.

Philips County Economic Development Corporation. (2004). Philips County, Colorado, at-a-glance. Available at: http://www.phillips countyco.org/pcglance.htm

Scheffler, R. M. (1996). Life in the kaleidoscope: The impact of managed care on the U.S. health care workforce and a new model for the delivery of primary care. In K. D. Yordy, K. N. Lohr, & N. A. Vanselow (Eds.), *Primary care: America's health in a new era* (pp. 312–340). Washington, DC: National Academy Press.

Shortell, S. M. (1985). The medical staff of the future: Replanting the garden. *Frontiers of Health Services Management*, 1(3), 3.

Showalter, J. S. (1999). *Southwick's the law of hospital and health administration*. Chicago: Health Administration Press.

Smith, H. L. (1955, March). Two lines of authority are one too many. *Modern Hospital*, 59–64.

Southwick, A. (1978). *The law of hospital and health administration*. Ann Arbor, MI: Health Administration Press.

Starr, P. (1982). *The social transformation of American medicine*. New York: Basic Books.

Stevens, R. (1971). *American medicine and the public interest*. New Haven, CT: Yale University Press.

Szilagyi, P. G., Rodewald, L. E., Humiston, S. G., Fierman, A. H., Cunningham, S., Gracia, D., et al. (1997). Effect of two urban emergency department immunization programs on childhood immunization rates. *Arch Pediatr Adolesc Med.*, 151(10), 999–1006.

U.S. Department of Agriculture. (2004). Rural utilities service. Accessed on-line at: http://www.usda.gov/rus/telecom/dlt/dltawards_co.htm

U.S. Department of Health and Human Services. (1995). Health, United States. (DHHS Publication No. PHS 96–1232). Washington, DC: U.S. Government Printing Office.

U.S. Department of Health and Human Services. (2000). Health, United States. (DHHS Publication No. PHS 01–1232). Washington, DC: U.S. Government Printing Office.

U.S. Department of Health and Human Services. (2003). Health, United States. Chartbook, Table 82.

U.S. Department of Veterans Affairs. Federal benefits for veterans and dependents. Accessed March 2004 at http://www.va.gov

Wilson, K. (1997). The VA healthcare system: An unrecognized national safety net. *Health Affairs*, 16, 200.

# 8

# CHRONIC CARE

Gerard Anderson and
James R. Knickman

- Quantify cost and prevalence of chronic conditions.
- Identify the overlap between chronic conditions and activity limitations.
- Recognize the problems faced by people with chronic conditions.
- Explore some of the options to change the delivery system to better meet the needs of people with chronic conditions.
- Examine changes that will be necessary to allow delivery systems to change.

TOPICAL OUTLINE

- Definition of and prevalence of chronic conditions
- Chronic conditions and activity limitations
- The cost of chronic care
- Insurance coverage and chronic care
- Dissatisfaction
- The evolving health care system
- Personal empowerment
- The Chronic Care Model
- Payment, coverage, information systems, medical education, and biomedical research
- Conclusion

KEY WORDS

Chronic condition, chronic care, care coordination, activity limitations

---

A LTHOUGH MOST AMERICANS think that the health care system spends most of its resources treating acute events like heart attacks and major traumas (as in the television show ER), in reality most medical care resources are spent treating chronic conditions such as asthma, diabetes, hypertension, Alzheimer's, congestive heart failure, and depression. However, because the health care system is oriented towards the treatment of acute care episodes, unfortunately many times people with one or more chronic conditions are not receiving appropriate medical care. Individuals with chronic conditions were responsible for most of the visits to doctors, hospitals, nursing homes, and other health care providers, and were associated with over three quarters of health care spending in 2000.

The 125 million Americans with one or more chronic conditions encompass the entire spectrum of ages, income levels, and geographic regions (Anderson and Knickman, 2001). Many people with chronic conditions also have activity limitations. In the next several decades, both the cost and the prevalence of chronic conditions are projected to increase. By 2030, almost half of all Americans will have one or more chronic conditions. These numbers alone suggest why the health care system should be oriented to treating people with chronic conditions. Unfortunately, clinical data as well as the perceptions of the public, clinicians, and policymakers suggest that the current system is not meeting the needs of people with chronic conditions. Specific changes are needed, which will require changes in how clinical research is conducted, clinicians are educated, health care is financed, payments are made, benefits are designed, and care is delivered.

Consider, for example, the case of a patient we will call Mary B. She is a 78-year-old Medicare beneficiary with diabetes, coronary heart disease, asthma, hypertension, and the initial stages of Alzheimer's. It is likely that she is seeing at least six different doctors and numerous other health care providers who treat her multiple chronic conditions. However, since her doctors and other providers are unable to communicate easily with each other, clinicians will develop her treatment protocol without knowing what the other clinicians are doing. Such a situation can lead to duplicate tests, advice from one clinician that contradicts the advice of another clinician, drugs prescribed by one doctor that adversely interact with drugs prescribed by another doctor, unnecessary and preventable hospitalizations and nursing home stays, and other events that only increase health spending and lower the quality of care for this patient. It is likely that at least one time during the year she will arrive at the pharmacist only to be told that the prescription she is trying to fill could cause an adverse drug reaction with other medications she is taking. Inadequate care coordination is only one problem that people with chronic conditions face every day.

This chapter began with a brief overview of chronic conditions and our present health care system. The chapter focuses on recent initiatives designed to help people educate themselves about treatment options. It introduces a model of a health care delivery system designed to improve care for people with chronic conditions. The chapter concludes with a discussion of how changes in health insurance coverage, provider payments, medical education, and biomedical research will be necessary in order to transform the health care system from having an orientation of providing acute, episodic care to having an orientation of providing ongoing, chronic care.

## DEFINITION OF AND PREVALENCE OF CHRONIC CONDITIONS

Chronic conditions are broadly defined as chronic illnesses or impairments that are expected to last a year or longer, limit what one can do, and/or require ongoing medical care. By this definition, an estimated 125 million Americans (45% of the U.S. population) had a chronic condition in 2000. This number is projected to increase to 161 million Americans (49% of the population) by 2030. Other definitions, and other projection methods may produce slightly different numbers. All of the estimates, however, show that 40 to 50% of the American population has at least one chronic condition.

Another approach is to examine the prevalence of specific chronic conditions. FIGURE 8.1 shows the most common chronic conditions in the U.S. in 2000 across all age groups. Hypertension (high blood pressure) is the most common chronic condition, occurring in more than 1 in 4 Americans. Over half of all people over age 65 have hypertension. When several different mental conditions (depression, schizophrenia, dementia, etc.) are combined, they form the second most common chronic condition. Mental illness occurs in all age groups.

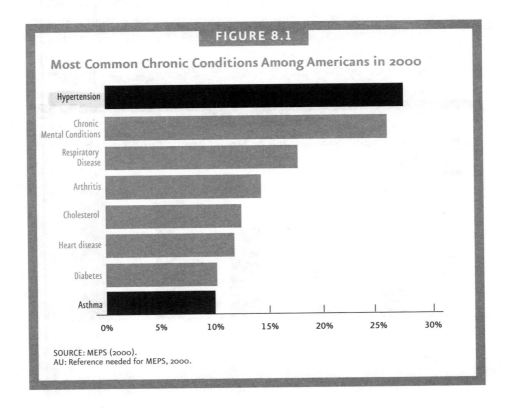

### FIGURE 8.1

**Most Common Chronic Conditions Among Americans in 2000**

SOURCE: MEPS (2000).
AU: Reference needed for MEPS, 2000.

Not all chronic conditions have the same impact on individuals. Chronic conditions vary considerably in how much they limit what one can do and the amount and type of ongoing care that is required. There is also wide variation in how much a person will be limited or the level of treatment required. For example, people with diabetes have a wide range of limitations and treatment regimens. Some diabetics have to only monitor their blood glucose daily, while it affects eye sight and mobility in others. Alzheimer's can cause people to momentarily forget names or completely deprive them of their memory.

As people age they are more likely to develop a chronic condition. For example, chronic conditions related to heart disease and conditions such as Alzheimer's disease all tend to be much more common among the elderly. Approximately 1 in 5 children ages 0–19 have a chronic condition compared to 4 in 5 people over age 65 (see FIGURE 8.2). Given the increasing average age of the U.S. population, this relationship will become increasingly evident as the baby boomers begin to pass age 65. The proportion of the population age 65 and older is projected to increase from 12.7% in 2000 to 20.0% in 2030.

Most of the clinical and media attention tends to focus on a single chronic condition. It is difficult to pick up a newspaper without reading a report of a new way to prevent or treat hypertension, diabetes, depression, asthma, or some other chronic condition. Because of this focus on single chronic conditions, it is not well understood by the public that half of all people with a chronic con-

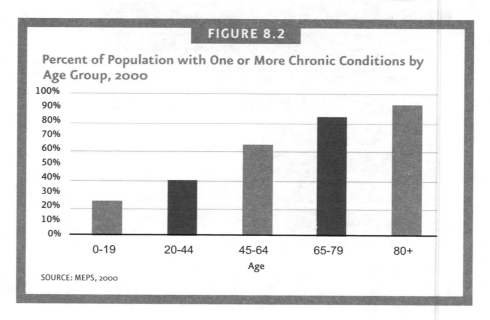

**FIGURE 8.2**

Percent of Population with One or More Chronic Conditions by Age Group, 2000

SOURCE: MEPS, 2000

dition have multiple chronic conditions. People with multiple chronic conditions are the heaviest utilizers of medical care services and are the most expensive to treat on an annual basis. They are also the people who frequently have the most problems with the medical care system.

Consider Mary B. who was introduced earlier. Because she has five different chronic conditions, it is likely that she will see five different specialists as well as a primary care physician. If she is hospitalized (1 in 3 chances) she will see even more doctors and other health professions. If she enters a nursing home (a 40% chance), she will encounter a different set of providers. She will fill on average one prescription per week. Unfortunately, there is no easy way for all these doctors and other clinicians to communicate with each other regarding Mary B.'s conditions. Someone needs to sort out the conflicting advice she is receiving. Because of her initial stages of Alzheimer's, she is unable to remember what the other doctors have told her. It is likely that her daughter (women are much more likely to be caregivers) will need to intervene and attempt to coordinate her care. This could become a full time job for the daughter.

The prevalence of multiple chronic conditions increases with age. Approximately 1 in 3 children with a chronic condition will have one or more other chronic conditions. In adults ages 18 to 64, approximately 2 in 3 with a chronic condition also have multiple chronic conditions. Almost 90% of people over age 65 with a chronic condition have multiple chronic conditions. The percentage of Americans with multiple chronic conditions is projected to increase, from 22% in 2000 to 26% in 2030. People with multiple chronic conditions were more likely to be hospitalized, have more physician visits, see more different physicians, utilize more medical services, and have higher medical expenditures. The cost and utilization increases with the number of chronic conditions. People with multiple chronic conditions are many of the people who fill our doctor's offices and hospital beds.

## CHRONIC CONDITIONS AND ACTIVITY LIMITATIONS

Individuals with chronic conditions may also have activity limitations. There are many different ways to define activity limitations. Each definition will result in a different number of people with activity limitations. For the purpose of calculating the overlap between chronic conditions and activity limitations, the following definitions are used. A chronic condition is an illness or impairment that is expected to last a year or longer, limits what one can do, and/or requires ongoing medical care. People with activity limitations need help or supervision with one or more activities of daily living (ADLs) or instrumental activities of daily living (IADLs).

By these definitions, 125 million Americans had a chronic condition in 2000 (Anderson & Knickman, 2001). Of these, approximately 92 million had a chronic condition but did not have an activity limitation in 2000. However, 33 million Americans (1 out of 4 Americans with a chronic condition) did have an activity limitation. Individuals with both chronic conditions and activity limitations were much worse off than people with chronic conditions only. They were much more likely to be hospitalized, had significantly more physician and home health visits, took more prescription drugs, had lower incomes, and were less likely to be going to school or to be working. Many of them are in need of some type of long term care. Activity limitations are a strong predictor of nursing home admissions. Frequently, these are people whose chronic condition (or more likely chronic *conditions*) have become so debilitating that they are having difficulty walking, cooking, or performing other routine activities and may need to enter a nursing home or assisted living facility.

## THE COST OF CHRONIC CARE

Individuals with chronic conditions are the heaviest users of medical services. They were associated with 96% of all home care visits, 88% of all prescriptions, 76% of inpatient stays, and 72% of physician visits in 2000. Overall, people with chronic conditions were associated with 78% of all medical care expenditures in 2000. As the prevalence of chronic conditions increases in the next several decades, these percentages will likely increase.

The more chronic conditions a person has the more expensive their health care is likely to be on an annual basis. FIGURE 8.3 shows the relationship between the percent of the population with 0, 1, 2, 3, 4, 5+ chronic conditions and the percent of spending by each group. The data show that 56% of the population does not have a chronic condition and were associated with only 20% of health care spending in 2000. At the other end of the spectrum, just 12% have 3 or more chronic conditions, and yet these individuals

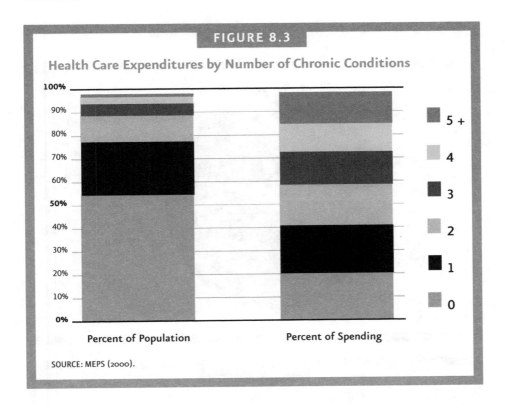

**FIGURE 8.3**

Health Care Expenditures by Number of Chronic Conditions

SOURCE: MEPS (2000).

accounted for 40% of the health care spending in 2000 (Wolff, Starfield, & Anderson, 2002).

As noted earlier, the prevalence of chronic conditions, especially multiple chronic conditions, increases with age. As shown in FIGURE 8.4, two thirds of Medicare expenditures were for Medicare beneficiaries with five or more chronic conditions in 1999. As a result, policymakers should address the needs of people with multiple chronic conditions when considering reform of the Medicare system. The greatest potential for cost savings and quality improvement is by the 15% of Medicare beneficiaries with 5 or more chronic conditions that represent two thirds of Medicare spending. The Medicare program has recently initiated a series of demonstrations and research initiatives on this population.

## INSURANCE COVERAGE AND CHRONIC CARE

Insurance status and age are strong predictors of who has chronic conditions. In this analysis, the population is first sorted by age (less than 65, greater than 65) and then by insurance status (see

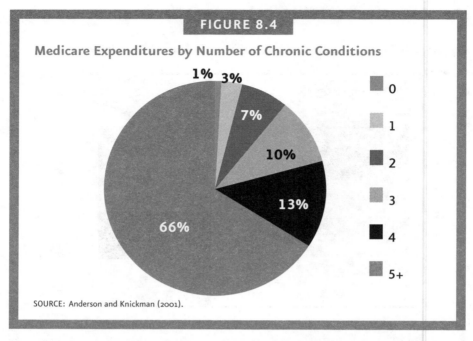

FIGURE 8.4

Medicare Expenditures by Number of Chronic Conditions

SOURCE: Anderson and Knickman (2001).

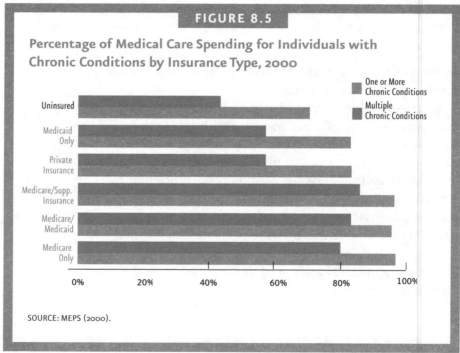

FIGURE 8.5

Percentage of Medical Care Spending for Individuals with
Chronic Conditions by Insurance Type, 2000

SOURCE: MEPS (2000).

FIGURE 8.5). People under age 65 who are uninsured, privately
insured, or covered by Medicaid are less likely to have one or more
chronic conditions than people over age 65 with Medicare only cov-

erage, Medicare and supplemental coverage, or Medicare and Medicaid coverage.

Among those under age 65, the uninsured are the least likely to have a chronic condition. Nevertheless, over half of all medical care spending by the uninsured is by people with a chronic condition and a third is by uninsured people with multiple chronic conditions. For these individuals, the lack of health insurance coverage severely compromises their ability to receive ongoing care. Almost two thirds of private health insurance spending for people under age 65 involves people with chronic conditions. Individuals over age 65 with chronic conditions represent nearly all of Medicare spending.

Private industry has recently become aware of their investment in chronic care and is looking to improve the delivery system primarily through disease management. It makes little difference if the Medicare beneficiary also has private supplemental insurance, is also insured by Medicaid (dual eligibles), or only has Medicare coverage. Over 80% of Medicare spending is by people with multiple chronic conditions. The Medicare program has thus become a program for people with multiple chronic conditions.

## DISSATISFACTION WITH THE CURRENT SYSTEM

Individuals with chronic conditions report considerable difficulty obtaining appropriate services (Anderson, 2003). There are numerous reasons for these access problems, which can influence the health status of people with chronic conditions. FIGURE 8.6 shows the results of a poll conducted of a cross section of adults in 2000. It shows that the American public generally recognizes that people with chronic conditions do not have access to adequate health insurance coverage or access to appropriate medical services. The level of dissatisfaction is much lower, however, when the same questions are asked about acute care services.

Almost 9 in 10 Americans recognize that people with chronic conditions have difficulty obtaining adequate health insurance. Three reasons are often given for this difficulty. First, some services are not covered by some health insurance plans. Uncovered services, however, are not the major concern since most health insurers cover most services to some extent.

A second issue that has received less public and policy attention is the criterion of medical necessity. For example, some people who believe they need ongoing rehabilitation services after a stroke

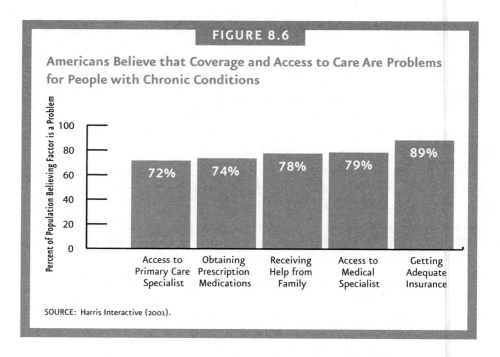

**FIGURE 8.6**

Americans Believe that Coverage and Access to Care Are Problems for People with Chronic Conditions

SOURCE: Harris Interactive (2001).

often find that insurers refuse to approve treatment after a set number of weeks. For people with chronic conditions, who have health insurance coverage, medical necessity rules are probably a bigger problem than inadequate health insurance coverage. Medical necessity criteria are used to deny payment even when the service is covered. One medical necessity criterion typically applied to some chronic conditions is that a specific service can only receive reimbursement if the services actually can improve the insured's condition. While this makes sense from an acute care perspective, it usually does not make sense from a chronic care orientation. Maintenance of functioning or health status is often the goal of the treatment plan for someone with a chronic condition though not necessarily improvement. Many claims for services used to treat chronic conditions are denied under the medical necessity criterion.

Consider Mary B. again. She may have difficulty getting Medicare to pay for treatment for her Alzheimer's condition. Mary is unlikely to "improve," and in fact her condition is likely to deteriorate over time as the Alzheimer's begins to take over. On medical necessity grounds, payment for her treatment will be denied. In response, many doctors have become good at coding something other than Alzheimer's in order to get payment for patient's care. In other areas, such as physical therapy, this subterfuge may not be as easy.

A third common problem with health insurance is cost-sharing.

To prevent excessive or unnecessary treatment, insurers generally require beneficiaries to bear some portion of the cost for care, through deductibles, coinsurance, or copays. This makes sense in an acute care context. However, cost-sharing can be a financial burden for those with chronic conditions. Out-of-pocket spending nearly doubles with each additional chronic condition, especially those who are seeing multiple clinicians for multiple conditions (see **FIGURE 8.7**).

Again, consider the circumstances of Mary B. As someone with five chronic conditions, she is likely to have over 30 doctors' visits, 2 hospitalizations, and 50 prescriptions during the year. Even if each of these services requires only a $10 copay, Mary will have $820 in out-of-pocket expenses for the year. If she needs to go to a nursing home, the cost could exceed $50,000 per year. The probability of entering a nursing home or needing home health services increases directly with the number of chronic conditions. It is not surprising that people with five or more chronic conditions spent over $10,000 out of pocket for medical care, on average in 2000.

In addition to difficulty obtaining adequate insurance coverage, the American public also recognizes that people with chronic conditions have health care access problems. Almost 3 in 4 people with chronic conditions have difficulty getting access to primary care

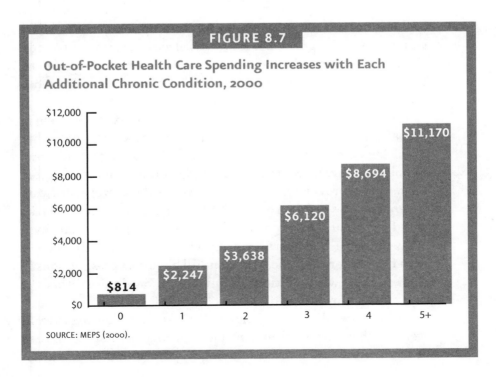

**FIGURE 8.7**

**Out-of-Pocket Health Care Spending Increases with Each Additional Chronic Condition, 2000**

SOURCE: MEPS (2000).

and specialty physicians (see Figure 8.6). These complaints about access problems are almost as great for people with health insurance coverage as for those without coverage. One possible explanation for these reported access problems is that most people with chronic conditions utilize multiple providers and have difficulty with care coordination.

Care coordination is needed to help providers decide on a treatment regimen that reflects the patient's multiple chronic conditions (Wagner et al., 2001). Mary B's proposed new treatment for diabetes could conflict with her ongoing treatment for congestive heart failure. It will be necessary for her endocrinologist to work with her cardiologist to resolve any treatment differences. Who arranges this and how the information is shared has not been resolved. Most likely it will not happen. The issue often includes coordination across medical providers and between medical and long-term, rehabilitation, and other care providers. Individuals with chronic conditions and activity limitations often have to navigate both the medical care and long-term care systems. These and other problems have led to considerable dissatisfaction with the current system by people with chronic conditions, their caregivers, and the general public. Physicians, other health professionals, and policymakers are becoming aware of and looking for solutions.

As a result, changes to the current system are beginning to occur. Probably the most important change is the development of data systems that link providers. Known as electronic medical records, these data systems allow clinicians access to a common set of data, including all medical records, results of clinical studies, and a listing of prescription drugs for a patient.

The Veteran's Administration already has this type of system in operation. Within the VA system, physicians know what other physicians are doing and can easily share laboratory results and radiologic images. People with multiple chronic conditions often see multiple providers. For example, while the average Medicare beneficiary sees between 6 and 7 different physicians, beneficiaries with five or more chronic conditions see almost 14 individual physicians in a year and average 37 physician visits annually. People with five or more chronic conditions fill almost 50 prescriptions in a year. People with multiple chronic conditions indicate that the care among providers is often uncoordinated.

Consider two different scenarios for Mary B. Under the current scenario, her various clinicians have minimal contact with each other. The endocrinologist treating her diabetes does not know what the cardiologist treating her congestive heart disease has prescribed. None of her doctors know the advice the other clinicians are giving or what drugs she is taking. Under an alternative scenario there is an integrated electronic medical record. All clinicians submit clinical data on a common format; lab test results are incorporated, drugs are recorded, and other necessary information is available to each clinician treating Mary B. All the clinician needs to do is to sit down at a computer terminal and find the information available. Currently, this alternative scenario is only available in a few locations, most notably in all the Veteran's Administration hospitals and clinics.

However, lack of this kind of coordination can lead to potentially adverse outcomes for patients, and inefficient or wasteful health care spending. A national survey of the American public found that over 60% of caregivers of people with chronic conditions report that they received conflicting medical advice from different providers, as did about 45% of people with serious chronic conditions. Over 50% of people with serious chronic conditions and caregivers reported that they received different diagnoses for the same set of conditions from different providers. Almost half of Americans with multiple chronic conditions went to a pharmacy last year only to be told that taking the prescription they were having filled could lead to an adverse drug reaction because of other medications they were taking. In a recent survey (Mathematica Policy Research, 2001), physicians reported that they found it difficult to coordinate care for people with chronic conditions and recognized that poor care coordination was leading to adverse outcomes such as unnecessary hospitalizations and nursing home stays.

Studies are beginning to report the number of adverse outcomes generated by lack of care coordination. For instance, one study found that among Medicare beneficiaries with one chronic condition, 7 out of 1,000 will have an inpatient hospital stay for an ambulatory care sensitive condition (preventable hospitalization), whereas among those with five chronic conditions, 95 out of 1,000 will have an ambulatory care sensitive condition. The number rises to 261 for those with 10 or more chronic conditions. Because beneficiaries with multiple conditions do not experience good care coordination, they are more likely to experience a hospitalization that could have been prevented. This adds up to more health care spending and reduces health care quality.

With five chronic conditions, Mary B has nearly a 20% chance of having an unnecessary hospitalization. At over $6,000 per hospitalization, the potential savings from eliminating or reducing the probability of an unnecessary hospitalization are considerable. If the number of duplicate tests and the probability of having an adverse drug reaction due to drug/drug interaction can be reduced, the potential savings from better care coordination are even greater.

## THE EVOLVING HEALTH CARE SYSTEM

The evolution of the health care system in the twentieth century reflects the changing demographics, mortality, and morbidity of the American population. During the first half of the 20th century, the emphasis of the health care system was on treating infectious diseases, reflecting the impact of destructive epidemics such as the Spanish influenza outbreak of 1918–1919. Smallpox, typhoid, cholera, tuberculosis, and other infectious diseases drove the design and implementation of the health care system. This era culminated with the successful development of a variety of vaccines and improved public sanitation and environmental standards, vastly reducing mortality and morbidity rates.

Having developed mechanisms to reduce the prevalence of infectious diseases, the health care system shifted its focus from infectious diseases to the treatment of acute illnesses by the middle of the twentieth century. Hospitals and physicians focused on treating acute health problems—trauma, heart attacks, etc. In response, the medical system evolved and the delivery, financing, educational, and biomedical research systems focused on providing acute, episodic care. Treatment for these acute conditions improved dramatically in the later half of the 20th century. Thus, the American health care system became oriented towards the treatment of acute events such as heart attacks.

By the end of the 20th century a third transformation had begun. Because Americans were living longer, and treatment and prevention for infections and acute care was improving, care for people with chronic conditions has become an increasingly important issue. While our health care system is still designed to provide acute, episodic care, our medical care utilization and expenditures increasingly center on people with ongoing, chronic conditions.

This transformation will require significant changes in personal responsibilities as well as changes to the health care system. In an attempt to provide a roadmap for these changes, this chapter groups the ongoing changes into three areas. The first involves changes in patient empowerment, that is, getting the person to take more responsibility for their own health status. The second involves reforms to the health care delivery system. This requires fundamental changes in how care is organized and delivered. The third involves changes in how medical care is paid for, how health professionals are trained, and how biomedical research is conducted.

## PERSONAL EMPOWERMENT

Individuals, clinicians, and policymakers can undertake health care activities that would help prevent chronic conditions (Lorig et al., 2000). A number of studies have shown that most chronic conditions are preventable through behavior change. Other studies have shown specific interventions that are successful in promoting these behavior changes. Initiatives to reduce the number of people who smoke, to reduce the level of obesity, and to promote exercise are just three examples. Many of these initiatives are designed to encourage the person to take actions to improve their behavior. Improvements in motivating individuals to adopt healthy lifestyles are expanding, but it takes persistent attention to motivational issues to encourage individuals to eat better, exercise more, and avoid social isolation—all key factors in avoiding the first, second, or tenth chronic condition.

However, even if these actions are successful and the number of people with chronic conditions does not increase as fast as forecast, it is still necessary to help those who already have chronic conditions. The first step is personal empowerment. The personal empowerment movement began with disabled people. Often they required long-term care services. Publicly funded programs began to subsidize personal assistance programs, covering everything from bathing and dressing to shopping and housekeeping, acknowledging the need to provide direct support for people with long-term health problems who require aid outside of the episodic care model. This development in the health care system, allowing recipients to arrange and supervise their own services, is also known as consumer direction. A number of factors led to this change, among them cost considerations, legal direction (such as the Supreme Court's 1999 Olmstead decision), and the aggressive advocacy of disabled interest groups.

A number of programs have been designed to foster personal empowerment for people with chronic conditions. For example, the Robert Wood Johnson Foundation has operated a program with state Medicaid agencies entitled "Cash and Counseling." It gives people who are nursing home eligible the option to receive cash benefits instead of receiving direct services whereby they can use the cash in conjunction with counseling to purchase services on their own. Findings from this program suggest higher satisfaction with services received when people receive cash and use it to purchase the services they think they really need. And, people who have the chance to manage their own services appear to be doing well on avoiding further declines in chronic conditions. If Mary B. were nursing home eligible, she and her family would have a choice. She would get public funding to allow her to remain in her home, or as her Alzheimer's causes deterioration, choose to enter a nursing home.

This growing awareness of the importance of patient activation expanded from the disabled and people with activity limitations to include people with chronic conditions. Reforming the health care system to accommodate people with chronic conditions began in earnest with a focus on the patient level of care. Providers began to recognize the importance of making people with chronic conditions "partners" in their care.

One example of this type of consumer-directed care for people with chronic conditions was developed at Stanford University by Hal Holman. Dr. Holman and his colleagues at Stanford emphasize the importance of the role of the patient in effecting positive outcomes for patients with chronic conditions, in what they called the "Health Partners" approach to care. This system of care relies on provider-patient interaction beyond the traditional hospital/office setting, a practice that was designed for acute care delivery, not for chronic care management. This approach involves the patient by informing them of the nature of the disease and what he/she can do to improve their quality of life. As Dr. Holman says,

> a one-on-one interaction between doctor and patient was an appropriate management tool when acute disease was the dominant problem. This works with something like a broken leg or a bout of pneumonia that is new to the patient. But with chronic disease, we should be exploring a new model, because patients have time to become 'smart' about what's happening. (Medical Staff Update, 2000)

Our chronic care recipient Mary B. wants to participate in her treatment choices. She recognizes that she is going to need to make accommodations as her Alzheimer's becomes worse and she becomes increasingly dependant on others. She also wants to choose different ways to treat her diabetes, asthma, coronary heart disease, and hypertension. She will need help from a variety of caregivers.

## THE CHRONIC CARE MODEL

The patient empowerment model pioneered by Dr. Holman represents an important departure from traditional patient care, but it does not address the need to reorient health care providers toward caring for people with chronic conditions. Dr. Edward Wagner and his colleagues at Group Health of Puget Sound in Seattle, Washington, have developed a chronic care model that integrates various aspects of the provider-patient interaction, including the community, the overall health system, patient self-management, health care delivery system design, decision support, clinical information systems, informed and activated patients, and prepared and proactive practice teams (Bodenheimer, Wagner, & Grumbach, 2001). A simplified version of the model is shown in FIGURE 8.8.

As shown in Figure 8.8, there are six components that lead to better care for people with chronic conditions in the chronic care model. First, community programs can play an important role in chronic care. Nutrition and exercises classes at senior centers, for

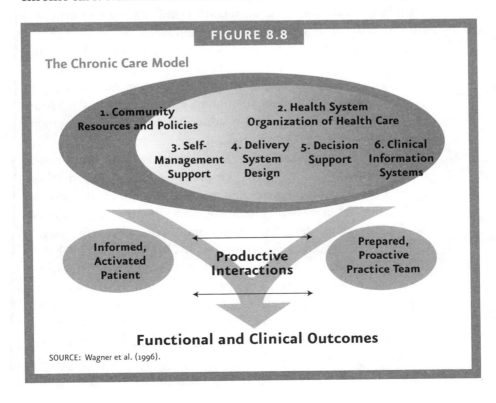

FIGURE 8.8

The Chronic Care Model

1. Community Resources and Policies
2. Health System Organization of Health Care
3. Self-Management Support
4. Delivery System Design
5. Decision Support
6. Clinical Information Systems

Informed, Activated Patient

Productive Interactions

Prepared, Proactive Practice Team

**Functional and Clinical Outcomes**

SOURCE: Wagner et al. (1996).

example, can reinforce healthy behaviors. Mary B may want to go to the social center for interaction with people her own age. Second, the organization of the overall health care system is critical to improving chronic illness care. Helping people with chronic conditions means changing a health care system that is designed to be reactive—acting when people are injured or sick—to one that is proactive, acting to keep people as healthy as possible. Mary B's health plan may offer a wellness program.

Third, a crucial aspect is the patient's own self-management; patients who properly take care of themselves can minimize complications, symptoms, and disabilities. Engendering a sense of personal responsibility for health outcomes encourages people to assume the central role in their care. Using established programs to provide basic information, emotional support, and strategies for living with chronic conditions is an important part of self-management support. Care decisions must be based on clearly established guidelines rooted in clinical research, and these guidelines need to be explained to people so that they understand the principles underlying their care. People making their own treatment decisions need ongoing training to make fully-informed choices, using improved models of provider education that are more effective than traditional "continuing medical education." Mary B will need continuing counseling to help her as her condition changes.

This leads naturally into the fourth component of the Chronic Care Model, the health care delivery system design. In order to alter practices, guidelines must be integrated into reminders, feedback, and standing orders to make them more evident as clinical decisions are made. To this end, involving supportive specialists in primary care is an increasingly common part of chronic care. Keeping providers focused on maintaining health rather than simply restoring it requires a combination of case management, aggressive follow-up, and ensuring that information is relayed to patients in ways that are compatible with their culture and background. Mary B's doctors need to know the latest clinical information on how to treat her.

The fifth and sixth components of the Chronic Care Model, decision support and clinical information systems, respectively, are inextricably tied to one another. Managing chronic care effectively requires access to information not only on individual patients, but on populations as well. A comprehensive clinical information system helps providers issue timely reminders about needed services, and allows for health care data to be followed easily and effectively. Data on all individuals can help point to groups needing additional attention, as well as aid in monitoring the performance of partic-ular providers and, thereby, efforts at quality improvement. Access to this data allows providers to develop evidence-based guidelines for their practices, and to share these evidence-based methods with their patients, so that they can understand the principles under-lying their care. As noted earlier, Mary B's doctors need to be able to communicate with each other.

The Chronic Care Model emphasizes that patients who are informed about their conditions and who assume an active role in managing their care, working in tandem with providers who are prepared and supported with time and resources at their disposal, are more likely to have more productive health care interactions (Bonomi, Wagner, Glasgow, & VonKorff, 2002). For example, acute episodes for diabetics and asthmatics decrease when engaged patients work closely with proactive providers. These interactions are not restricted to face-to-face encounters, but run the gamut from telephone conferences to group visits to email exchange. Such alternative communication methods are examples of new forms of self-management support that have developed.

Mary B. now has found a delivery system that allows her to par-ticipate in the decision making process. She knows her different clinicians who openly communicate with her and with each other, and the community in which she lives is supportive of her needs. The next question is how this can be sustained. This will require major changes in how clinical research is done, how clinicians are trained, how care is reimbursed, what services are covered, and better information technology.

## PAYMENT, COVERAGE, INFORMATION SYSTEMS, MEDICAL EDUCATION, AND BIOMEDICAL RESEARCH

Individuals can assume greater personal responsibility and be given information to help them manage their behavior and treat-ment. Delivery systems can improve the way they provide care. However, it will be difficult to sustain these activities if other com-ponents of the health care system are not oriented towards pre-vention or the delivery of ongoing, chronic care. In this final sec-tion, necessary changes to the payment system, coverage policy, information systems, medical education training, and biomedical research are briefly outlined.

Our current fee-for-service payment system encourages episodic care—promoting a 'silo' approach to individual facilities or providers, and encouraging cost shifting among these same entities and across different payers (Vladeck, 2001). Many experts highlight how capitation would be ideal for promoting the type of crosscutting, integrated delivery systems that good chronic care ultimately requires. However, enrollment in staff model and other health maintenance organization models that stress care coordination are on the decline due to the complexity of managing these organizations, the difficulty of recruiting physicians to work in such settings, and the reluctance of many individuals, especially those without chronic conditions, to enroll in the plans.

Health plans that operate through exclusive provider networks often have payment systems that do not foster care coordination. Most health plans do not have information systems that allow clinicians to communicate with each other, particularly across diverse networks or groups. Often health plan providers, if they are capitated, are capitated within their own specialty spheres and are responsible only for the utilization of their own services. As a result, they have no need to be aware of utilization outside their specialty and may have incentives to move costs and services onto other providers and other parts of the system. Insurers and managed care plans faced with rising programs are reluctant to pay for services such as information systems or care coordination.

If there is a desire to change the way care is practiced, financial incentives at the practitioner level will need to change so that practice patterns can be changed (Berenson & Horvath, 2002). One approach is to adopt the clinical care manager model. In this model, a patient with multiple chronic conditions, who is having difficulty self-managing care, would designate a clinician to be his/her clinical care manager. This physician would receive a monthly administrative payment for care. The fee would remunerate for additional office staff time required to take on this role. The point of this model is to assign the task of treatment coordination to a single clinician and reimburse accordingly. The ultimate responsibility for treatment and, therefore resource utilization, rests with practicing physicians. The majority of physicians are probably not trained to take on this role at this time. They may hire individuals to perform this function. However, if payment tied to process and outcome standards is established, the field can respond over time.

Under this model, Mary B, because she has 5 chronic conditions, would qualify for a clinical care manager. Perhaps the clinical care manager would receive $100 per month to help her manage her care and to coordinate with other clinicians. Mary B. (likely with the help of her caregiver) would designate one clinician or one clinical team to perform this function and to get paid for performing this service.

Coverage would need to address three areas. First, certain benefits would need to be added to insurance policies to cover services needed by people with chronic conditions. Second, the medical necessity criterion would need to be clarified to allow claims to be paid if the purpose of the visit is not improvement but maintenance of the health status of the individual. Third, coinsurance would need to be restructured so that people with multiple chronic conditions do not incur large financial burdens each year.

In Mary B's case, her services are mostly covered by Medicare. However, when she goes to her geriatrician for advice and treatment for her Alzheimer's disease, it is often the case that care is denied on medical necessity grounds. Mary is increasingly having difficulty remembering to perform certain tasks, and her doctor and the nurse are helping her. However, many of these services are denied on medical necessity grounds. In addition, each time she goes to the doctor, she must pay 20% of the doctor's bill. This means that she has a very large out-of-pocket payment because of the number of doctor visits she has during the year.

Clinical information systems that allow clinicians to know what other clinicians are doing when they treat a patient will need to become more common. As noted in the discussion of care coordination, people with multiple chronic conditions often see multiple clinicians. If the same person has activity limitations, then encounters with long-term care and other providers are possible. Information systems that allow communication across clinicians and providers are needed to improve quality of care; reduce unnecessary hospitalizations, eliminate duplicate tests, and reduce the amount of contradictory advice; and to lower medical care costs.

Clinicians need to be trained to work cooperatively. Providing appropriate care in isolation may not be appropriate for people with multiple chronic conditions. Clinicians will need to learn to work with other clinicians to treat people with multiple chronic conditions. This will require a relatively fundamental change in how doctors are trained because it will require different specialties to work together, especially in the outpatient setting.

Even biomedical research will need to change. Currently most clinical trials have exclusions that limit the enrollment of people with multiple chronic conditions. This can make it difficult for practicing physicians to know whether a drug, device, or procedure is appropriate for their patient with multiple chronic conditions. Changes in clinical trials will be necessary if information on how patients with multiple chronic conditions will respond is considered important data to collect.

How likely is it that such types of insurance coverage and changes in information systems and clinical training will emerge? Because private insurers have little incentive to recruit high-cost, chronically ill patients with multiple chronic conditions, such new approaches to coverage, information, and training would need to be induced by public interventions. And such interventions probably would only be likely if stresses in the health care system force a rethinking of our approach to insurance coverage and health care delivery more generally. Because the Medicare program spends two thirds of its budget on people with five or more chronic conditions, the Medicare program is a logical starting point.

## CONCLUSIONS

The American health care system needs to focus on the management of chronic conditions, especially multiple chronic conditions. Policymakers, clinicians, and the public are aware that substantial reform is needed if the 125 million Americans with one or more chronic conditions are to receive appropriate medical care. It is important to think how the current system will need to change in order to provide better care. Insurance rules and the way health care providers think about organizing services need to be tailored better to meet the needs of people with chronic conditions.

The growing number of Americans with chronic conditions, especially those with multiple chronic conditions, will necessitate changes in how individuals view their own personal health care responsibility, how the medical care system is organized, and what incentives and information the medical care system is given to operate.

## DISCUSSION QUESTIONS

Health leaders during the period of the aging of America need to be familiar with the important role chronic conditions play, and will continue to play in the delivery of health care. This chapter

## CASE STUDY

Three options:

1. Assume you have just been hired by a large multi-specialty group practice and they are interested in designing a care management system for patients who have multiple chronic conditions:
   a. Who would you involve in this process?
   b. How would you go about determining which model to use?
   c. Once designed, how would you go about convincing the leadership of the group practice that it should be adopted (i.e., what would the "business case" for changing the care model be?)?
   d. How would you convince the physicians and other clinicians to participate actively?

2. Assume you have just accepted a position in the federal government at the Centers for Medicare & Medicaid Services (which oversees the Medicare and Medicaid programs from policy, reimbursement, and regulatory perspectives) and you are asked to come up with policy options available to the federal government (through legislation or administrative rules) to encourage health care providers to better coordinate and manage the service needs of Medicare enrollees who have multiple chronic conditions:
   a. Who would you involve in this process?
   b. How would you go about determining which policy options to pursue?
   c. Once the policy is designed, how would you go about convincing the leadership of the Centers for Medicare & Medicaid Services that your plan is worth pursuing and has a chance to make it through political and bureaucratic processes?
   d. What would you communicate to beneficiaries with multiple chronic conditions?

3. Assume you have just accepted a position with a major private insurance company that offers managed care products in its employer-based insurance markets and they have asked you to develop reimbursement approaches that would encourage

(Continued)

## CASE STUDY (Continued)

physicians to better coordinate and managed services for the people covered by your company's managed care insurance policies:

    a. Who would you involve in this process?

    b. How would you go about determining which reimbursement approaches to pursue?

    c. Once designed, how would you go about convincing the leadership of the insurance company that your approach should be adopted (i.e., what would the "business case" be for changing the reimbursement approach?)?

    d. How would you market this product to subscribers?

attempts to make the reader familiar with the definitions and epidemiology of chronic care in America. Important in this descriptive purpose of the chapter is to make clear that many people have concurrent multiple chronic conditions and that this subset of people represents the greatest challenge to the U.S. health care system, which has been organized around episodic medicine for the past 40 years. The chapter also familiarizes the reader with current efforts to improve the management of chronic conditions in order to reorient the organization and financing of health care to meet the needs of people with chronic conditions. Consider these possible discussion questions:

1. What are the major problems faced by people with multiple chronic conditions?
2. What are the distinctions and interrelations among the following: chronic conditions, frailty, activity limitations, and disability?
3. Discuss how features of current insurance coverage may not encourage the best type of health care for people with chronic conditions?
4. Why do people with chronic conditions have difficulty obtaining adequate health insurance coverage?
5. What is meant by "medical necessity criteria" in the health insurance field, and how do they affect reimbursements for care needed by people with chronic conditions?
6. What is meant by "care coordination?" Who should be involved in care coordination?
7. How important is an electronic medical record to improve care coordination?

8. Various approaches to organizing the delivery of care for chronic conditions have been suggested. How do you think services should be organized?

9. What would have to happen to encourage implementation of your suggestions? Would implementation of these changes decrease or increase expenditures across the health care system?

## REFERENCES

Anderson, G. (2003). Physician, public, and policymakers perspectives on chronic conditions. *Archives of Internal Medicine*.

Anderson, G., & Knickman, J. (2001). Changing the chronic care system to meet people's needs. *Health Affairs, 20,*146–159.

Berenson, R. & Horvath, J. (2002–2003). Barriers to chronic care management in Medicare. *Health Affairs*, Web-exclusive.

Bodenheimer, T., Wagner, E.H., & Grumbach, K. (2002). Improving primary care for patients with chronic illness. *Journal of the American Medical Association, 288,*1775–1779.

Bonomi, A.E., Wagner, E.H., Glasgow, R, & VonKorff, M. (2002). Assessment of chronic illness care: A practical tool for quality improvement. *Health Services Research, 37,* 791–820.

Harris Interactive Inc. (2001). *Survey on chronic illness and caregiving.* New York: Author.

Lorig, K., Holman, H., Sobel, D., Laurent, D., Gonzalez, V., & Minor, M. (2000). *Living a healthy life with chronic conditions* (2nd ed.). Bull Publishing.

Mathematica Policy Research Inc. (2001). *National Public Engagement Campaign on Chronic Illness—Physician Survey, Final Report.* Princeton, NJ: Author.

Medical Staff Update. (2000). Fact file, questions and answers. Interview with Joseph R. Hopkins & Halstead R. Holman. *Stanford Hospital and Clinics, 24* (2).

MEPS. (2002). *The Medical Expenditure Panel Survey, Household Component Data.* Washington, DC: The Agency for Health Care Research and Quality.

Vladeck B. (2001). You can't get there from here: Obstacles to improving care of the chronically ill. *Health Affairs, 20,* 6, 175–179.

Wagner, E.H., Austin, B.T., & Von Korff, M.(1996). Organizing care for patients with chronic illness. *Milbank Quarterly, 74,* 511–544.

Wagner, E.H., Austin, B.T., Davis, C., Hindmarsh, M., Schaefer, J., & Bonomi A. (2001). Improving chronic illness care: Translating evidence into action. *Health Affairs, 20,* 64–78.

Wolff, J., Starfield, B., & Anderson, G. (2002). Prevalence, expenditures, and complications of multiple chronic conditions in the elderly. *Archives of Internal Medicine*.

# 9

# LONG-TERM CARE

Penny Hollander Feldman,
Pamela Nadash, and
Michal D. Gursen

- Define the key components of long-term care (LTC) and discuss the factors that contribute to need and demand for service.
- Describe the principal users and the principal sources of payment for LTC.
- Discuss the differences and similarities between individual and societal-level goals for the LTC system.
- Distinguish among the principal paid providers of LTC and the populations they serve.
- Identify the major cost, quality, and access issues in LTC and discuss the strengths and weaknesses of alternative policy options.

KEY WORDS

Long-term care, chronic health conditions, activities of daily living, instrumental activities of daily living, formal and informal services/paid and unpaid caregivers, nursing homes, home and community based services (HCBS), home care, home health care, certified home health agency (CHHA), hospice services, adult day care, respite services, assisted living facilities, continuing care retirement communities (CCRCs), financing mechanisms—public/private financing; integrated long-term and acute care financing; private LTC insurance, access, quality, consumer choice

> Nearly every American will encounter the need for long-term care, either for themselves or a loved one. The rapidly increasing cost of long-term care is one of the largest expenses facing states and their spiraling Medicaid budgets. We need to change the culture of long-term care to help our seniors age healthier and our states more efficiently provide the dignified care our citizens deserve.
>
> —NGA Chairman Gov. Dirk Kempthorne of Idaho

THE NEED FOR long-term care (LTC) is growing. The American population is aging, and the fastest population growth is among the "oldest old"—those people 85 years or older who are most likely to be affected by chronic, disabling conditions. Moreover, technological advances are enabling virtually everyone with a disabling condition—young or old—to live longer. Today, hardly any human being, no matter how handicapped or disabled, is beyond some rehabilitation (Callahan, 1990). As a result, family caregivers, community service providers, health care experts, policymakers, and consumers of care themselves are struggling on a daily basis to identify the kinds of service and supports needed to optimally address the challenges of those who live with disability.

All too often, the public equates LTC with care in a nursing home or another institution. However, LTC is a broad constellation of services provided in diverse settings to a heterogeneous population with diverse needs (Stone, 2000). "Supportive" services form the core of LTC. These services include personal assistance with basic daily activities such as bathing, eating, walking, or going to the toilet. In the LTC literature, such activities are commonly referred to as activities of daily living or "ADLs." Supportive services also include help with household chores and related activities such as shopping, cooking, managing money and paying bills, or traveling to and from one's home. In the LTC literature, these activities are commonly referred to as instrumental activities of daily living or "IADLs."

In order to control the symptoms and progression of their disease, millions of individuals with chronic disabling conditions also require ongoing medical monitoring and intervention in addition to routine help with ADLs or IADLs. Others require rehabilitative services to recover physical or mental function or to delay a decline. Thus LTC often has a medical or rehabilitative as well as a supportive component.

In addition, people suffering from chronic disabling disease can benefit from palliative care, defined as the "comprehensive management of physical, social, spiritual, and existential needs of patients" (Kaplan & Urbina, 2000). Although palliative care is most commonly associated with the decision to give up active medical treatment in the last weeks, days or hours of life, a number of experts are now seeking to incorporate palliative care principles "upstream" in the LTC continuum (Kaplan & Urbina).

## TABLE 9.1

### Range of Long-Term Care Services

| TYPE OF SERVICE | EXAMPLE |
| --- | --- |
| Housekeeping and other IADL support | Cleaning, cooking, laundry, shopping, home maintenance, financial management |
| Companionship and social support | Visiting, calling, counseling, advising, case management |
| Transportation | Arranging, accompanying, providing transportation and escort services |
| Personal care | Hands-on, supervision or standby assistance with ADLs (bathing, dressing, walking, transferring, feeding, toileting) |
| Nursing and health care procedures | Assessment, care planning, promotion of optimum health status including recovery from acute illness and relief of symptoms |
| Rehabilitative services | Exercises and programs to improve or restore functioning (motion, speech, bowel, bladder) |
| Palliative care | Comfort care, symptom management, and medication management at the end of life |
| Care management | Planning and arranging appointments, equipment, transportation, and provider communication |

ADAPTED FROM: Kane, R. A. (1999). Goals of Home Care: Therapeutic, Compensatory, Either, or Both? *Journal of Aging and Health*, 11(3), 299–321, Tables 2 and 3.

In this chapter we adopt a *broad definition of LTC that encompasses a range of supportive, rehabilitative, nursing and palliative services provided to people—young or old—whose capacity to perform daily activities is restricted due to chronic disease or disability.* **TABLE 9.1** outlines the range of services we include in our definition of LTC and provides examples of each. LTC may be provided in institutions, congregate settings, or individual homes or apartments to people of all ages suffering from physical and mental disabilities. Family, friends, neighbors and other unpaid caregivers provide most LTC. Among paid providers, individual service providers include nurses, aides, therapists, social workers, case managers, physicians, and others. Organized providers include home health agencies, nursing homes, adult day centers, and a variety of community-based residential facilities including board and care homes and assisted living facilities. Service purchasers include individuals and families, as well as third parties such as state Medicaid agencies, area agencies on aging, private insurers, and managed LTC plans.

## LONG-TERM CARE NEEDS AND DEMANDS

In general, people who need help in carrying out one or more ADLs or IADLs due to physical disability, cognitive impairment, or both, are considered candidates for LTC. However, disabled individuals differ considerably in the severity of their limitations and their need for assistance. Some individuals may require direct "hands-on" assistance or supervision in order to meet their basic daily needs, while for others, special equipment or training can enable them to function relatively independently. Disability can be present from birth, as in the case of individuals with developmental disabilities; it may occur as the result of injury or disease; or it may manifest itself as a part of the aging process (General Accounting Office [GAO], 1999a).

Of the 9.5 million Americans who reported need for LTC services in 2000, approximately 63% were 65 years or older, and 37% were less than 65 (Rogers & Komisar, 2003). More than 4 out of 5 lived in the community, while just fewer than 1 in 5 were in institutions (Rogers & Komisar). TABLE 9.2 illustrates the wide range of conditions and impairments that regardless of age may lead to the need for LTC.

The body of work on "successful aging" shows that the majority of older Americans are generally healthy and that even among the "oldest old"—people aged 85 or older—44% are fully functional (Gibson et al., 2003). Nevertheless, as people age, they do become more dependent. They are at increased risk of the chronic diseases of old age—arthritis, hypertension and heart disease, diabetes, hearing and visual impairments, and Alzheimer's disease. They require help with tasks such as cleaning, shopping, and preparing meals. They also become more reliant on others for transportation and for assistance in activities of daily living, such as bathing, dressing, eating and moving from bed to chair. In 2003, adults age 85 or older were more than seven times as likely as adults age 65 to 74 to need personal assistance with activities of daily living (The Centers for Disease Control and Prevention [CDC], 2004b). (See FIGURE 9.1.)

Moreover, while a relatively small number (1.56 million) and percentage (4.5%) of people 65 and over live in nursing homes, the percentage increases dramatically with age, ranging from 1% of

## TABLE 9.2

**Examples of Conditions and Impairments Requiring Long-Term Care Services**

| CHRONIC ILLNESS | DEVELOPMENTAL DISABILITIES |
| --- | --- |
| Cancer | Cerebral palsy |
| Heart disease | Genetic or congenital defects |
| Emphysema | Seizure disorders |
| Alzheimer's disease | |
| Cystic fibrosis | |

| IMPAIRMENTS | INJURIES |
| --- | --- |
| Blindness | Paralysis from head and spinal cord injuries |
| Hearing loss | Burns |
| Paralysis | |

SOURCE: Richardson, H., Raphael, C., & Barton, B. (1998). Long-Term Care: Health, Social and Housing Services for Those with Chronic Illness. In A. R. Kovner & S. Jonas (Eds.), *Jonas and Kovner's Health Care Delivery in the United States* (6th ed., p. 209). New York: Springer Publishing Co.

## FIGURE 9.1

**Percentage of Adults Aged 65 Years and Over Who Need Help with Personal Care, by Age Group and Sex, January–September 2003**

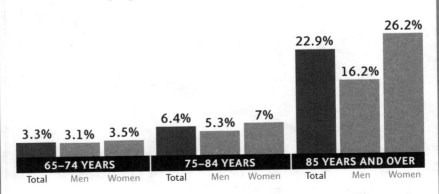

SOURCE: Centers for Disease Control and Prevention. (2004b). *Early Release of Selected Estimates Based on Data from the January–September 2003 National Health Interview Survey.* Available: http://www.cdc.gov/nchs/about/major/nhis/released200403.htm#12

persons 65 to 74 years to about 5% of persons 75 to 84 years and 18% of persons 85+. In addition, approximately 5% of the elderly live in self-described senior housing of various types, many of which have supportive services available to their residents (Administration on Aging [AoA], 2004b).

The demand for LTC is expected to grow in the coming years as both the absolute numbers and the proportion of older persons in the population increase. The absolute number of people age 65 and older will double between 2000 and 2030, from 35 million to 71.5 million (AoA, 2004a). Their share of the population will increase from 12% in 2000 to nearly 20% in 2030. The most significant growth will be among people 85 or older, who are at highest risk for disability and institutionalization. The absolute number of people age 85 and older will grow from about 4.2 million in 2000, to 9.6 million by 2030, when the first of the baby boomers reach their 85th birthday. By 2050, the number of people 85 and over will more than double again to over 20.8 million, or nearly 5% of the total population (AoA, 2004a). (See FIGURE 9.2.)

This exponential growth of the older population will almost certainly increase the absolute numbers of Americans who are

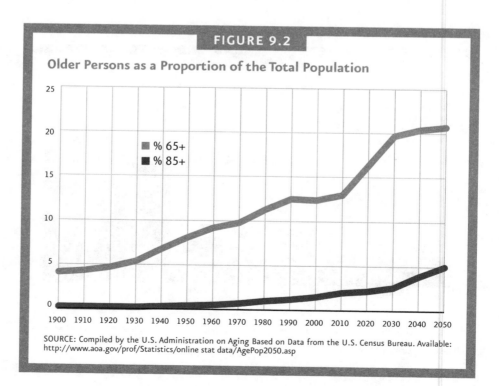

FIGURE 9.2

Older Persons as a Proportion of the Total Population

SOURCE: Compiled by the U.S. Administration on Aging Based on Data from the U.S. Census Bureau. Available: http://www.aoa.gov/prof/Statistics/online stat data/AgePop2050.asp

affected by chronic conditions and who experience related functional impairments. However, a number of recent studies suggest that increased demand for LTC may not be directly proportionate to increases in absolute numbers. This is because older people today tend to be less disabled than they were 10 or 20 years ago (Freedman, Martin, & Schoeni, 2002; Manton, Corder, & Stallard, 1997; Manton & Gu, 2001). For example, from 1989 to 1999, the number of persons 65 and older who reported any need for assistance rose from 6.6 to only 6.8 million—1.5 million fewer than would have been expected had disability rates stayed at the 1984 level (Gibson et al., 2003).

## U.S. SPENDING ON LONG-TERM CARE AND ITS FINANCING

In 2002, personal health care spending in the United States stood at more than $1.6 trillion. Determining how much of this enormous figure went toward LTC is difficult, because the national chart of health accounts does not clearly separate out LTC dollars from dollars that may be spent on post-hospital, subacute,[1] or end-of-life care. Moreover, the national system of accounting does not take into account the value of unpaid LTC services provided by family, friends, and neighbors.

Many estimates of formal LTC spending in the U.S. simply sum expenditures for nursing home and home health services. Thus, in 2002, a total of $139.3 billion was spent on nursing home and home health care—$103.2 billion or 74% went to pay for nursing home care and $36.1 billion or 26% went to home health services (Centers for Medicare & Medicaid Services [CMS], 2004b). Not all care provided by home health agencies and nursing homes, however, is long-term care. Virtually all home health agencies and many nursing homes also serve short-stay patients. Furthermore, LTC is provided by a wide variety of other organizations, such as local housekeeping agencies, aide registries, and "meals-on-wheels" programs, as well as community-based residences including "board and care" homes, assisted living facilities, and many others. A fuller estimate of LTC expenditures suggests that the U.S. spent at least $160 bil-

---

1 While post-acute care refers to care following a hospital stay, subacute refers to "a vague treatment modality that may bypass hospitals altogether or that focuses on longer-term rehabilitation, ventilation care, and the like" (Stone, 2000, p. 4).

lion on LTC in 2002—two thirds of this on nursing home care.[2] In addition, it has been estimated that the economic value of unpaid caregiving in the U.S. is close to $257 billion—nearly twice the annual cost of both nursing home and home care, an amount equivalent to 20% of all health care spending in the year the calculation was made (Arno, 2002).

The three major sources of financing for formal (i.e., paid) LTC services are Medicaid, Medicare, and personal out-of-pocket spending. According to estimates of the Congressional Budget Office (CBO), Medicaid accounted for approximately 35% of all LTC spending in 2004, followed by out-of-pocket expenditures (33%) and Medicare (25%) (Congressional Budget Office [CBO], 2004). Medicaid covered proportionately more nursing home than home care, while Medicare covered proportionately more home health than nursing home care. Although between them, Medicaid and Medicare cover about 60% of LTC spending, private out-of-pocket payments for LTC are quite substantial. Private health insurance covered less than 5% of LTC spending in 2004. (See FIGURE 9.3.)

Medicaid, the federal-state entitlement program that covers medical and other health-related services for selected low-income families and individuals, is the one national program with a clear mandate to cover long-term care. Within broad federal guidelines, each state determines the type, amount, duration, and scope of services its Medicaid program will cover, sets the rate of payment for services, and administers its own program (U.S. Department of Health and Human Services [USDHHS], 1999). The states are free to regulate the supply of nursing home beds in their respective jurisdictions and to determine rates of payment for Medicaid residents. However, federal rules are quite explicit with regard to eligibility for nursing home coverage. These rules stipulate that states must cover nursing home care for disabled individuals 65 and older with income up to three times the limit—$564 per month in 2004–for the federal Supplemental Security Income (SSI) program (CMS, 2004c). Furthermore, individuals may qualify by "spending down" their income and assets as a result of their institutionalization. In turn, they must contribute all of their income to their nursing

2 The $160 billion figure is the authors' calculation based on data from CMS, http://www.cms. hhs.gov/statistics/nhe/historical/tables.pdf plus Eiken, Burwell, & Schaefer (2003). Author's calculation: LTC costs = out of pocket HH and NH + other private HH and NH + private health insurance HH and NH + Medicare HH and NH + other federal HH and NH + Eiken et al. total Medicaid LTC.

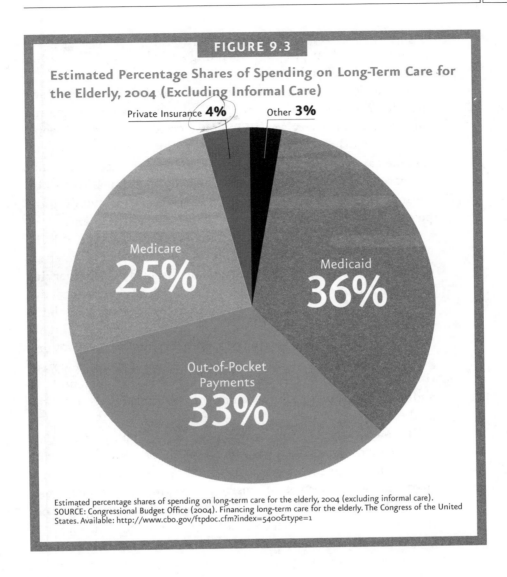

**FIGURE 9.3**

**Estimated Percentage Shares of Spending on Long-Term Care for the Elderly, 2004 (Excluding Informal Care)**

Private Insurance **4%**    Other **3%**

Medicare
**25%**

Medicaid
**36%**

Out-of-Pocket
Payments
**33%**

Estimated percentage shares of spending on long-term care for the elderly, 2004 (excluding informal care). SOURCE: Congressional Budget Office (2004). Financing long-term care for the elderly. The Congress of the United States. Available: http://www.cbo.gov/ftpdoc.cfm?index=5400&type=1

home care, except for a small personal needs allowance determined by the state. In 2002, federal, state, and local Medicaid dollars together accounted for 49% of all nursing home expenditures (CMS, 2004a), and Medicaid was the principal source of coverage for about two thirds of current nursing home residents (American Health Care Association [AHCA], 2003d).

Under federal guidelines, state Medicaid programs also are required to cover home health care ordered by a physician for people who are eligible for skilled nursing services. Under the "optional" category, they may choose to cover personal care for all eligibles. As of 2002, 32 states offered personal care as an optional benefit under their program, spending a total of $5.5 billion (Burwell, Sredl, & Eiken, 2004).

In addition, states may apply for a federal waiver that allows them to provide a broad array of medical and supportive home and community-based services (HCBS) to selected subgroups of people who would otherwise require nursing home care. Services can include case management, homemaker/chore services, and adult day care, as well as personal care. The waiver option allows states to limit the number receiving HCBS services, thus avoiding the potential liability conferred by an open-ended entitlement.

All states and the District of Columbia offer some type of HCBS waiver. By 2002, there were 250 approved waivers that targeted six eligibility groups, including the frail and disabled elderly, working age individuals with disabilities, people with developmental disabilities, persons with AIDS, children with a variety of disabling conditions, and individuals with serious mental illness (Eiken, Burwell, & Schaefer, 2003). In 2002, spending on HCBS waiver programs was $16.3 billion, about double the amount spent in 1997. Of this, about three quarters was for persons with developmental disabilities and about 20% for aged and other disabled persons (Eiken et al., 2003).

The Medicare program, which pays for skilled nursing home care (up to 100 days after a hospitalization for people who need continued nursing or therapy services) and home health services (on a "part-time" or "intermittent" basis), was originally intended to provide a finite, post-acute care benefit. Nevertheless, during the 1990s the Medicare home health benefit became an important source of LTC, especially in states with the least generous state and local-funded home care programs. Three main factors account for this phenomenon. First, settlement of a 1988 federal court case (Duggan v. Bowen, 1988) resulted in a relaxation of Medicare rules that had denied home health benefits to beneficiaries who did not show the potential for rehabilitation. Second, once a Medicare beneficiary qualifies for part-time or intermittent skilled nursing or rehabilitation services, a significant amount of home health aide-provided personal care also can be covered by Medicare payments. Third, while both Medicare payment and managed care created pressure on hospitals to reduce lengths of stay and move patients to other settings, payment for home health care continued to be based on per visit costs, providing an incentive for home health agencies to admit all types of patients and provide care generously. Between 1990 and 1997, the combination of these factors led to increases in both the proportion of Medicare beneficiaries receiving home health care and the number of visits per person. Over that period, the number using home health rose from 57 to 109 per 1,000 beneficiaries served. Similarly, the average number of visits went from 36 to 73 per user (GAO, 2000).

Although Medicare remains the major governmental payer of home health care, spending decreased to about $7.5 billion in 2003 from its peak of $18 billion in 1997 (USDHHS, 2003), due to changes in Medicare payment embodied in the Balanced Budget Act of 1997 (BBA) (P.L. 105–33, title IV, Chapter I). The BBA set forth an Interim Payment System (IPS), effective on October 1, 1997, that imposed an annual per beneficiary cap on the amount of money a home health agency could be reimbursed by Medicare. This was followed by a Prospective Payment System (PPS), effective on October 1, 2000, that introduced a fixed case-mix adjusted payment rate for each 60-day episode of home health care. Because both IPS and PPS eliminated fee for service payment and with it the incentive for home health agencies to provide as many visits as needed over as a long a time period as necessary, LTC experts were concerned that Medicare beneficiaries might be denied needed services. In fact, both the IPS and the PPS resulted in lower service use: the proportion of Medicare beneficiaries receiving home health care declined by nearly one third between 1997 and 2001, and the number of visits dropped even more dramatically—from 79 per user in 1997 to 32 per user in 2001, with the greatest drop in visits occurring for home health aid services (Murtaugh, McCall, Moore, & Meadow, 2003). Counteracting the declines in Medicare service use—at least over the short run—was a dramatic increase in the share of all home care services funded by Medicaid and by other state and local programs (Spector, Cohen, & Pesis-Katz, 2004). Information on the impact of PPS service reductions is still incomplete. However, analyses of the IPS found no clear evidence of harm to Medicare beneficiaries (McCall, Komisar, Petersons, & Moore, 2001; McCall, Korb, Petersons, & Moore, 2002). In general, the shrinking of services under Medicare home health has made the coordination of public and private, as well as state and local-funded, post-acute and LTC services more critical than ever (Murtaugh, McCall, Moore, & Meadow, 2003).

Given the limits of both Medicaid and Medicare LTC coverage, it is not surprising that out-of-pocket payments constitute a significant share of spending for both nursing home and HCBS users (Feder, Komisar, & Niefeld, 2000). The CBO estimated such spending, which does not include premium payments for private LTC insurance, at $44.5 billion in 2004, or about 33% of the total $135 billion spent on nursing home and home health care. The bulk of these payments went to cover the costs of nursing home care, as individuals contributed to the high yearly costs of those institutions—nearly $66,000 on average (CBO, 2004)—often depleting their assets and "spending down," thereby becoming eligible for Medicaid. Other out-of-pocket costs went to cover home-based services that were not covered by Medicare, Medicaid, or private insurance.

Purchase of private LTC insurance policies has grown rapidly. The industry claims an 18% increase for each year between 1987 and 2001 (Coronel, 2003). Much of this growth is likely due to an increased ability to purchase policies from employers, including the federal government, which made long-term care insurance available to federal employees in 2002. Nearly a quarter of all policies bought in 2001 were purchased through employers (Coronel, 2003). Nevertheless, private health insurance payments still covered only 7.5% of nursing home expenditures in 2002, down from the 8.4% of nursing home expenditures they covered in 1999 (CMS, 2004a). The CBO predicts that this share will rise to 17% by 2020 (CBO, 2004).

Because annual premiums tend to be high—from $1,000 to $2,300 at age 65 or $4,200 to $7,000 at age 79 (Coronel, 2003)—policies tend to be bought by more affluent individuals. (Premium ranges depend on whether or not the policy includes inflation protection or a nonforfeiture benefit.) Although premiums are significantly lower for younger purchasers, younger people are often unaware of the risks of LTC. Moreover, those who are more informed may be skeptical about the value of such policies, given uncertainty about both future service costs and future public LTC coverage policies. Although there is no consensus on the future importance of private insurance as a vehicle for covering LTC costs, some experts have estimated that over the next 20 years, 10 to 20% of retirees could have sufficient financial resources to enable them to purchase such policies (Tilly, Goldenson, Kasten, O'Shaughnessy, Kelly, & Sidor, 2000).

## TABLE 9.3

### Individual and Societal Goals for LTC

| INDIVIDUAL | SOCIETAL |
|---|---|
| Meet needs for care and assistance | Provide an adequate level of services to meet basic needs |
| Ensure comfort, safety, and freedom from pain | Target those most in need |
| Remain "at home" as long as possible in the face of disability and dependence | Promote the efficient production of cost-effective services |
| Maximize function; prevent or delay deterioration of functional abilities | Maximize individual responsibility |
| Access services readily | Promote a fair and equitable distribution of services |
| Maintain and improve physical, psychological, and social health and well-being | Provide comprehensive services |
| Improve self-knowledge and self-care abilities | Encourage reliance on "informal" systems of family provided care |
| Maximize independence, autonomy and individual choice | Facilitate consumer choice |
| Receive highest quality care | Ensure acceptable quality of services |
| Find information easily | Integrate and coordinate services |
| Minimize out-of-pocket costs | Contain costs to government and taxpayers |

## THE GOALS OF LONG-TERM CARE

We have discussed what LTC services are, who needs and gets them, and how they are financed. The goals of LTC, however, are less straightforward, primarily because LTC is not an end in itself but rather a means to multiple ends, depending on whose perspective is being considered. TABLE 9.3 lists some LTC goals expressed from the point of view of the *individual* consumer and from a broader *societal* perspective (Benjamin, 1999; Feldman, 1999; Kane, 1999).

These goals matter, because it is the balancing of individuals' goals with society's goals that determines the shape of LTC services. Clearly set, consistent goals could better guide providers' practices; they could also facilitate a more rational allocation of public LTC resources. However, setting clear goals is difficult. Government regulators, for example, aim to balance individual goals against societal goals but also need to consider providers' needs and interests. Legislators aim to satisfy their constituents by providing more alternatives to institutional care, while responding to other claims on the public purse, such as education and prisons.

In some cases, societal and individual goals correspond well. For example, both aim to facilitate individual choice. Often, however, individual goals expressed as desired outcomes for a single person receiving services or supports conflict with societal goals that define desired outcomes for financing and delivery systems, a step removed from the direct impact on an individual consumer (Benjamin, 1999).

In Table 9.3, virtually every individual goal embodies an element of subjective judgment.[3] For example, the definitions of "comfort," "safety," "function," "health," "well-being," "independence," "autonomy," and "choice" will vary from individual to individual and, for any one individual, over time, depending on conditions and circumstances. The very subjectivity of individual preferences and tastes suggests that individual choice and service direction will be important in any LTC service system that seeks to maximize goals that are important to consumers.

Some of the individual goals are *therapeutic goals*, in that they entail an effort to achieve measurable improvement—or to forestall measurable deterioration—in an individual's physical, psychological, or social health. In contrast, others are *compensatory goals*, in that they aim to compensate for an individual's functional impairments by facilitating comfort, safety, and autonomy in spite of disability. Therapeutic goals are generally associated with "medical models" of care, which tend to rely on professional assessment of clinical problems and clinical guidelines for treatment of specific conditions. In contrast, compensatory goals are generally associated with "social models" of care, which are more likely to emphasize consumer satisfaction and choice as indicators of success.

Third, some of the individual goals listed in Table 9.3 are contradictory. In recent years, the contradiction between safety and autonomy probably has received the most attention. Family members' concerns about safety often directly contradict their loved ones' desire to remain alone in their own homes. Yet safety concerns often win out over autonomy, particularly when families or

---

3 Much of the following discussion of goals is adapted from Feldman (1999).

public authorities assume legal or financial responsibility. Nevertheless, aging experts and consumer advocates increasingly make the case for informed risk-taking that would allow vulnerable individuals to stay at home with less protection than judged optimal to prevent harm or injury. In general, the greater priority given to individual autonomy as a goal of care, the greater the possibility that the individual's choice of services or supports to promote his or her well-being will clash with the recommendations of family or the expert judgments of an outside professional.

The list of societal goals also contains much subjectivity and many potential contradictions. For example, "adequate," "equitable," "acceptable," and even "cost effective" are all subject to widely different interpretations depending upon the discipline, philosophy, politics, socio-economic status, or institutional vantage point of those defining the terms. Furthermore, potential contradictions among goals abound. For example, depending on how "adequacy" and "basic" are defined, providing an adequate level of services to meet basic needs may imply providing services to a population different from those "most in need." Promoting a "fair and equitable" distribution of services may run counter to relying on informal, family provided care, while the latter may conflict with facilitating consumer choice. Facilitating consumer choice could raise system costs, depending on the range of choices provided, and thereby conflict with the goal of containing costs to government and taxpayers. Similarly, ensuring adequate quality of care across a diversity of settings and services may require increased government spending. These examples illustrate the challenges facing policymakers who struggle to finance LTC that is distributed equitably, with quality standards and proven efficiency, while promoting consumer choice and controlling costs. We return to some of these policy issues at the end of this chapter.

## PROVIDERS OF LONG-TERM CARE
A wide variety of agencies, facilities, and individuals including formal and informal caregivers provide long-term care in various settings, as described in the following sections.

### Unpaid Caregivers
The vast majority of long-term care in the U.S. is provided by family, friends, neighbors, and other unpaid caregivers. Unpaid care

provided by these individuals is usually referred to as "informal care." However, many advocates object to the term "informal," which seems to belie the amount of time, effort, organization, and coordination dedicated to carrying out such activities.

In 1994, approximately 57% (2.2 million) of elderly LTC users who lived in the community relied solely on unpaid caregivers for assistance, with at least one ADL or IADL. Over a third (1.4 million) relied on a mix of unpaid caregivers and paid services, while only 5% (256,000) relied solely on paid help. Among the 5.9 million unpaid caregivers, approximately two thirds were the spouses or children of care recipients. Furthermore, approximately 30% were over 65 years old themselves. More than a third of unpaid caregivers were female, and a little more than half were married. Although they were more likely to assist persons limited in IADLs only, 32% cared for persons with at least 3 ADL limitations (Spector, Fleishman, Pezzin, & Spillman, 1998). Recent data from a large national survey covering all adults 18 years and older found that 13.2 million adults received 21.5 billion hours of personal assistance services per year, of which 18.7 billion or 87% were provided by unpaid caregivers (LaPlante, Harrington, & Kang, 2002).

Most experts would agree that family care has been undervalued in our society. First, there has been no official governmental effort—comparable, for example, to the national health accounting system—to calculate the dollar value of unpaid services, which, as noted above, has been estimated to be over $250 billion. Second, despite an abundant literature on caregiver burden and stress, systematic efforts to provide information, training, support, and respite to family caregivers are quite recent and not well funded. The range of short-term respite services—which may be supplied at home, in adult day care centers, or in institutions (e.g., nursing homes, hospitals, or foster care homes)—varies across states (Kane & Kane, 1987; Meltzer, 1982; Richardson, Raphael, & Barton, 1998) and suffers from limited funding dispersed among a wide variety of sources.

The undervaluing of family care is all the more remarkable given nearly universal acknowledgment that the availability of families willing to care for their loved ones is probably the pivotal factor in preventing or postponing nursing home placement, thus limiting government's financial responsibility for the institutional care of indigent elders. Although lawmakers continue to propose a variety of initiatives, including tax deductions, tax credits, and federal appropriations designed to support informal care giving, only one significant initiative has been approved. Through the Older Americans Act, Congress has funded a National Family Caregiver Support Program (P.L.–106–501) authorized to establish support networks providing: (a) information about the availability of support services for family caregivers, (b) assistance in gaining access to these services, (c) individual counseling to help make decisions and solve problems, (d) respite care, and (e) supplemental services. Funding for this program rose from $125 million in its first year (FY 2001) to $155.2 million in FY 2003.

## Paid Caregivers

Since the Medicare and Medicaid programs were signed into law in 1965, the supply of LTC services has been heavily influenced by the primary payer of those services—government. The two major types of organizations that have evolved to provide LTC in the U.S. are home care agencies and nursing homes. Many more people receive home care than nursing home care, although expenditures for the latter are much higher, due to the more complicated range of services provided and the inclusion of housing costs in the nursing home payment. In addition, a small but growing number of individuals receive LTC services in adult day centers, while many more are being served by a large and growing number of "alternative" community-based residential settings, such as assisted living facilities, board and care or adult family homes, and—for the very affluent—continuing care retirement communities.

### Home Care Agencies

In 2002, nearly 7,000 home health agencies were certified to provide medically related services to Medicare beneficiaries (MedPAC, 2004), while a larger but unknown number of agencies—generally unlicensed—provided nonmedical personal care, housekeeping, or chore services (including, for example, meals on wheels) in individual homes and congregate residential settings. Medicare-certified home health agencies (CHHAs) provide skilled nursing, rehabilitation, and home health aide services to individuals in their place of residence to promote, maintain, or restore health and/or to maximize independence while minimizing the effects of disease and disability (Haupt, 1998). Individuals receiving Medicare services from CHHAs must be homebound and demonstrate medical necessity for intermittent, part-time, skilled nursing or therapy services ordered by a physician. Medicare requirements often influence states' Medicaid programs, in that their Medicaid home health eligibility rules often match Medicare's, although care recipients must meet a state's definition of *indigence* to be eligible for service. To fund long-term home and community-based services outside the home health rubric, all states also operate some type of Medicaid home and community-based waiver program (as previously discussed in the section on LTC spending).

Since the introduction of the Medicare program, the home health industry has changed considerably in both composition and size. Although community-based visiting nurse associations were historically the predominant provider of home health services, both hospital-based and proprietary agencies have assumed a significant role in the industry. Today voluntary nonprofit agencies, including VNAs and nonprofit-hospital-based agencies, account for approximately a third of all CHHAs, while public agencies account for approximately 15%, and proprietary agencies, which were nonexistent in 1967, account for half (MedPAC, 2004). Overall, the number of Medicare-certified agencies increased from fewer than 2,000 in 1967 to about 6,000 in 1985, to over 9,000 in 1997, before declining

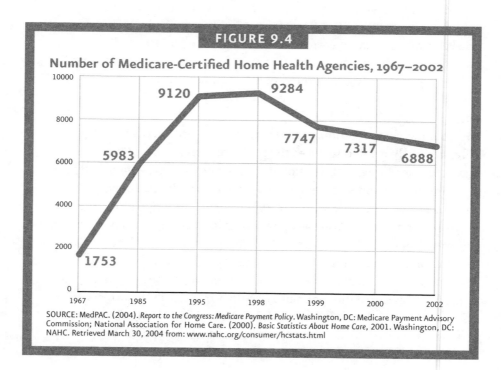

**FIGURE 9.4**

**Number of Medicare-Certified Home Health Agencies, 1967–2002**

SOURCE: MedPAC. (2004). *Report to the Congress: Medicare Payment Policy.* Washington, DC: Medicare Payment Advisory Commission; National Association for Home Care. (2000). *Basic Statistics About Home Care,* 2001. Washington, DC: NAHC. Retrieved March 30, 2004 from: www.nahc.org/consumer/hcstats.html

to 7,104 in 2003 (CMS, 2003a). (See **FIGURE 9.4**.) Multiple and complex reasons are behind the rapid growth, changing composition, and recent decline in the number of CHHAs. However, the responsiveness of the proprietary sector to changes in Medicare entitlement and payment policy has played a significant role (GAO, 2000). For example, in 1998 and 1999, after implementation of the payment changes mandated by the BBA of 1997, more than 1,800 or 36% of for-profit agencies closed, compared to 14 to 15% of nonprofits (National Association for Home Care, 2000).

Among the array of LTC services, home health services touch the greatest number of people. In 2000, U.S. home health agencies discharged approximately 7.2 million people. An estimated 1.4 million—most of them Medicare beneficiaries—were receiving home health services at any one time (the sources for this figure and others in this paragraph are CDC, 2004a, 2004c). The typical home health patient is 65 years of age or older (71%), female (65%), white (76%), and married or widowed (67%). Individuals with primary diagnosis of diseases of the circulatory system—most often some type of heart disease—comprise the single largest share of home health patients (23.6%). Those with cancer, diabetes, chronic obstructive pulmonary disease, fractures, and osteoarthritis and related conditions comprise an additional 26%. More than half (51%) received help with ADLs; 43% received help with IADLs.

Most home health patients enter care after a hospitalization, and approximately a third have just had a surgical or diagnostic procedure. In 2000, nearly two thirds of home health patients were discharged either because they had recovered or their condition had stabilized (27%), or because services were no longer needed or their treatment plan was complete (36.6%). Another 23% were discharged because their care was being provided by another source (family or friends, transferred to another agency, or admitted to a hospital or nursing home) (CDC, 2004c).

Insofar as home health care focuses on helping patients learn how to better self-manage complex chronic conditions such as diabetes, heart failure or chronic lung disease, it is generally viewed as an economical way to prevent unnecessary hospitalizations or rehospitalizations (Haupt, 1998; Rich, 2003). In 2001, for a home health patient with heart failure, the average Medicare payment was approximately $4,265 and the average number of visits 41; for a patient with diabetes, the corresponding figures were $5,229 and 64, respectively; while for a patient with chronic airway obstruction they were $3,859 and 37. The average yearly cost for home health patients across all conditions was $3,557, encompassing 32 visits[4] (Murtaugh et al., 2003). In contrast, Medicare paid on average $10,817 for a single hospital discharge, while it paid $8,528 for a heart failure discharge, $9,820 for diabetes and $10,320 for respiratory disease[5] (USDHHS, 2001).

*Hospice Services*

Hospice care is defined as a program of palliative care that provides physical, psychological, social, and spiritual services to terminally ill individuals, as well as support to their families and other loved ones (Haupt, 1998). Hospices are staffed by interdisciplinary teams that include physicians, nurses, medical social workers, therapists, and counselors, complemented by volunteers, who develop and implement a coordinated plan of care that is sensitive to the personal and cultural values of individual care recipients and their families. The main goals of palliative care, which need not be confined to formal hospice programs, are to sustain the highest quality of life attainable through the control of pain and symptoms and to maintain care recipients' independence, comfort, and dignity through the period of terminal illness, whether short- or long-term (Hospice Association of America, 2001; Kaplan & Urbina, 2000; Richardson et al., 1998).

Medicare has significantly shaped the hospice industry. Since it began funding hospice services in 1983, it has become their primary source of financing, and providers, patients, and program expenditures have increased dramatically. For the terminally ill beneficiaries who enroll, the Medicare hospice benefit encompasses a wide range of medical and palliative services, including medications, medical supplies, and hospitalization if necessary. Medicare hospice expenditures rose from $205.4 million in 1989 to more than $3.6 billion in 2001 (Hospice Association of America, 2002), while the proportion of decedent Medicare beneficiaries who were enrolled in hospice grew from fewer than 1 in 10 to more than 1 in 5 (Campbell, Lynn, Louis, & Shugarman, 2004).

The Medicare program certified nearly 2,300 participating hospices in the U.S. in 2002. The Hospice Association of America esti-

---

4 Figures are in nominal 2001 dollars, calculated from the inflation-adjusted figures presented in Murtaugh et al. (2003).

5 Dollar figures were derived by inflation-adjusting the 1999 figures presented in U.S. Department of Health and Human Services (2001), Table 27, to 2001 dollars.

mated that, in addition, approximately 200 volunteer hospices were in operation that year. Little information is available about hospices that do not participate in Medicare or Medicaid, as rules for licensure and regulation vary state to state. Among Medicare-certified hospices, about 45% are freestanding, mostly nonprofit organizations. Approximately 30% are owned and operated by home health agencies (both nonprofit and proprietary), 25% are hospital-based, and fewer than 1% are operated by nursing homes (Hospice Association of America, 2002).

In fiscal year 2000, about 620,000 people received hospice services (CDC, 2004d), nearly 10 times the number of hospice recipients in 1989 (Hospice Association of America, 2002). About 80% received care from a voluntary, nonprofit hospice organization (CDC, 2004d). Half of hospice patients were female, 80% were 65 or older, 84% white, 47% married, and 33% widowed. Although the most common admission diagnosis for hospice patients remains cancer (58%), its prevalence has been reduced significantly from 1992, when it accounted for more than three quarters of hospice recipients. The average hospice patient spent about 50 days in care, and 86% were discharged due to death. Another 3% were discharged because someone else took over their care (CDC, 2004d).

Medicare hospice services are generally viewed as cost effective. A recent study of Medicare program expenditures associated with hospice use found hospice to be "cost-neutral to cost-saving" for people who die of cancer but cost-adding for those who die of other causes (Campbell et al., 2004). There was also some evidence that early entry to hospice could reduce added costs for people with terminal illnesses other than cancer. The study concluded that even though in some cases hospice care might cost Medicare somewhat more than conventional care, its quality of life benefits for both patients and caregivers might well merit those costs (Campbell et al., 2004). Nevertheless, several barriers have prevented expansion of palliative care either among the terminally ill or to those who are at an earlier stage of illness. These include: (a) Medicare's relatively strict eligibility rules, which require a life expectancy of six months or less, (b) the lack of systematic training of physicians in palliative care principles, and (c) the widespread perception on the part of both professionals and lay persons that opting for palliative care means "giving up" (Kaplan & Urbina, 2000). As the end-of-life care movement gains momentum, and with it a broader understanding that hospice and hospice-like services are a humane and compassionate way to deliver health care and supportive services to the terminally ill, some of these obstacles may give way to wider financing and broader accessibility.

### Nursing Homes

Nursing homes in the U.S. vary significantly in ownership, size, services, and the population served. For purposes of classification, the federal government defines nursing homes as facilities with three or more beds that routinely provide nursing care services (Gabrel, 2000). They may be free standing or a distinct unit of a larger facility or chain. In 2003, the industry consisted of approximately 16,400 homes with approximately 1.7 million beds (American Health Care Association [AHCA], 2003a). For-profit nursing homes accounted for nearly two thirds of all facilities and beds, while nonprofit homes comprised 28% and government homes 6% of total facilities (AHCA, 2003c; CMS, 2003b). Forty-eight percent of nursing homes functioned independently, while 53% operated as part of a chain (i.e., a group of facilities under one general authority or ownership) (AHCA, 2003b). In 1999, the average size nursing home had 105 beds. Only 8% of homes had more than 200 beds, while 11.5% had fewer than 50 (Jones, 2002).

The nursing home industry is heavily dependent on Medicare and Medicaid reimbursement, which requires facilities to meet federal standards enforced through annual inspections and complaint investigations conducted by the states. Approximately 80% of nursing homes are certified by both Medicare and Medicaid, another 16% by one of the two programs, while just 2% operate with state licensure only (Jones, 2002). All employ paid staff to provide basic medical and personal care to address the long-term needs of frail residents.

Over the last 20 years, U.S. nursing homes have experienced significant changes in the services they provide and the populations they serve. Where the sole purpose of many institutions was once to provide a permanent residence for frail individuals, especially elders, to live out the last years of their lives, today nursing homes serve a more varied population. Many facilities provide medically intensive, rehabilitative services to patients who stay for a short time only, and a number have added special care units for patients with special needs (e.g., Alzheimer's disease, AIDS, brain injury, ventilator-dependency, or hospice care) (Rhoades & Krauss, 1999). A major concern for nursing homes is the increasing cost of liability insurance and malpractice claims. Altogether, liability costs have risen at an average of 24% since 1991 (CMS, 2003b).

The shift to providing more medically-oriented services to a short-stay population can be seen in nursing home revenue trends. In 1980, Medicare accounted for less than 2% of nursing home expenditures, whereas it accounted for over 12.5% in 2002 (CMS, 2004a). Even with increased provision of Medicare-reimbursed services, however, Medicaid still accounts for half of nursing home payments (CMS, 2004a). Furthermore, at any one time, about 60% of nursing home residents have Medicaid as their primary source of expected payment (Jones, 2002).

Nursing homes residents are typically the oldest old, and the average age of the residential population has been rising. In 1999, nearly 8 out of 10 residents were 75 years of age or older, while nearly half were 85 or older, and just 10% were under 65 (Jones, 2002). Seventy-two percent of nursing home residents were female, while just over a quarter were male. More than 8 out of 10 residents (86%) were white, while the remainder were black or "other" (Jones, 2002). The under-representation of minorities has been attributed to their greater reliance on informal care, as well as to the discriminatory practices of some nursing homes (Richardson et al., 1998).

Marital status is one of the two most important predictors of whether an individual enters a nursing home. Among those who are disabled, the availability of a spouse to provide supportive help is a key factor in averting or delaying nursing home entry. According to one recent quantitative study, the presence of a spouse more than halves the probability of nursing home entry, and other studies have shown that the death of a spouse is the life event most likely to trigger nursing home entrance (Lakdawalla & Philipson, 2000). Thus, it is not surprising that among elderly nursing home residents in 1999, only 18% were married, while the rest were widowed, divorced, or never married (Jones, 2002).

Disability is the major predictor of nursing home entry, and by virtually any measure, nursing home residents are extremely disabled. In 1999 three quarters of residents needed assistance with three or more ADLs, including 11% who needed help with five ADLs (Jones, 2002) (see **FIGURE 9.5**). About 3 out of 5 residents used a wheelchair and another quarter used a walker. Nearly one half were visually and/or hearing impaired. Nearly 60% had difficulty controlling bowel and/or bladder, including 44% who had difficulty

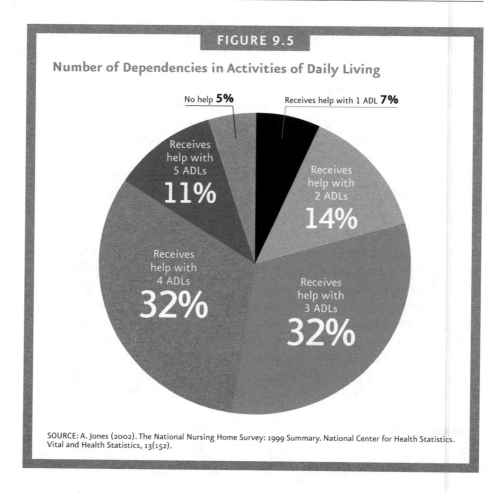

### FIGURE 9.5

## Number of Dependencies in Activities of Daily Living

No help **5%**

Receives help with 1 ADL **7%**

Receives help with 5 ADLs
**11%**

Receives help with 2 ADLs
**14%**

Receives help with 4 ADLs
**32%**

Receives help with 3 ADLs
**32%**

SOURCE: A. Jones (2002). The National Nursing Home Survey: 1999 Summary. National Center for Health Statistics. Vital and Health Statistics, 13(152).

controlling both. Among those residents discharged from a nursing home in the year ending September 1999, only 13% were discharged because they had recovered, whereas another 20% were discharged after stabilization. More than a third were admitted to a hospital or another nursing home, and 24% died (Jones).

The future need for nursing home beds in the U.S. will depend on a number of factors, including demographic changes resulting in a rapidly aging population, patterns of marriage and disability, public and private financing policies, and the availability of nursing home alternatives. Caution is required in projecting future nursing home use based on past utilization patterns, lest projections yield overestimates of needed facility beds. In the mid-1970s, for example, the nursing home population grew at a 4.8% annual rate. By the early 1980s, however, this rate had fallen to 1.7%, and in the late 1980s to early 1990s, the growth rate dropped even further, to about 0.4% per year. Furthermore, this drop occurred even though the average annual increase in the older population remained at a roughly constant annual rate of 2.7%. Improvements in older persons' health almost certainly played a part: first, age-specific disability rates declined for all older people, and second, longer living male spouses were available to support their wives at home (Lakdawalla & Philipson, 2000). Rising obesity and resulting illnesses and disabilities might slow the rates of improvement in future years (Sturm, Ringel, & Andreyeva, 2004). Nevertheless, increases in the use of home health and other alternatives to institutional care suggest that elders' LTC needs will increasingly be met outside of nursing homes, whatever their underlying patterns of disability.

### Adult Day Services

Adult day services (ADS) are community-based group programs that are becoming an important component of the overall mix of home and community-based LTC. These programs, which are mainly non-profit (78%), provide a variety of health, social, and other support services in a protective setting during any part of a day, but for less than 24 hours. The aim is not to supplant, but rather to support informal services, enabling chronically ill people to stay at home. ADS are particularly suited to the needs of informal caregivers who work during the day, although these centers can also provide respite for nonworking caregivers.

Normally, clients visit adult day centers for a full day a few days a week. Centers serve a variety of populations, such as those with memory impairment (the most significant category, at 52% of participants), frail elders with no dementia (41%), persons with mental retardation/developmental disabilities (24%), and those with physical disabilities (23%). (All figures on ADS come from Partners in Caregiving 2003, which provides the results of a national survey of ADS in the United States.)

There are three primary forms of ADS: one, comprising 21% of all centers, is known as adult day health services. These "medical model" centers seek to provide a full array of health and health-related services, including nursing services and medication management. Another is known as adult day care or "social model" ADS. These, which make up 40% of all centers, provide a range of nonmedical support services. The remainder comprises a third form, which combines features of the other two. In 2002, there were 3,407 centers operating across the country, mostly located in more densely populated parts of the country. However, both urban and rural areas likely could support more ADS. Partners in Caregiving (2003) estimated that 3,991 new adult day centers are needed in urban areas and 1,424 in rural areas.

Nearly all adult day centers provide some types of therapeutic activities (97%) and personal assistance—help with meals, walking, and toileting—(96%); most provide meals (84%) and social services (82%). Among the other services provided, 74% are health-related services, 70% medication management, 68% transportation, 64% help with bathing and grooming, 47% nursing, 28% rehabilitation therapy, 12% medical services, and only 7% provide hospice.

ADS centers charge an average of $46 a day—although it costs an average of $56 per day to serve a client—making subsidies an important part of center financing. Public programs account for 38% of revenues, while private pay participants account for a little over a third (35%). Another 14% of centers' funding comes from nonoperating revenue such as grants and donations. The final 13% comes from other operating revenue, including managed care. Despite (or perhaps because of) this array of funding sources, 44% of centers reported a deficit in 2002.

Quality control for ADS is still under development. Currently, about three quarters of centers are licensed or certified by their state, while the rest either operate in states where certification and licensure do not exist, or where they are not required. In addition, although centers can be accredited through CARF (the Commission on Accreditation of Rehabilitation Facilities), relatively few are currently accredited or plan to apply for accreditation.

## Community-Based Residential Alternatives to Institutional Care

Many adults experiencing or anticipating some disabling condition are seeking noninstitutional residential settings that will allow them to live independently of family but will provide necessary assistance with personal care, meals, and other household activities. Proponents of community-based residential care maintain that these settings provide a better quality of life compared to nursing homes. Many state policymakers also are hopeful that shifting LTC spending from nursing homes to residential alternatives will result in a more affordable system.

Responding to the demand for a range of supported housing options, community-based residential care and assisted living facilities (ALFs) provide housing, food, supervision or protective oversight, and personal assistance to individuals who wish to receive LTC services in a setting other than in a nursing facility or their own home. These residential nursing home alternatives are marketed, reimbursed, and regulated under various labels and definitions across and within states. Their labels include "board and care," "adult family homes," "personal care homes," "assisted living facilities," and some 20 others. Even the single category "assisted living" can encompass a wide range of residential settings-with-services, depending on whether or not a state chooses to license these facilities and how it defines their essential features.

Ardent proponents of home-like settings argue that the defining features of an ALF should be private rooms and bathrooms, lockable doors, and individual cooking facilities or appliances. In addition, these proponents argue that ALFs should have available a range of services, including assessment and care planning, personal care, medication assistance, the option of three meals per day, and 24-hour staffing and access to nursing services. However, a recent survey of facilities that self-identified as ALFs suggests that the great majority of these residential settings for older persons do not fit the assisted living model put forward by proponents. When facilities were classified along two dimensions—privacy and services—only a small percentage (11%) were found to offer both a high level of services and a high level of privacy (Hawes, Rose, & Phillips, 1999). Thus only a small portion of self-identified ALFs nationwide meet the definition of what many consider "assisted living."

Depending on the state and the services provided, residential care settings may or may not be licensed. Thus, an estimate of their numbers is necessarily imprecise. One recent estimate concluded that there were approximately 36,000 *licensed* residences for older adults in the U.S. in 2002, with approximately 910,000 "beds" (Mollica, 2002). Other sources have estimated that more than a million people over 65 reside in some kind of community residential setting (American Association of Homes and Services for the Aging [AAHSA], 2000b). Although current residents of alternative settings are less disabled, on average, than nursing home residents, they often have significant disabilities. One national survey found that almost one fourth of residents in ALFs[6] received help with at least three ADLS, and approximately one third had moderate to severe cognitive impairments (Hawes et al., 1999).

The variation among community residential facilities is enormous. Some of these settings are designed to be like small family homes; others may house up to 1,000 individuals in semi-private rooms; while others, such as some ALFs, are designed as apartment-like residences with private bathrooms, cooking facilities, and lockable doors. The services provided range from light housekeeping to assistance with medications or activities of daily living to daily nursing care on an "as needed" basis (Hawes et al., 1999). Some facilities provide these services themselves, while others arrange for outside service providers, while still others require residents to arrange for services beyond a bare minimum.

The cost of living in a residential care facility ranges from a few hundred dollars to more than $3,000 per month based on the type of services available. Residences usually use one of four payment models. Some use an all-inclusive rate model that charges residents a flat fee for housing and all other services. Others use a "basic/enhanced model" that provides a pre-defined group of services (including housing) for a flat fee, and charges residents an additional fee for all other services utilized. A third group of facilities uses a fee-for-service model that charges residents for each service used. Finally, a fourth "service level model" charges residents a fixed fee based on a predetermined level of care (AAHSA, 2000a).

While individuals' monthly SSI or social security payments may be sufficient to cover the housing, room and board costs in low-price, low-service facilities, such payments are usually insufficient to cover the costs in facilities located in expensive urban areas or offering a high level of services or amenities. Acting on the assumption that savings can be realized by diverting individuals in need of LTC services from nursing homes to less costly residential settings, many states have begun to fund the nonresidential service component of alternative community care settings through the Medicaid program. By the end of 2002, some 40 states funded at least some LTC services in ALFs or other supportive housing settings, primarily

---

6 The study's three basic eligibility criteria were that a facility had to have more than 10 beds and serve a primarily elderly population. In addition, the facility had to either represent itself as an assisted living facility or offer at least a basic level of services, which were: 24-hour staff oversight, housekeeping, at least two meals a day, and personal assistance, defined as help with at least tow of the following: medications, bathing, or dressing.

through their Medicaid home and community-based waiver programs (Mollica, 2002). Still, public financing of LTC services in ALFs and other residential settings is relatively modest (Stevenson, Murtaugh, Feldman, & Oberlink, 2000). Even so, the most common source of payment is out-of-pocket payments by residents or family members. In addition, private LTC insurance may be used to cover some costs (AAHSA, 2000a).

State efforts to expand residential LTC options have been tempered by concerns about quality of care (Stevenson et al., 2000), and their reduced ability to support the expansion of infrastructure due to recent budget crises. One particular area of concern is the retention of individuals as they grow more frail and disabled. Two somewhat contradictory fears about retention policies lead to quality concerns. On the one hand is the concern that residents will be discharged as soon as their care needs increase, preventing individuals from aging in place. Indeed, available information indicates that many board-and-care homes and ALFs reject applicants with wheelchairs, incontinence, cognitive impairments, or who need their medications dispensed to them. Residents who incur such disabilities may be relocated to another facility. According to one survey, for example, only one quarter of ALFs will retain residents who have behavioral problems (e.g., wandering or mild dementia) (Hawes et al., 1999). On the other hand, those responsible for monitoring quality are concerned that residents will not be discharged to a more intensive setting if their needs outstrip what a community residence can provide. The incentive to hold onto residents may be strongest in areas where the market for residential alternatives to nursing homes is relatively saturated, making high occupancy (and profitability) more difficult to maintain. The difficulty of balancing these two concerns has made it especially difficult for states to develop uniform regulatory policy in this area.

### Continuing Care Retirement Communities

Continuing Care Retirement Communities (CCRCs) are a type of community residential care facility that has explicitly addressed the resident retention issue in its model of care, which is designed to meet the changing health and personal care needs of occupants over the remainder of their lifetime. The model offers more than one level of care, ranging from independent living in a housing and/or apartment complex, to assisted living, to nursing home care. Among the services offered by CCRCs are meals, transportation, social services and nursing services, as well as recreational and educational activities. In addition, many CCRCs are equipped with amenities such as banks, barber shops, fitness centers, and gardening facilities.

The Continuing Care Accreditation Commission (CARF-CCAC), an independent, third-party accreditation system acquired in 2003 by the Commission on Accreditation of Rehabilitation Facilities, estimates that in 2004 approximately 2,500 CCRCs were in operation in the 50 states and the District of Columbia. However, most are situated in just a few states: Pennsylvania, California, Florida, Illinois, and Ohio. The number of CCRCs increased by about 75% from 1996 to 2000, with a corresponding increase in the number of residents, from 350,000 to 625,000 (AAHSA, 2000b; Richardson et al., 1998). The average age of CCRC residents is over 80 years, and three quarters of residents are female. About 30% of residents are married couples living together, a feature that distinguishes CCRCs from other types of residential facilities (AAHSA, 2000b).

Residents can choose from a variety of coverage options and a range of payment plans. Coverage can include unlimited access to specified health services, or the resident can opt to pay for these on a fee-for-service basis. Similarly, the resident can pay for accommodation on a rental basis, or purchase real estate or membership in the CCRC.

Despite variation in rates based on region, size, and amenities, most CCRCs are costly and not widely affordable. In the year 2000, entrance fees, which may be fully or partially refundable, ranged from $45,000 to $108,000, depending on the size of the living unit. Monthly rates ranged from approximately $1,100 for a studio to $1,800 for a two-bedroom dwelling, although additional fees could be required, depending on the payment plan (AAHSA, 2000b). Moreover, there has been concern about their financial viability and capacity to provide heavy nursing care to residents who will eventually require it. Thus, they are not viewed as a mainstream solution to the demand for affordable community-based residential care facilities.

## CHALLENGING ISSUES

Containing costs, promoting access, and assuring quality of needed services—the classic triumvirate of U.S. health care policy problems—pose a set of challenges for current and future LTC policymakers. On the cost side, LTC looms as a large and growing component of health care expenditures, particularly of overstressed state budgets. On the access side, the institutional bias of the LTC system has limited development of and access to affordable community-based alternatives to nursing home care. Furthermore, reliance on Medicaid and personal savings as the two main sources of LTC financing means that many people forego necessary or beneficial services until the need becomes urgent, when they risk impoverishment if they avail themselves of LTC. Meanwhile, the future availability of an adequate range of LTC services (including the necessary infrastructure for home-based services) is uncertain. Finally, on the quality side, increased regulation has yielded some measurable improvements in nursing home care—the principal target of improvement efforts. Nevertheless, serious quality issues remain for all service settings. Clearly, innovative payment, quality, and financing policies—drawing on a mix of public and private responsibility—will be needed to sustain and expand a viable LTC system that can meet the needs of a rapidly growing older population.

## Containing Costs While Improving Access

For many years policymakers, particularly state policymakers, have been concerned about the rising costs of LTC, a concern that can only heighten as the disabled and elderly population grows in size. LTC expenditures constituted approximately 12% of U.S. personal health care spending in 2002,[7] and the burden on state and local Medicaid spending was twice as heavy. Of $95.4 billion that state and local governments spent on Medicaid out of their own coffers, $24.2 billion or 25% went to cover nursing home and home health services (CMS, 2004d).

In general, states have employed three broad strategies to control their LTC expenditures: (a) substituting private or federal dollars for state dollars, (b) shifting the cost control burden to providers by controlling nursing home bed supply or cutting provider payment rates, and (c) attempting to reform the health care delivery system, through some combination of integrating

7 This percentage was calculated by dividing $160 billion in LTC costs for 2002 by $1.340 trillion in personal health care expenditures (Levit, Cowan, Lazenby, Sensenig, McDonnell, Stiller, et al., 2000). (The $160 billion figure is the authors' calculation based on data from CMS, http://www.cms.hhs.gov/statistics/nhe/historical/tables.pdf, plus Eiken, Burwell and Schaefer, 2003. Author's calculation: LTC costs = out of pocket HH and NH + other private HH and NH + private health insurance HH and NH + Medicare HH and NH + other federal HH and NH + Eiken et al. total Medicaid LTC.)

acute and LTC services and/or increasing the availability of HCBS alternatives to institutional care (Wiener & Stevenson, 1998). The first strategy includes the creation of incentives for individuals to purchase private LTC insurance, for example, by allowing pur-chasers of such insurance to keep more assets than generally required to qualify for Medicaid coverage when their insurance benefits run out. It also includes "musical chairs" initiatives designed to shift as many LTC costs as possible from state Medicaid budgets to the federal Medicare program. The second, "provider burden" strategy, based on the assumption that "a bed built is a bed filled," includes the use of state "certificate of need" laws to control the building of nursing beds. It also includes tight reimbursement controls on Medicaid nursing home rates, a practice made possible by repeal of a federal law that required states to pay nursing homes "reasonable costs."

The third strategy, system reform, has two variants. One involves experimenting with ways of consolidating Medicare and Medicaid funding streams and capitating payments to managed care entities that assume responsibility for providing LTC, as well as acute and primary care services, to dually eligible Medicare/Medicaid beneficiaries. The second variant involves using a host of state incentives to foster the growth of HCBS and community-based residential care options, which can then be used to divert individuals from nursing homes.

None of the three strategies has produced unmitigated, resound-ing success; however, several show promise. Efforts to increase pri-vate resources going toward LTC by encouraging individuals to pur-chase LTC insurance policies have been associated with increased private purchase of LTC insurance policies, which have grown at the rate of about 18% per year over the last decade (Coronel, 2003). Much of this growth is probably attributable to forces other than state initiatives per se. Nevertheless, states can benefit if pur-chasers are drawn from the group of middle income elders with few informal supports who might otherwise divest themselves of assets or spend down to qualify for Medicaid coverage.

Systems reforms that focus on pooling financing for long-term, primary and acute care services have also shown promise. Advo-cates of this approach argue that integrated funding for people dually eligible for Medicare and Medicaid not only will be less expensive due to reductions in cost-shifting, but also will lead to gains in service effectiveness and efficiency through better care management. Several models have received widespread attention. One is the Arizona Long Term Care System (ALTCS), which had enrolled 38,591 individuals as of February 2004 (Arizona Health Care Cost Containment System [ALTCS], 2004). ALTCS, a statewide program, capitates Medicaid acute and LTC services, which are generally provided alongside but not financially integrated with Medicare-covered services. While outside evaluators agree that ALTCS has saved money, there is some disagreement about the extent to which savings are attributable to the effective management of LTC services or to the program's restrictive eligibility requirements (Sparer, 1999; Weissert, 1997). A second model is the social HMO, or SHMO, in which a limited LTC benefit is included in a traditional Medicare HMO's capitated rate and service package. SHMOs had difficulty, however, encouraging physicians to work cooperatively with social workers and LTC providers to create a coordinated system of care (Harrington, Lynch, & Newcomer, 1993), resulting in a second generation of SHMOs that has attempted to address these problems more fully. Meanwhile, evidence on the model's cost-effectiveness is still being awaited. A third model is PACE, the Program of All-Inclusive Care for the Elderly, where Medicare and Medicaid premiums are pooled to finance a staff-model HMO that focuses on elderly health issues and relies heavily on multidisciplinary care management teams to coordinate and provide services, including a rich package of LTC benefits. Although the PACE sites provide excellent care and do appear to save money (White, 1998), so far they have been successful on a very small scale. By the end of 2004, some 90 sites across the country cared for approximately 9,000 individuals (CBO, 2004). Questions have been raised, therefore, about the model's potential to lead to widespread LTC systems reform.

Uncertainty about the cost-savings potential of integration stems from the difficulty of implementing integrated care, which has limited the amount of experimentation.[8] Difficulties arise from both the need for states to strike agreements with the federal government (waivers are needed to diverge from standard policy affecting Medicare and Medicaid beneficiaries) and the need for managed care entities to work with unfamiliar patient populations, providers, and services. Such difficulties have motivated a number

---

8 It has also proven difficult to design rigorous evaluations of innovative approaches due to problems in identifying appropriate comparison groups.

of states—for example, New York, Texas, and Wisconsin—to experiment with less comprehensive but nevertheless ambitious models. New York's managed LTC (MLTC) model differs from PACE or SHMO by excluding hospital, physician, and related services from the capitation umbrella. While this model, like PACE and SHMO, requires LTC plans to coordinate acute care services, it does not require them to pay for or provide them. Consequently, members of Medicaid-only MLTC plans need not give up their existing primary care providers when they enroll. Texas's STAR+PLUS program, like ALTCS, capitates all Medicaid acute and LTC services, and emphasizes care coordination with uncovered Medicare services (Border, Morrison, Dyer, & Blakely, 2002). Unlike ALTCS, however, it is not statewide. The "jury is still out" on the care coordination and cost savings impact of this new generation of state LTC initiatives.

Meanwhile, a body of evidence suggests that state-initiated system reforms aimed at increasing the availability of HCBS resources can serve more individuals without significantly raising total LTC costs. For 20 years or more, the LTC literature has been replete with articles debating whether or not increasing the availability of HCBS resources will result in lowering total LTC costs. Many researchers have argued that it will not, for the simple reason that expanding HCBS options can result in a "woodwork" effect, whereby community-residing individuals with unmet LTC needs emerge to increase the total demand for LTC (Weissert & Hedrick, 1994). The result can then be large increases in the use of HCBS, which more than offset the cost of small decreases in nursing home use. Nevertheless, recent experience in Oregon, Washington, and Colorado suggests that the woodwork effect need not result in increasing total LTC costs if entry to nursing homes is tightly controlled and a variety of lower cost residential care and home-based service options are targeted to those most in need of supportive care (Alecxih, Lutzky, Corea, & Coleman, 1996; GAO, 1994).

Accordingly, states are increasingly focusing on developing home and community-based alternatives to nursing homes. In fact, spending on HCBS has increased much faster than spending on nursing home care, with much of the growth in HCBS spending being due to the implementation and/or expansion of Medicaid HCBS waiver programs. From 1990 through 2002, the compound annual rate of growth for Medicaid-funded HCBS waiver services (including HCBS for the mentally retarded/developmentally disabled population) was 24%, while the rate of growth for nursing

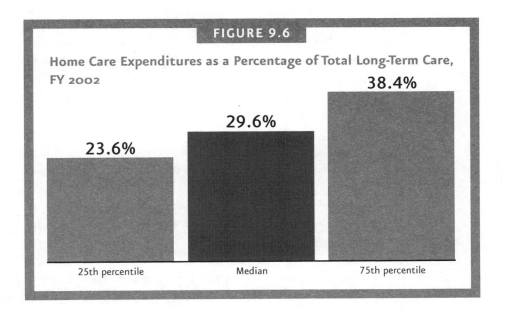

**FIGURE 9.6**

**Home Care Expenditures as a Percentage of Total Long-Term Care, FY 2002**

| 25th percentile | Median | 75th percentile |
|---|---|---|
| 23.6% | 29.6% | 38.4% |

homes was only 8.2% (Eiken et al., 2003). Even so, HCBS expansion is uneven among states, and most Medicaid dollars for LTC continue to go to nursing homes. In 2002, half of all states spent less than 30% of their LTC dollars on HCBS (including HCBS for the developmentally disabled), and a quarter spent less than 25%. At the high end, the top quarter of states spent an average of 38% of their LTC dollars on HCBS.[9] (See **FIGURE 9.6**.)

## Assuring Quality in Long-Term Care

Assuring quality in LTC is an inexact science. On the one hand, the attempt to assure quality in nursing homes has resulted in a welter of monitoring requirements and complicated regulations, which address everything from the width of hallways to the length of time between residents' meals. Despite these efforts and recent improvements, there is general agreement that many nursing homes still deliver sub-standard care. On the other hand, alternatives to the highly regulated approach used for nursing homes are comparatively untested. Although it is hoped that the mistakes of nursing home regulators can be avoided in some of the newer alternative residential settings such as assisted living facilities, little consensus exists as to how this can be done.

9 Author's calculation based on data from Eiken et al. (2003).

The landmark Nursing Home Reform Act of 1987 sought to upgrade the quality of nursing home care by instituting a broad set of regulatory changes aimed at improving resident assessments, resident rights, care processes, staffing, inspection procedures, and the enforcement of inspection findings (Wunderlich & Kohler, 2001). Nevertheless, a 2003 GAO report concluded,

> The proportion of nursing homes with serious quality problems remains unacceptably high, despite a decline in the incidence of such reported problems. Actual harm or more serious deficiencies were cited for 20 percent or about 3,500 nursing homes during an 18-month period ending January 2002, compared to 29 percent for an earlier period. (GAO, 2003b, p. 1)

The types of deficiencies cited included insufficient attendance to residents' pressure sores, failure to provide supervision or avert accidents, as well as failure to properly conduct resident assessments and prepare appropriate care plans. Additional deficiencies included inadequate nutrition, improper management of incontinent residents, failure to sustain residents' dignity, and inappropriate utilization of physical and chemical restraints.

Monitoring nursing homes to enforce the standards laid down by law is a joint responsibility of state and federal governments. This includes regular surveys to evaluate compliance with regulations and measures to assure that shortcomings are rectified (GAO, 1999b). Nursing homes found out of compliance may be subject to sanctions that include monetary penalties, state-assigned substitute management, staff training in problem areas, and correction of deficiencies in specified time intervals (GAO, 1999b). The ultimate sanction is applied when Medicare or Medicaid withdraws certification and payment from a provider.

However, investigations of the effectiveness of these quality enforcement mechanisms routinely turn up serious flaws. For example, a 2003 GAO investigation of homes that had a history of quality of care problems but whose current survey was clear found that 39% of the 76 homes investigated had documented problems—such as (residents') serious, avoidable pressure sores—that should have been classified as actual harm or higher (GAO, 2003b). The understatement of problems of providing quality care has been attributed at least in part to the inability or unwillingness of surveyors to detect and/or document problems (Wunderlich & Kohler,

2001). Unwillingness to comply may in turn be attributable to concern that imposing heavy fines or closing an institution could actually make things worse for residents, by reducing the resources available to improve care, or forcing residents to be moved to another facility.

The government also supports the Long Term Care Ombudsman Program through the Older Americans Act. In contrast to regulators, whose role is to apply laws and regulations, ombudsmen are appointed on a local basis to help identify and resolve problems on behalf of residents in order to improve their overall well-being. Ombudsmen's reports provide an additional source of information on the quality of long-term care institutions.

More recently, as part of the Nursing Home Quality Initiative (NHQI), the federal government launched a new Web site, "Nursing Home Compare" (http://www.medicare.gov/NHCompare/home.asp), which provides comparative information on nursing home quality indicators for all Medicare and Medicaid certified nursing homes in the country. The hope is that consumers will use such information to choose among nursing homes, thereby fostering improved quality through market mechanisms. The indicators are derived from resident assessment data (referred to as the Minimum Data Set) that nursing homes routinely collect on all residents at specified intervals during their stay, and include measures such as percent of residents with moderate to severe pain, percent with pressure sores, and percent who have deteriorated in their ability to perform activities of daily living. The website also incorporates quality information from other sources, including state surveys, so that consumers can obtain information about a nursing home's staffing levels and its performance when surveyed by quality inspectors.

Although many are supportive of the goals of the NHQI—and nursing homes appear attentive to their comparative rankings—it is not clear that consumers will be able to act readily on the quality indicators, given limited nursing home bed availability in some areas and the crisis situation that often precipitates a nursing home placement. Moreover, the indicators have been criticized for their omission of important aspects of quality, such as residents' self-reported quality of life, or self-perceived psychological and social well-being. These, in turn, are partly a function of consumers' self-perceived autonomy and choice.

A key element of quality, therefore, is whether a system of care responds to individuals' preferences. Here the finding is clear: most people prefer care at home, and many elders say they would rather die than live permanently in a nursing home (Mattimore et al., 1997). When staying in one's own home is not feasible due to LTC needs, people generally prefer moving to places as homelike as possible that provide needed supports. However, assuring quality in environments other than nursing homes brings with it a host of equally difficult issues.

Home care, the preferred mode of LTC, presents a series of quality assurance challenges. First and most obvious, care delivered at home is more difficult to observe and supervise than care delivered in an institution. Second, the quality and outcomes of home care are significantly influenced by a wide variety of difficult-to-control factors, such as the physical environment and family circumstances of the person needing care, which can be more readily controlled in an institutional setting. Third, even among Medicare certified home health agencies, most services are provided by paraprofessional aides, whose training requirements are minimal and whose supervision is often the responsibility of professionals who work for an entirely separate agency or organization. In addition, injuries, heavy workloads, and low wages among aides often result in burnout and turnover, which create discontinuities in care and lower the morale of remaining staff (Feldman, 1994; Richardson et al., 1998; Stone, 2000).

Because home care is funded through a patchwork of federal, state, and local programs, the regulatory regimen differs considerably from program to program and across locales. To address quality issues in Medicare-funded home health, the federal government has launched a Home Health Quality Initiative (http://www.cms. hhs.gov/quality/hhqi/) (GAO, 2002)—similar to the NHQI described earlier—which provides comparative information on the patient outcomes achieved by Medicare CHHAs across the country. As in the NHQI, consumers can access a website (http://www. medicare.gov/HHCompare) containing a range of information based on a standard patient assessment (the OASIS [Outcomes Assessment and Information Set]) mandated by the federal government and regularly administered. Among the published indicators are the percentage of patients who improve at bathing, the percentage who improve at walking, the percentage experiencing less pain, the percentage admitted to the hospital, and the percentage who needed urgent care while receiving home care. Like the Nursing

Home Quality Indicators, these are intended to inform consumer choice. However, as in the case of Nursing Home Compare, their impact may turn more on the ways that providers use them to inform their internal quality improvement efforts than on the choices made by consumers in the health care "market place." It therefore remains to be seen whether this approach will be effective in improving quality and whether it will spread to state- and locally-administered home care programs, where the level of oversight is uneven across states and low overall (GAO, 2003a), reflecting a lack of consensus on what information should be required from providers.

Assisted living facilities—often cited as a home-like alternative to nursing homes—are not without their own quality problems and also suffer from a lack of consensus on how best to assure quality. Lack of federal regulation of residential facilities has resulted in wide variation and lack of uniform definitions, making them difficult to compare and assess. Facilities vary in size, cost, privacy, staff-resident ratio, and available services. States may set their own standards for licensure, staffing, physical design, and resident population characteristics (AAHSA, 2000a; Mollica, 2002; Richardson et al., 1998), but there is little consensus on what those standards should be. A number of states are currently debating whether to license and how best to regulate these facilities. On one side are providers and some consumer advocates who are concerned about excessive regulation, fearing that the homelike atmosphere of these new residential models of care will be diminished if nursing home-like regulations are implemented. On the other side of the debate are policymakers and other consumer advocates who are more concerned about safety and quality of care than innovation (Stevenson et al., 2000).

The quality assurance regimes for nursing homes, on the one hand, and community-based options such as assisted living and home care, on the other, represent very different approaches to quality assurance. The nursing home industry, while highly regulated and well researched, has not always been successful in maintaining minimum quality standards. Community-based options, which are less regulated and less well-researched, are characterized by services of largely undetermined quality. Thus the optimum degree of regulation is left open to question.

## Choices for Long-Term Care Consumers

Today in the U.S., there is wide agreement that consumers should have significant choice over their long-term care arrangements. This argument is made on the grounds of ethical, psychological, and quality considerations. First, it is agreed that the ability to exercise autonomy is an important element of most Americans' moral experience and their sense of self (Cohen, 1988). Second, a broad psychological literature speaks to the health impacts of self-efficacy and the ability to control one's environment, particularly among older persons (Rodin & Timko, 1992). Lastly, it is argued that enhanced consumer choice will introduce market mechanisms into the LTC service environment, thus improving the quality of services.

The consumer-directed movement in long-term care arose out of resistance to the "medicalization" of everyday life that people with chronic or disabling conditions sometimes experience. Consumers pointed out that the role of medical professionals in their everyday lives could be limited, particularly given the low-tech nature of many LTC services. They felt that consumers of LTC services, regardless of age, should be able to take responsibility for and control those aspects of services they feel capable of managing. In their view, the role of professionals is to assist users of LTC services in assessing and managing their own care, not in determining what they need and when.

Consumer choice first requires that the conditions for choice exist. At minimum, this means that (a) consumers are considered the primary decisionmakers regarding the services they receive, unless they choose to delegate that responsibility; (b) a range of service options is available to them; (c) information about these options is available to them; and (d) consumers participate meaningfully in service allocation and systems design (National Institute on Consumer-Directed Long-Term Services, 1996). Some distinguish between *consumer-directed care*, when consumers take responsibility for all aspects of care including hiring, firing, training, supervising, and evaluating their own caregivers, and *consumer-centered care*, when care managers aim to involve consumers and incorporate their preferences into care plans. In one form or another, consumer choice is relevant to all LTC recipients, including those with developmental disabilities, mental illnesses, and cognitive impairments such as Alzheimer's disease.

Inevitably, respecting consumers' choice involves tradeoffs with professional judgments and may, in some cases, compromise patients' safety (Benjamin, 1999). However, advocates of consumer choice argue that it is an individual's right—in LTC as it is in other areas of life—to take risks in order to lead a preferred lifestyle, although there is considerable debate as to how risky LTC consumer choice is. A recent study found that outcomes of a consumer-directed program serving a large proportion of older people were actually better than those of a comparable group receiving usual care (Foster, Brown, Phillips, Schore, & Carlson, 2003). Nevertheless, family members and service providers are often uncomfortable with anything that is seen to threaten the safety of those receiving services. Service providers are also concerned about their potential liability for any adverse events that occur as a result of increased patient risk-taking.

Currently, efforts to increase choice in LTC are hampered by the institutional bias of the LTC system, which limits the options available for those who need care and ignores their preference for care at home. Although policymakers have been wary of creating choice by providing community-based alternatives to nursing homes because of their fear of expanding LTC expenditures, a number of federal initiatives and the 1999 Olmstead decision from the Supreme Court have encouraged the development of consumer-directed options across the states. Following the Supreme Court decision *Olmstead vs. L.C. 98–536, 9* (1999), which confers a duty on states to serve people with disabilities in the "most integrated setting," President Bush's "New Freedom" initiative is a nationwide effort to remove barriers to community living for people of all ages with disabilities and long-term illnesses.

## Financing Long-Term Care in the Future

For numerous reason discussed earlier in this chapter, policy experts agree that significant additional resources will be required to meet the future LTC needs of the U.S. population. To recap, the reasons include:

- Rapid aging of the population
- Prevalence of disabilities among older adults
- Increasing demand for home care services and residential alternatives to nursing homes

■ Rising costs of both institutional and community-based LTC
■ Heavy burden of consumer out-of-pocket costs for LTC services not covered by public programs

Many experts also agree that the need for LTC is an insurable risk, i.e., an uncertain occurrence that carries with it substantial, even catastrophic financial consequences for individuals, but affects a relatively small and predictable proportion of the total population. Such events make a strong case for insurance mechanisms that spread the risk of financial loss among a large group of people (Chen, 2003). Beyond consensus on the need for additional resources and the applicability of insurance principles, however, considerable disagreement exists on the policy options that should be pursued (Chen, 2003; Feder, 2001; Feder et al., 2000).

At one extreme are those who believe that LTC should first and foremost be the responsibility of government and should be financed by a social insurance mechanism that provides universal benefits and spreads the risks and costs across the public at large. Wiener and colleagues, for example, have recommended a social insurance model that would provide LTC coverage for all who need services, regardless of income. The insurance would pay for home and community-based care options, along with nursing home care. As social insurance programs are costly, financing would derive from several sources including federal taxes, state sources and recipients (i.e., the elderly) (Wiener, Illston, & Hanley, 1994). At the other extreme are those who believe that paying for LTC should be primarily a private responsibility, that public policy should focus on improving the market for purchase of private LTC insurance and that government's role in direct financing of services should be limited to providing a welfare safety net for the truly destitute. Policies that might improve the market for private LTC insurance include standardizing private policies, allowing consumers to supplement Medicaid benefits with private coverage, and expanding the tax deductibility of LTC insurance premiums (CBO, 2004). In between are those who argue out of principle and/or pragmatism for "mixed" approaches that combine public and private dollars and accommodate both insurance and welfare mechanisms. Recognizing the high costs of private LTC insurance policies, Chen, for example, proposes a system modeled on a "three-legged stool," consisting of social insurance, private insurance, and personal savings. In this model, the social insurance component would be funded by diverting a small portion of Social Security benefits and would provide a basic level of coverage to everyone. Private insurance—or Medicaid, in the case of indigent individuals in need of LTC—would then supplement this basic provision (Chen, 2003).

Enacting LTC financing reform has proved more successful in other countries than in the United States. For example, in 1994, Germany instituted mandatory, universal social insurance for LTC that covers both community-based and institutional care. Benefits, which people can choose to receive in the form of either cash or services, are financed by a premium set at 1.7% of salary, paid jointly by German employees and employers (Cuellar & Wiener, 2000). Similarly, in 2000, Japan introduced a universal LTC insurance program that covers both institutional and community-based care, half of which is paid through general revenue and the other half through premiums levied on those over the age of 40 (Campbell & Ikegami, 2000). Japan's move is surprising for a country with strong social norms regarding family care and a reputation for lagging as a "welfare state" (Campbell & Ikegami), but its experience may show how major demographic shifts can move policy.

For the time being, however, LTC financing reform in the U.S. appears to be stalled. For a brief period during the Clinton Administration's health care reform initiative, publicly financed LTC insurance was on the policy agenda, along with national health insurance. Since the demise of the proposed Clinton Health Security Act of 1993, LTC insurance has received little attention except from a few ardent advocacy groups. Although LTC is a necessary service, it is one that has been largely ignored by those not directly affected by the need for care. Many reasons for this have been suggested. Some say it is because the health care system is focused on cure rather than on care: LTC is ignored because it is a low-status service within health care. Others argue that the drawbacks of expanding publicly financed LTC outweigh the benefits because increased public spending would diminish personal responsibility and worsen the fiscal problems that future demographic changes are expected to produce (CBO, 2004). Yet others argue that social attitudes about disability at the end of life prevent us from thinking hard about the need for care and facing up to the problems involved in providing it. All of these arguments doubtless contain a grain of truth. However, the growing need for services will make confrontation with these hard issues unavoidable in the future.

## CONCLUSIONS

This chapter has reviewed key facts about LTC: what it is, who receives it, who provides it, and who pays. The most important fact, however, is the growing number of people who will need LTC services and the unpreparedness of the current system to meet that demand in ways that consumers would prefer and need. This chapter has also covered some of the pressing issues around service provision and the challenges involved in financing care—none of which is likely to be resolved soon. Much work needs to be done before there is agreement on the goals of LTC and the best ways of meeting these goals.

## CASE STUDY

Joe Ambitious has just been sworn in as governor of Heartland, U.S.A. He ran on a twofold ticket of fostering the growth of jobs in the state's still lagging economy and investing in the workforce of the future by improving the accountability of local school districts, increasing their internet connectivity, and keeping elementary schools open 9 to 5 across the state. Suddenly he finds himself besieged with a host of LTC issues that seem to require immediate attention.

The incoming state Medicaid Director tells him that the state's LTC budget is already over spent, and next year's budget must be formulated quickly. Nursing homes want higher payment rates and the association of assisted living providers is clamoring for more generous Medicaid payments for assisted living residents who are eligible for Medicaid services. The consumer advocacy community is waging a major campaign to improve regulation of nursing homes as well as assisted living facilities. Consumer advocates also are arguing vociferously for more Medicaid "waiver" slots to open up community-based LTC options to poor citizens, along with a more generous "needs"-based policy to make home care services more readily available to the citizenry at large, and more state dollars to expand respite services for unpaid caregivers. It seems likely that LTC "business as usual" will not fly. However, Governor Ambitious knows next to nothing about LTC. As the governor's chief of staff, you have been asked to give him a short immersion course in LTC. His questions are listed on the following page.

## DISCUSSION QUESTIONS

1. Who are the main users of LTC and who pays for their care?
2. Who are the main providers of care and how do their interests differ?
3. What are his options for containing LTC costs, and what are the risks of a tight cost containment policy?
4. Why are the consumer advocates "up in arms," and what should he do about their demands?
5. Assuming Governor Ambitious is in office for two terms, what should be his larger goals for LTC in the state and why?

## REFERENCES

Administration on Aging. (2004a). *Older population by age: 1900 to 2050.* Available: http://www.aoa.gov/prof/Statistics/online_stat_data/AgePop2050.asp

Administration on Aging. (2004b). *A profile of older Americans: 2003.* Available: http://www.aoa.gov/prof/Statistics/profile/2003/6.asp

Alecxih, L. M., Lutzky, S., Corea, J., & Coleman, B. (1996). *Estimated cost savings from the use of home and community-based alternatives to nursing facility care in three states.* Washington, DC: AARP.

American Association of Homes and Services for the Aging. (2000a). *Assisted living.* Washington, DC: Author.

American Association of Homes and Services for the Aging. (2000b). *Continuing care retirement communities.* Washington, DC: Author.

American Health Care Association. (2003a). Nursing facility beds by certification type. Available: http://ahcaweb.org/research/oscar/rpt_certified_beds_200312.pdf

American Health Care Association. (2003b). *Nursing facility control.* Available: http://www.ahca.org/research/oscar/rpt_control_200312.pdf

American Health Care Association. (2003c). *Nursing facility ownership.* Available: http://www.ahca.org/research/oscar/rpt_ownership_200312.pdf

American Health Care Association. (2003d). *Nursing facility patients by payor—percentage of patients: CMS OSCAR data current surveys.* Available:http://www.ahca.org/research/oscar/rpt_payer_200312.pdf

Arizona Health Care Cost Containment System (2004, February). Available:http://www.ahccca.state.az.us/Statistics/Enrollment/ALTCS/2004/altcenr1022004.asp

Arno, P. S. (2002, February 24). *Economic value of informal caregiving.* Annual Meeting of the American Association of Geriatric Psychiatry, Orlando, FL.

Benjamin, A. E. (1999). A normative analysis of home care goals. *Journal of Aging and Health, 11*(3), 445–468.

Border, S., Morrison, H., Dyer, J., & Blakely, C. (2002). Medicaid Managed Care Waiver Study: An independent assessment of access, quality, and cost-effectiveness of the STAR+PLUS Program. Prepared for The Texas Department of Human Services by the Public Policy Research Institute, Texas A&M University.

Burwell, B., Sredl, K., & Eiken, S. (2004, May). *Medicaid long-term care expenditures in FY 2003.* Memorandum. Cambridge, MA: Medstat.

Callahan, D. (1990). *What kind of life.* New York: Simon & Schuster.

Campbell, J. C., & Ikegami, N. (2000). Long–term care insurance comes to Japan. *Health Affairs, 19*(3), 26–39.

Campbell, D. E., Lynn, J., Louis, T. A., & Shugarman, L. R. (2004). Medicare program expenditures associated with hospice use. *Annals of Internal Medicine, 140,* 269–277.

Centers for Disease Control & Prevention. (2004a). *Current home health care patients.* Available: http://www.cdc.gov/nchs/data/nhhcsd/cur homecare.pdf

Centers for Disease Control & Prevention. (2004b). *Early release of selected estimates based on data from the January–September 2003 National Health Interview Survey.* Available: http://www.cdc.gov/nchs/about/major/ nhis/released200403.htm#12

Centers for Disease Control & Prevention. (2004c). *Home health care discharges.* Available: http://www.cdc.gov/nchs/data/nhhcsd/home caredischarges.pdf

Centers for Disease Control & Prevention. (2004d). *Hospice care discharges.* Available: http://www.cdc.gov/nchs/data/nhhcsd/hospicecare discharges.pdf

Centers for Medicare & Medicaid Services. (2003a). *Health care industry market update: Home health.* Baltimore, MD: U.S. Department of Health and Human Services, Centers for Medicare & Medicaid Services. Available: http://www.cms.hhs.gov/reports/hcimu_09222003.pdf

Centers for Medicare & Medicaid Services. (2003b). *Health care industry market update: Nursing facilities.* Baltimore, MD: U.S. Department of Health and Human Services, Centers for Medicare & Medicaid Services. Available: http://www.ahca.org/research/cms_market_ update_030520.pdf

Centers for Medicare & Medicaid Services. (2004a). Table 7: *Nursing home care expenditures aggregate and per capita amounts and percent distribution, by source of funds: Selected calendar years 1980–2002.* Baltimore, MD: U.S. Department of Health and Human Services, Centers for Medicare & Medicaid Services. Available: http://www.cms.hhs.gov/statistics/ nhe/historical/tables.pdf

Centers for Medicare & Medicaid Services. (2004b). Table 3: *National health expenditures, by source of funds and type of expenditure: Selected calendar years 1997–2002.* Baltimore, MD: U.S. Department of Health and Human Services. Available: http://www.cms.hhs.gov/statistics/nhe/historical/tables.pdf

Centers for Medicare & Medicaid Services. (2004c). *2004 SSI FBR, resource limits, 300% cap, break-even points, spousal impoverishment standards.* Baltimore, MD: U.S. Department of Health and Human Services, Centers for Medicare & Medicaid Services. Available: http://www.cms.hhs.gov/medicaid/eligibility/ssi104.asp

Centers for Medicare & Medicaid Services. (2004d). Table 9: *Personal health care expenditures, by type of expenditure and source of funds: Calendar years 1995–2002.* Baltimore, MD: U.S. Department of Health and Human Services, Centers for Medicare & Medicaid Services. Available: http://www.cms.hhs.gov/statistics/nhe/historical/tables.pdf

Chen, Y. (2003). Funding long-term care: Applications of the trade-off principle in both public and private sectors. *Journal of Aging and Health, 15*(1), 15–44.

Cohen, E. S. (1988). The elderly mystique: Constraints on the autonomy of the elderly with disabilities. *The Gerontologist, 28*(Suppl.), 24–31.

Congressional Budget Office. (2004). *Financing long-term care for the elderly.* The Congress of the United States. Available: http://www.cbo.gov/ftpdoc.cfm?index=5400&type=1

Coronel, S. (2003). *Long-term care insurance in 2000–2001.* Washington, DC: Health Insurance Association of America Center for Disability and Long-Term Care.

Cuellar, A. E., & Wiener, J. M. (2000). *Can social insurance for long-term care work? The experience of Germany.* Washington, DC: The Urban Institute.

*Duggan v. Bowen:* U.S. District Court for the District of Columbia, Number 87–0383, August 1, 1988.

Eiken, S., Burwell, B., & Schaefer, M. (2003, May 15). *Medicaid LTC expenditures in 2002.* Cambridge, MA: The MEDSTAT Group, Memorandum.

Feder, J. (2001). Long-term care: A public responsibility. *Health Affairs, 20*(6), 112–113.

Feder, J., Komisar, H., & Niefeld, M. (2000). Long-term care in the United States: An overview. *Health Affairs, 19*(3), 40–56.

Feldman, P. (1994). 'Dead end' work or motivating job? Prospects for front-line paraprofessional workers in LTC. *Generations, 23*(2), 5–10.

Feldman, P. (1999). 'Doing more for less': Advancing the conceptual underpinnings of home-based care. *Journal of Aging and Health, 11*(3), 261–276.

Freedman, V. A., Martin, L. G., & Schoeni, R. F. (2002). Recent trends in disability and functioning among older adults in the United States. *Journal of the American Medical Association, 288*(24), 3137–3146.

Foster, L., Brown, R., Phillips B., Schore J., & Carlson, B. L. (2003). *Does consumer direction affect the quality of Medicaid personal assistance in Arkansas?* Princeton, NJ: Mathematica Policy Research.

Gabrel, C. S. (2000). An overview of nursing home facilities: Data from the 1997 national nursing home survey. In *Advance Data from Vital and Health Statistics* (No. 311). Hyattsville, MD: National Center for Health Statistics.

General Accounting Office. (1994). *Medicaid long-term care: Successful state efforts to expand home services while limiting costs.* (GAO/HEHS-94–167). Washington, DC: U.S. Government Printing Office.

General Accounting Office. (1999a). *Adults with severe disabilities: Federal and state approaches for personal care and other services.* (GAO/HEHS-99–101). Washington, DC: U.S. Government Printing Office.

General Accounting Office. (1999b). *Nursing homes: Additional steps needed to strengthen enforcement of federal quality standards.* (GAO/HEHS-99–46). Washington, DC: U.S. Government Printing Office.

General Accounting Office. (2000). *Medicare home health care: Prospective payment could reverse recent declines in spending.* (GAO/HEHS-00–176). Washington, DC: U.S. Government Printing Office.

General Accounting Office. (2002). *Medicare home health agencies: Weaknesses in federal and state oversight mask potential quality issues.* (GAO-02–382). Washington, DC: U.S. Government Printing Office.

General Accounting Office. (2003a). *Long-term care: Federal oversight of growing Medicaid Home and Community-Based Waivers should be strengthened.* (GAO-03–576). Washington, DC: U.S. Government Printing Office.

General Accounting Office. (2003b). *Nursing home quality: Prevalence of serious problems, while declining, reinforces importance of enhanced oversight.* (GAO-03–561). Washington, DC: U.S. Government Printing Office.

Gibson, M. J., Freiman, M., Gregory, S., Kassner, E., Kochera, A., Mullen, F., et al. (2003). *Beyond 50.03: A report to the nation on independent living and disability.* Washington, DC: AARP Public Policy Institute. Accessible: http://www.research.aarp.org/il/beyond_50_il.html

Harrington, C., Lynch, M., & Newcomer, R. J. (1993). Medical services in social health maintenance organizations. *The Gerontologist, 33*(6), 790–800.

Haupt, B. J. (1998). An overview of home health and hospice care patients: 1996 National Home and Hospice Care Survey. In *Advance Data from Vital and Health Statistics* (No. 297). Hyattsville, MD: National Center for Health Statistics.

Hawes, C., Rose, M., & Phillips, C. D. (1999). *A national study of assisted living for the frail elderly: Results of a national survey of facilities* (prepared for the U.S. Department of Health and Human Services, Assistant Secretary for Planning and Evaluation). Beachwood, OH: The Myers Research Institute.

Hospice Association of America. (2001). *Basic statistics about hospice.* Washington, DC: National Association of Home Care. Available: http://www.nahc.org/Consumer/hpcstats.html

Hospice Association of America. (2002). *Hospice facts and statistics.* Available: http://www.nahc.org/Consumer/hpcstats.html

Jones, A. (2002). The national nursing home survey: 1999 summary. National Center for Health Statistics. *Vital and Health Statistics,* 13(152), 1–116.

Kane, R. A. (1999). Goals of home care: Therapeutic, compensatory, either, or both? *Journal of Aging and Health,* 11(3), 299–321.

Kane, R. A., & Kane, R. L. (1987). *Long-term care: Principles, programs and policies.* New York: Springer.

Kaplan, K., & Urbina, J. (2000). *Moving palliative care upstream: Addressing questions, controversies, practicalities and possibilities regarding integrating curing and caring paradigms along the long term care spectrum.* New York: Partnership for Caring: America's Voices for the Dying.

Lakdawalla, D., & Philipson, T. (2000, June). Public financing and the market for long-term care in NBER. In A.M. Garber (Ed.), *Frontiers in health policy research* (Vol. 4). (Forthcoming monograph). Cambridge: National Bureau of Economic Research.

LaPlante, M., Harrington, C., & Kang, T. (2002). Estimating paid and unpaid hours of personal assistance services in activities of daily living provided to adults living at home. *Health Services Research,* 37(2), 397–416.

Levit, K., Cowan, C., Lazenby, H., Sensenig, A., McDonnell, P., Stiller, J., et al. (2000). Health spending in 1998: Signals of change. The Health Accounts Team. *Health Affairs,* 19(1), 124–132.

McCall, N., Komisar, H., Petersons, A., & Moore, S. (2001). Medicare home health before and after the BBA. *Health Affairs,* 20(3), 189–198.

McCall, N., Korb, J., Petersons, A., & Moore, S. (2002). Constraining Medicare home health reimbursement: What are the outcomes? *Health Care Financing Review,* 34(2), 57–76.

Manton, K., Corder, L., & Stallard, E. (1997). Chronic disability trends in elderly United States populations: 1982–1994. *Proceedings of the National Academy of Science,* 94, 2593–2598.

Manton, K. G., & Gu, X. (2001). Changes in the prevalence of chronic disability in the United States black and nonblack population above age 65 from 1982 to 1999. *Proceedings of the National Academy of Sciences (PNAS),* 98(11), 6354–6359.

Mattimore, T. J., Wenger, N. S., Desbiens, N. A., Teno, J. M., Hamel, M. B., Liu, H., et al. (1997). Surrogate and physician understanding of patients' preferences for living permanently in a nursing home. *Journal of the American Geriatrics Society,* 45(7), 818–824.

MedPAC. (2004). *Report to the Congress: Medicare payment policy.* Washington, DC: Medicare Payment Advisory Commission.

Meltzer, W. (1982). *Respite care: An emerging family support service.* Washington, DC: Center for the Study of Social Policy.

Mollica, R. (2002). *State assisted living policy: 2002.* Portland, ME: National Academy for State Health Policy.

Murtaugh, C. M., McCall, N., Moore, S., & Meadow, A. (2003). Trends in Medicare home health care use: 1997–2001. *Health Affairs, 22*(5), 146–156.

National Association for Home Care. (2000). *Basic statistics about home care.* Washington, DC: NAHC. Available: http://www.nahc.org/consumer/hcstats.html

National Institute on Consumer-Directed Long-Term Services. (1996). *Principles of consumer-directed home and community-based services.* Washington, DC: National Council on the Aging.

Partners in Caregiving. (2003). *National study of adult day services, 2001–2002.* Winston-Salem, NC: Partners in Caregiving: The Adult Day Services Program, Wake Forest University School of Medicine.

Rich, M. W. (2003). Heart failure in the elderly: Strategies to optimize outpatient control and reduce hospitalizations. *American Journal of Geriatric Cardiology, 12*(1), 19–27.

Richardson, H., Raphael, C., & Barton, B. (1998). Long-term care: Health, social, and housing services for those with chronic illness. In A. R. Kovner & S. Jonas (Eds.), *Jonas and Kovner's health care delivery in the United States* (6th ed., pp. 206–242). New York: Springer.

Rhoades, J. A., & Krauss, N. A. (1999). *Nursing home trends, 1987 and 1996.* Rockville, MD: Agency for Health Care Policy and Research. (MEPS Chartbook No. 3. AHCPR Publication No. 99–0032.)

Rodin, J., & Timko, C. (1992). Sense of control, aging, and health. In M. G. Ory, R. P. Abeles, & P. D. Lipman (Eds.), *Aging, health and behavior* (pp. 174–206). Newbury Park, CA: Sage.

Rogers, S., & Komisar, H. (2003). *Who needs long-term care?* Policy brief. Washington, DC: Georgetown University Long-Term Care Financing Project. Available: http://ltc.georgetown.edu/pdfs/whois.pdf

Sparer, M. S. (1999). *Health policy for low-income people in Arizona.* Washington, DC: The Urban Institute.

Spector, W. D., Cohen, J., & Pesis-Katz, I. (2004). Home care before and after the Balanced Budget Act of 1997: Shifts in financing and services. *The Gerontologist, 44*(1), 39–47.

Spector, W. D., Fleishman, J. A., Pezzin, L. E., & Spillman, B. C. (1998). *The characteristics of long-term care users.* Paper prepared for the Institute of Medicine, Committee on Improving Quality in Long-Term Care, Washington, D.C.

Stevenson, D. G., Murtaugh, C. M., Feldman, P. H., & Oberlink, M. R. (2000). *Expanding publicly financed assisted living and other residential alternatives for disabled older persons: Issues and options.* New York: Center for Home Care Policy and Research, Visiting Nurse Service of New York. Available: http://www.vnsny.org/research/publications/pdf/No3_AssLivBrief.pdf

Stone, R. I. (2000). *Long-term care for the disabled elderly: Current policy, emerging trends and implications for the 21st century* [On-line]. Available: http://www.milbank.org/sea/jan2000/index.html

Sturm, R., Ringel, J. S., & Andreyeva, T. (2004). Increasing obesity rates and disability trends. *Health Affairs, 23*(2), 199–205.

Tilly, J., Goldenson, S., Kasten, J., O'Shaughnessy, C., Kelly, R., & Sidor, G. (2000). *Long-term care chart book: Persons served, payors, and spending.* Congressional Research Service.

U.S. Department of Health and Human Services. (1999). *Health care financing review: Medicare and Medicaid statistical supplement, 1999.* Baltimore, MD: Author.

U.S. Department of Health and Human Services. (2001). *Health care financing review: Medicare and Medicaid statistical supplement, 2001.* Baltimore, MD: Author.

U.S. Department of Health and Human Services. (2003). *2003 CMS statistics.* CMS Publication No. 03445.

Weissert, W. G. (1997). Cost savings from home and community-based services: Arizona's capitated Medicaid long term care program. *The Journal of Health Politics, Policy, and Law, 22*(6), 1329–1357.

Weissert, W. G., & Hedrick, S. C. (1994). Lessons learned from research on effects of community-based long-term care. *Journal of the American Geriatrics Society, 42*(3), 348–353.

White, A. J. (1998). *The effect of PACE on costs to Medicare.* Cambridge, MA: Abt Associates.

Wiener, J. M., & Stevenson, D. G. (1998). State policy on long-term care for the elderly. *Health Affairs, 17*(3), 81–100.

Wiener, J. M., Illston, L. H., & Hanley, R. J. (1994). *Sharing the burden: Strategies for public and private long-term care insurance.* Washington, DC: The Brookings Institution.

Wunderlich, G., & Kohler, P. (2001). *Improving the quality of long-term care.* Washington, DC: Institute of Medicine, Committee on Improving Quality in Long-Term Care.

# 10

# HEALTH-RELATED BEHAVIORS

C. Tracy Orleans and
Elaine F. Cassidy

- Describe the contributions of personal health practices to individual and population health status (e.g., tobacco use, risky drinking, physical activity, diet, obesity).
- Describe how strategies for changing individual and population health behaviors have evolved, and identify the targets and characteristics of effective interventions.
- Summarize new clinical and community practice guidelines for health behavior change.
- Describe how strategies for improving the delivery of primary care health behavior change interventions have evolved, and identify the targets and characteristics of effective interventions.
- Summarize new models and prospects for addressing behavioral risk factors through national health care quality improvement efforts.

- Behavioral risk factors: Overview and national goals
- Changing health behaviors: Individual-oriented and population-based interventions for achieving national health objectives
- Changing provider behavior: Provider-oriented and system-based interventions for achieving national health care quality objectives

KEY WORDS

Behavioral risk factors, prevention, tobacco use, risky drinking, diet and physical activity, obesity, health disparities, patient self-management, stages of change, clinical practice guidelines, paradigm shift, social ecological models, health care quality improvement, chronic care model.

---

HEALTH CARE PROFESSIONALS, who live in a world in which often-heroic efforts are needed to save lives, can easily believe that medical care is the key instrument for maintaining and assuring the health of Americans. This chapter explains, however, that behavioral choices—how we live our lives—are the key instruments that determine Americans' health and well-being. To some extent, the task of helping people choose healthy lifestyles falls into the realm of behavioral psychology and sometimes social marketing. However, emerging theories of how to encourage healthy lifestyles include major roles for medical providers. Therefore, clinicians, health care payers, managers of provider organizations, and health care policymakers need to understand the dynamics of behavioral choices that affect health status.

The chapter begins with a brief overview of the major behavioral risk factors that contribute to the growing burden of preventable chronic disease in the United States, namely, tobacco use, alcohol abuse, sedentary lifestyle, and unhealthy diet, related obesity, and overweight. It then describes the extraordinary progress that has been made over the past three decades to help adults modify these risk factors, by intervening both at the individual level—with educational and behavioral treatments that can be delivered in clinical settings—and at the broader population level—with environmental and policy changes that help to support and maintain healthy behavior. Theoretical advances (e.g., social learning theory, stage-based and social ecological models) leading to a major "paradigm shift" in understanding the need for broad spectrum, multilevel ecological approaches are described. In addition, new science-based clinical and community practice guidelines developed to guide these broad spectrum approaches are summarized with reference to heuristic models for primary care and population interventions that can be applied to all of the risk factors. The chapter goes on to summarize similar developments in efforts to promote the wider delivery of proven health behavior change protocols in primary care settings—by combining individual, provider-focused interventions (education, training) with broader changes in health care systems and policies to guide and support provider efforts. Many parallels can be drawn between what we have learned about the processes, principles, and paradigms for effective health promotion (i.e., patient behavior change) and what we have learned about the processes, principles, and paradigms for effective health care quality improvement (i.e., provider behavior change). The significant progress made in both areas has created unprecedented potential for breakthrough improvements in national health status and health care quality.

## BEHAVIORAL RISK FACTORS: OVERVIEW AND NATIONAL GOALS

Acute and infectious diseases are no longer the major causes of death, disease, and disability in the United States. Today, chronic diseases, such as coronary heart disease, cancer, diabetes, asthma, and cancer are the leading causes of death and disease. Chronic diseases and conditions affect more than 100 million Americans and account for three quarters of the nation's annual health care costs (Institute for Health and Aging, 1996). Given the continued aging of the population, both the prevalence and costs of chronic illness care will continue to rise. Yet, much of the growing burden of chronic disease is preventable. More than a decade ago, McGinnis and Foege (1993) estimated that 50% of mortality from the 10 leading causes of death was attributable to lifestyle behaviors that cause or complicate chronic disease. A recent analysis by Mokdad, Marks, Stroup, and Gerberding (2004) confirmed this estimate, finding that the four leading behavioral risk factors—tobacco use, alcohol abuse, sedentary lifestyle, and unhealthy diet—together accounted for more than 900,000 deaths in the year 2000. Moreover, research findings over the past two decades have established that modifying these risk factors leads to improved health and quality of life, and to reduced health care costs and burden (Halvorson & Isham, 2003; Institute of Medicine [IOM], 2000; Orleans, Ulmer, & Groman, 2004).

Today, almost 90% of Americans report that they engage in at least one of these risk factors, and 52% report engaging in two or more, with the highest prevalence of individual and multiple behavioral risks occurring in low-income and racial/ethnic minority populations (Coups, Gaba, & Orleans, in press; IOM, 2000). Given these statistics, it is not surprising that half of the leading health indicators tracked by *Healthy People 2010*, which sets forth the nation's primary objectives for promoting longer, healthier lives, and eliminating health disparities, relate to healthy lifestyles (U.S. Department of Health and Human Services [USDHHS], 2000). Selected indicators for tobacco use, alcohol abuse, diet, physical activity, obesity are shown in **TABLE 10.1**.

## Tobacco Use

Tobacco use causes more preventable deaths and diseases than any other behavioral risk factor, including 435,000 premature deaths from several forms of cancer, heart, and lung disease (Mokdad et al., 2004), and it accounts for annual health care costs of $75 billion (Centers for Disease Control and Prevention [CDC], 2004a). Smoking represents the single most important modifiable cause of poor pregnancy outcomes, accounting for 20% of low-birth-weight

## TABLE 10.1

### Selected Healthy People 2010 Objectives: Behavioral Risk Factors

| | BASELINE[a] (%) | 2010 GOALS (%) |
|---|---|---|
| **Tobacco use** | | |
| Cigarette smoking | | |
|     Adults (18 years and older) | 24.0 | 12.0 |
|     Adolescents (grades 9–12) | 35.0 | 16.0 |
| Exposure to secondhand smoke | | |
|     Children (6 years and younger) | 27.0 | 10.0 |
| **Alcohol misuse/risky drinking** | | |
| Proportion of adults who exceed guidelines for low-risk drinking | 72 (Females); 74 (Males) | 50 |
| Binge drinking | | |
|     Adults (18 years and older) | 16.6 | 6.0 |
|     Adolescents (12 to 17 years) | 7.7 | 2.0 |
| Deaths from alcohol-related auto crashes | 5.9 | 4.0 |
| **Physical activity** | | |
| Regular moderate physical activity (At least 5 days/wk for 30 mins.) | | |
|     Adults (18 years and older)[b] | 15.0 | 30.0 |
|     Adolescents (grades 9–12)[c] | 27.0 | 35.0 |
| Vigorous physical activity (At least 3 days/wk for 20 mins.) | | |
|     Adults (18 years and older) | 23.0 | 30.0 |
|     Adolescents (students in grades 9 through 12) | 65.0 | 85.0 |
| **Diet and overweight** | | |
| Proportion of people over 2 years of age eating recommended daily fruit consumption[d] | 28.0 | 75.0 |
| Proportion of people over 2 years of age eating recommended daily vegetable consumption[e] | 3.0 | 50.0 |
| Proportion of people over 2 years of age eating recommended daily grain consumption[f] | 7.0 | 50.0 |
| Overweight and obesity | | |
|     Obesity among adults (aged 20 years and older) | 23.0[d] | 15.0 |
|     Overweight and obesity among children and adolescents(aged 6 to 19)[g] | 11.0[d] | 5.0 |

[a]Baseline data extracted from sources between the years 1988–1999.
[b]At least 30 minutes per day.
[c]At least 30 minutes 5 or more days per week.
[d]At least 2 daily servings of fruit.
[e]At least 3 daily servings of vegetables (at least one third being dark green or orange).
[f]At least 6 daily servings of grain products (at least 3 being whole grains).
[g]Includes both overweight and obesity.
FROM: U.S. Department of Health and Human Services (2000c).

deliveries, 8% of preterm births, and 5% of perinatal deaths. For infants and young children, parental smoking is linked to SIDS, respiratory illnesses, middle ear infections, and decreased lung function, with annual direct medical costs estimated at $4.6 billion (Orleans, Barker, Kaufman, & Marx, 2000). Smoking cessation, even after 50 years of smoking, can produce significant improvements in health and health care utilization (U.S. Public Health Service [USPHS], 2000).

Although the adult smoking prevalence rate has dropped 40% since the first surgeon general's report in 1964, nearly 1 in 4 adults still smokes, with the highest rates (33%) in low-income populations (USPHS, 2000). Rates of smoking during pregnancy also have dropped in the past decade, but 12% of women reported in 1999 that they smoked during pregnancy (CDC, 2001). Each day, more than 3,000 children and teens become new smokers, 30% of whom will become addicted (National Center for Health Statistics [NCHS], 1999). Also, 28% of high school and college students, and 33% of young adults not attending college, smoke cigarettes. Nearly 8 million Americans, mostly adolescent and young adult males, report smokeless tobacco use, which is linked to oral cancer, gum disease, and tooth loss. In addition, 27% of children aged 6 and younger are exposed to harmful environmental tobacco smoke (ETS) at home, and 37% of nonsmoking adults are exposed to ETS at home or in the workplace (Grantmakers in Health [GIH], 2004).

## Alcohol Use/Misuse

Alcohol abuse or misuse includes alcohol dependence and risky or harmful drinking. About 5% of the U.S adult population meet the criteria for alcoholism or alcohol dependence, and another 20% of U.S. adults engage in harmful or risky drinking, defined as drinking more than 1 drink per day or 7 drinks per week for women, more than 2 drinks per day or 14 drinks per week for men, periodic binge drinking (5 or more drinks on a single occasion), drinking while driving, or drinking during pregnancy (Babor, Aguirre-Molina, Marlatt, & Clayton, 1999; Whitlock, Polen, Green, Orleans, & Klein, 2004). Approximately 40% of college students and young adults engaged in binge drinking from 1975 to 2002, a rate well above the *HP 2010* goal of 6% (Johnston, O'Malley, & Bachman, 2003b). Alcohol misuse is most common in young adults, particularly White and Native American males (Babor et al., 1999). Moderate levels of alcohol use in adults (below those defined as risky) have been linked to modest health benefits, such as lowered risk for heart disease (Whitlock et al., 2004)

Alcohol misuse is associated with 60 to 90% of cirrhosis deaths, 40 to 50% of auto-related fatalities, and 16 to 67% of home and work injuries (McGinnis & Foege, 1993) and with fetal alcohol syndrome. It was estimated to have caused 85,000 deaths in 2002 (Mokdad et al., 2004). The total annual costs of alcohol misuse, including costs related to health care, lost wages, premature death, and crime, were estimated at $185 million in 1998 (National Institute on Alcohol Abuse and Alcoholism [NIAAA], 2001). The health benefits of treatment of alcohol dependence are well established (Babor et al., 1999), and the U.S. Preventive Services Task Force (USPSTF) (1996) recently found that brief behavior change interventions to modify risky drinking levels and practices produced positive health outcomes detectable four or more years post-intervention.

## Physical Activity

The health risks associated with physical inactivity and sedentary lifestyle are numerous, including heart disease, Type 2 diabetes, stroke, hypertension, osteoarthritis, colon cancer, depression, and obesity (USPSTF, 2002). In addition to its relationship to physical health, physical activity helps maintain healthy bones, muscles, joints, and healthy weight. It has been shown to yield positive psychological benefits, including lower levels of stress and depression, and increased self esteem (USDHHS, 2000b). U.S. medical costs associated with sedentary lifestyle were estimated at nearly $76.6 billion in the year 2000 (CDC, 2004a).

*Healthy People 2010* guidelines recommend that adults and adolescents engage regularly in moderate physical activity (such as walking or biking) for at least 30 minutes at least 5 days a week, and that they engage in vigorous physical activity that promotes the development and maintenance of cardiorespiratory fitness three or more days per week for 20 or more minutes per occasion. As Table 10.1 shows, most American adults and adolescents do not get enough physical activity to meet public health recommendations. The populations most at risk for inactivity include those with lower income and education levels, those living below the poverty line in all racial and ethnic groups, members of several racial/ethnic minority groups (e.g., African Americans, Hispanics), and those with disabilities (Powell, Slater, & Chaloupka, 2004). Increasing physical activity levels yields a range of positive health outcomes, including substantial reductions in risks for heart disease and diabetes.

## Diet

In conjunction with sedentary lifestyle, unhealthy eating is linked to an estimated 400,000 deaths each year in the U.S. (Mokdad et al., 2004). Together, inactivity and unhealthy diet are associated with 25 to 30% of cardiovascular deaths, 30 to 35% of cancer deaths, and 50 to 80% of Type 2 diabetes cases (McGinnis & Foege, 1993). They have also contributed jointly to a surge in overweight and obesity that has reached epidemic proportions over the last 20 years, particularly within low-income and minority populations.

Four of the 10 leading causes of death—coronary heart disease, some cancers, stroke, and Type 2 diabetes—are associated with unhealthy diet. The relationships between dietary patterns and health outcomes have been examined in a wide range of observational studies and randomized trials with patients at risk for diet-related chronic disease. The majority of studies suggest that people consuming diets that are low in fat, saturated fat, trans-fatty acids, and cholesterol, and high in fruits, vegetables, and whole grain products containing fiber have lower rates of morbidity and mortality from coronary heart disease and several forms of cancer (USPSTF, 2003a). Moreover, dietary change has been found to reduce risks for many chronic diseases, as well as for overweight and obesity (USPSTF, 2003b).

Dietary Guidelines for Americans age two and older recommend 3 to 5 daily servings of vegetables and vegetable juices, 2 to 4 daily servings of fruits and fruit juices, and 6 to 11 daily servings of grain products, with no more than 30% of total calories from fat and 10% from saturated fat (USPSTF, 2003a). But, as Table 10.1 shows, there are enormous gaps between the recommended guidelines and actual diets for American children and adults. More than 80% of Americans, especially those in low-income populations, do not meet these guidelines (Powell et al., 2004; USPSTF, 2003a).

## Obesity

As poor dietary habits and physical inactivity have become endemic, national obesity rates have soared. Nearly 70% of all American adults are overweight or obese, an increase from 12% just one decade ago (Mokdad et al., 2004). These trends in adults are alarming given the strong links between obesity and many chronic diseases, including Type 2 diabetes, coronary heart disease, some cancers, gall bladder disease, and osteoarthritis (Must et al., 1999). Total expenditures related to overweight- and obesity-related problems were estimated at nearly $92.6 billion in 2002 (Finkelstein, Fiebelkorn, & Wang, 2003), numbers that will likely continue to rise unless effective interventions are put in place. New findings show that even modest weight loss (e.g., 5 to 10% of body weight) over a period of 12 to 24 months can reduce these risks and can prevent diabetes onset among adults with impaired glucose tolerance (Tuomilehto et al., 2001).

Even more alarming is the prevalence of overweight and obesity among children and adolescents (ages 6 to 19), which has nearly tripled over the past two decades (Flegal, Carroll, Ogden, & Johnson, 2002). Like adults, overweight youth are at risk for coronary heart disease, hypertension, certain cancers, and even Type 2 diabetes early in life (Rees, Neumark-Sztainer, Kohn, & Jacobson, 2000; USDHHS, 2000b). The highest and fastest rising rates of childhood obesity are seen among children and adolescents of African American or Latino descent and children from low-income backgrounds, particularly girls (Mei, Scanlon, et al., 1998)—making efforts to reach these groups a public heath priority.

## CHANGING HEALTH BEHAVIORS: INDIVIDUAL-ORIENTED AND POPULATION-BASED INTERVENTIONS

The landmark Institute of Medicine (IOM) report, *Health and Behavior*, published almost 25 years ago, was one of the first scientific documents to convincingly establish the links between behavioral risk factors and disease, and to identify the basic bio-psycho-social mechanisms underlying them (IOM, 1982). It recommended intensified social and behavioral science research to develop interventions that could help people change their unhealthy behaviors and improve their health prospects. This section presents a broad overview of the behavior change interventions that have emerged from the past two to three decades of research to address this challenge and close the gaps between current population health practices and the health objectives set for the nation, or, put differently, between "what we know" and "what we do" when it comes to adopting healthy lifestyles. This review describes the major theories used to guide this research, stressing the evolution from educational interventions to multi-component cognitive-behavioral interventions, and from individually-oriented and clinical treatment programs to broader public health approaches—an evolution which culminated in a major "paradigm shift" in understanding what the targets of effective interventions needed to be. New research-based practice guidelines for each of the behavioral health risks covered in this chapter are discussed with reference to both a unifying 5-A framework for primary care interventions and to a generic model for broad spectrum multi-level population health promotion efforts (McKinlay, 1995).

## A Brief History of Behavior Change Interventions

Early behavior change efforts in the 1970s and 1980s relied primarily on public education campaigns and individually-oriented health education interventions. They were guided by the Health Belief Model and similar theories (the Theory of Reasoned Action, the Theory of Planned Behavior) that emphasized the cognitive and motivational determinants of health behavior change and sought to raise awareness of the harms of unhealthy behaviors versus the benefits of behavior change, as a primary intervention strategy (e.g., Elder, Ayala, & Harris, 1999; Glanz, Rimer, & Lewis, 2002; Whitlock, Orleans, Pender, & Allan, 2002). These cognitive/decisional theories were based on a "rational man" model of human behavior change, with an underlying premise that people are rational beings whose intentions and motivations to perform a behavior strongly predict its actual performance (i.e., "if you tell them, they will change"). Since raising health risk awareness and motivation was a primary goal, the doctor-patient relationship was seen as a "unique and powerful" context for effective health education (e.g., Glynn & Manley, 1989; Orleans, 1993).

In fact, both population-level and individual clinical health education efforts based on these theories achieved initial successes. For instance, tens of thousands of smokers quit in response to the publication of the first U.S. Surgeon General's Report on Smoking and Health in 1964 and the multiple public education campaigns that followed (Warner, 2000). By the mid-1980s, most U.S. smokers said they wanted to quit and were trying to do so, mostly for health reasons (Fiore et al., 1990). Recent findings confirm that physician advice can be a powerful "catalyst" for health behavior change efforts—boosting the number of patients who quit smoking for at least 24 hours or who made some changes in their diet and activity levels (Kreuter, Cheda, & Bull, 2000). But a growing body of research on health education strategies found these successes to be modest—important and perhaps *necessary* for changing people's health knowledge, attitudes and beliefs and broader social norms, but *not sufficient* to produce lasting behavior change. Cumulative findings have made it clear that people need not only motivation but also new skills and supports to succeed in changing deeply ingrained health habits and to sustain those changes (e.g., Orleans, 1993; Whitlock et al., 2002).

These findings spurred the development and testing of expanded multi-component, cognitive-behavioral treatments designed not only to (a) raise perceptions of susceptibility to poor health outcomes and benefits of behavior change but also to (b) help patients learn the actual skills required to replace ingrained unhealthy habits with healthy alternatives and make changes in their natural (home, work, social) environments to help them successfully establish and maintain these new behaviors. Bandura's (1986) social learning theory, which emphasized interactions between intrapersonal and external environmental determinants of behavior, provided the primary theoretical basis for this evolution, and it remains the dominant model for effective cognitive-behavioral health behavior change interventions (e.g., Elder et al., 1999; Glanz et al., 2002; Whitlock et al., 2002).

Health lifestyle change interventions derived from social learning theory combined educational and skill-based strategies, including techniques such as modeling and behavioral practice, to help patients learn not just "why" but "how" to change unhealthy habits. For instance, these interventions taught effective self-management or behavior change skills such as goal-setting, self-monitoring, and the development of new stress management skills for those who had relied on smoking, eating, or drinking as coping tactics. Self-management skill training included teaching patients skills for re-engineering their immediate environments, replacing environmental cues and supports for unhealthy behaviors with new cues and supports for healthy ones (e.g., removing ashtrays, replacing unhealthy high-calorie foods with healthy alternatives, finding exercise buddies, and avoiding high-risk events such as office parties at which risky drinking was normative and expected). Another principle was that individualized behavioral problem-solving should start with helping patients set realistic, personal behavior change goals, and go on to address the unique barriers and relapse-temptations they faced. The expectation was that setting and meeting achievable goals would lead to a heightened self-efficacy and confidence in their self-change abilities. Finally, new social learning theory treatments taught patients to take a long-range problem solving perspective, viewing repeated attempts over time as part of a cumulative learning process, rather than as signs of failure (Orleans, 1993).

Effective multicomponent treatments were initially delivered and tested in multi-session, face-to-face group or individual clinic-based programs, typically offered in clinical or medical settings, and usually led by highly trained (e.g., MD, PhD) professionals (Lichtenstein & Glasgow, 1992). Results were extremely encouraging, with substantial behavior change (e.g., smoking quit rates as high as 40%) maintained 6 to 12 months post-treatment. However, participants were typically self-referred or recruited based on high readiness or motivation for change, and thus represented only a small fraction of those who could benefit. And treatment costs were high. As Lichtenstein and Glasgow indicate, once the effective treatment elements had been discovered, the next push was to distill core elements into lower-cost formats with much wider reach (e.g., paraprofessional-led worksite-based clinics, self-help manuals and programs, brief primary care counseling). Absolute treatment effects were smaller (e.g., 20% long-term quit rates for primary care tobacco interventions), but potential population impacts were much greater (e.g., Orleans & Alper, 2003). For instance, only 5 to 10% of smokers might ever attend intensive clinics, but a brief effective tobacco intervention reaching the 70% of U.S. smokers who saw their providers each year would double the nation's annual quit rate (Kottke, Battista, DeFriese, & Brekke, 1988).

The development of the "stages of change model" in the mid-1980s accelerated the shift from individual to population intervention models and has had a profound, lasting impact on the design and delivery of health behavior change programs. Though naturalistic studies of how people went about changing on their own, Prochaska and DiClemente (1983) discovered that health behavior change was a multistage process, with six sequential stages:

- *Precontemplation*—not planning to change behavior, behavior is not seen as a problem
- *Contemplation*—seriously planning to change behavior within next

6 months, weighing the pros and cons, and building supports and
confidence

- *Preparation*—plans to change are imminent, small initial steps are
taken
- *Action*—active attempts are made—to quit smoking, drink less,
become more active, or change to a healthier diet—and sustain for
up to 6 months
- *Maintenance*—change is sustained beyond 6 months
- *Relapse*—individual returns to any earlier stage and begins again to
recycle through the earlier stages

Prochaska et al. also discovered that different skills and knowledge, and different types of treatment, were needed to help people
in each stage; motivational and educational interventions were
helpful to people in precontemplation and contemplation stages,
and active cognitive-behavioral interventions were needed for
those in preparation, action, and maintenance stages (Prochaska,
DiClemente, & Norcross, 1992). Moreover, many population surveys
found that, at any given time, the vast majority of people (80%)
with any particular risk factor were in the precontemplation and
contemplation stages, which helped to explain why so few people
enrolled in weight loss or quit smoking clinics, even when they
were free and accessible.

Stage of change models have been successfully applied to each
of the behavioral health risks covered in this chapter and others
(e.g., cancer screening adherence, sun protection). It also has been
used to help people with multiple risk factors make progress in
changing several of them at the same time (Prochaska et al., in
press). This model helped to propel a shift away from "one-size-fits-
all" approaches to individualized stage-tailored strategies that
could be effectively applied to entire populations—in communities, worksites, and health care settings—assisting people at *all*
stages of change (not just the motivated volunteers in action stages,
but also those needing motivation and support to reach action
stages). It stimulated the development and wider use of effective
motivational interventions for clinical settings, especially motivational interviewing (Emmons & Rollnick, 2001). Originating as they
did in the study of successful self-change, stage of change models
also fueled a burgeoning movement towards low-cost self-help tools
and treatment formats. Stage-based interventions capitalized on
the revolution in computer-based and interactive communication

technologies for designing and delivering computer-tailored print materials, interactive video, computer, web-based and telephone interventions that were designed to fit not only the individual's stage of change but also address many other variables important for tailoring treatment methods and improving treatment outcomes (e.g., degree of nicotine addiction, unique behavior change assets, barriers, and cultural norms) (Glasgow, Bull, Piette, & Steiner, in press; Orleans et al., 2004; Prochaska et al., in press).

A final force in the evolution from individual to population-based approaches was the emergence of social marketing strategies which applied the concepts and tools of successful commercial marketing to the challenge of health behavior change (Elder et al., 1999; Whitlock et al., 2002). Basic marketing principles and methods (e.g., market analysis, audience segmentation, the use of focus groups) played an especially important role in the development of culturally appropriate communication and intervention strategies for reaching underserved and high-risk low income and racial/ethnic minority populations for whom the prevalence of behavioral health risks is highest (e.g., Maibach, Rothschild, & Novelli, 2002). For instance, social marketing strategies were used to tailor a state of-the-art self-help quit smoking guide to the needs of African American smokers and to develop messages for Black-format radio that promoted the use of the guide as well as free telephone quit-line counseling (Boyd et al., 1998). Results included a higher quit-line call rate from African American smokers and a higher quit rate among those receiving the tailored (vs. generic) guide.

## The Role and Impact of Primary Care Interventions

The progress in health behavior change research and treatment described above set the stage for the development of brief, individually-oriented, primary care health interventions that could be widely offered to all members of a practice, health plan, or patient population. These efforts were based on a strong rationale for primary care intervention to address behavioral health risks. Over 80% of American adults report having a usual source of care, visiting their doctor's offices on average about three times each year (NCHS, 2003). Patient surveys have repeatedly found that patients expect and value advice from their providers about their personal diet, exercise, and substance use behaviors, and are motivated to act on this advice (Kreuter et al., 2000; Stange, Woolf, & Gjeltema, 2002; Vogt et al., 1998). Similarly, most primary care providers describe health behavior change advice and counseling as an essential part of their role and responsibilities (Wechsler, Levine, Idelson, Schor, & Coakley, 1996). The unique extended relationship that is the hallmark of primary care provides multiple opportunities over time to address healthy behavior in a "string of pearls" approach, capitalizing both on "teachable moments" (e.g., introducing physical activity or diet counseling when test results show elevated cholesterol levels) and a therapeutic alliance that often extends beyond the patient to include key family members (Crabtree, Miller, & Stange, 2001; Stange et al., 2002). This vision has prompted a tremendous amount of work to identify brief, effective interventions that could be integrated into routine practice.

As noted above, once effective multicomponent behavior change treatments had been identified, attention shifted to distilling their core elements into briefer, lower-cost interventions that could be packaged as self-help programs or modules and/or so-called "minimal contact" primary care counseling interventions (Lichtenstein & Glasgow, 1992; Orleans, 1993). In these minimal-contact models, the physician was seen as the initial "catalyst" for change, providing brief motivational advice, social support, and follow-up, with referral to other staff members or community resources for more intensive behavior change assistance (e.g., Kreuter et al., 2000). The use of stage-based and social marketing approaches brought the potential to reach and assist entire populations of patients, including those not yet motivated for change and those in underserved and high-risk groups. Computer-based, patient-tailored and population-targeted interventions provided new ways to reduce provider burden. And the emergence of managed care as the dominant health care model brought new incentives and demand for population-based preventive clinical services, and more centralized systems for delivering them (e.g., Thompson, Taplin, McAfee, Mandelson, & Smith, 1995).

Progress in developing effective minimal-contact, primary care interventions occurred first in the area of smoking cessation, culminating in the development of an evidence-based "practice-friendly" intervention model now known as the "the 5-A's"—Ask, Advise, Agree, Assist, Arrange Follow-up (USPHS, 2000). The 5-A's model, outlined in TABLE 10.2, was developed through a review and meta-analysis of hundreds of controlled studies, and has been widely promoted through government-approved clinical practice guidelines (Agency for Health Care Policy and Research [AHCPR],

---

**TABLE 10.2**

## The 5-A's Model for Treating Tobacco Use and Dependence

| STEP | EXAMPLE OF PROVIDER BEHAVIOR |
|------|------------------------------|
| 1. Assess | Ask every patient about tobacco use and smoking at every visit |
| 2. Advise | Advise every tobacco user to quit in a clear, strong personalized manner |
| 3. Agree | Assess willingness or readiness to make a quit attempt and establish an agreed-upon goal and quitting plan |
| 4. Assist | Assist the patient willing to make a quit attempt with proven counseling strategies (problem-solving skills training, intra-treatment social support, counseling to develop extra-treatment social support) and include pharmacotherapy if appropriate (e.g., nicotine replacement, bupropion). Assist the patient not yet ready to quit with brief motivational counseling |
| 5. Arrange | Arrange follow-up contact and adjust treatment plan as needed, including offering or referring to more intensive treatments and/or community resources and programs, if appropriate |

Adapted from USPHS, U.S. Prevention Service 2000.

---

1996; USPHS, 2000). The model was found to be effective when used by a variety of health care providers (physicians, nurses, dentists, dental hygienists), with as few as 2 to 3 minutes of in-office provider time, starting with a routine *assessment* of tobacco use status. In this model, provider *advice* seeks to raise personal quitting motivation and self-efficacy, and ends with an offer to help quit. The *agree* step starts with assessing patient readiness to quit and goes on to establish a goal and quitting plan. For those not ready to quit, *assistance* includes a recommended motivational intervention. For those ready to quit, *assistance* is combined with brief behavior change counseling with FDA-approved pharmacotherapy (e.g., nicotine gum, patch, nasal spray or inhaler, and/or Zyban), unless contraindicated (e.g., pregnancy). Behavioral counseling was found to be most effective when provided through multiple formats (e.g., self-help materials, face-to-face and/or telephone counseling), with a clear dose-response relationship between the intensity of counseling (# minutes/sessions) and quit rates. Effective follow-up *arrangements* include planned visits, calls, or contacts to reinforce progress, adjust the quitting plan to better meet individual needs, and/or to refer for more intensive help. One-year quit rates for patients receiving these interventions are typically 2 to 3 times higher than the 7% quit rates of patients who try quitting on their own (USPHS, 2000), and as noted previously, could double the nation's annual quit rate (Kottke et al., 1988). The Centers for Disease Prevention and Control (CDC) and Partnership for Prevention found the 5-A primary care smoking cessation counseling intervention to be one of the two most effective and cost-effective of all evidence-based clinical preventive services (Coffield et al., 2001).

The 5-A model was recently adopted by the U.S. Preventive Services Task Force as a unifying conceptual framework for primary care preventive behavioral counseling interventions for *all* behavioral health risks. New USPSTF guidelines for risky drinking, physical activity, diet and obesity are briefly summarized in **TABLE 10.3**. In most cases, the USPSTF found evidence for counseling interventions that could produce clinically meaningful, population-wide health improvements that were sustained for at least 6 to 12 months. Though there are many common elements, the specific intervention components and intensity of recommended strategies vary from behavior to behavior, as does their effectiveness with unselected versus high-risk patients. Primary care providers may intervene more forcefully with healthy patients when they are known to be at high-risk for chronic disease (e.g., elevated cholesterol, blood pressure, familial-history risks); and patients at high risk may feel more vulnerable and motivated to act on the advice and assistance they receive.

The first step is always to *assess*, not only the relevant behavior(s) (using a standard health risk appraisal or brief screening that can easily be administered in a busy practice setting) but also the individual factors that are helpful in tailoring the intervention (e.g., medical and physiologic factors, motives, barriers, patient's stage of change, social support, cultural values). Based on this information, and ideally with reference to the patient's immediate health concerns and symptoms, the clinician provides brief, personalized *advice*, expressing confidence in the patient's ability to change and soliciting his his/her thoughts about the recommended changes. The next critical step is to negotiate and *agree* on a collaboratively defined behavior change goal and/or treatment plan, which commonly includes practical behavioral, problem-solving to *assist* the patient to address personal change barriers and build social support, and to help patients develop a more supportive, immediate social and physical environment, and secure adjunctive behavior change resources and pharmacologic aids (e.g., nicotine replacement). Adjunctive resources could also include face-to-face coun-

## TABLE 10.3

### USPSTF Recommendations for Addressing Primary Risk Behaviors

■ **Risky or harmful alcohol use:** The USPSTF has recommended routine screening and brief behavioral intervention for patients engaging in risky drinking based on evidence showing clinically significant reductions in harmful alcohol consumption levels sustained over 6 to 12-months or longer. All interventions that showed statistically significant improvements in alcohol outcomes included screening with feedback, personal advice, and goal-setting, while several employed individually-tailored behavior change counseling elements (USPSTF, 2004; Whitlock et al., 2004). They were delivered wholly or in part in the primary care setting, and involved one or more members of the health care team, including physician and nonphysician providers. Alcohol dependent patients who were identified were not included in these studies but referred to more intensive treatments.

■ **Physical activity:** The USPSTF found insufficient research evidence to determine intervention efficacy but identified a number of promising, brief 5-A type primary care interventions meriting further investigation (Eden, Orleans, Mulrow, Pender, & Teutsch, 2002; USPSTF, 2002). Promising interventions often included patient goal-setting, written exercise prescriptions, individually-tailored physical activity regimens, mailed or telephone follow-up provided by specially trained staff, and linking patients to community-based, physical activity and fitness resources. The USPSTF recommended the use of proven community-level interventions, ranging from community-based, individually-adapted self-help and behavior change programs (which tailor interventions to individual interests, preferences and stage of change, and help patients build needed social supports for changes in their exercise and activity levels) as well as proven policy and environmental changes, such as strengthening school-based physical education requirements and improving community resources for physical activity (e.g., sidewalks, bike paths, fitness facilities) along with administering social marketing campaigns to promote their use (CDC, 2001).

■ **Unhealthy diet:** The USPSTF recommended intensive 5A-type interventions delivered by specially trained primary care clinicians or by other specialists (e.g., nutritionists, dietitians, health educators) for healthy adults known to be at high risk for obesity-related chronic diseases based on evidence of clinically significant, long-term changes in daily intake of saturated fat, fiber, fruits, and vegetables. Effective primary-care initiated interventions included helping patients to set their own goals, teaching diet self-monitoring and skills to overcome common barriers to selecting a healthy diet, providing training in food shopping and preparation, role playing, enlisting family involvement, and providing intra-treatment social support. The USPSTF found insufficient evidence to judge the efficacy and long-term health impacts of routine low- to moderate-intensity dietary counseling with unselected (i.e., primary care) patients (Pignone et al., 2003; USPSTF, 2003a). But, two such approaches were found to be promising: (a) medium intensity face-to-face dietary counseling (2–3 group or individual sessions) by a dietitian or specially trained primary care physician or nurse and (b) lower-intensity interventions involving five minutes or less of primary care provider counseling supplemented by patient self-help materials, telephone counseling, or personally tailored computer-generated newsletters.

■ **Obesity:** The USPSTF recommended routine obesity screening using BMI (Body Mass Index) and high-intensity behavioral counseling (about diet, exercise, or both) for healthy obese adults seen in primary care settings based on evidence of modest, but clinically significant weight loss (3 to 5 kg or 5 to 10% of bodyweight) maintained for 6 to 12 months or longer (McTigue et al., 2003; USPSTF, 2003b). Effective primary care screening and counseling interventions involved more than one person-to-person (individual or group) session per month for at least the first three months of treatment and were delivered by a variety of providers, including physicians, dietitians, exercise instructors, and multi-disciplinary teams. They were similar in design and impact to those found in the Diabetes Prevention Trial to prevent the onset of Type 2 diabetes in adults with impaired glucose tolerance (e.g., Tuomilehto et al., 2001). However, the USPSTF found insufficient evidence to evaluate the long-term efficacy of moderate- or low-intensity primary care counseling for obese adults, or for behavioral counseling of any intensity (low, moderate or high) with overweight, but nonobese, adult primary care patients.

seling from medical or community-based programs, telephone counseling, tailored or generic self-help materials (e.g., mailings, manuals), and newer web-based and other interactive tools that are personally tailored (e.g., based on gender, age, racial/ethnic or cultural group, health status or condition, stage of change, and other relevant variables) and can be used before, during, and after the office visit (Glasgow et al., in press). The final step is to *arrange* follow-up support and assistance, including referral to more intensive or customized help.

These new guidelines provide unprecedented scientific evidence and support for the UPSTF assertion that "the most effective interventions available to clinicians for reducing the incidence and severity of the leading causes of disease and disability in the U.S. are those that address patients' personal health practices" (1996, p. iv). However, several important limitations and gaps must be noted. The greatest limitation is the lack of long-term maintenance following successful behavior change in primary care or more intensive cognitive-behavioral interventions (Orleans, 2000; Whitlock et al., 2002). The literature is replete with evidence of difficulty in maintaining successful behavior change for 12 months or longer. This is not surprising given that patients return to the environments that shaped and supported their unhealthy lifestyles and choices. Higher maintenance rates were achieved in clinic-based programs that offered extended booster or maintenance sessions (providing ongoing social support and behavior change assistance) or helped patients to create an enduring "therapeutic micro-environment" to shield them from wider "unhealthy" influences (e.g., implementing an in-home smoking ban, arranging for the delivery of recommended diet foods, arranging ongoing behavior change buddies) (Orleans).

Major research and evidence gaps include the following:

- There have been few studies to develop and test primary care interventions for children and adolescents, for any of the behavioral risk factors discussed in this chapter (tobacco, alcohol, physical activity, diet, obesity) (Barlow & Dietz, 2002; USPSTF, 2002, 2003a, 2003b, 2004).
- Similarly, few studies have been done to develop and test behavior change interventions for underserved populations, especially those in low-income and racial/ethnic minority groups (e.g., USPSTF, 2002; Whitlock et al., 2002).

- Except for obesity, little is known about how best to address multiple behavioral risk factors in the same individual or population (Goldstein, Whitlock, & DePue, in press; Prochaska et al., in press).

- And, despite growing evidence that effective chronic illness care often revolves around helping patients change the behavioral risks that cause or complicate their disease (Wagner, Austin, & Von Korff, 1996), formal evidence reviews and recommendations, such as those issued by the USPSTF, have focused mainly on primary prevention in healthy populations. Therefore, a rapidly expanding evidence base (e.g., Glasgow et al., 2002), the heightened demand for evidence-based behavioral counseling guidelines to help manage the nation's skyrocketing burden of chronic disease (Institute for Health and Aging, 1996), and recent use of the 5-A's framework as a template for the key steps in behavioral chronic illness self-management (Glasgow, Goldstein, Ockene, & Pronk, in press) may stimulate more research and guidelines for secondary prevention.

### The Emergence of Broad Spectrum Multi-Level Models for Population-Based Health Behavior Change

As previously noted, beginning in the early 1980s, a "paradigm shift" began to occur—from an almost exclusive emphasis on individually oriented and clinical models of health behavior change to broader population-based models of health promotion and disease prevention. Some of the seeds for this evolution were the successes of effective, brief, and intensive social learning theory-based interventions, which gave greater prominence to the external, environmental determinants of healthy and unhealthy behaviors, and the emergence of new stage-based and social marketing models for population-wide interventions (Sallis & Owen, 2002). However, the disappointing reach and long-term effectiveness of even the most successful cognitive-behavioral treatments were another catalyst. This was especially the case given the contrast with new evidence from public health research that far-reaching and lasting health impacts were slowing because of environmental and policy changes that eliminated the need for individual decision-making (e.g., the development of safer roads and more crashworthy automobiles, combined with shifts in laws and norms regarding seatbelt use, and drinking and driving, which dramatically reduced auto accident deaths and injuries) (IOM, 2000). With the stage well set, the final push for this "paradigm shift" came in the 1990s with the

development of social ecological models of health behavior (McKinlay, 1995; Sallis & Owen, 2002).

Based on an integration of behavioral science, clinical and public health approaches, social ecological models redefined what the
targets of successful health interventions need to be—not just individuals but also the powerful social contexts in which they live and
work. Social emerging ecological models of health behavior emphasized that it is determined by multiple levels of influence—interpersonal factors (e.g., physiologic factors, knowledge, skill, motivation), social factors (e.g., social-cultural norms, supports, and
networks), organizational and community factors, and broader
environmental influences and public policies. And proponents of
the ecological model recommended that multi-level strategies were
needed to address all these levels of influence (IOM, 2000; McKinlay, 1995; Sallis & Owen, 2002). More specifically, they proposed that
educational and clinical interventions to improve the motivations,
skills, and supports for behavior change at the individual level
(e.g., for permanently quitting smoking or risky drinking, or adopting and maintaining healthier activity and eating patterns) would
be more successful when policies and influences in the wider environment supported healthy behaviors (e.g., through clean indoor
air laws, access to safe and attractive places to walk or bike, or to
healthy, affordable food choices).

A strong proponent of the ecological approach, McKinlay (1995)
proposed a template for more effective population health promotion strategies that linked individual-level, clinical health behavior change strategies with broader population-level health promotion efforts, including "upstream" policy and environmental
interventions. As early as 1975, McKinlay had indicated the need
to "refocus upstream," recounting his conversation with a physician weary of treating preventable diseases:

> "You know," [the doctor] said, "sometimes it feels like this. There I
> am standing by the shore of a swiftly flowing river, and I hear the
> cry of a drowning man. So I jump into the river, put my arms
> around him, pull him to shore, and apply artificial respiration. Just
> as he begins to breathe, someone else cries out for help. So I jump
> into the river again, reach him, pull him to shore and apply artifi-
> cial respiration, and then as he begins to breathe, there's another
> cry for help. So back into the river again, reaching, pulling, apply-
> ing, breathing, and then another yell. I'm so busy jumping in and

pulling them to shore that I have no time to see who the hell upstream is pushing them in." (McKinlay, 1975, p. 7)

The model McKinlay proposed in 1995 (see **TABLE 10.4**) recommended interventions across a broad spectrum of factors, linking "downstream" individual clinical approaches with "midstream" interventions aimed at health plans, schools, worksites, and communities, with "upstream" macro-level public policy and environmental interventions, strong enough to subvert or redirect strong societal, economic and industry counter forces. In essence, McKinlay argued that success in achieving lasting population-wide health behavior change required a "full court press"—using broad spectrum, multi-level approaches.

In a review of the past three decades of progress in population health promotion, the most recent IOM report on health and behavior reached the same conclusion (IOM, 2000). It used McKinlay's broad-spectrum, multilevel model for describing the balance needed between the dominant clinical and individually-oriented approaches to disease prevention and the population-level approaches address-

---

### TABLE 10.4

### Overview of McKinlay's (1995) Population-Based Intervention Model

| DOWNSTREAM INTERVENTIONS | MIDSTREAM INTERVENTIONS | UPSTREAM INTERVENTIONS |
|---|---|---|
| Individual-level interventions aimed at those who possess a behavioral risk factor or suffer from risk-related disease. Emphasis is on changing rather than preventing risk behaviors. | Population-level interventions that target defined populations in order to change and/or prevent behavioral risk factors. May involve mediation through important organizational channels or natural environments. | State and national public policy/environmental interventions that aim to strengthen social norms and supports for health behaviors and redirect unhealthy behaviors. |
| • Group and individual counseling<br>• Patient health education/cognitive behavioral interventions<br>• Self-help programs and tailored communications<br>• Pharmacologic treatments | • Worksite and community-based health promotion/disease prevention programs<br>• Health plan-based primary care screening/intervention<br>• School-based youth prevention activities<br>• Community-based interventions focused on defined at-risk populations | • National public education/media campaign<br>• Economic incentives (e.g., excise taxes on tobacco products, reimbursement for effective primary care, diets, and extensive counseling)<br>• Policies reducing access to unhealthy products (e.g., pricing, access, labeling)<br>• Policies reducing the advertising and promotion of unhealthy products and behaviors |

ing the generic social and behavioral determinants of disease, injury, and disability. Observing that "it is unreasonable to expect that people will change their behavior easily when so many forces in the social, cultural and physical environment conspire against such change" (IOM, 2000, p. 2), the authors of the IOM report recommended population-based health promotion efforts that:

- [U]se multiple approaches (e.g., education, social support, laws, incentives, behavior change programs) and address multiple levels of influence simultaneously (i.e., individuals, families, communities, nations) . . .
- [T]ake account of the special needs of target groups (i.e., based on age, gender, race, ethnicity and social class) . . .
- [T]ake the long view of health outcomes, as changes often take many years to become established; and
- [I]nvolve a variety of sectors in society that have not traditionally been associated with health promotion efforts, including law, business, education, social services and the media. (IOM, 2000, p. 6)

The last three decades of progress in national tobacco control, hailed by some as one of the greatest public health successes of the second half of the twentieth century, is the example most often used to illustrate the power and promise of ecological approaches for health intervention (IOM, 2000; Warner, 2000). In response to comprehensive tobacco control programs and policy changes in health care settings, worksites, schools, and communities and in all 50 states, adult smoking prevalence in the U.S. has dropped by almost 40% since the first Surgeon General's report in 1964, and the prevalence of teen smoking has declined steadily since 1998 (Orleans & Cummings, 1999; Warner, 2000). The interventions have been multilevel and broad spectrum—including changes in laws and regulations (clean indoor air laws, worksite smoking bans, changes in minimum age of purchase laws, advertising regulation, increased public and private insurance coverage for tobacco dependence treatment), economic disincentives (increases in tobacco prices and cigarette excise taxes), effective mass communication and counter-advertising campaigns, as well as increased access to effective quit smoking interventions (widening access to nicotine replacement through over-the-counter products, the proliferation of national, state, and health plan quit lines). Although major disparities in tobacco use and its addiction remain, regressive tobacco tax and

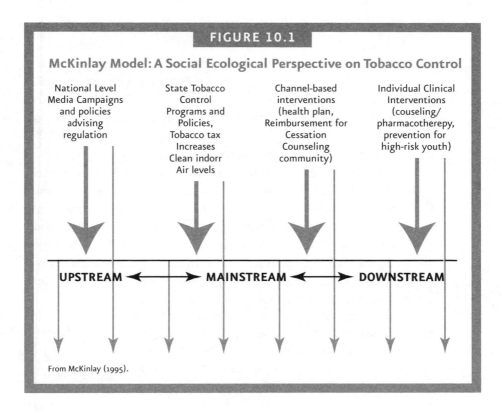

**FIGURE 10.1**

**McKinlay Model: A Social Ecological Perspective on Tobacco Control**

National Level Media Campaigns and policies advising regulation

State Tobacco Control Programs and Policies, Tobacco tax Increases Clean indorr Air levels

Channel-based interventions (health plan, Reimbursement for Cessation Counseling community)

Individual Clinical Interventions (couseling/ pharmacotherepy, prevention for high-risk youth)

UPSTREAM ← → MAINSTREAM ← → DOWNSTREAM

From McKinlay (1995).

price increases have proven especially effective in certain high-risk and underserved populations—including adolescents, pregnant and low-income smokers—and telephone quit lines have expanded the reach of evidence-based individual counseling to traditionally under-served low-income and minority populations (Boyd et al., 1998; Orleans & Alper, 2003). FIGURE 10.1 illustrates the application of McKinlay's model in tobacco control just described.

Reflecting the growth in research evaluating the population-impacts of "midstream" and "upstream" interventions for tobacco control, the Centers for Disease Control and Prevention (CDC) Task Force for Community Preventive Services now conducts systematic evidence reviews for community-based and policy interventions to change health behaviors that are similar to those conducted by the USPSTF for "downstream" clinical interventions. Based on its review of the evidence for 14 different interventions to reduce exposure to environmental tobacco smoke (ETS), reduce youth tobacco use initiation, and increase tobacco use cessation (CDC, 2001), it recommends: smoking bans and restrictions to reduce ETS exposure;

tax and price increases and mass media campaigns both to reduce youth initiation and promote cessation; and patient telephone quit line support as well as a number of health care system interventions to increase cessation (provider reminder systems plus provider education, and reducing out-of-pocket costs for effective cessation therapies). Figure 10.1 links these and related interventions to individual clinical and behavior change strategies, using McKinlay's model for full-court press interventions. Behavior-specific ecological models similar to the one shown in Figure 10.1 for tobacco control have been described and proposed for each of the other major behavioral risk factors discussed in this chapter—including risky drinking (Babor et al., 1999), physical activity (Marcus & Forsyth, 1999), dietary behavior change (Glanz, 1999), and obesity (Sallis & Owen, 2002). And soon CDC Community Task Force guidelines will be developed in each of these areas, concentrating initially on physical activity promotion and obesity prevention and control.

In fact, there is a great sense of urgency about the need to identify evidence-based "full-court press" strategies that can halt the nation's current obesity epidemic (Mokdad et al., 2004). The dramatic rise in the prevalence of overweight and obesity among youth and adults over the past several decades is primarily due to environmental and economic changes affecting behaviors on both side of the energy balance equation (Booth et al., 2001; Sallis & Owen, 2002). The cumulative effects of technology (e.g., automobile-dependent transportation, more sedentary jobs, and less recreation), changes in our lifestyle and environment (e.g., the shift from traditional neighborhoods where people could walk and bike to work and to shop, to suburban sprawl), and a decline in the number of children who walk or bike to school or take part in active physical education classes have all reduced the physical activity in our everyday life. At the same time, increased access to low-cost, sugar-laden, and high-fat foods and beverages, larger portion sizes, increased consumption of foods when away from home, an exodus of grocery stores and other sources of fresh fruits and vegetables from the cites to the suburbs, and the rising cost index for fresh fruits and vegetables relative to soda and snack foods have helped to promote excessive caloric intake, especially in low-income and racial/ethnic minority populations. As Booth et al. (2001) observe,

> Americans live in environments that do not favor a healthy balance between physical activity and food intake . . . Limited adoption of

healthful behaviors and poor maintenance of behavior change frequently observed in individually-based interventions may be partially explained by a failure to alter environments in which it is difficult to make healthy choices. In addition, environmental supports for healthy eating and physical activity are distributed unevenly throughout the population. (p. S22)

Rapid progress is being made in understanding the environmental and policy determinants of physical activity and in identifying promising multi-level, broad-spectrum interventions (Lavizzo-Mourey & McGinnis, 2003; Sallis & Owen, 2002). The CDC Community Preventive Services Task Force (CDC, 2001) reviewed research on interventions and found evidence for recommendations spanning the full McKinlay model. These include *downstream* health behavior change programs that increase social supports for physical activity and exercise (e.g., walking clubs); *midstream* requirements for school physical education classes that increase the time students spend in moderate or vigorous physical activity, and the use of "point of decision" prompts on elevators and escalators to encourage people to use nearby stairs; and more *upstream* efforts to create, or increase access to, safe, attractive, and convenient places for physical activity (e.g., parks, trails, bike lanes, sidewalks), along with informational outreach to change knowledge and attitudes about the benefits of and opportunities for physical activity. These recommendations sparked a recent study of socio-economic differences in access to community physical activity settings (sports areas, parks, and green space, public pools and beaches, and bike paths/lanes), which found predicted disparities in facilities, favoring the wealthy over low-income and minority communities (Powell & Chaloupka, 2004). A second set of CDC Task Force physical activity recommendations will soon be issued, addressing multi-level transportation and land use policies—ranging from zoning guidelines to improved federal, state, and community projects for walking and bicycling. Together, these guidelines provide an unprecedented science-based blueprint for multiple efforts (e.g., public health, urban planners, transportation agencies, parks and recreation, architects and landscape designers, public safety, local government, and mass media) both to close the gaps between recommended and actual physical activity levels for children and adults and to address pervasive environmental disparities (Lavizzo-Mourey et al., 2003).

As we learned from the success of tobacco control, highly credible scientific evidence can persuade policymakers and withstand the attacks of those whose interests are threatened. But the difficulty of implementing effective broad-spectrum approaches should not be underestimated (Isaacs & Schroeder, 2001; Sallis & Owen, 2002; Warner, 2000). Powerful political barriers include the sale, promotion, and marketing of unhealthy products, legislative lobbying by industry groups, limited public support for healthy public policies, and inadequate funding for and enforcement of effective policies and programs. Examples include poor enforcement of youth tobacco and alcohol access laws, the use of Tobacco Master Settlement Agreement funds for state budget deficits rather than for evidence-based tobacco control, and subsidies for unhealthy food products. Creating a favorable political climate requires using advocacy to instill broad public pressure and support for change, clear well-communicated evidence of public demand and/or support for change, and evidence of the beneficial health and economic impacts of proposed programs and policies. Sustaining this progress and effectively targeting special needs populations requires systematic surveillance to monitor the prevalence of both behavioral risk factor and effective programs and policies (Sallis & Owen; Warner). Such surveillance systems, which already exist for tobacco control and are rapidly developing for physical activity, establish a national baseline that makes it possible to assess the effects of specific interventions and to evaluate important local, state, and national intervention efforts. Finally, while some events and political changes may create opportunities for rapid change (e.g., the Master Settlement Agreement), a long-term view is essential. Most successful health promotion and social change efforts have required decades of hard work (Isaacs & Schroeder).

## CHANGING PROVIDER BEHAVIOR: PROVIDER-ORIENTED AND SYSTEM-BASED INTERVENTIONS FOR ACHIEVING NATIONAL HEALTH CARE QUALITY OBJECTIVES

One of the most basic measures of national health care quality is the extent to which patients receive recommended, evidence-based care (IOM, 2001). Now that evidence-based government guidelines exist for primary care interventions to help patients modify their primary behavioral risks for preventable death and chronic diseases, putting these guidelines into practice has become an important objective for national health care quality improvement efforts. The IOM's (2001) report *Crossing the Quality Chasm* has set forth a bold national agenda for improving the health care quality across the full spectrum of care from prevention to acute and chronic illness and palliative care, including health behavior change. A follow-on report (IOM, 2003) selected health behavior change interventions for tobacco and obesity as two of the top 20 priorities for national action.

This section presents a brief overview of past and present efforts to close the gaps between "what we know" and "what we do" when it comes to helping patients change serious lifestyle risks and health behaviors. It describes the major approaches that have been used and the evolution that has taken place from individual provider-focused strategies to broader health care systems-based approaches—mirroring similar shifts in population health promotion. New science-based guidelines and protocols for systems changes to improve the delivery of primary care interventions for each of the behavioral risks covered in this chapter are presented with reference to a generic model for planned proactive preventive and chronic illness care.

## Understanding and Closing the Gaps Between "Best Practice" and "Usual Care" for Primary Care Health Behavior Change Counseling and Intervention

Despite strong evidence for behavioral prevention in primary care, there are gaps between recommended and actual care, which are consistently greater than those for other evidence-based medical treatments and procedures (Glasgow, Orleans, Wagner, Curry, & Solberg, 2001a). For instance, in a recent study of the quality of outpatient health care for U.S. adults, McGlynn et al. (2003) found that U.S. adults, on average, received only about *half* the recommended medical care they needed overall, and even less (only 18%) of the lifestyle screening and counseling services they needed (McGlynn et al.). In fact, based on these studies, it is safe to say that most patients, especially those from low-socioeconomic (SES) and racial/ethnic minority backgrounds, who could benefit from health behavior change counseling are not receiving it. In most studies, patients were only asked about *assessment* and *advice*:

- *Tobacco use.* Only 50 to 60% of current smokers report being asked about tobacco use or advised to quit, and only about half report any assistance (counseling, pharmacotherapy) or follow-up (Orleans & Alper, 2003). Brief primary care tobacco use counseling has been ranked the single highest priority clinical preventive service to be received by fewer than half of the patients who need it (Coffield et al., 2001).

- *Alcohol use.* McGlynn et al. (2003) found that only 10.5% of adults seen in primary care settings were screened for alcohol misuse and referred for treatment when alcohol-dependent.
- *Physical inactivity and unhealthy diet.* In a 1992 survey, 40% of internists and 30% of nurse practitioners reported routinely assessing the physical activity levels of their patients, but only about half of each group reported developing physical activity plans for their patients (Francis, 1999). A 1997 survey found that only 42% of adult patients reported receiving advice from their primary care providers to increase their activity levels (Eden et al., 2002). Data from the 2000 National Health Interview Survey found that 25% and 21% of adults who had seen a doctor in the past 12 months reported receiving physician advice on diet and activity, respectively (Honda, 2004). And in a 1999–2000 survey of U.S. adults, only 33% reported past-year medical advice to eat more fruits and vegetables and only 29% reported receiving advice to reduce their fat intake (Glasgow, Eakin, Fisher, Bacak, & Brownson, 2001).
- *Obesity.* Fewer than half (42%) of obese adults (BMI of 30 or greater) surveyed in 1996 reported that their primary care provider had advised them to lose weight. Patients who were sicker (e.g., with diabetes, higher BMIs) and better educated were more likely to report receiving weight loss advice (Galuska, Will, Serdula, & Ford, 1999).

Early efforts to improve provider adherence to recommended clinical practices mirrored early efforts to boost patient adherence to recommended healthy personal practices. They emphasized individually-focused educational strategies, including educational materials and continuing medical education (CME) to change provider motivation, knowledge, attitudes, and self-efficacy (e.g., Davis, Thomson, Oxman, & Haynes, 1992; Hulscher, Wensing, Grol, Weijden, & Weel, 1999). This was true for evidence-based clinical practice guidelines generally, and for prevention and health behavior change guidelines specifically (e.g., Dickey, Gemson, & Carney, 1999; Hulscher et al., 1999). However, these efforts, like the parallel patient-focused efforts, were met with only modest success. Systematic evidence reviews conducted in the 1990s found these results: limited evidence for the efficacy of most educational approaches, including traditional CME; somewhat stronger evidence for more interactive and skill-based educational efforts, based on principles of adult learning and consonant with the principles of social learning theory (including modeling by respected peer "opinion leaders"); and strongest evidence for multicomponent interventions which addressed the multiple intrapersonal and environmental barriers to provider adherence, especially system barriers (Bero et al., 1998; Davis et al., 1992; Hulscher et al., 1999). Reflecting on these findings, and foreshadowing the "paradigm shift" that was to follow, John Eisenberg (Greco & Eisenberg, 1993), then director of the Agency for Healthcare Research and Quality, made the following observation:

> The faith that education can induce change in physicians' practices assumes that doctors' decisions are based on rational behavior and that poor decisions are simply the result of inadequate information. Give physicians information that is adequate and they will change their behavior. This is reasonable, but it does not work in practice. (p. 559)

The limited success of "if you tell them, they will change" educational strategies drew greater attention to the multiple system-level barriers to guideline adherence, including the lack of time (in the face of more urgent medical issues), office-level system supports, provider and patient resources, and financial incentives (e.g., Dickey et al., 1999: Solberg et al., 1998; Whitlock et al., 2002). Follow-up studies confirmed (a) that clinician training was most effective when combined with efforts to create office supports to prompt, facilitate, and reward the delivery of preventive interventions, especially behavioral counseling and (b) that the most successful interventions were those which were not "one-size-fits-all" but tailored to the unique barriers present in any particular office practice setting (e.g., Hulscher et al., 1999).

## The Emergence of Broad-Spectrum, Multilevel Approaches for Improving the Delivery of Effective Clinical Interventions

Collectively, these findings led to a shift in understanding what the targets of interventions to change *provider* health care practices need to be. This shift was almost identical to the one that took place in understanding how best to change *patients'* personal health practices. In fact, Crabtree and colleagues (2001) introduced a "practice ecological model" to describe the need to address not just the behavior of individual providers, but also the powerful health care systems in which they practice. They and other proponents of a broader view of health care improvement emphasize the need for *broad-spectrum* strategies addressing *multiple* levels of influence— from ("downstream") intrapersonal/individual provider-level factors, to ("midstream") interpersonal/practice team, office micro-systems and health plan influences, to ("upstream") macro-level health care systems and policies (e.g., Berwick, 2002; Dickey et al., 1999; Solberg et al., 1998). This paradigm shift was described in the IOM's *Crossing the Quality Chasm* report (2001), a charter for national health care quality improvement, as follows: "The current care systems cannot do the job. Trying harder will not work. Changing systems of care will" (p. 4). The *Quality Chasm* report went on to recommend a fundamental re-engineering of the nation's health care system—moving from a system designed primarily to support and pay for the delivery of reactive acute illness care, to one that would support and pay for the planned proactive (and behavioral) care needed to manage and prevent chronic disease.

Several systematic evidence reviews have been done to identify effective systems supports and policy changes needed to improve preventive care (see FIGURE 10.2). Again, work in the area of tobacco has led the way. The CDC Community Preventive Services Task Force (2000) reviewed research on the effectiveness of multiple interventions (e.g., provider training/feedback, organizational, administrative, and reimbursement changes) to improve the delivery of primary care tobacco interventions. It recommended reducing patient copays for proven tobacco dependence treatment services, and reminder systems to help providers identify patients who use tobacco products and to prompt them to implement the 5-As (e.g., chart stickers, stamps including tobacco use as a "vital sign," medical record flow sheets, checklists). Provider training (e.g., through CME seminars, lectures, videos, written materials for providers and patients) was recommended in conjunction with reminder systems, but not on its own. Similarly, the USPSTF found that training plus office-level system supports (prompts, reminders, and counseling algorithms) significantly improved the delivery of screening and counseling for unhealthy diet and risky

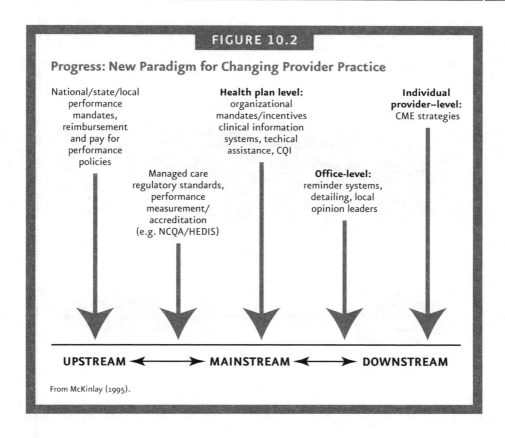

**FIGURE 10.2**

**Progress: New Paradigm for Changing Provider Practice**

National/state/local performance mandates, reimbursement and pay for performance policies

Managed care regulatory standards, performance measurement/ accreditation (e.g. NCQA/HEDIS)

**Health plan level:** organizational mandates/incentives clinical information systems, techical assistance, CQI

**Office-level:** reminder systems, detailing, local opinion leaders

**Individual provider–level:** CME strategies

**UPSTREAM** ←——→ **MAINSTREAM** ←——→ **DOWNSTREAM**

From McKinlay (1995).

drinking (Ockene, Hebert, & Ockene, 1996; USPSTF, 2003a, 2003b, 2004; Whitlock et al., 2004).

In response to these findings, it has often been said that "an ounce of prevention takes a ton of office system change." Until recently, we lacked a coherent model for what this "ton of change" included. Filling this void, Wagner, Austin, and Von Korff (1996) reviewed the research on effective chronic illness care and prevention and devised just such a model for the multiple inter-locking systems supports required for effective planned, proactive chronic illness care—called the "Chronic Care Model" (see **FIGURE 10.3**). This model appears to apply equally to the *prevention* and *treatment* of chronic disease, both of which require helping patients to change the behavioral risk factors that cause or complicate chronic disease (Glasgow et al., 2002).

The six key elements of the model in Figure 10.3 can be implemented at the level of the office practice and/or larger health care

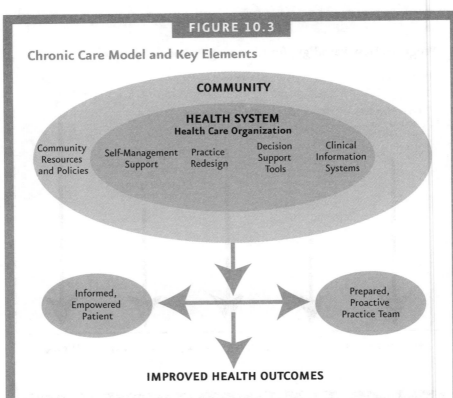

**FIGURE 10.3**

Chronic Care Model and Key Elements

- **Health care organization**—leadership and incentives that provide financial and nonfinancial incentives for providers to adhere to evidence-based guidelines and visible commitment to guideline-based health care and care improvement

- **Clinical information systems**—reminder and feedback systems for clinicians, patient tracking systems, and registries of targeted patient groups (e.g., patients with specific behavioral risk factors, heart disease, diabetes, obesity), plus other tools to help both providers and patients adhere to recommended practices

- **Decision support tools**—provider training and point-of-care prompts that give primary care practitioners timely access to relevant patient status information and clinical practice guidelines or algorithms

- **Practice redesign**—new formats for planned patient care that minimize provider burden, effectively use the entire health care team and/or deliver care outside of office visits (e.g., telephone counseling, personalized computer-generated mailings, web-based interventions, counseling from lay health advisors, group visits)

- **Self-management support**—interventions and resources that improve patients' knowledge, motivation, skills, confidence and psychosocial (including family) support to manage their care and adopt healthier lifestyles

- **Community resources and policies**—community-level programs, policies and resources that facilitate or support adherence to prescribed medical care and lifestyle modification, especially important in low-income and medically underserved populations (e.g., peer support, community and worksite programs, and policies to prevent or modify behavioral risk factors, access to opportunities for physical activity and to healthy, affordable, culturally-appropriate foods)

Glasgow et al., 2001a; Wagner et al., 1996

delivery system. The common principles that apply to each of these elements include interventions that are (a) planned (rather than reactive); (b) patient-centered and informed by individually-relevant patient data; (c) proactive (involving scheduled outreach and follow-up); and (d) population-based (focused on an entire panel of patients with a specific behavioral risk factor, disease, or condition, not just those who present for care). As noted, these core principles apply equally to the prevention and treatment or management of chronic disease. Since both require regular (nonsymptom-driven) screening and counseling for health behavior change, both involve ongoing planned care with proactive follow-up, and both depend on active patient involvement in decision-making and adherence, and both require linkages to supportive community resources and services (Glasgow et al., 2001a).

The Chronic Care Model was recently used to describe an organization-wide initiative at Group Health Cooperative of Puget Sound to integrate screening and treatment for tobacco use and dependence with routine primary care for all its members (Glasgow et al., 2001a; IOM, 2003). This successful plan applied all six model elements as follows:

- *Health care organization* health plan leaders made reducing tobacco use their top prevention priority, provided financial and other incentives to providers (including hiring of dedicated clinic counselors) and eliminated patient copays for counseling.
- *Clinical information systems* were used to create a registry of the tobacco users enrolled in the health plan, track their use of treatment resources and programs, and generate proactive telephone quitline calls for patients with feedback reports for providers.
- *Decision support tools* included extensive provider training, ongoing consultation, automated patient assessment and guideline algorithms, and reminder tools.
- *Practice redesign and self-management support* included self-help materials and a telephone quitline to deliver counseling and/or pharmacotherapy without burdening the provider.
- *Community resources and policies* included referral to community and worksite quit smoking clinics and related healthy lifestyle change programs (e.g., stress management exercise, weight loss) as well as support for worksite cessation campaigns and smoking restrictions and expanded state funding for tobacco prevention and control programs.

These integrated "full-court press" provider education, systems, and policy change efforts dramatically reduced the prevalence of smoking from 1985 to 1993 (from 25 to 15.5%) and led to substantial reductions in smokers' inpatient and outpatient health care services.

The Chronic Care Model provides a unifying approach to health care quality improvement that cuts across health behaviors and chronic conditions. As such it promises to provide a more efficient, sustainable, and cost-effective approach to health care quality improvement (Glasgow et al., in press). This is especially the case given the development of several successful continuous quality improvement (CQI) techniques and processes for putting Chronic Care Model-based systems changes into place. Promising "mid-stream" CQI approaches involve systematically experimenting with office system changes to find ways to eliminate the barriers and strengthen the supports for recommended care, often through a series of practice "rapid cycle" (plan-do-study-act) improvement efforts (Chin et al., 2004; Glasgow et al., in press).

Successful collaborative CQI interventions have been delivered through learning collaboratives involving multiple health care teams from multiple organizations who meet and work over a 12 to 18-month period with faculty who are expert in CQI techniques and in the type of care targeted for improvement (e.g., treating diabetes, tobacco dependence, obesity). Individual practice-level, chronic care model-based improvements involve planning, implementing, evaluating, and refining changes in their individual practices to address each practice's unique delivery problems, barriers, resources, and preferences (Chin et al., 2004; Glasgow et al., 2002). These collaboratives have substantially increased the proportion of patients, including those in most disadvantaged populations, receiving evidence-based care, and for whom individual behavior change plans were developed and implemented (e.g., dietary changes, smoking cessation) (Chin et al., 2004; Glasgow et al., 2002).

Effective individual practice consultation models for CQI have also been developed, making changes quite similar to those prescribed by the Chronic Care Model. The best example comes from the STEP-UP (Study To Enhance Prevention by Understanding Practice) trial conducted by Goodwin et al. (2001) and Stange, Goodwin, Zyzanski, and Dietrich (2003). This randomized, controlled trial tested a brief practice-tailored approach to improving preventive service delivery, which had an emphasis on improving rates of health habit counseling. Intervention practices received a 1-day practice assessment, an initial practice-wide consultation, and several brief follow-up visits to assess and address practice-specific barriers to and opportunities for improving the delivery of preventive services recommended by the USPSTF. All interventions were delivered by a specially trained nurse facilitator who helped practices identify promising changes and presented a menu of tools for implementing them (e.g., reminder systems, flow sheets, patient education materials, clinical information systems), including a practice improvement manual. An average of 4 follow-up visits took place in the 9 months following the initial consultation, during which the nurse facilitator helped practices to further individualize and implement their chosen tools and approaches and adjust their practice-led change efforts as needed. Follow-up discussions were used to assess the effectiveness and acceptability of each individual practice's improvement efforts and revise them as needed, and were informed by repeated assessment and mailed feedback on preventive service delivery rates every 6 months over a 2-year period. This brief CQI intervention resulted in significant improvements at 6 and 12 months that were maintained at a 24-month follow-up. Improvements in behavioral counseling services were especially dramatic. The investigators attributed these lasting results to the maintenance of the practice/system changes that were made, changes that may have been easier to institutionalize because they were tailored to the unique characteristics of each practice.

The STEP-UP trial has furnished compelling evidence that even a brief tailored intervention can increase providers' and practices' abilities to help their patients adopt healthier lifestyles, despite the often competing demands and pressures and toxic reimbursement systems of the larger health care system in which they operate (Goodwin et al., 2001; Stange et al., 2003). The parallels between the STEP-UP and individual health behavior change counseling and maintenance are striking. As Glasgow et al. (in press) have pointed out, "The same basic processes or principles of behavior change apply at both the *patient* level and the practice setting and *health system* levels" (p. 19). The same issues are important for individual behavior change and practice-level provider behavior change—i.e., using practice *assessment* and feedback, *advising* on strategies to address the barriers and opportunities in each practice, *agreeing* on a mutually negotiated, achievable, and specific action plan tailored to each practice's resources, problems, and readiness for change; *assisting* with tools and ongoing incremental problem-solving strategies, and *arranging* for follow-up support and resources to refine and maintain successful improvements.

In the long run, just as upstream macro-level societal and policy change is needed to sustain individual behavior change, upstream macro-level health system and policy change will be needed to support and spread the kinds of midstream and downstream-level provider and systems-level changes that can improve care at the office-practice and health plan levels (e.g., Berwick, 2002). Such changes include: quality performance measurement and public reporting; "pay-for-performance" initiatives that reward providers based on the quality of care they offer; and improved information technology (IT) to support case improvement processes (IOM, 2001). Schauffler and Chapman (1998), for instance, found that health plan providers were more likely to offer health behavior change counseling when a portion of their capitation payment was based on their doing so. And McMenamin et al. (2004) found that providers in physician organizations were more likely to offer proven health promotion services if they publicly reported performance measures and/or received public recognition or economic benefit from doing so, and if they had greater clinical IT capacity.

## CONCLUSIONS

Health-related behaviors, as this chapter is titled, represent a prime target for improving national health and health care. At no time in the history of public health and medicine have we known more about the importance of addressing the health lifestyle factors and health-related behaviors that represent the most serious threat to the nation's health, and make the greatest contributions to its health care burden and cost. The growing burden of chronic disease, a national epidemic of obesity, and escalating health care costs (at a time when health care spending already outstrips the growth of the U.S. gross domestic product) creates an urgent need to establish a stronger preventive orientation in the U.S. health care and public health systems (Mokdad et al., 2004). Likewise, we have never known as much about how to motivate, support, and assist individuals to make lasting lifestyle changes, using evidence-based primary care treatments as part of a broader population-based strategy to build healthy environments, with special efforts to target underserved and high-risk populations. And finally, we have never known as much about how to support and assist health care professionals to deliver evidence-based behavioral preventive care, implementing changes in health care systems and policies that will improve care for the management and prevention of chronic disease. The tremendous parallel gains made in what we have learned about the processes, principles, and paradigms for effective health promotion (i.e., patient behavior change) and what we have learned about the processes, principles, and paradigms for effective health care quality improvement (i.e., provider behavior change) have created unprecedented potential for change. The stage is already set for breakthrough improvements in national health status and health care quality, but the urgency of work to achieve these improvements has never been greater. However, real-

## CASE STUDY

You have just been hired as the Director of Strategic Planning for a health plan that insures of 30% of the residents in a metropolitan area with 500,000 residents. Those insured by this health plan are mostly employed by large companies in the metropolitan area, and these companies pay for their employees' health insurance. Other insurance companies and health plans are active in this metropolitan area, so there is strong competition to keep the costs employers pay for health plan charges as low as possible, which in turn should keep costs down for the plan's enrollees.

In your new role as Director of Strategic Planning, you are asked to create a "business case" for investing more of the health plan's resources into interventions that might influence behavioral choices related to smoking, diet, and physical activity. This business case will need to consider whether the benefits of undertaking new interventions will offset the costs of the interventions to the health plan. How would you go about preparing this business case? What types of information will be important to have? Write a report to your manager that lays out your plan for completing this business case.

izing this potential depends entirely on how we use this knowledge. To quote Goethe, "Knowing is not enough; we must apply.
Willing is not enough; we must do" (cited in IOM, 2000).

## DISCUSSION QUESTIONS

1. What types of interventions at the national level might make it possible to reach the ambitious *Healthy People 2010* national goals (as
   described in Table 10.1)?
2. How have behavior change interventions changed over the past 20
   years?
3. What are some examples of individual-level change interventions
   (compared to population-level change interventions)?
4. What types of interventions can primary care providers undertake
   to change behavioral health risks among individuals?
5. What are examples of multilevel models for population-based behavior change?

## REFERENCES

Agency for Health Care Policy and Research (AHCPR). (1996). *Smoking Cessation*. Clinical Practice Guideline, No. 18. AHCPR Publication No.
96–0692. Rockville, MD: U.S. Department of Health and Human
Services.

Babor, T. F., Aguirre-Molina, M., Marlatt, G. A., & Clayton, R. (1999). Managing alcohol problems and risky drinking. *American Journal of Health
Promotion, 14*(2), 98–103.

Bandura A. (1986). *Social foundations of thoughts and actions*. Englewood Cliffs,
NJ: Prentice Hall.

Barlow, S. E., & Dietz, W. H. (2002). Management of child and adolescent
obesity: Summary and recommendations based on reports from
pediatricians, pediatric nurse practitioners, and registered dietitians. *Pediatrics, 110*(1), 236–238.

Boyd, N. R., Sutton, C., Orleans, C. T., McClatchey, M., Bingler, R., et al.
(1998). "Quit Today"—A targeted communications campaign to
increase use of the Cancer Information Services as a quit smoking
resource among African American smokers. *Preventive Medicine, 27*,
S50–60.

Bero, L., Grilli, R., Grimshaw, J. M., Harvey, E., Oxman, A. P., & Thomson, M. A. (1998). Closing the gap between research and practice: An
overview of systematic reviews of interventions to promote implementation of research findings by health care professionals. *British
Medical Journal, 316*, 465–468.

Berwick, D. (2002). A user's manual for the IOM's 'Quality Chasm' report. *Health Affairs, 21*(3), 80–90.

Booth, S. L., Sallis, J. F., Ritenbaugh, C., Hill, J. O., Birch, L. L., Frank, L. D., et al. (2001). Environmental and societal factors affect food choice and physical activity: Rationale, influences, and leverage points. *Nutrition Reviews, 59*(3), S21–S39.

Centers for Disease Control and Prevention. (2000). Strategies for reducing exposure to environmental tobacco smoke, increasing tobacco use cessation, and reducing irritation in communities and health-care systems. *Morbidity & Mortality Weekly Report, 49*(RR12), 1–11.

Centers for Disease Control and Prevention (CDC). (2001). Increasing physical activity: A report on recommendations of the Task Force on Community Preventive Services. *MMWR Recomm Rep, 50*(RR-18), 1–14.

Centers for Disease Control and Prevention (CDC). (2002). The guide to community preventive services: Tobacco use and prevention. Reviews, recommendations, and expert commentary. *American Journal of Preventive Medicine, 20*(Suppl.).

Centers for Disease Control and Prevention (CDC). (2004a). *Chronic disease overview,* http://www.cdc.gov/nccdphp/overview.htm Accessed on June 23, 2004.

Centers for Disease Control and Prevention (CDC). (2004b). *The 2004 Surgeon General's Report: Health consequences of smoking,* http://www.cdc.gov/tobacco/sgr/sgr_2004/Factsheets/2.htm Accessed on June 23, 2004.

Chin, M. H., Cook, S., Drum, M. L., Jin, L., Guillen, M., Humikowski, C. A., et al. (2004). Improving diabetes care in Midwest community health centers with the health disparities collaborative. *Diabetes Care, 27*(1), 2–8.

Coffield, A. B., Maciosek, M. V., McGinnis, J. M., Harris, J. R., Caldwell, M. B., Teutsch, S. M., et al. (2001). Priorities among recommended clinical preventive services. *American Journal of Preventive Medicine, 21*(1), 1–9.

Coups, E. J., Gaba, A., & Orleans, C. T. (in press). Physician screening for multiple behavioral health risk factors. *American Journal of Preventive Medicine.*

Crabtree, B. F., Miller, W. L., & Stange, K. C. (2001). Understanding practice from the ground up. *The Journal of Family Practice, 50*(10), 881–887.

Davis, D. A., Thomson, M. A., Oxman, A. D., & Haynes, R. B. (1992). Evidence for the effectiveness of CME. A review of 50 randomized controlled trials. *Journal of the American Medical Association, 268,* 1111–1117.

Dickey, L. J., Gemson, D. H., & Carney, P. (1999). Office system interventions supporting primary care-based health behavior change counseling. *American Journal of Preventive Medicine, 17*(4), 299–308.

Eden, K. B., Orleans, C. T., Mulrow, C. D., Pender, N. J., & Teutsch, S. M.

(2002). Does counseling by clinicians improve physical activity? A summary of the evidence for the U.S. Preventive Services Task Force. *Annals of Internal Medicine, 137*(3), 208–215.

Elder, J. P., Ayala, G. X., & Harris, S. (1999). Theories and intervention approaches to health-behavior change in primary care. *American Journal of Preventive Medicine, 17,* 275–284.

Emmons, K. M., & Rollnick, S. (2001). Motivational interviewing in health care settings: Opportunities and limitations. *American Journal of Preventive Medicine, 20,* 68–74.

Finkelstein, E. A., Fiebelkorn, I. C., & Wang, G. (2003, May 14). National medical spending attributable to overweight and obesity: How much, and who's paying? Available: http://eletra.com/bio analogics/e_article000172535.cfm

Fiore, M. C., Novotny, T. E., Pierce, J. P., Giovino, G. A., Hatziandreu, E. J., Newcomb, P. A., et al. (1990). Methods used to quit smoking in the United States: Do cessation programs help? *Journal of the American Medical Association, 263,* 2760–2765.

Flegal, K. M., Carroll, M. D., Ogden, C. L., & Johnson, C. L. (2002). Prevalence and trends in obesity among U.S. adults, 1999–2000. National Center for Health Statistics, *Journal of the American Medical Association, 288*(14), 1723–1727.

Francis, K. T. (1999). Status of the year 2000 health goals for physical activity and fitness. *Phys Ther, 79*(4), 405–414.

Galuska, D. A., Will, J. C., Serdula, M. K., & Ford, E. S. (1999). Are health care professionals advising obese patients to lose weight? *Journal of the American Medical Association, 282*(16), 1576–1578.

Glanz, K. (1999). Progress in dietary behavior change. *American Journal of Health Promotion, 14*(2), 112–117.

Glanz, K., Rimer, B. K., & Lewis, F. M. (2002). Theory, research, and practice in health behavior and health education. In K. Glanz, B. K. Rimer, & F. M. Lewis (Eds.), *Health behavior and health education: Theory research and practice* (3rd ed., pp. 22–39). San Francisco: Jossey-Bass.

Glasgow, R. E., Bull, S. S., Piette, J. D., & Steiner, J. (in press). Interactive behavior change technology: A partial solution to the competing demands of primary care. *American Journal of Preventive Medicine.*

Glasgow, R. E., Eakin, E. G., Fisher, E. B., Bacak, S. J., & Brownson, R. C. (2001). Physician advice and support for physical activity: Results from a national survey. *American Journal of Preventive Medicine, 21*(3), 189–196.

Glasgow, R. E., Funnell, M. M., Bonomi, A. E., Davis, C., Beckham, V., & Wagner, E. H. (2002). Self-management aspects of the improving chronic illness care Breakthrough Series: Implementation with diabetes and heart failure teams. *Annals of Behavioral Medicine, 24*(2), 80–87.

Glasgow, R. E., Goldstein, M. G., Ockene, J. K., & Pronk, N. P. (in press).

Translating what we have learned into practice: Principles and hypotheses for addressing multiple behaviors in primary care. *American Journal of Preventive Medicine.*

Glasgow, R. E., Orleans, C. T., Wagner, E. H., Curry, S. J., & Solberg, L. I. (2001). Does the Chronic Care Model serve also as a template for improving prevention? *Milbank Quarterly, 79*, 579–612.

Glynn, T. J., & Manley, M. W. (1989). How to help your patients stop smoking: A manual for physicians. (NIH publication No. 89–3064.) Bethesda, MD: National Cancer Institute.

Goldstein, M. G., Whitlock, E. P., & DePue, J. (in press). Multiple behavioral risk factor interventions in primary care: Summary of research evidence. *American Journal of Preventive Medicine.*

Goodwin, M. A., Zyzanski, S. J., Zronek, S., Ruhe, M., Weyer, S. M., Konrad, N., et al. (2001). A clinical trial of tailored office systems for preventive service delivery: The Study to Enhance Prevention by Understanding Practice (STEP-UP). *American Journal of Preventive Medicine, 21*, 20–28.

Grantmakers in Health (GIH). (2004). Healthy behaviors: Addressing chronic disease at its roots. Issue Brief No. 19, February 2004, Based on a Grantmakers in Health Issue Dialogue. Washington, DC: Grantmakers in Health.

Greco, P. J., & Eisenberg, J. M. (1993). Changing physicians' practices. *New England Journal of Medicine, 329*(17), 1271.

Halvorson, G. C., & Isham, G. J. (2003). *Epidemic of care: A call for safer, better, and more accountable health care.* San Francisco: Jossey-Bass.

Honda, K. (2004). Factors underlying variation in receipt of physical advice on diet and exercise: Applications of the behavioral model of health care utilization. *American Journal of Health Promotion, 18*(5), 370–377.

Hulscher, M., Wensing, M., Grol, R., Weijden, T., & Weel, C. (1999, May). Interventions to improve the delivery of preventive services in primary care. *American Journal of Public Health, 89*(5), 737–746.

Institute for Health & Aging & University of California San Francisco. (1996). *Chronic care in America: A 21st century challenge.* Princeton, NJ: The Robert Wood Johnson Foundation.

Institute of Medicine. [IOM]. (1982). *Health and behavior: Frontiers of research in the biobehavioral sciences.* D. A. Hamburg, G. R. Elliott, & D. L. Parron, Eds. Division of Mental Health and Behavioral Medicine. Washington, DC: National Academy Press.

Institute of Medicine. [IOM]. (2000). *Promoting health: Intervention strategies from social and behavioral research.* B. D. Smedley & S. L. Syme, Eds. Washington, DC: National Academy Press.

Institute of Medicine. [IOM]. (2001). *Crossing the Quality Chasm: A new health system for the 21st century.* R. Briere, Ed. Washington, DC: National Academy Press.

Institute of Medicine. [IOM]. (2003). *Priority areas for national action: Transforming health care quality. Quality Chasm* series. K. Adams & J. M. Corrigan, Eds. Washington, DC: National Academies Press.

Isaacs, S. L., & Schroeder, S. A. (2001). Where the public good prevailed: Lessons from success stories in health. *American Prospect, 12*(10), 26–30.

Johnston, L. D., O'Malley, P. M., & Bachman, J. G. (2003a). *Monitoring the future national survey results on drug use, 1975–2002: Vol. 2. Secondary students.* (NIH Pub. No. 03–5375). Bethesda, MD: National Institute of Drug Abuse.

Johnston, L. D., O'Malley, P. M., & Bachman, J. G. (2003b). *Monitoring the future national survey results on drug use, 1975–2002: Vol. 2. College students and young adults.* (NIH Pub. No. 03–5376). Bethesda, MD: National Institute of Drug Abuse.

Kottke, T. E., Battista, R. N., DeFriese, G. H., & Brekke, M. L. (1988). Attributes of successful smoking cessation interventions in medical practice. A meta-analysis of 39 controlled trials. *Journal of the American Medical Association, 259*(19), 2883–2889.

Kreuter, M. W., Chheda, S. G., & Bull, F. C. (2000). How does physician advice influence patient behavior? *Archives of Family Medicine, 9*(5), 426–433.

Lavizzo-Mourey, R., & McGinnis, J. M. (2003). Making the case for active living communities. *American Journal of Public Health, 93*(9), 1386–1388.

Lichtenstein, E., & Glasgow R. E. (1992). Smoking cessation: What have we learned over the past decade? *Journal of Consulting and Clinical Psychology, 60*(4), 518–527.

Maibach, E. W., Rothschild, M. L., & Novelli, W. D. (2002). Social marketing. In K. Glanz, F. M. Lewis, & B. Rimer (Eds.), *Health behavior and health education* (3rd ed., pp. 437–461). San Francisco: Jossey-Bass.

Marcus, B. H., & Forsyth, L. H. (1999). How are we doing with physical activity? *American Journal of Health Promotion, 14*(2), 118–124.

Marcus, B. H., Goldstein, M. G., Jette, A., Simkin-Silverman, L., Pinto, B. M., Milan, F., et al. (1997). Training physicians to conduct physical activity counseling. *Preventive Medicine, 26*(3), 382–388.

McGinnis, J. M., & Foege, W. H. (1993). Actual causes of death in the United States. *Journal of the American Medical Association, 270*, 2207–2212.

McGlynn, E. A., Asch, S. M., Adams, J., Keesey, J., Hicks, J., DeCristofaro, A., et al. (2003). The quality of health care delivered to adults in the United States. *New England Journal of Medicine, 348*(26), 2635–2645.

McKinlay, J. B. (1975). A case for re-focusing upstream: The political economy of illness. In A. J. Enelow & J. B. Henderson, (Eds.), *Applying behavioral science to cardiovascular risk* (pp. 7–18). Seattle, WA: American Heart Association.

McKinlay, J. B. (1995). The new public health approach to improving physical activity and autonomy in older populations. In E. Heikkinen (Ed.), *Preparation for aging* (pp. 87–103). New York: Plenum.

McMenamin, S. B., Schmittdiel, J., Halpin, H., Gillies, R., Rundall, T. G., & Shortell, S. M. (2004). Health promotion in physician organizations: Results from a national study. *American Journal of Preventive Medicine, 26*(4), 259–264.

McTigue, K. M., Harris, R., Hemphill, B., Lux, L., Sutton, S., Bunton, A. J., et al. (2003). Screening and interventions for obesity in adults: Summary of the evidence for the U.S. Preventive Services Task Force. *Annals of Internal Medicine, 139*(11), 933–949.

Mei, Z., Scanlon, K. S., Grummer-Strawn, L. M., Freedman, D. S., Yip, R., & Trowbridge, F. L. (1998). Increasing prevalence of overweight among U.S. low-income preschool children: The Centers for Disease Control and Prevention pediatric nutrition surveillance, 1983 to 1995. *Pediatrics, 101*(1), E12.

Mokdad, A. H., Marks, J. S., Stroup, D. F., & Gerberding, J. L. (2004). Actual causes of death in the United States, 2000. *Journal of the American Medical Association, 291*(10), 1238–1245.

Morbidity Mortality Weekly Report (MMWR). (1997). Medical care expenditures attributable to cigarette smoking during pregnancy—United States. *Morbidity Mortality Weekly Report, 46,* 1048–1050.

Must, A., Spadano, J., Coakley, E. H., Field, A. E., Colditz, G., & Dietz, W. H. (1999). The disease burden associated with overweight and obesity. *Journal of the American Medical Association, 282*(16), 1523–1529.

National Center for Health Statistics (NCHS). (1999). *Healthy People 2000 Review, 1998–1999.* Hyattsville, MD: Public Health Service.

National Center for Health Statistics (NCHS). (2003). *Health, United States, 2003.* Hyattsville, MD: National Center for Health Statistics.

National Institute on Alcohol Abuse and Alcoholism (NIAAA). (2001, January). *Economic perspectives in alcoholism research: Alcohol Alert No. 51.* Washington, DC: National Institute on Alcohol Abuse and Alcoholism.

Ockene, I. S., Hebert, J. R., & Ockene, J. K. (1996). Effect of training and a structured office practice on physician-delivered nutrition counseling: The Worcester-Area Trial for Counseling in Hyperlipidemia (WATCH). *American Journal of Preventive Medicine, 12*(4), 252–258.

Orleans, C. T. (1993). Treating nicotine dependence in medical settings: A stepped-care model. In C. T. Orleans & J. Slade (Eds.), *Nicotine addiction: Principles and management* (pp. 145–161). New York: Oxford University Press.

Orleans, C. T. (2000). Promoting the maintenance of health behavior change: Recommendations for the next generation of research and practice. *Health Psychology, 19*(1), (Suppl.). 76–83.

Orleans, C. T., & Alper, J. (2003). Helping addicted smokers quit. In S. L.

Isaacs & J. R. Knickman (Eds.), *To improve health and health care* (Vol. 6, pp. 125–148). San Francisco: Josey-Bass.

Orleans, C. T., Barker, D. C., Kaufman, N. J., & Marx, J. F. (2000). Helping pregnant smokers quit: Meeting the challenge in the next decade. *Tobacco Control, 9*(Supp. III), iii6–iii11.

Orleans, C. T., & Cummings, K. M. (1999). Population-based tobacco control: Progress and prospects. *American Journal of Health Promotion, 14*(2), 83–91.

Orleans, C. T., George, L. K., Houpt, J. L., & Brodie, K. H. (1985). Health promotion in primary care: A survey of U.S. family practitioners. *Preventive Medicine, 14,* 636–647.

Orleans, C. T., Gruman, J., Ulmer, C., Emont, S. L., & Hollendonner, J. K. (1999). Rating our progress in population health promotion: Report card on six behaviors. *American Journal of Health Promotion, 14,* 75–83.

Orleans, C. T., Ulmer, C., & Groman, J. (2004). The role of behavioral factors in achieving national health outcomes. In R. G. Frank, A. Baum, & J. L. Wallander (Eds.), *Handbook of clinical health psychology* (Vol. 3: Models and Perspectives in Health Psychology). Washington, DC: American Psychological Association.

Pignone, M. P., Ammerman, A., Fernandez, L., Orleans, C. T., Pender, N., Woolf, S., et al. (2003). Counseling to promote a healthy diet in adults: A summary of the evidence for the U.S. Preventive Services Task Force. *American Journal of Preventive Medicine, 24*(1), 75–92.

Powell, L. M., Slater, S., & Chaloupka, F. J. (2004). The relationship between community physical activity settings and race, ethnicity, and socioeconomic status. *Evidence-Based Preventive Medicine, 1*(2), 135–144.

Prochaska, J. O., & DiClemente, C. C. (1983). Stages and processes of self-change of smoking: Towards an integrative model of change. *Journal of Consulting and Clinical Psychology, 51,* 390–395.

Prochaska, J. O., DiClemente, C. C., & Norcross, J. C. (1992). In search of how people change: Applications to addictive behaviors. *American Psychologist, 47,* 1102–1114.

Prochaska, J. O., Velicer, W. F., Rossi, J. S., Redding, C. A., Greene, G. W., Rossi, S. R., et al. (in press). Impact of simultaneous stage-matched expert system interventions for smoking, high fat diet and sun exposure in a population of parents. *Health Psychology.*

Rees, J. M., Neumark-Sztainer, D., Kohn, M., & Jacobson, M. (2000). Improving the nutritional health of adolescents. Society for Adolescent Medicine Position Statement. *Journal of Child and Family Nursing, 3*(1), 80–81.

Research Triangle Institute. (2004, January 21). *Researchers estimate states spend billions in medical costs of obesity,* www.rti.org/printpg.cfm?objectid=4CDB8DC2–6720–4FBF-806A064BB32DD00B Accessed July 7, 2004.

Sallis, J. F., & Owen, N. (2002). Ecological models of health behavior. In K. Glanz, F. M. Lewis, & B. Rimer (eds.), *Health behavior and health education* (3rd ed., pp. 462–484). San Francisco: Jossey-Bass.

Sallis, J. F., & Owen, N. (2004). Ecological models of health behavior. In K. Glanz, B. Rimer, & F. M. Lewis (Eds.), *Health behavior and health education: Theory research and practice* (3rd ed., pp. 462–484). San Francisco: Jossey-Bass.

Schauffler, H. H., & Chapman, S. A. (1998). Health promotion and managed care: Surveys of California's health plans and population. *American Journal of Preventive Medicine, 14*, 161–171.

Solberg, L. I., Kottke, T. E., Brekke, M. L., Conn, S. A., Magnan, S., & Amundson, G. (1998). The case of the missing clinical preventive services systems. *Effective Clinical Practice, 1*, 33–38.

Stange, K. C., Goodwin, M. A., Zyzanski, S. J., & Dietrich, A. J. (2003). Sustainability of a practice-individualized preventive service delivery intervention. *American Journal of Preventive Medicine, 25*(4), 296–300.

Stange, K. C., Woolf, S. H., & Gjeltema, K. (2002). One minute for prevention: The power of leveraging to fulfill the promise of health behavior counseling. *American Journal of Preventive Medicine, 22*(4), 320–323.

Thompson, R. S., Taplin, S. H., McAfee, T. A., Mandelson, M. T., & Smith, A. E. (1995). Primary and secondary prevention services in clinical practice: Twenty years' experience in development, implementation, and evaluation. *Journal of the American Medical Association, 273*, 1130–1135.

Tuomilehto, J., Lindstrom, J., Eriksson, J. G., Valle, T. T., Hamalainen, H., Ilanne-Parikka, P., et al. (2001). Prevention of Type 2 Diabetes Mellitus by changes in lifestyle among subjects with impaired glucose tolerance. *New England Journal of Medicine, 344*(18), 1343–1350.

U.S. Department of Health and Human Services (USDHHS). (1990). *The health benefits of smoking cessation. A report of the Surgeon General, 1990.* Rockville, MD: Public Health Service, Centers for Disease Control, Office of Smoking and Health, 1990. (DHHS Publication No. (cdc) 90–8416).

U.S. Department of Health and Human Services (USDHHS). (2000). Nutrition and your health: Dietary guidelines for Americans (5th ed.). Available: http://www.health.gov/dietaryguidelines/

U.S. Department of Health and Human Services (USDHHS). (2000a). *Healthy People 2010* (2nd ed., Vol. 1). Washington, DC: USDHHS.

U.S. Department of Health and Human Services (USDHHS). (2000b). *Treating tobacco use and dependence.* Update of 1996 *Smoking Cessation Clinical Practice Guideline No. 18.* Washington, DC: USDHHS.

U.S. Department of Health and Human Services (USDHHS). (2000c). *Healthy people 2010: Understanding and improving health.* Washington, DC: USDHHS.

U.S. Preventive Services Task Force (USPTF). (1996). *Guide to clinical preventive services* (2nd ed.). Baltimore: Williams & Wilkins.

U.S. Preventive Services Task Force (USPTF). (2002). Behavioral counseling in primary care to promote physical activity: Recommendation and rationale. *Annals of Internal Medicine, 137*(3), 205–207.

U.S. Preventive Services Task Force (USPTF). (2003a). Behavioral counseling in primary care to promote a healthy diet: Recommendations and rationale. *American Journal of Preventive Medicine, 24*(1), 93.

U.S. Preventive Services Task Force (USPTF). (2003b). Screening for obesity in adults: Recommendations and rationale. *Annals of Internal Medicine, 139*(11), 930–932.

U.S. Preventive Services Task Force (USPTF). (2004). Screening and behavioral counseling interventions in primary care to reduce alcohol misuse: Recommendation statement. *Annals of Internal Medicine, 140*(7), 554–556.

U.S. Public Health Service (USPHS). (2000). Treating tobacco use and dependence: A clinical practice guideline. (AHRQ Publication No. 00–0032). U.S. Department of Health and Human Services. Available: www.ahrq.gov

Vogt, T. M., Hollis, J. F., Lichtenstein, E., Stevens, V. J., Glasgow, R., & Whitlock, E. (1998). The medical care system and prevention: The need for a new paradigm. *HMO Practitioner, 12*, 5–13.

Wagner, E. H., Austin, B. T., & Von Korff, M. (1996). Organizing care for patients with chronic illness. *Milbank Quarterly, 74*, 511–544.

Wagner, E. H., Curry, S. J., Grothaus, L., Saunders, K. W., & McBride, C. M. (1995). The impact of smoking and quitting on health care use. *Archives of Internal Medicine, 155*(16), 1789–1795.

Wagner, E. H., Glasgow, R. E., Davis, C., Bonomi, A., Provost, L., McCulloch, D., et al. (2001). Quality improvement in chronic illness care: A collaborative approach. *Joint Commission Journal on Quality Improvement, 27*, 63–80.

Warner, K. E. (2000). The need for, and value of, a multi-level approach to disease prevention: The case of tobacco control. In B. D. Smedley & S. L. Syme (Eds.), Institute of Medicine *Promoting health: Intervention strategies from social and behavioral research* (pp. 417–449). Washington, DC: National Academy Press.

Wechsler, H., Levine, S., Idelson, R. K., Schor, E. L., & Coakley, E. (1996). The physician's role in health promotion revisited: A survey of primary care practitioners. *New England Journal of Medicine, 334*(15), 996–998.

Whitlock, E. P., Orleans, C. T., Pender, N., & Allan, J. (2002). Evaluating primary care behavioral counseling interventions: An evidence-based approach. *American Journal of Preventive Medicine, 22*(4), 267–284.

Whitlock, E. P., Polen, M. R., Green, C. A., Orleans, C. T., & Klein, J. (2004). Behavioral counseling interventions in primary care to reduce risky/harmful alcohol use by adults: A summary of the evidence for the U.S. Preventive Services Task Force. *Annals of Internal Medicine, 140*(7), 557–568.

Windle, M. (1999). *Alcohol use among adolescents.* Thousand Oaks, CA: Sage.

Yi, H., Williams, G. D., & Dufour, M. C. (2003). *Trends in alcohol-related fatal traffic crashes, United States, 1977–2001.* (Surveillance Report No. 65). Washington, DC: National Institute on Alcohol Abuse and Alcoholism.

# 11

# PHARMA-CEUTICALS AND MEDICAL DEVICES

Robin J. Strongin and
Ron Geigle

- Compare and contrast the U.S. pharmaceutical and medical device industries.
- Understand the drug discovery and development processes.
- Describe the FDA drug and device approval processes.
- Analyze pharmaceutical marketplace dynamics.
- Highlight landmark legislation.
- Understand the role of Medicare in device reimbursement.
- Describe the growing focus on "value" in drugs and devices.
- Analyze the new standards for evidence for devices.

- Discovery and development
- Research and development: The price of innovation
- Patents and generics
- Pharmaceutical marketplace dynamics
- The Medicare Prescription Drug, Improvement and Modernization Act of 2003
- Medical devices industry overview
- FDA premarket review
- Medicare coverage and payment
- Private sector coverage, payment, and cost control
- The value of medical technology
- Conclusions

Clinical trials, drug, pharmacogenomics, pharmaceutical equivalence, bioequivalence, therapeutic equivalence, generics, Medicare prescription drug legislation, prescription, patents, research and development, formulary, rebates, pharmaceutical, pharmacy benefit manager, reimportation, coverage, payment, user fees, premarket approval, medical device, medical diagnostic, medical technology, value, evidence, innovation, Food and Drug Administration

P RESCRIPTION DRUGS AND medical devices are integral parts of the U.S. health care delivery system. Both have revolutionized the prevention, diagnosis, and treatment of disease. But the price tag of this medical progress is staggering—not only in terms of dollars, but in the degree of risk companies must take, and the complex regulatory responsibilities they must bear to balance safety on the one hand with experimental development on the other.

These two health care industries, along with the biotechnology industry, share many traits: they each invest billions of dollars into research and development (R&D); they are regulated by the Food and Drug Administration (FDA); they represent, for many patients, a critical lifeline to better health; they each face challenges in both the private and public sectors of the marketplace, as coding, coverage, payment, and reimbursement decision-making require increasingly more sophisticated levels of analysis; and they each face the troubling reality that not all individuals who need these products are able to access them—because of insurance denials, affordability, or politics. Finally, both industries have been challenged by increasing demands from payers, regulators, and others to prove that their products improve health outcomes, and do so in a cost-effective manner.

While drugs and medical devices share much in common, they represent two very distinct industries with important and fundamental differences. Although the FDA approves both drugs and devices for marketing, the approval processes are very different. Due to the very nature of how innovation occurs for drugs and devices, the timing, number granted, patent life, and overall importance of patents are markedly different. Innovation in the pharmaceutical sector is, to a greater degree than in the medical device industry, supported by taxpayer funded NIH (National Institutes of Health) research.

Because the nature of innovation is unique in each industry, it is not surprising that the two industries are configured very differently. Generally, the medical device industry is comprised of a greater number of small and start-up companies as compared to the major pharmaceutical companies. Although an impressive number of drug discoveries occur in smaller life sciences and pharmaceutical companies, the majority of successfully marketed drugs are products of the larger drug firms—where the infrastructure, experience, capital, and vast resources necessary to finance and market innovation are more plentiful. On the other hand, the developers of innovative devices tend to be smaller companies, where scientists work side by side with practicing physicians to create, modify, and improve new and existing technologies. Often these companies partner with larger companies to bring these products to market.

With scientific advances, a number of exciting new therapies are on the horizon. Some of these are drugs; some are devices. Some are a combination of both, while still others are defining entirely new technologies. The areas of genomics, nanotechnology, robotics, information systems, vaccines, and pharmacogenomics all hold the promise of further breakthroughs in medical science.

The road from the laboratory to the patient is a long and challenging one, however. Many obstacles and challenges lie along the route. But miraculous achievements in public health and scientific achievement do as well. Yet the question remains—and answering it may grow even more difficult in the future: Will patients who need these drugs and medical devices be able to get them?

# PHARMACEUTICALS

The process of developing, testing, and marketing pharmaceutical drugs is described in the first section of this chapter. The section also includes information on patients and generic drugs.

## Drug Discovery and Development

In 1928, a Scottish bacteriologist inadvertently left a culture of staphylococci uncovered in his London laboratory. A mold grew in the culture. He noticed later that a space had formed between the bacteria and the mold and realized that something in the mold was destroying the bacteria. Alexander Fleming eventually named his discovery penicillin. While the process of drug discovery today can still be as serendipitous, it is not haphazard. The discovery and subsequent development of new drugs occur within a structural framework and require heavy investments of time and resources.

### The Preclinical Phase

Drug discovery and development consists of both a preclinical and a clinical phase. A great deal of work must take place before the clinical phase of R&D can begin. The medical scientist, working with chemists, must learn how to make the drug in quantities larger than a test tube, while insuring that the substance is stable. A company usually files one or more patent applications at this time and begins toxicological tests as well as short- and long-term animal testing.

Depending upon the outcomes of the these tests, a manufacturer must then decide whether or not to move ahead to clinical trials—

the beginning of the clinical phase of R&D. Before a company can begin its U.S. clinical trials of testing a new drug in humans to evaluate the safety and effectiveness of a pharmaceutical product, the Food and Drug Administration requires a sponsor to apply to the agency for permission to initiate human testing with an investigational new drug application, known as an IND.

### The Drug Approval Process: Testing for Safety and Efficacy

The regulatory process begins when an IND is submitted to the FDA. It is important to keep in mind that the FDA itself does not investigate new drugs or conduct any trials. Rather, it reviews the procedures a manufacturer follows and analyzes the data submitted by the company.

*Phase I Trials.* INDs are "in effect" 30 days after submission to the FDA, unless they are placed on clinical hold—typically, as a result of a safety concern. As long as there is not a clinical hold, a manufacturer can proceed with its clinical trials, continuing its animal studies at the same time. In Phase I trials, initial human safety studies are conducted. This generally involves between 20 and 100 healthy volunteers. Phase I studies are designed to determine the metabolism and pharmacologic actions of the drug in humans.

The objective in this phase is to provide information on toxicity and to identify potential side effects. The drug is administered at very low doses, much below the dose that had an effect in the animal studies. If no side effects occur, the dose is gradually increased until a dosage range—establishing toxic levels—is determined.

Regulations issued by the FDA in 1981 require that all research involving FDA-regulated products be reviewed by an Institutional Review Board before human testing can begin. These review boards, known as IRBs, exist in research institutions, academic health centers, and hospitals. They are made up of experts and lay persons whose job it is to make certain that participants are well informed and willing to participate before the studies get underway. A key element in participant protection is informed consent, which the IRB ensures is obtained and documented from each subject.

*Phase II Trials.* Phase II trials are controlled efficacy studies, which attempt to determine optimal dosage levels and to detect short-term side effects. They tend to be double-blinded, randomized control trials (RCTs). In a randomized control trial, patients are randomly assigned to a treatment group, which receives the experimental drug, or a control group which receives a placebo, standard treatment, or no treatment. This phase takes approximately two years to complete and involves a few hundred patients.

One of the most difficult aspects of clinical trials, which usually occurs during Phase II, involves the selection of clinical endpoints. That is, focusing a study on intermediate endpoints, such as changes in biochemical, physiological, or anatomical parameters, or including clinical endpoints such as effect on mortality, morbidity, or quality of life. These decisions are critical and have enormous impact on the development process. Testing treatments for AIDS provides a good example, in that a number of drugs being developed today are not necessarily designed to cure this syndrome but rather to target associated symptoms of the disease. The issue of endpoint selection is gaining considerable attention today as more and more drugs are being developed to treat chronic, degenerative diseases.

*Phase III Trials.* Most of the drugs that make it to Phase III have a very good chance of going to market. During this phase, which takes from one to three years, the drug is studied in 2,000 to 3,000 human subjects having the disease or condition in order to analyze long-term safety, efficacy, and toxicity effects. Many of the studies in this phase involve multi-center trials. Also occurring at the same time as Phase II and Phase III—although not part of the trials—are efforts by chemists and engineers to "scale up," that is to produce, as efficiently as possible, large quantities of the compound.

*Expedited Drug Reviews: Treatment INDs.* For patients with serious or immediately life-threatening diseases, the drug approval process presents a difficult dilemma. On the one hand, the process is designed to insure the safety of investigational new drugs. On the other hand, if a new drug appears promising as a treatment for a terminal illness, time becomes crucial, resulting in a balancing act for the government. The FDA has responded by developing stopgap mechanisms to provide broader availability of drugs between the time a drug looks promising and before it is approved. One such mechanism is the Treatment IND.

The use of investigational new drugs are usually limited to subjects enrolled in clinical trials. In 1987, new regulations, known as Treatment Use of Investigational New Drugs, changed all that.

Known as Treatment INDs, compassionate use approvals, or Group C drugs (in the case of the National Cancer Institute), these regulations enable physicians to use an investigational new drug for desperately ill patients, provided no comparable or satisfactory alternative drug or therapy is available.

*New Drug Applications.* At the completion of Phase III trials, a sponsor summarizes its study findings, as well as the formulation and chemistry of the drug, quality control procedures, and manufacturing practices, and submits a new drug application (NDA) to the FDA.

Once FDA approval is granted, the manufacturer may market the new drug for the specific indications that are approved. It is important to note that although the FDA gives permission to market drugs which it believes to be safe and effective, it does not regulate the practice of medicine. Physicians can, therefore, prescribe a drug for "off-label" uses not sanctioned by the FDA.

*Phase IV.* Phase IV, which takes place after an NDA has been approved, consists of post-marketing studies and takes place over the life of a drug. Its main objective is to examine the long-term safety and effectiveness of a drug and includes the reporting of adverse drug reactions (ADRs) to the FDA.

In addition to the submission of ADR reports by manufacturers and health professionals, large-scale, randomized controlled trials may also be conducted—often by such agencies as the National Heart, Lung, and Blood Institute, rather than the sponsor—to amass additional data. It is interesting to note that Phase IV activities are a much larger part of the drug approval process in Europe, where the philosophy is to get a product to market sooner and to monitor it more closely than in the United States.

### Increasing New Drug Approvals for Adults and Children

Analysts studying the pharmaceutical industry follow the FDA's record regarding how long it takes and how many new drugs are approved over a given time. One of the most meaningful indicators is the number of new molecular entities or NMEs annually approved by the FDA. NMEs are defined as compounds that have never been marketed in the U.S. before. The FDA also approves new drug applications (NDAs) for products that are not new molecular entities. Tracking NME approvals provides analysts with a good indication of the pharmaceutical industry's level of innovation.

Accelerated review times have been bolstered by the passage of two key pieces of federal legislation. The first, entitled the Prescription Drug User Fee Act (PDUFA), which Congress passed in 1992, authorized the FDA to collect user fees from pharmaceutical companies to be used to hire more drug reviewers and to improve the computer infrastructure necessary to hasten the review process. In exchange for the money, the FDA was required to meet annual performance targets. In 1997, when the PDUFA legislation was to sunset, Congress passed Public Law 105–115, the Food and Drug Administration Modernization Act (FDAMA). Among other things, FDAMA provided for an additional five years of user fee legislation, expanding PDUFA's emphasis on faster approval times. Faster approval times and access to markets serve to stimulate further pharmaceutical research and development.

Another important element of FDAMA was the creation of the *pediatric exclusivity provision*—the aim of which was to stimulate drug research in the pediatric population. The legislation provides a pharmaceutical manufacturer or sponsor with an additional six months of marketing exclusivity for the drug product in exchange for pediatric study data.

In addition to the pediatric exclusivity provision, another effort to further encourage pharmaceutical research in the pediatric field resulted in the April 1999 Pediatric Rule—which stipulates that applications for new active ingredients, new indications, new dosage forms, new dosing regimens, and new routes of administration must contain a pediatric assessment unless the sponsor (manufacturer) has obtained a waiver or deferral of pediatric studies.

A pediatric assessment is defined as:

> The data set (results of studies) adequate to characterize the safety and effectiveness of a drug or biological product for the claimed indication in all relevant pediatric subpopulations and to support dosing and administration for each pediatric subpopulation for which the drug is safe and effective. (www.fda.gov)

## Research and Development: The Price of Innovation

Drug products in the early part of the twentieth century consisted mainly of patent medicines, home remedies, and folk cures. The sophisticated, science-based pharmaceutical industry that exists today did not start to develop until the 1930s, when the first sulfa drug was introduced. This discovery set the stage for the development of penicillin and ushered in the "Age of Antibiotics" that lasted from the late 1930s until the early 1950s. The biotechnology industry, born in the late 1970s, moved the industry even further along with the advent of monoclonal antibody technology, cell culture technology, and genetic modification technology, among others.

In many ways, companies today are being forced to rethink their R&D portfolios as the very nature of R&D itself is changing. As the biotechnology revolution advances, the very essence of our understanding of disease and therapy is undergoing a profound shift. Scientists today now realize that many diseases are actually a collection of several different diseases, each with a unique molecular cause. It is clear that as the secrets of genomics are demystified, promising new miracle products (drugs may no longer be the correct term) will become available.

As a result of sophisticated new tools, such as computer modeling, 3-D computer-visualization techniques, combinational chemistry, and x-ray crystallography, the process of discovery, while still somewhat serendipitous, is much less haphazard than it was 20 years ago. Nevertheless, research and development in the pharmaceutical arena remains a risky business.

- In 2003, U.S. pharmaceutical companies spent $33.2 billion in research and development, a 7% increase over the previous year.
- It costs an average of $800 million to discover and develop just one new medicine.
- It takes nearly 15 years from the time a drug is discovered in the laboratory until it reaches patients.
- New medicines generated 40% of the two-year gain in life expectancy achieved in 52 countries between 1986 and 2000.
- In the 1990s, the U.S. surpassed Europe as the leading site for pharmaceutical research and development.

(*Source*: PhRMA, *Pharmaceutical Industry Profile 2004*, Washington, DC, www.phrma.org)

Research and development are only part of the risk for a company. The ability to recoup R&D investments is another. Patent protection is the life preserver around the company R&D pipeline.

## Patents and Generics
Patent protection is essential for companies investing in pharmaceutical R&D. Unlike many other technological advances, a drug

product, once discovered, is relatively easy to reproduce. Without the period of market exclusivity that patents provide, companies would not have the opportunity to recoup their R&D investments. The 20-year patent "clock" starts ticking immediately, although the effective patent life—that is, the time from FDA marketing approval to loss of patent protection—is actually much shorter, averaging only 11 to 12 years.

Some argue that patents provide a monopoly, a barrier to market entry for competing products. The other side of that has been articulated by the Congressional Budget Office (CBO):

> Patents do not grant complete monopoly power in the pharmaceutical industry. The reason is that companies can frequently discover and patent several different drugs that use the same basic mechanism to treat an illness. The first drug using the new mechanism to treat that illness—the breakthrough drug—usually has between one and six years on the market before a therapeutically similar patented drug (sometimes called a 'me-too' drug) is introduced. (p. xi)

As the future of medical research itself changes, patent policy will face interesting challenges. For example, the area of genetic research has raised significant issues, such as what is patentable (that is, are gene sequences bona fide inventions?) While the future of patenting and biotechnology is still unfolding, past patent legislation and regulation are still affecting today's pharmaceutical market. This is true both domestically and abroad, where patent piracy costs the industry hundreds of millions of dollars a year, despite various provisions agreed to in NAFTA (the North American Free Trade Agreement) and GATT (the General Agreement on Tariffs and Trade).

### The 1984 Drug Price Competition and Patent Term Restoration Act

Approximately one half of the prescriptions filled annually are for generic drug products. These substitutes typically enter the market priced at 70 to 80% of the relevant brand-name drug, with such prices dropping to 40% or less as the market becomes more competitive (Employee Benefits Research Institute [EBRI], 2004).

Domestically, the prescription drug market was radically altered with the passage of the 1984 Drug Price Competition and Patent

Term Restoration Act (commonly referred to as the Hatch-Waxman Act after its authors, Sen. Orrin G. Hatch (R-Utah) and Rep. Henry A. Waxman (D-California). The act was "intended to strike a balance between promoting innovation (by guaranteeing makers of brand-name drugs a certain number of patent years) and ensuring that consumers have timely access to lower-cost generic medicines (by guaranteeing makers of generic drugs that those patents would eventually end)" (Serafini, 2000, p. 548).

More recently, the Greater Access to Affordable Pharmaceuticals (GAAP) Act of 2001, commonly referred to as the McCain-Schumer bill after senators John McCain (R-Arizona) and Charles Schumer (D-New York), who co-sponsored the legislation, was enacted to further ease the ability of quality generic equivalent products to enter the market sooner.

Since the 1980s, the use of generics has continued to increase. Along with the passage of the Hatch-Waxman and McCain-Schumer measures, the passage of drug-product substitution laws (at the state level) allowing pharmacists to dispense a generic, even in the case of a brand-name prescription, and the active promotion of generic substitution by government health programs and private health plans have all spurred an increase in generic sales.

As a result, the Generic Pharmaceutical Association (GPhA) projects global sales of generic drugs to rise from $29 billion in 2003 to $49 billion in 2007. Beyond 2004, GPhA expects generic drug sales to increase an average of 14% a year. A number of factors contribute to the increase in their growth, not the least of which are patent expirations on major brand name drugs, as seen in **TABLE 11.1**.

### Generic Equivalence: Today and Tomorrow

The FDA uses three terms to describe generic drug products: pharmaceutical equivalence, bioequivalence, and therapeutic equivalence. Each is defined below.

> *Pharmaceutical equivalence:* Drug products are considered pharmaceutical equivalents if they have the same active ingredient(s), the same dosage form, and are identical in strength as the brand-name product. Even if a generic has a different color, a different taste, or comes in a different shape or package, the FDA considers the product to be equivalent if it meets the same standards for strength, quality, purity, and identity as the branded product.

## TABLE 11.1

### Top 20 Prescription Drugs and Patent Expiration Dates

| BRAND DRUG | GENERIC NAME | PATENT HOLDER | INDICATION | PATENT EXPIRES | 1998 U.S. SALES (in millions of $) |
|---|---|---|---|---|---|
| Prilosec | omeprazole | Astra Merck | duodenal ulcers | 4/1/01 | 2,933 |
| Prozac | fluoxetine HCL | Lilly | depression | 2/2/01 | 2,271 |
| Zocor | simvastatin | Merck | hypercholesterolemia | 12/24/05 | 2,170 |
| Claritin | loratadine | Schering-Plough | allergies | 4/21/04 | 1,800 |
| Vasotec | enalapril maleate | Merck | hypertension | 2/22/00 | 1,010 |
| Biaxin | clarithromycin | Abbott | respiratory infection | 5/23/03 | 624 |
| Pravachol | pravastatin | Bristol-Myers Squibb | hypercholesterolemia | 10/20/05 | 1,022 |
| Pepcid | famotidine | Merck | duodenal ulcers | 10/17/00 | 1,005 |
| Cipro | ciprofloxacin HCL | Bayer | infection | 12/9/03 | 779 |
| Mevacor | lovastatin | Merck | hypercholesterolemia | 6/15/01 | 595 |
| Zithromax | azithromycin | Pfizer | infection | 10/14/05 | 775 |
| Glucophage | metformin HCL | Bristol-Myers Squibb | diabetes | 3/3/00 | 854 |
| Hytrin | terazosin | Abbott | hypertension | 2/17/00 | 546 |
| Zestril | lisinopril | Zeneca | hypertension | 12/30/01 | 549 |
| Relafen | nabumetone | SmithKline Beecham | arthritis | 12/13/02 | 449 |
| Zofran | ondansetron | Glaxo-Wellcome | nausea | 6/25/05 | 442 |
| Buspar | buspirone | Bristol-Myers Squibb | anxiety disorder | 5/22/00 | 490 |
| Axid | nizatidine | Lilly | duodenal ulcers | 4/12/02 | 301 |
| Ceftin | cefuroxime axetil | Glaxo-Wellcome | infection | 5/12/00 | 365 |
| Diflucan | fluconazole | Pfizer | infection | 1/29/04 | 440 |

SOURCE: Generic Pharmaceutical Industry Association. Accessed April 27, 2000, at http://www.gpia.org/edu_top20drugs.html (now www.gphaonline.org).

*Bioequivalence:* A generic drug is considered bioequivalent if it is absorbed in the bloodstream at the "same rate and extent" as the brand drug.

*Therapeutic equivalence:* A generic drug is considered therapeutically equivalent to the comparable brand when the FDA determines the generic is safe and effective, pharmaceutically equivalent, and bioequivalent. (Generic Pharmaceutical Association, 2000)

Because biologics (for example, human growth hormone) are difficult to produce and because the FDA currently has no mechanism for measuring the equivalency of generic biotech-based drug products, producing generics in the future will become more complicated. The overall effect of this on the market, on competition, and on price, sales, and expenditures remains to be seen.

## Pharmaceutical Marketplace Dynamics

There is no single pharmaceutical marketplace. There is no single price for a specific drug product. There are, however, multiple customers, multiple distribution channels, multiple prescription drug reimbursement systems, multiple purchasing arrangements, multiple pricing methodologies, multiple marketing techniques, and multiple cost control tools.

The economics of the pharmaceutical marketplace are extremely complex: the companies themselves range in size from newly merged behemoths to very small one-product start-ups; some of the manufacturers are multinational, spanning the globe, while others are domestic, and still others are foreign companies seeking to do business in America.

In addition to the availability of new products, consumers are noticing other changes and trends. Products once requiring prescriptions, for example, are now being sold over the counter; more and more products are being marketed directly to consumers, and a large number of top selling products have or are due to come off patent very soon, enabling consumers to purchase the generic version of these products at a greatly reduced cost.

### Drug Expenditures

Three factors have contributed to the recent increases in pharmaceutical budgets: *unit cost inflation*, *utilization* (that is, increases in the absolute number of prescriptions), and *intensity* (that is, availability of new drug technologies and therapeutic mix—substituting newer, higher cost products for older less expensive products, including generics). The best evidence appears to suggest that while pure price inflation has played a smaller role, especially on existing (older) prescription drug products, utilization growth has played a major role (Brandeis University/Schneider Institute for Health Policy, 2000).

Fueling the increase in utilization is the explosion of direct-to-consumer (DTC) advertising by the pharmaceutical companies.

The National Institute for Health Care Management's July 1999 study, "Factors Affecting the Growth of Prescription Drug Expenditures," reported that "the 10 drugs most heavily advertised directly to consumers in 1998 accounted for $9.3 billion or about 22 percent of the total increase in drug spending between 1993 and 1998" (p. iii). The study, citing data from the Scott-Levin Source Prescription Audit Data, found that in 1998, pharmaceutical companies spent $8.3 billion promoting their products in the United States, of which approximately $1.3 billion was spent on DTC advertising and $7.0 billion on advertising and detailing to health care professionals.

Other nonprice factors explaining the growth in total drug expenditures include demographic changes (a growing elderly population, changing chronic disease prevalence patterns); the growth in third-party drug coverage, which tends to drive demand; record sales of new products; new product formulations; changing mix of products used; patient noncompliance; and underutilization of prescription drugs and inappropriate prescribing.

### Prescription Drug Pricing: Multiple Markets, Multiple Prices

As indicated above, pricing alone does not account for the total growth in drug expenditures. But it does, of course, play a role, especially for newer products, many of which are currently working their way through the R&D pipeline. As external market forces change, internal pricing strategies also change.

Defining and comparing pharmaceutical prices is complicated and not always consistent—many terms are used and many methodologies are employed. There is no one way to price a product. A variety of factors are considered in drug pricing, among them: the relative commercial success of the agent; the prices, product features, and past actions of the competition; specific patient characteristics; the economic and social value of the therapy itself; the decision-making criteria of prescribers and those who influence that decision; company needs in terms of market position, revenue, and other considerations; the current and anticipated insurance reimbursement environment; company abilities, including available budgets and willingness to support the project; and the type of manufacturer supplying the drug (Kolassa, 1997).

Three basic pricing strategies, each chosen to maximize a competitive edge are described below.

*Skimming:* The product, anticipating little direct competition, is priced above prevailing levels to maximize profits. Prilosec, the first proton pump inhibitor, was priced in this manner, substantially above the price of the H2 antagonists.

*Parity:* The product is viewed internally as being little or no different from current competitors and is priced equivalent to the prevailing levels. The nonsedating antihistamine Claritin and the ACE inhibitor Accupril were priced at parity to the market leaders at the times of their launches.

*Penetration:* A product is viewed as equal to or slightly inferior to current or anticipated offerings and is priced below prevailing levels in hopes of gaining market share with its low price or of erecting a barrier to entry for anticipated future competitors. Lescol appears to be the only pharmaceutical product to have successfully employed a penetration pricing strategy. (*Source:* E. M. Kolassa, 1997)

Manufacturers use these various pricing methods depending on internal strategies, external forces, distribution channels, and specific purchasers. The price a manufacturer sets often changes as it makes its way through the distribution chain and onto the negotiating table. It is not unusual for one specific product to be priced differently in different markets, thereby creating a dazzling array of prices paid for the same product. For example, someone with insurance that includes a prescription drug benefit will almost always pay less for the same drug as someone without insurance because employers (or their designated representative such as a pharmacy benefit manager, which is described later in this chapter) will negotiate a volume discount on behalf of their beneficiaries. Similarly, different government programs negotiate a variety of prices, based on different legislative and regulatory requirements. (See TABLE 11.2.)

### International Comparisons

Many cross-national drug pricing comparisons have been made over the years. While these findings are significant, they merit caution as to how the comparisons are made and how the conclusions are drawn. Because markets, demographics, and values vary, and because medical practices and economic circumstances also vary, it is difficult simply to transfer one country's pricing methods to another. Nevertheless, for many reasons, price differentials

| TABLE 11.2 |
| :---: |

## Illustrative Example of Pricing for Brand Name Prescription Drugs

| | CASH CUSTOMERS (NO 3RD-PARTY PAYMENT AT POINT OF SALE) | INSURERS AND PBMS | HMO* | MEDICAID | FEDERAL SUPPLY SCHEDULE |
| --- | --- | --- | --- | --- | --- |
| List price (AWP#) | | | $50 | | |
| Manufacturer's price (manufacturer to wholesaler or other entity) | $40 (AWP – 20%) | $40** (AWP – 20%) | $34 (AWP – 33%) | $40** | $24 (AWP – 52%) |
| Acquisition price (wholesaler to pharmacy) | $41 | $41 | n/a | $41 | n/a |
| Retail price at pharmacy (total of amounts paid by customer and reimbursed by 3rd-party payer) | $52 (AWP + 4%) | $46** (AWP – 13% + $2.50) | n/a | $41 + $2.50 | n/a |
| Retail price, less typical manufacturer rebate | n/a | $30 to $44 (5% to 35% rebate) | n/a | $30 to $37 (15.1% to 30% rebate) | n/a |
| Ultimate (net) amount paid by final purchaser and/or consumer | $52 | $30 to $44 | $34 (avg.) | $30 to $37 $34 (avg.) | $24 |

SOURCE: Assistant Secretary for Planning and Evaluation, Report to the President: Prescription Drug Coverage, Spending, Utilization, and Prices, Department of Health and Human Services, April 2000, 98.
n/a = not applicable
*This column refers only to HMOs that buy directly from manufacturers.
**without rebate
#Average Wholesale Price
NOTES:
1. Prices are based on a composite of several commonly prescribed brand-name drugs for a typical quantity of pills. For some cells in the table, the relative relationships have been calculated based on relationships reported in *How Increased Competition from Generic Drugs Has Affected Prices and Returns in the Pharmaceutical Industry* (CBO, 1998) and on other relationships widely reported by industry sources.
2. These prices are used for illustrative purposes only and do not represent any type of overall average.
3. Prices reported in this table include both amounts paid by third-party payers and amounts paid by the consumer as cost-sharing.

between products purchased in the U.S. and other countries are often substantial.

An October 1999 Alliance for Health Reform document, *Prescription Drugs, A Primer for Policymakers,* reported that

> U.S. Government Accounting Office studies found U.S. drug prices for specific drugs were, on average, one-third higher than in Canada

(1991), and 60 percent higher than in the United Kingdom (1992). Patricia Danzon of the University of Pennsylvania finds that drug prices vary by country, some are higher abroad and some are higher in the U.S. (April 1999, p. 2)

### Cost-Control Tools

Prescription drug benefits, once viewed as a relatively small expenditure by employers and purchasers, have come under tighter cost controls. While the clinical benefits of many of these new products are significant, their high prices place a heavy burden on payers and patients. As new products make their way into the market, the market has responded with new tools to control drug costs. One of the most dramatic responses has been the growth of pharmacy benefit managers, or PBMs.

*PBMs.* By acting as intermediaries between pharmaceutical manufacturers and third-party payers (that is, employers, managed care organizations, labor unions, and state-funded pharmaceutical assistance programs for the elderly), PBMs administer prescription drug benefits. In addition to offering their core services—claims processing, record keeping, and reporting programs—PBMs offer their customers a wide range of services, including drug utilization review, disease management, consultative services, and most recently, Internet fulfillment. PBMs also assist clients with establishing their benefit structure. Options for plan design include developing and maintaining a network of pharmacy providers, providing a mail service component, and developing and maintaining a drug formulary. In an effort to save plan sponsors money, PBMs negotiate with pharmaceutical manufacturers for rebates on products selected for the formulary (Strongin, 1999).

To counter the rise in prescription drug prices, employers and third-party payers have begun instituting various benefit restrictions and cost control measures, some of which are used more than others. In addition to the more traditional methods—formulary compliance; generic substitution; prior authorization; beneficiary cost-sharing (i.e., the recent move by most third-party plans to triple-tiered copays); prescribing and dispensing limits; drug utilization review; disease management, and the use of mail service pharmacies for maintenance drugs—additional cost control tools are being utilized. Some of these include:

*Negotiated Discounts.* Negotiating discounts for pharmaceuticals is a common practice (although senior citizens without drug coverage generally do not enjoy the benefits of "preferred pricing"). PBMs and managed care plans, for example, negotiate discounts in exchange for the ability to move market share, while the federal government (for example, the Veterans Health Administration, the Public Health Service, and the Indian Health Service) mandates discounts.

*Drug Interchange Programs.* The use of various drug interchange programs, such as generic substitution, therapeutic substitution (which requires pharmacists to give patients chemically different, less costly drugs that may accomplish the same thing as the ones their doctors prescribe), and step therapy (which requires doctors to begin by prescribing lower-cost drugs whenever possible. If they prove ineffective, physicians can prescribe more expensive medications)—has sparked a good deal of controversy. At issue is the question of whether these programs compromise patients' access to necessary therapies, thereby contributing to negative health outcomes. On the other hand, proponents are of the opinion that these programs hold great promise in slowing the growth rate of drug expenditures by promoting clinically appropriate and cost-effective products.

*Other Initiatives—Reimportation.* Additional cost control strategies employed include restrictive formularies, preferred drug lists, prior authorization, and disease management programs.

One of the more controversial cost control tools to be utilized by individuals, states, and other purchasers is the importation and reimportation of pharmaceutical products. Proponents of this approach are urging the federal government to find a way to bring cheaper drugs safely into the country while critics point out that not only is the practice potentially dangerous and life-threatening but that reimportation will ultimately erode the drug development pipeline in this country.

Congress mandated the establishment of a 13-member Task Force on Importation when it enacted the Medicare Prescription Drug, Improvement, and Modernization Act of 2003 (Public Law 108–173). The Task Force was to have held six "listening sessions" and issue its report to Congress no later than December 1, 2004.

When analyzing the success—or failure—of all these cost control measures, it is important to examine their effect on the over-all cost and quality of health care.

### Private and Public Prescription Drug Markets

Americans spent over $140 billion on prescription drugs in 2001, about 10% of the country's health care bill. More than 3 in 5 Americans fill at least one prescription annually, and more than half of those older than 75 fill more than 15 prescriptions (including refills) annually (EBRI, 2004).

Domestically, the pharmaceutical market can be broken down into two broad categories: private markets and government programs.

*Private Markets.* The private marketplace includes retail (such as traditional drug store chains, mass merchandisers, independent pharmacies, supermarket pharmacies, and mail order pharmacies), wholesale, hospital, managed care organizations and providers (such as clinics, long-term care facilities, including nursing homes, outpatient facilities and physician offices), and the Internet.

*Public Markets and Government Programs.* The federal government spends billions of dollars a year providing pharmaceutical products to beneficiaries through its Federal Employee Health Benefit Program, Department of Veterans Affairs (VA) and federal supply schedule (FSS), Medicaid, and various public health service programs such as the Indian Health Service and the Coast Guard. Until 2003, however, the Medicare program had been noticeably absent from this list.

That all changed with the passage of Public Law 108–173, the Medicare Prescription Drug, Improvement and Modernization Act of 2003, which ushered in sweeping changes, including the establishment of prescription drug coverage under the Medicare program.

*Medicare Prescription Drug, Improvement, and Modernization Act of 2003.* On December 8, 2003, President George W. Bush signed this landmark piece of legislation that among other things creates a voluntary Part D drug benefit for Medicare beneficiaries beginning in January 2006. During the transition between when the law was enacted and when it is to begin in 2006, Medicare beneficiaries can sign up for a Medicare-endorsed drug discount card. The government will provide low-income beneficiaries (beneficiaries with incomes below 135% of poverty) without private or Medicaid drug coverage, $600 per year for drug expenses in 2004 and 2005 in addition to paying for the annual enrollment fee.

Once the actual outpatient prescription drug benefit begins, beneficiaries will:

- Pay the first $250 in drug costs (deductible);
- Pay 25% of total drug costs between $250 and $2,250;
- Pay 100% of drug costs between $2,250 and $5,100 in total drug costs (the $2,850 gap or so called "doughnut hole"), equivalent to $3,600 out-of-pocket; and
- Pay the greater of $2 for generics or $5 for brand drugs, or 5% coinsurance after reaching the $3,600 out-of-pocket limit ($5,100 catastrophic threshold).

The new Medicare drug benefit will be delivered through private risk-bearing entities under contract with the U.S. Department of Health and Human Services (USDHHS). Drug benefits will be provided through stand-alone prescription drug plans (PDPs) or comprehensive plans, with government fallback plans authorized to serve areas without sufficient plan choices.

While this legislation has been a long time coming—Medicare has operated without an outpatient prescription drug benefit since its enactment in 1965—the policy implications, costs, and benefits are being hotly debated in academic circles, on Capitol Hill, and in advocacy communities across the country. It is too early to predict what effect the new benefit will have on retiree health benefits, the long-term effect on Medicare's financial future, and the overall health of seniors and the disabled.

*The VA Federal Supply Schedule.* In Fiscal Year 1999, the Department of Veterans Affairs spent more than $1.8 billion or approximately 11% of its health care budget in order to provide pharmacy benefits for U.S. veterans. The VA negotiates FSS contracts with individual manufacturers according to a set statutory and regulation framework. The Veterans Health Care Act of 1992 established a mandatory federal ceiling price (beyond those of the FSS) on a manufacturer's sales of innovator medicines to four federal agencies: the VA, the Department of Defense, the Public Health Service (including the Indian Health Service), and the Coast Guard. The formula establishes an upper limit on all procurements by any of the four agencies equal to 76% of the weighted average nonfederal selling price for the product, limited to annual increases of no more than the increase in the consumer price index-urban (CPI-U). The FSS generally limits annual increases in any pharmaceutical price over the life of a contract (typically five years) to the increase in the CPI-U over the same period.

*Medicaid Rebates.* The Omnibus Budget Reconciliation Act of 1990 (OBRA) established the Medicaid rebate program. The basic formula requires that, in exchange for having their products reimbursed (that is, on the formulary), pharmaceutical manufacturers rebate to the states the greater of (a) 15.1% of the average manufacturer price (AMP)[1] paid by wholesalers for brand-name drugs that Medicaid beneficiaries purchase as outpatients or (b) the difference between AMP and the manufacturer's "best price." The best price is the lowest price offered to any other customer, excluding FSS prices and prices to state pharmaceutical assistance programs. Similarly, manufacturers pay a rebate equal to 11% of the AMP on generic and over-the-counter drugs.

> If a brand-name drug's AMP increases faster than the inflation rate, an additional rebate is imposed so that manufacturers cannot offset the basic rebate by raising their AMP. The additional rebate is equal to the difference between the current AMP and a base-year AMP increased by the inflation rate as measured by the consumer price index. (CBO, 1996, p. xi)

OBRA 93 changed the pricing schedule of single-source and innovator multiple-source drugs approved by the FDA after October 1990.

> In general, OBRA 93 had an impact on the computation of the unit rebate amount for covered outpatient drugs. The effective date for implementation of OBRA 93 was October 1, 1993. Presently, more than 500 manufacturers have rebate agreements with the Federal

---

1 Average manufacturer price is the weighted average price to wholesalers for product distributed to the retail pharmacy class of trade, whereas a wholesaler is defined as any entity to whom the manufacturer sells (except relabelers) and where the retail pharmacy class of trade excludes hospitals and HMOs.

Government which, in turn, address approximately 55,000 drug products. (Baugh, Pine, & Blackwell, 1999, p. 80)[2]

## MEDICAL DEVICES

The medical device industry operates much like the pharmaceutical industry. Medical devices are used in many of the same settings and for the same purpose—to meet patients' health care needs. They are used by the same kinds of practitioners, undergo FDA premarket regulation, and—like drugs—seem to be in a constant state of innovation and evolution.

Yet medical devices are an industry unto themselves, with a unique character and place. Medical device producing firms are often much smaller than pharmaceutical companies; their financing is less predictable and flows in different patterns, and the products themselves undergo a distinctive form of innovation that is highly interactive with, and dependent upon, medical practitioners.

Many complex policy issues influence medical device development and innovation, from how the Food and Drug Administration regulates medical products to how insurance companies decide whether to pay for particular technologies. But underscoring virtually all of these issues is a very clear and unmistakable policy question—that is, to what extent do medical devices improve patient health and offer value to patients, consumers, and medical providers? As medical devices proceed from the idea stage to the physician or patient's use, this fundamental question is posed in many ways and in many forms—by regulators, payers, investors, and providers. How well companies answer it factors heavily into whether their products, and their companies, succeed.

To begin, it is important to understand the nature and structure of the medical device industry.

### Medical Device Industry Overview

Patients and consumers encounter medical devices every day—in hospitals, physician offices, outpatient clinics, and other treatment settings. In effect, medical devices are the medical instruments that doctors and nurses use to treat or diagnose a medical condi-

2 The figures in this quotation that concern the number of manufacturers with rebate agreements with the federal government were received in a personal communication by the authors with S. Gaston, Baltimore, March 11, 1999.

tion or injury. Devices can range from relatively simple products, such as surgical gloves, tongue depressors, eyeglasses, or hearing aids, to highly sophisticated technologies, such as cardiac defibrillators, fiberoptic surgical instruments, or artificial joints. Diagnostic products are medical devices that help diagnose illnesses or injuries, such as CT scanners, blood tests, or ultrasound machines.

Wall Street analysts often separate the industry into two groups: hospital supply companies, which manufacture the routine supplies patients see in hospitals—from wound dressings to surgical gowns—and medical device companies, whose main products are items such as pacemakers and heart bypass machine (U.S. Centers for Medicare & Medicaid Services [CMS], 2003). In many cases, however, all products in the industry—as well as the device and diagnostic industry itself—are simply referred to as "medical technology."[3]

### Strong Financial Performance

Developing and marketing such products has resulted in strong financial performance for the U.S. medical device industry. Annual sales in 2002 were projected at $77 billion—making the U.S., by far, the leading producer in the world—with average annual revenue growth over the past decade of about 15%. The median net income, or profit margin from 1998 to 2002 was 18% for device companies and 14% for supply firms, well above the average in the U.S. industry as a whole.

Despite the industry's financial strength, many companies are quite small. Of the 6,000 firms in the industry, some 5,000 have fewer than 50 employees. These firms, together, are responsible for 10% of overall industry sales (The Lewin Group, 2000). In contrast, many of the large firms in the industry are multinational corporations, some with more than 100,000 employees. In fact, the top 2% of large companies generate almost half of sales in the industry.

Device markets are also generally much smaller than those of the pharmaceutical industry. While an individual pharmaceutical product could easily generate annual revenues topping $1 billion, no device product can boast revenues on that scale.

---

3 This term is also used frequently to encompass all medical interventions, including devices, pharmaceuticals, and medical procedures. In this chapter, however, "medical technology" refers only to medical devices and diagnostic products.

## Intensive Commitment to R&D

Much of the device industry's success can be attributed to the rapid pace of innovation, reflected, in part, by the strong commitment to research and development. R&D spending as a percentage of the medical device industry sales increased from 5.4% in 1990 to 12.9% in 1998. That brings the industry's R&D investment in line with the percentage invested by the pharmaceutical industry—and well above most other industries.

The most R&D intensive sectors are companies producing laboratory tests and related diagnostic products, followed by firms making surgical and medical instruments. Another R&D standout is the small company sector generally. According to the Lewin Group, companies with sales under $5 million in 1998 spent 252% of sales on R&D, while those with sales between $5 million and $20 million invested 50%. Though such companies might employ only a handful of workers, they are often powerhouses of innovation—taking on projects that larger companies find too risky. As such, small and emerging companies are often responsible for some of the most dramatic advances—such as angioplasty catheters, artificial hips, mechanical heart valves, IV pumps, and blood glucose monitors (Wilkerson, 1995; Strongin & Geigle, 1993).

At the same time, small medical technology firms are highly vulnerable. They must negotiate the complex regulatory and payment requirements, which takes time and money. They must also depend upon funding from venture capital firms. Such funding may be available—or not—depending on many factors, not the least of which is the time required for regulatory approval and payment for a new product. Venture capitalists continue to be cautious, reducing investment in the medical device industry from $2.5 billion in 2000 to about $1.5 billion in 2003 (PriceWaterhouseCoopers/Thomson Venture Economics, 2004).

Large companies have little trouble with capital, relying upon cash from their own operations or turning to public equity or debt offerings when necessary (CMS, 2002). They also can count on a history of strong performance in the stock market to help generate capital. Since 1994, such companies have performed well ahead of the S&P 500 index.

Acquisitions are common in the industry, a reflection of two forces: first, the need among larger firms to expand financial clout and product breadth in meeting payer demands and competition from other firms; second, the need among smaller firms for the marketing and regulatory expertise of larger firms, along with their financial resources to navigate regulatory and payment hurdles.

## "Dialogue of Innovation"

Another defining characteristic of the medical device/technology industry is the unique process of innovation. Whereas the traditional model of innovation—proceeding from concept, to prototype, to production, to market adoption—certainly occurs with medical technology, the process is often more dynamic, interactive, and unpredictable. The reason is that a vast amount of innovation occurs *after* medical devices reach the market and are used in real-world care by clinicians.

There is a kind of "dialogue of innovation" between clinicians and manufacturers, whereby medical technologies undergo near continuous improvement and adjustments—perhaps adding a new capacity, speed, or use for another patient group—as clinician experience grows and they see new possibilities and applications. For many products, this dynamic translates into near-continuous incremental adjustments and improvements. Though breakthrough innovation often occurs in the industry, innovation in medical device technology is more often marked by incremental change. Examples include improvements in the materials, design, and fixation of artificial hips; the power source, size, and capability of pacemakers; and the size and ability of fiberoptic endoscopes (Strongin & Geible, 1973).

One of the effects of this process is short product life—sometimes as short as a few months to a few years. Products can be outdated within a matter of months, making the role of patents much less important than in other industries. Over time, generations of incremental change can translate into major transformation in a product line. A good example is the implantable cardiac defibrillator, which can correct life-threatening and often fatal heart arrhythmias. Originally introduced in the late 1980s, the device required open-chest surgery, general anesthesia, and a stay in the hospital of 12 days. The mortality associated with surgery was about 4%, with hospital costs in the range of $100,000. Over the past two decades, multiple generations of incremental advances have resulted in a dramatic transformation in the device. It is now one-sixth the size of the early versions, lasts three times as long, and treats a number of additional conditions. Its smaller size means that open-chest procedures are no longer required and some procedures can be performed in the outpatient setting. The mortality associated with the operation is now well under one percent (Collins, 2003).

Another important aspect of device innovation is that the ultimate value of a product in improving patient care often does not become clear until the product is well along in the process of incremental change. Angioplasty was introduced in the early 1980s as a less-invasive alternative to coronary artery bypass surgery. Only after multiple generations of incremental improvements, and growing physician experience, did the technology become the primary method for reestablishing blood flow in blocked arteries (Cutler & Huckman, 2002; Gelijns & Rosenberg, 1994; Jacobs, 2003).

## FDA Premarket Review

Before medical devices and diagnostic products can reach patients and medical providers, they must undergo premarket review by the Food and Drug Administration. The degree of review is based on the degree of potential risk posed by the products, which are classified into three groups.

- Class I products pose the least degree of risk, such as bandages and enema kits. They must meet general regulatory controls, such as labeling and manufacturing requirements.
- Class II products pose moderate risk, such as catheters and syringes. The safety of these products can reasonably be ensured through product performance standards and general controls.
- Class III products are those in which safety and effectiveness can be ensured only by premarket review. These include high-tech products such as heart valves, diagnostic imaging scanners, and implantable stents (Munsey, 1995).

In general, products requiring premarket review reach the market on one of two tracks—a 510(k) premarket review notification or a premarket approval application, called a PMA. The 510(k) is, by far, the easier track, requiring manufacturers to show that the new device is substantially equivalent to an earlier, legally marketed product. In some cases, the FDA requires the company to submit clinical data in support of its claim, but usually not (U.S. Food and Drug Administration [FDA], 2003b).

In contrast to 510(k)s, PMA applications require the applicant to prove that the product is safe and effective—a much higher standard. Usually this requires the company to submit clinical data on how well the product has performed in clinical studies on patients. The FDA scrutinizes the data submitted by the company, often asking for additional information and sometimes asking for new clinical studies.

In neither case, however, does FDA test the actual product itself. Its assessment is based upon materials from the company that explain how the product works, the results of any testing, and how it will be manufactured.

### Delays in Product Approvals

The primary controversy involving FDA review of medical devices over the past two decades has revolved around the review process, particularly delays in review of both PMAs and 510(k)s. Though Congress required the FDA to complete a 510(k) review in 90 days and a PMA review in 180 days, the review times soared in the 1990s. The primary reason was the tougher review and enforcement policies under the leadership of FDA Commissioner David Kessler, appointed in 1990.

Under Kessler, the FDA significantly increased its demands for scientific rigor in the clinical studies supporting device applications. Increasingly, it asked the industry to conduct randomized controlled clinical trials—long considered the gold standard of evidence and widely used to evaluate the performance of pharmaceutical products (DeMarinis, 2003). The agency said that payers, medical providers, and, most of all, patients could not be assured that medical technologies were truly effective without this type of rigorous evidence. The challenge for the industry was that such trials are costly, difficult, and often very slow—sometimes taking years to complete. More significant, however, was that—in taking this approach—the FDA had clearly started shifting the definition of "safety and effectiveness," the standard that PMA products had to meet to get approved. The agency was now demanding that manufacturers show how products, especially PMA products, improved the health outcomes for patients—such as lengthening lives or improving quality of life—rather than simply showing that the product performed as its label indicated.

The effect of this transformation in what the FDA expected of medical devices was two fold—much longer review times and intense political jockeying. In 1993, for example, the average total elapsed time for final approval of a PMA was 799 days—a full 19 months beyond the six-month review time required by law—and 195 days for 510(k)s, well above the 90 days set by the law. The industry strongly criticized such delays, often citing the detrimental impact on patient access to medical technologies. Yet virtually no outcry arose from consumer groups, many of which had argued—as far back as the 1980s—that the FDA went too easy on medical technology.

### FDA Modernization

With the Republican sweep of Congress in 1994 and increasing political action by the technology industry to dramatize what it considered to be serious problems with the FDA, the agency's delays and evaluation criteria received growing political attention—and action. The result was the FDA Modernization Act of 1997, perhaps the most important legislation since Congress first regulated medical devices. The new law required the FDA to out-source certain 510(k) reviews, eliminate pre-market review requirements for many low-risk products, expedite reviews of breakthrough technologies, and—most important—use the "least burdensome" method of product approval (DeMarinis, 2003).

With implementation of the new law came improvements in product review times and, generally, a more collaborative relationship between the FDA and the device industry. Review times for PMAs were cut in half between 1999 and 2003 (see FIGURE 11.1). Yet to achieve further improvements, the industry reversed a long-held position and, in 2002, finally embraced "user fees" for medical device submissions to FDA. It concluded that the agency had made about as many reforms as it would—or perhaps could—and further improvements in review times would only come from new reviewers (DeMarinis, 2003). As a result, the industry agreed to pay fees for PMA and 510(k) reviews, with special provisions to reduce the burden on small companies. For fiscal year 2004, the standard fee for a PMA was $206,811; for a 510(k) $3,480. For small businesses, the fees were $78,588 and $2,784, respectively. In exchange for such fees, the agency also stated its commitment to further reduce review times through greater efficiencies and by encouraging higher-quality applications.

Though difficulties and controversies continue to develop in the complex interactions between the FDA and the medical device industry—on issues ranging from evidence to review times—the state of relations between the two is generally agreeable.

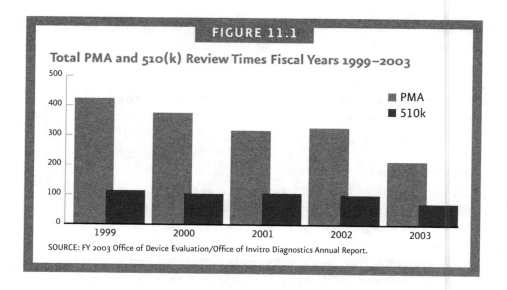

FIGURE 11.1

Total PMA and 510(k) Review Times Fiscal Years 1999–2003

SOURCE: FY 2003 Office of Device Evaluation/Office of Invitro Diagnostics Annual Report.

## Medicare Coverage and Payment

Once products are approved by the FDA, they are available for use throughout the U.S. health care system. In reality, however, many patients must await access to certain products until after their insurance companies have reviewed and approved them for reimbursement. Insurers decide whether or not these products meet the insurer's standards of effectiveness and value. Often, an insurance company's focus is on products that raise costs significantly or introduce a technological breakthrough.

Perhaps the best example of this process is Medicare, which provides coverage for some 40 million beneficiaries. Its coverage and payment decisions carry added importance because they often influence the decisions of private insurance companies. Often, Medicare's systems for reviewing and paying for medical technology work very quickly; other times, they drag on for years.

### Coverage

The first judgment Medicare makes is whether it will cover a new medical technology—that is, whether a new product or medical service is eligible for payment. In the vast majority of cases, this judgment is made as a routine part of the billing and payment process by local Medicare contractors.[4] Technologies handled in

4 These are private insurance companies that handle billing and payment on behalf of Medicare throughout the country.

this way receive no special scrutiny and are, in effect, covered and paid for automatically (U.S. Medicare Payment Advisory Commission [USMPAC], 2003).

In some cases, however, Medicare undertakes a more formal, "premarket" type of coverage review. It does so when the product raises questions of cost or clinical efficacy, or if the product is a breakthrough innovation. The purpose is to determine whether the product is "reasonable and necessary"—the standard for Medicare coverage—for the Medicare population.

Such reviews can be conducted at the local level by Medicare's contractors, in which case the decision applies only to the local contractor's region of jurisdiction. Or coverage can be conducted nationally by Medicare—in which case the determination applies to all regions. In many ways, explicit coverage evaluations of this kind are the Medicare equivalent of a PMA evaluation at the FDA: the agency seeks clinical data, literature, and often the views of experts on whether the product qualifies for coverage, much as the FDA requires such information for PMA product submissions.

One of the flashpoints between manufacturers and Medicare is how and when such coverage decisions are made—and the criteria that are used. In the past, such decisions were made behind closed doors. But in 1998, Congress forced the agency to open up the process, giving the public greater opportunity to participate in and understand what Medicare was doing.

What industry saw, it did not like: demands for higher levels of evidence, particularly from randomized controlled clinic trials. This was essentially the very same battle the industry had just fought at the FDA. Now it was Medicare saying that it wanted the same deep, rigorous studies that showed whether or not products improved net health outcomes for patients. Medicare also made it clear that the kind of evidence often developed by the device industry—nonrandomized studies using historical data—was of considerably less value (Tunis & Kang, 2001).

As might be expected, Medicare's efforts encountered intensive opposition from the industry. It argued that this higher level of clinical data would be very costly to develop, particularly for small device companies. It also said that randomized controlled clinical trials were often not appropriate for medical devices because the real value of such products emerges over time, through real-world use by clinicians.

The industry also pointed to long delays in the Medicare cover-

## MEDICARE'S VIEW OF THE HIERARCHY OF EVIDENCE

Excerpt from discussion materials for Medicare Coverage Townhall Meeting, Centers for Medicare and Medicaid Services (previously called the Health Care Financing Administration, or HCFA)
September 25, 1998

In making coverage decisions, HCFA weighs the medical and scientific evidence in accordance with a fairly standardized hierarchy that ranks the relative authority given to various types of studies. This hierarchy of evidence is as follows, ranked with the most authoritative first:

- Controlled clinical trials* published in peer-reviewed medical or scientific journals;
- Controlled clinical trials completed and accepted for publication in peer-reviewed medical or scientific journals;
- Assessments initiated by [Medicare];
- Evaluations or studies initiated by Medicare contractors;
- Case studies published in peer-reviewed medical or scientific journals that present treatment protocols.

*A controlled clinical trial is one in which one group of patients is given the treatment being evaluated, while another (the control group) receives no treatment, a "usual" or "standard" treatment, or a placebo. To make the comparison as valid as possible, the composition of the control group should resemble that of the treatment group as closely as possible. . . .

age processes—delays that it said would only increase as the burden of evidence grew. According to an industry-funded study by The Lewin Group in 2000, Medicare coverage took from 15 months to 5 years, figures that the industry continues to cite widely. A USD-HHS report to Congress in June 2002 said that Medicare took an average of 383 days to fully implement the 10 coverage decisions in Fiscal Year 2001,[5] with individual decisions ranging from 195 to 733 days. When the GAO examined the coverage process, it found that 55 national coverage policies from January 1999 through July 2002 took Medicare an average of about 7.5 months to make a national coverage judgment. If Medicare sought an external technology assessment or requested the advice of its primary advisory group, the GAO found that it is added another 8 months to the process.

In essence, these have been the battle lines between industry and Medicare since the late 1990s—Medicare's rising demands for

5 This figure eliminates two "emergency" coverage decisions on organ transplantation at one hospital.

evidence, and industry's criticism of the lengthy delays and what it believes are Medicare's often excessive demands. Though Medicare introduced a public advisory committee on clinical evidence issues in 1998, it became a lightning rod in its own right. Its meetings have often become the forum for intensive debate over what evidence is truly necessary and whether Medicare demands are reasonable.

Another overlay in the evidence debate has been the issue of costs. When Congress first created Medicare, it gave the program authority to cover only treatments that were deemed "reasonable and necessary" for Medicare patients. These criteria were traditionally interpreted as referring to patient medical need. But as health spending rose in the U.S. through the 1980s and 1990s, Medicare increasingly argued that the overall cost impact of a new technology should be a factor in "reasonable and necessary," particularly for technologies that would have a large budgetary impact. Though CMS was never successful in its efforts to make cost considerations an official part of coverage criteria, Medicare made it very clear, informally at least, that cost was definitely considered.

In 2003, Congress added new dynamics to the Medicare coverage process by imposing time limits on coverage decisions—6 months for decisions without an external technology assessment; 9 months for those with such an assessment—and by directing the agency to explain the criteria it uses in making decisions. Congress also urged the agency to reduce inconsistencies in local coverage decisions and to explore how more local decisions could be made nationally—a clear threat to the faster, technology-friendly local Medicare coverage process. It is unclear how, or if, these requirements will change the debate over Medicare coverage, but it is safe to say that the debate is far from over.

### Payment

Once products are covered by Medicare, they face another challenge: they must be paid for under Medicare's reimbursement systems.

In most cases, Medicare provides a fixed payment to providers to cover all the costs associated with a particular condition, procedure, or episode of care (such as an admission, day, or visit)[6] (Lewis,

---

6 The exception is some home health products, durable medical equipment, and laboratory tests, which are reimbursed on a fee schedule basis.

2000a). Hospitals, physicians, and other providers can then use these bundled payments to purchase the materials they need to provide care for their patients. Thus, Medicare does not pay directly for products used in the hospital or physician's office; the provider uses the bundled payment to purchase what it desires (USMPAC, 2003).

Most medical technologies flow smoothly into this system and receive payment from physicians, hospitals, and other providers. That is particularly true for cost-reducing technologies, or those that only modestly increase costs. The pre-set payment levels are adjusted every year to reflect changes in costs, including changes in medical technology.

As in any administered-price system, complexities arise. Payment levels are sometimes inadequate for higher-cost technologies; for other technologies, they may be excessive. Reliable data on resource use among providers—the basis for Medicare payment adjustments—often develop slowly, creating an inherent lag in how quickly payment rates can reflect real-world practice. In addition, the system of coding—which providers use to record the treatments they provide and seek reimbursement from insurers—can be very slow to accommodate new technologies. Complicating this picture is the fact that the stream of new treatments is fast-paced and nearly continuous.

Medicare argues that, generally speaking, medical technologies do just fine in its payment systems. Yes, the payment systems are sometimes bulky and slow, says Medicare, but they are generally sound and generally provide adequate—sometimes excessive—reimbursement. In an analysis of the medical device industry that CMS released in 2002, the agency said that,

> while bundled payment amounts may not always fully reflect new technology cost, new devices and procedures can be reflected in and adjustments made to these bundled payments in as little as 12 months for the inpatient PPS [prospective payment system] and as little as 4 months in the outpatient PPS. (CMS, 2002, p. 13)

Countering this view, the industry's primary trade association, AdvaMed, points to a Lewin Group study it funded in 2000, which concluded that, "A manufacturer may be required to successfully negotiate multiple, distinct, and complex processes to obtain adequate payment for a single device. Each process can take years to complete" (p. 2). One example the industry points to is the coding process. Under Medicare's rules, new codes are published only once a year. Thus, if a coding request for a new technology is submitted by Medicare's April 1 deadline of any given year, Medicare will not have the new code ready for publication until January 1 of the following year. If the request arrives after the April 1 deadline, however—say on April 15 or May 1—it will have to wait yet another 12 months—almost two years from the time it was first submitted (CMS, 2004).

At the urging of industry, Congress created new mechanisms to provide special payments for new, higher-cost technologies in the hospital inpatient and outpatient prospective payment systems (see **TABLE 11.3**). In the outpatient setting, Congress created two systems—one provides a pass-through payment for high-cost technologies that are used as part of an established medical service; the other creates new payment categories for technologies that are, in

## TABLE 11.3

### Stakeholder Interests in Health Care Delivery

| DESIGN ELEMENT | INPATIENT ADD-ON PAYMENT | MEDICAL DEVICES | DRUGS/BIOLOGICS | OUTPATIENT NEW TECHNOLOGY APC |
|---|---|---|---|---|
| What kinds of new technologies can receive additional payment? | New technologies that represent a new procedure or are an input to an existing DRG | New technologies that are an input to an existing service | New technologies that are an input to an existing service | New technologies that represent a new service |
| What criteria are applied by Medicare? | Eligibility based on clinical benefit, newness, and cost | Eligibility based on clinical benefit, newness, and cost | Eligibility based on newness and cost. | Eligibility based on newness. |
| What is the unit of payment? | Based on additional costs of treating a case using the technology | Based on the cost of the new technology | Payment based on the cost of the new technology | Payment based on the cost of providing the service. |
| How are payments determined? | Payment equal to 50% of the additional costs; capped at 50% of the estimated costs of the new technology | Payment equal to 100% of reported costs minus device costs already built into the base payment rate | Payment equal to 95% of average wholesale price. | Payment equal to the midpoint of the payment range for the new technology APC group. For example, a service in the APC that pays $1,000 to $2,000 is $1,500. |

SOURCE: Adapted from *Report to Congress: Medicare Payment Policy*, U.S. Medicare Payment Advisory Commission, March 2003, p. 181.

themselves, a complete service or procedure that is not reflected in existing payment groups. In the inpatient setting, Congress allowed add-on payments for new technologies if they significantly improved diagnosis and treatment and met certain cost thresholds.

While the industry and investors greeted such provisions, some observers charged that the special payments were expensive and unnecessary. The U.S. Medicare Payment Advisory Commission, which is the primary advisory group to Congress on Medicare, criticized the outpatient pass-through for new technology: "As currently structured, the pass-through payments provide manufacturers and hospitals with incentives to raise their prices and charges, potentially resulting in overpayment" (USMPAC, 2002, p. III).

## Private Sector Coverage, Payment, and Cost Control

Obviously, private sector insurance companies also play a key role in determining whether new medical technologies will be available for patients. As with Medicare, private payers have become more demanding in recent years for high-quality clinical data, usually from randomized controlled clinical trials that show whether new technologies improve net health outcomes for patients.

One of the primary insurers, Blue Cross and Blue Shield, maintains a special technology assessment program that examines, among other things, how well a medical technology improves ultimate patient outcome, such as disease, pain, or death. It also demands data from well-designed and carefully-conducted investigations published in peer-reviewed journals—in effect, the same level of data that Medicare and the FDA seek. In fact, Blue Cross officials have indicated that one randomized controlled trial will likely no longer suffice for obtaining coverage; companies will have to provide more than one and ensure that it is of a very high caliber.

Other techniques in use by private payers to curb what they perceive as excessive use of medical technologies include:

- Tracking the development of new technologies, including cost, performance, and clinical value;
- Using negotiations or competitive bidding to secure the best prices;
- Employing coverage policies that restrict use of new technologies or limit use to specific circumstances; and
- Seeking cost-effectiveness data to more effectively understand long-term value (USMPAC, 2003).

Payers can also employ indirect methods of influencing the use of medical technologies. The Blue Cross and Blue Shield Association announced in 2003 that it was undertaking a national public affairs campaign to highlight the impact of medical technology in driving health cost increases. This strategy led to press briefings, news articles, and published studies that blamed medical technology as a cost driver, though the campaign also acknowledged the significant clinical improvements from many technologies.

To a large extent, the effort by payers to rein in what they see as excessive spending on medical technology reflects a broader movement, led primarily by scholars and researchers, that questions the value of large amounts of such spending. The view usually is not that such devices are unsafe—though that claim crops up at times—but that they do not confer enough added value for the additional cost. Ever since the 1980s, when cost concerns truly took hold in the U.S., this theme has reverberated through countless reports, conferences, news articles, peer-reviewed journals, and congressional hearings. To be sure, many reports, hearings, and studies have strongly demonstrated the life-giving and life-improving qualities of medical technologies, but with rising health costs and approximately 45 million Americans uninsured, the concerns over costs have been highly visible and gaining increasing attention.

## The Value of Medical Technology

Facing the growing criticism of the cost of medical technologies, the medical device industry, as noted earlier, has accelerated its efforts since the late 1990s to underscore the economic, not just clinical, value of its products. It is doing so by identifying, and then quantifying, the economic output and value from broad-based improvement of health—such as allowing workers to get back to work sooner, reducing disabilities, creating new efficiencies in health care delivery, and providing lower-cost treatments.

The industry is also working to identify the economic value of better health. It is doing so by pointed to the work of, among others, Cutler and current CMS commissioner Mark McClellan. They have argued that the benefits from medical technology, on average, far exceed the costs, pointing particularly to improvements in treating cardiovascular disease and low-birthweight babies (Cutler, 2004).

Two recent efforts reflect the industry's approach on the value of improvement in health care. In early 2004, the industry's primary trade association, the Advanced Medical Technology Association (AdvaMed), co-sponsored a report with other major medical groups that calculated the economic value of health improvements over the past two decades. The report found that each additional dollar spent on health care between 1980 and 2000 produced health gains valued at $2.40 and $3.00. Regarding the four major diseases studied, the AdvaMed report found that, in the year 2000,

- Mortality from heart attack was cut in half;
- Stroke deaths were reduced by a third;
- Mortality from breast cancer declined by 20%; and
- Diabetes management led to a 25% reduction in complications such as blindness, kidney failure, stroke, and death. (MEDTAP, 2004)

The leading trade association for the medical imaging industry, the National Electrical Manufacturers Association, introduced a website in 2004 that uses peer-reviewed literature to identify the economic and clinical value of imaging technologies.[7] The Web site www.medicalimaging.org shows how imaging detects disease early, enables less invasive therapies, introduces efficiencies in health care delivery, and improves worker productivity. Among other things, the site states that:

- Medical imaging eliminates half the futile surgeries for lung cancer; and
- Imaging-guided breast biopsies cost a third of what surgical biopsies do and take half the time.

Nonetheless, balancing the cost, quality, and access of both pharmaceutical and medical device products continues to be an ongoing challenge for regulators, payers, and providers of health care.

## CONCLUSIONS

**Drugs.** Although lawmakers seek to curb drug prices and reduce industry profits, it is difficult to say whether or not Americans pay too much for their prescription drugs. Critics of the pharmaceutical industry maintain that prices and profits are too high and that

---

7 MedicalImaging.org is sponsored by the National Electrical Manufacturers Association. Available: www.medicalimaging.org

this is indicative of monopoly power. Abuses, critics contend, include price discrimination (selling the same drugs for less to large purchasers), drugs priced at levels out of proportion to their cost of production, and a lack of price competition among companies.

In response to such accusations, members of the pharmaceutical industry and some in academia point to the extremely high costs of research and development, which include costs for the large number of "dry holes" that must be dug before a successful drug therapy is produced, as well as the high price of developing drug treatments for the complex diseases—such as cancer—that are still unconquered. Moreover, they note that drugs increase the quality of life by reducing mortality and morbidity and that drugs are less expensive forms of treatment for a number of diseases, such as ulcers and asthma, than are surgery and hospitalization. In order to measure more accurately the *value* of pharmaceutical products, decision-makers will need to move away from "silo budgeting"—analyzing prescription drug cost expenditures without accounting for total health care offsets.

**Devices.** The highly innovative and dynamic medical devices industry continues to generate significant innovations, along with clinical success. With an aging American population, demand for these products will clearly increase, ranging from cardiovascular technologies such as pacemakers to orthopedic products such as implantable hips and joints. Investment in research and development continues to be strong, along with industry revenues and earnings. The industry's success has occurred, in part, because it has dealt effectively with the changing demands of regulators and the increasing resistance by insurers to pay for these technologies. However, the industry has shifted and re-shaped itself to the contours of a more cost-conscious and restrictive payment environment. But concern over rising health costs remains a sobering backdrop for medical technology—and critics abound, questioning the value of many devices and demanding more rigorous proof that health benefits truly outweigh the costs. The successful companies will be those that can marshal the evidence, pinpoint value, and offer cost-effective technologies. Most likely, large medical device companies will have no trouble doing this, given their financial muscle, but whether (and how) small device companies—which constantly struggle to secure venture capital—succeed in this environment is much less certain.

## CASE STUDY

Implantable cardiac defibrillators are life-saving medical devices that are used to regulate patients' abnormal heart rhythms, which can lead to sudden cardiac death and which take the lives of 400,000 Americans each year.

In March 2002, the New England Journal of Medicine published a study that found that patients who had experienced a heart attack and whose heart-pumping capacity was roughly half of what it should be would benefit from ICDs. In fact, according to the study, the device had cut the relative mortality rate from sudden cardiac death in these patients by roughly 30%. This meant that patients no longer needed to go through an expensive and risky procedure known as electrophysiologic testing. Physicians have long assumed that this test is essential in identifying which patients are most likely to benefit from ICDs—though no study has ever proven it.

The study published in the New England Journal of Medicine was sponsored and paid for by Guidant Corporation, one of the largest cardiovascular technology companies in the world, and led by physician investigators from the University of Rochester.

Following the publication of the ICD study in the New England Journal of Medicine, the Blue Cross and Blue Shield Association evaluated the study, gave it high marks, and opened the way for plan coverage. Other payers followed. Also, the primary medical specialty associations reviewed the study and recommended that Medicare cover ICDs for this patient group—but they also urged that more data be developed on the application of the ICD in the specific patient group under study. Finally, an advisory committee to Medicare—whose advice Medicare sought—recommended that the device be covered for this patient group. The FDA had approved the device in 2002.

Medicare took a different view than these other groups and agencies. It said that the data were insufficient. Medicare said that the study might have been flawed because some of the patients had conditions that might have resulted in abnormally favorable results for the ICDs. To bolster its point, Medicare further analyzed the data, suggesting that the results of the original study were not as strong as proponents believed and that the data could be interpreted a way as to suggest much less benefit from the ICD

(Continued)

## CASE STUDY (Continued)

than the published study concluded. Medicare denied allegations that it was resisting covering the product because projected expenditures for the device for this population of patients—if covered on the basis of the study—could be enormous.

When Medicare finally issued its decision in June 2003, it granted coverage for a narrower group of patients than suggested by the original study, and narrower than the guidelines adopted by Blue Cross and the medical specialty societies. Some critics argued that Medicare based its finding on much less robust data than in the original study, and that its intent was to keep the patient population using the device small. Medicare disagreed.

Medicare said further data were needed before full coverage, as proposed by the initial study, could be provided. Medicare said it was also interested in learning the results of yet another trial, underway at NIH, that would shed further light on the performance of ICDs in this particular patient population. When the NIH announced the results of the next study in March 2004, Medicare officials stated that this data appeared to be more robust and that they might broaden the indications of the earlier decision on the basis of this new data.

1. If the FDA approves a product as safe and effective, as the ICD should Medicare be able to reject its coverage on the basis that the data on its clinical value are insufficient?
2. How much evidence is enough? What risks are there in delaying coverage while additional evidence is gathered? What risks are there in covering a product if insufficient evidence is available for coverage?
3. What would have been the impact of the CMS decision if a small company had funded the study?
4. What conclusion regarding efficacy would medical practitioners likely draw from this case study?

## DISCUSSION QUESTIONS

### Pharmaceuticals

1. How has the nature of pharmaceutical R&D changed over the past 20 years? What effect will biotechnology and the mapping of the human genome have on prescription drug research and development, and ultimately on patients? How will the practice of medicine change as R&D continues to change?

2. The FDA must walk a regulatory tightrope, balancing patient safety on the one hand with timely access to needed medications on the other. Is the FDA meeting its dual objectives? How will the increased pressure from the additional burdens of regulating DTC advertising, the reimportation of drug products, and Internet pharmacy activity affect the FDA's performance?

3. Much of today's political dialogue revolves around the notion of profitability and "public good," in the case of drug products. For the pharmaceutical industry, how much profit is too much? Who should decide?

4. Should the federal government regulate the price of drugs? If so, what marketplace dynamics could be expected?

5. How is the *value* of pharmaceuticals measured? How should it be measured?

### Medical Devices

1. What impact do you think that additional demands for extensive clinical data might have on the ability of a medical device or diagnostic company to develop a new product? What would be the impact on the industry or on innovation in light of the fact that so many device companies are small?

2. If the FDA approves a medical technology, should an insurance company, including a public insurer like Medicare, be allowed to say that the evidence is not adequate and that they will not pay for it?

3. Whose definition of the value of a medical technology should prevail? The FDA? Payers? Society? Investors?

4. What happens when the findings of various payers differ, as in the case of implantable cardiac defibrillators? How much credence should Medicare give to practice guidelines of physicians or other clinicians?

5. Should political action by the device industry be allowed to change the dimensions of what the FDA or Medicare demand in terms of the evidence of value or effectiveness?

6. What are the main differences between the medical technology
   industry and the pharmaceutical industry?


## REFERENCES

Baugh, D. K., Pine, P. L., & Blackwell, S. (1999). Trends in Medicaid prescription drug utilization and payments, 1990–97. *Health Care Financing Review, 20*(3), (Spring), 80.

Brandeis University/Schneider Institute for Health Policy Prescription
Drug Analysis Group. (2000). *Prescription drug policy: Background paper
for the Princeton Conference*, May 10, 2000.

Collins, A. (2003). *Patient access to medical technologies*. Speech by Chairman
and CEO, Medtronic, Inc., Cleveland Clinic, October, 2003.

Congressional Budget Office (CBO). (1996, January). *How the Medicaid rebate
on prescription drugs affects pricing in the pharmaceutical industry*. CBO
Papers.

Congressional Budget Office (CBO). (1998, July). *How increased competition
from generic drugs has affected prices and returns in the pharmaceutical industry*. Washington, DC.

Cutler, D. M., & Huckman, R. S. (2002, October). *Technological development
and medical productivity: Diffusion of angioplasty in New York State*. Working Paper 9311, National Bureau of Economic Research.

Cutler, D. M. (2004). *Your money or your life: Strong medicine for America's health
care system*. New York: Oxford University Press.

DeMarinis, A. J. (2003). Medical device regulation—then and now.
*Research Practitioner, 4*(4), 124–137.

Employee Benefits Research Institute (EBRI). (2004). Prescription drugs:
Recent trends in utilization, expenditures, and coverage, January
2004, No. 265.

Gelins, A., & Rosenberg, N. (1994). The dynamics of technological change
in medicine. *Health Affairs, 13*(3), 29–46.

Jacobs, A. K. (2003). Primary angioplasty for acute myocardial infarction—Is it worth the wait? *The New England Journal of Medicine, 349*(8),
798–799.

Kolassa, E. M. (1997). *Elements of pharmaceutical pricing*, Pharmaceutical Products Press.

The Lewin Group. (2000). Outlook for medical technology innovation:
Will patients get the care they need? Report 1: *The State of the Indus-
try*. First in a series of reports prepared for the Advanced Medical
Technology Association.

The Lewin Group. (2000a). Outlook for medical technology innovation:
Will patients get the care they need? Report 2: *The Medicare Payment
Process and Patient Access to Technology*. Second in a series of reports

prepared for the Advanced Medical Technology Association. July 21, 2000.

Medicare Prescription Drug, Improvement, & Modernization Act of 2003. (Public Law 108–173).

MEDTAP International (2004). *The value of investment in health care: Better care, Better lives.* Bethesda, MD. Available: http://www.medtap. com/Products/HP_FullReport.pdf

Munsey, R. (1995). Trends and events in FDA regulation of medical devices over the last fifty years. *Food and Drug Law Journal, 50*(Special Issue), 163–177.

National Institute for Health Care Management. (1999). *Factors affecting the growth of prescription drug expenditures.* Washington, DC: Author.

PriceWaterhouse/Coopers/Thompson Venture Economics/National Venture Capital Association. (2004). *Money Tree Survey: Medical Devices and Equipment, 1995–2003* [Online]. Available: http://www.pwcmoney tree.com/moneytree/nav.jsp?page=historical

Serafini, M. W. (2000). No easy prescription on no-name drugs. *National Journal,* February 19, 2000, 548.

Strongin, R. (1999). *The ABCs of PBMs.* National Health Policy Forum Issue Brief No. 749, October 27, 1999.

Strongin, R., & Geigle, R. (1993). *The dialogue of device innovation: An overview of the medical technology innovation process.* Health Care Technology Institute.

Tunis, S. R., & Kang, J. L. (2001, Sept/Oct). Improvements in Medicare coverage of new technology. *Health Affairs, 20*(5), 83–85.

U.S. Centers for Medicare & Medicaid Services (CMS), Medicare Coverage Advisory Committee. (2001, February). *Recommendations for Evaluating Effectiveness* [Online]. Available http://www.cms.hhs.gov/mcac/ 8bl-i9.asp

U.S. Centers for Medicare & Medicaid Services (CMS). (2002, October). *Health care industry market update: Medical devices & supplies* [Online]. Available: www.cms.hhs.gov/marketupdate

U.S. Centers for Medicare & Medicaid Services (CMS). (2003, December). *Health Care Industry Market Update: Medical Devices & Supplies* [Online]. Available: www.cms.hhs.gov/marketupdate

U.S. Centers for Medicare & Medicaid Services (CMS). (2004). *Medicare program; Procedures for coding and payment determinations for clinical laboratory tests and for durable medical equipment.* Available: http://www. cms.hhs.gov/medicare/hcpcs/codpayproc.asp

U.S. Department of Health and Human Services (USDHHS). (2002, June 4). *Report to Congress on National Coverage Determination.* Letter from Tommy G. Thompson, Secretary of Health and Human Services.

U.S. Food and Drug Administration (FDA). Center for Biologics Evaluation and Research; Center for Devices and Radiological Health. (2003). *Guidance for Industry and FDA: FY 2004 MDUFMA Small Business*

*Qualification Worksheet and Certification* [Online]. Available: http://www.fda.gov/cdrh/mdufma/guidance/1225.pdf

U.S. Food and Drug Administration (FDA), Center for Devices and Radiological Health. (2003b). *Office of Device Evaluation and Office of In Vitro Diagnostic Device Evaluation and Safety Annual Report: Fiscal Year 2003.*

U.S. General Accounting Office (GAO). (2003). Divided authority for policies on coverage of procedures and devices results in inequities. (GAO-03–175).

U.S. Medicare Payment Advisory Commission (USMPAC). (2002, March). *Report to Congress: Medicare Payment Policy*, p. 111.

U.S. Medicare Payment Advisory Commission (USMPAC). (2003, March). *Report to Congress: Medicare payment policy*. Chapter 4: Payment for new technologies in Medicare's prospective payment systems; Appendix B: An introduction to how Medicare makes payment decisions.

The Wilkerson Group. (1995, June). *Forces reshaping the performance and contribution of the U.S. medical device industry*. A report for the Health Industry Manufacturers Association, 17–18.

# 12

# THE
# HEALTH CARE
# WORKFORCE

Carol S. Brewer

MANY CHANGES HAVE occurred in our health care system over the last 10 years, with a dramatic impact on the number and types of workers needed, and where and how they will practice. Health care professions are evaluating their roles and relationships within the health care system and with other workers. Education and regulatory systems are responding and evolving as well.

The health care workforce is part of an industry that consumes a large portion of our nation's resources. Evidence of the size, growth, and complexity of that industry is presented in other chapters of this text. Over the last 50 years, health care employment has consistently grown at a faster rate than the overall employment in the American economy. From 1983 through 2002, there was a 58% increase in the number of people in health care occupations (U.S. Census Bureau [USCB], 2003). Even during national recessions, health care employment has risen. The health care workforce is large and diverse, and health services are labor intensive. This is true whether the services are provided in hospitals, in nursing homes, or in physicians' offices.

In spite of the slower growth of the health care economy in the 1990s that led to predictions of an oversupply of various health care personnel (Pew Health Professions Commission [PHPC], 1995), the aging of the population, and efforts to address specific health problems, such as high rates of infant mortality, are contributing to the need for additional health care personnel. In 2002, the 9.2 million people in the health occupations and professions were 6.8% of the total workforce in the U.S. (USCB, 2003). This number does not include the many affiliated workers in computer, janitorial, secretarial, and other occupations who work in health care settings. Another group of people not included in the formal health care workforce are family and volunteer caregivers. The emphasis on reducing hospital lengths of stay, which is a focus of managed care, has had the consequence of sending sicker patients into the home setting to recover. The increase in chronic illnesses has also resulted in care giving at home. An estimate of family care giving in New York State found that an average of 22 hours per week, worth between $7.5 and $11.2 billion dollars, was provided by family members (Farberman et al., 2003) and a study of depressed elderly patients in the U.S. found that 3 to 6 hours per week of care were provided them, valued was at $9 billion (Langa, Valenstein, Fendrick, Kabeto, & Vijan, 2004).

The U.S. Bureau of Labor Statistics projects that employment in health care settings will continue to rise over 30% between 2002 and 2012 (U.S. Bureau of Labor Statistics [USBLS], 2004a). The health occupations are among the fastest growing of all occupations, comprising half of the 20 fastest-growing occupations. More new jobs (3.5 million or 16% of all new jobs) will be created in the health services sector than in any other industry (USBLS, 2004b).

Health care employment can be analyzed in two ways: by work location or by occupation. Health care professionals and others workers are typically employed in settings such as hospitals, nurs-

### TABLE 12.1

**Percentage of Distribution of Wage and Salary Employment and Establishments in Health Services, 2002**

| ESTABLISHMENT TYPE | ESTABLISHMENTS | EMPLOYMENT |
|---|---|---|
| Health services, total | 100.0 | 100.0 |
| Hospitals, public and private | 1.9 | 40.9 |
| Nursing and residential care facilities | 11.7 | 22.1 |
| Offices of physicians | 37.3 | 15.5 |
| Offices of dentists | 21.6 | 5.9 |
| Home health care services | 2.8 | 5.5 |
| Offices of other health practitioners | 18.2 | 3.9 |
| Outpatient care centers | 3.1 | 3.3 |
| Other ambulatory health care services | 1.5 | 1.5 |
| Medical and diagnostic laboratories | 1.9 | 1.4 |

SOURCE: U.S. Bureau of Labor Statistics, 2004b, p. 81. Career Guide to Industries, 2004–2005, p. 81.

ing homes, and ambulatory care facilities. **TABLE 12.1** shows the distribution of the total health workforce by practice setting. Many health personnel work in settings that are not considered part of the health industry (where patient care is provided). For example, physicians teach at medical schools and pharmacists work for pharmaceutical firms. Counting members of the health workforce can also be problematic. Workers can be counted by the number of people in a setting or occupation (e.g., by licenses), by how much they work (full-time or part-time, with two part-time workers making one full-time equivalent, or FTE, worker), or by the number of paychecks or jobs (U.S. Department of Labor (USDOL). Thus, if part-time workers are substituted for full-time workers, the DOL data might show an increase and the FTE data might show a decrease. Also, counting the number of licenses may include both active and inactive professionals as well as those with multiple state licenses.

## SUPPLY AND DEMAND FACTORS

Because the workforce represents a large portion of health care resources, there is increasing concern that it be adequately pre-

## TABLE 12.2

**Factors Influencing Supply and Demand in the Health Care Workforce**

|  | SUPPLY | DEMAND |
|---|---|---|
| **Demographics** | Age, gender, race/ethnicity, family composition, attitudes, and beliefs | Age, epidemiology, race distribution |
| **Education** | Number and types of programs, articulation of programs, number of graduates, immigrants, funding | Faculty availability, clinical site availability |
| **Health care delivery system** | Location, flexibility of hours, benefits, working conditions | Services, technology, employee or professional substitution, patient acuity |
| **Economic system** | Inflation, unemployment, wages and other incentives | Payment systems, direct reimbursement, price controls |
| **Contextual factors** | Socio-cultural values, government, political systems | |

SOURCE: Adapted from Dumpe, Herman, and Young, 1998.

pared as well as effective and efficient. Five basic factors influence the supply and demand of the health care workforce: the health care delivery system, educational system, economic system, and demographics and contextual factors (see TABLE 12.2) (Dumpe, Herman, & Young, 1998). The contextual factors of our culture, government, and political system determine the range of options within which we can find solutions to workforce issues.

These factors have a complex interaction that results in the aggregate supply and demand for health care workers. If these factors are in balance, a market equilibrium exists, i.e., there are enough workers wanting the jobs employers are offering, at the wages they are offering. However, historically there have been a number of factors that have created a lack of equilibrium in one or more of the workforce markets. Most often workforce shortages are of concern, but sometimes there has been an oversupply of a particular group of workers (Brewer, 1997). Nurses and physicians, because they are the largest of the professions and politically well organized, are often the focus of labor supply policy.

An example of an economic factor that has influenced workforce policy is the managed care revolution that was implemented from about 1993 to 2000. Managed care had the effect of flattening the growth of nurses and physicians' incomes, reducing hospital stays, and causing other effects as discussed elsewhere in this text. For example, in the last half of the 1990s, RN inflation-adjusted income was essentially flat (Sprately, Johnson, Sochalski, Fritz, & Spencer, 2001). Physicians still are among the highest paid professionals in the U.S. as shown in TABLE 12.3 (USBLS, 2004a; Guglielmo, 2003) but also saw income growing more slowly than inflation from 1995 to 2000 (Crane, 2001; Guglielmo).

A report published in 1995 (Pew Health Professions Commission [PHPC], 1995) indicated the lower numbers of physicians and nurses being used by managed care organizations in California than elsewhere. It predicted that both nurses and physicians would be oversupplied and that the number of educational programs should be reduced. The study was repeated in 2004 with similar findings: the physician-population ratio was 22 to 37% lower in three very large managed care organizations than in the rest of the U.S. (Weiner,

## TABLE 12.3

### Physician Income

| PRIMARY CARE PHYSICIANS | 2002 TOTAL MEDIAN COMPENSATION[1] |
|---|---|
| Obstetric/gynecologists | 220,000 |
| Family practitioners | 150,000 |
| Internists | 150,000 |
| Pediatricians | 130,000 |
| General Practitioners | 116,000 |
| **OTHER SPECIALTIES** | |
| Cardiologists (invasive) | 360,000 |
| Gastroenterologists | 300,000 |
| Orthopedic surgeons | 300,000 |
| Cardiologists (noninvasive) | 250,000 |
| General surgeons | 230,000 |
| All respondents | 162,000 |

SOURCE: Guglielmo, W. J. (2003). Physicians' earnings: Our exclusive survey, p. 83.

1. Total compensation for unincorporated physicians refers to earnings after tax-deductible expenses but before income taxes. For physicians in professional corporations, compensation is the sum of salary, bonuses, and retirement/profit-sharing made on their behalf. All figures are medians. Data apply to individual office-based MDs and DOs.

2004). However, there are a number of problems in applying this approach to health care workforce policy. The method may not adequately account for population differences that include health differences, and the scope of work may be different (that is, less teaching, research, and more care for high-need patients). If managed care staffing systems are more efficient, we know very little about how the delivery and financing system should be changed to create these efficiencies, and whether they are replicable in the general health care workforce. Limiting the production of physicians or other health care professionals on the basis of a delivery and financing system that perhaps should—but does not—exist is thus not sound policy (Salsberg & Forte, 2004).

Historically however, shortages are more common. This is due in large part to the expansion of our health care spending, which has increased to 14.1% in 2001 or more of the GDP each year (USCB, 2003). Continued growth in health care spending that is faster than inflation creates a demand for a higher paid workforce to match. The resulting shortages (where demand outstrips supply through continuous growth) have created alarm because of underlying structural changes in the demographics of the workforce, a major factor shown in Table 12.2.

Nursing is a profession for which the changing demographics and other factors are expected to create a crisis in the workforce in the future (Buerhaus, Staiger, & Auerbach, 2000). Registered nurses are getting older, and had a mean age of 45.2 years in 2000 (Sprately et al., 2001). Only 18% of RNs were under 35 years of age. In 2000, the nursing shortage was estimated at 6% nationally. By 2020, it expected to grow to 29% unless demand is moderated. The supply of nurses is expected to grow until 2011, after which the number of retiring nurses leaving the profession is expected to outstrip the number entering (U.S. Department of Health and Human Services [USDHHS, 2002). These aging trends are influencing most of the health professions.

In part, this aging of the population has resulted from the older average age at graduation and reflects a trend, also seen in most of the health professions, of older students coming back for a career change. At the same time, the baby boom generation is aging and entering their sixties, and will be needing increasing amounts of health care. Characteristics of the health care delivery system, such as 24-hour and holiday staffing, have also been unappealing to many younger health care workers. Societal career options have broadened for women, who have been the mainstream of many health care occupations, and salaries have not kept pace with other professions. For example, elementary school teachers earned $4,400 more than RNs in 1983. In 2000, they made $13,600 more than the average RN (USDHHS, 2002). However, this workforce shortage does appear to be having a welcome effect on RN incomes, as 2001 saw a 14% rise in wages and 2003 saw a 10% increase (Bauer, 2003).

## Measuring Supply

Two fairly sensitive indicators of changes in the supply of health care workers are nursing school admission and enrollment figures. These data, supplied by accrediting organizations, may not be accurate or complete, however. For example, in nursing, the American Association of Colleges of Nursing and the National League for Nursing each keep different statistics. However, a downward trend in admissions and enrollments has always been translated into a decline in graduate 2 to 4 years later, and vice versa (see FIGURE 12.1). This illustrates a fundamental issue in predicting and explaining shortages; responses to current events by students

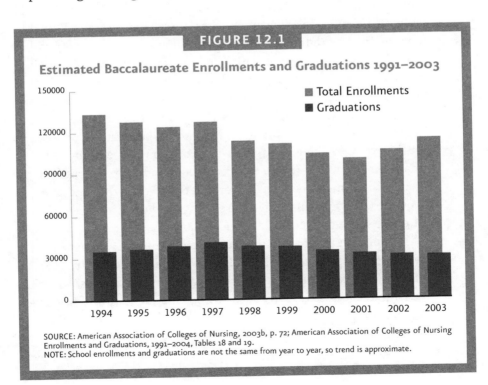

**FIGURE 12.1**

**Estimated Baccalaureate Enrollments and Graduations 1991–2003**

- Total Enrollments
- Graduations

SOURCE: American Association of Colleges of Nursing, 2003b, p. 72; American Association of Colleges of Nursing Enrollments and Graduations, 1991–2004, Tables 18 and 19.
NOTE: School enrollments and graduations are not the same from year to year, so trend is approximate.

| | | | TABLE 12.4 | | | |
|---|---|---|---|---|---|---|

## Ratio of Physicians to Population and Percentage Female

| | TOTAL NONFEDERAL PHYSICIANS | RATIO/ 100,000 | FEMALE PHYSICIANS | PERCENTAGE |
|---|---|---|---|---|
| **1975** | 356,560 | 169 | 35,626 | 10% |
| **2002** | 831,645 | 288 | 215,005 | 26% |

SOURCES: American Medical Association, 2004. Physician Characteristics and Distribution in the U.S. Department of Physician Practice and Communication Information, Division of Survey and Data Resources (p. 68); American Medical Association, 2003–2004 and prior editions; U.S. Census Bureau, Current Population Reports, Series P-25, No. St-99-2, 1044, 1045, 1106, 1127.

entering schools and making career choices is not reflected in the workforce until they graduate, 2 to 8 years later, depending on the discipline. Licensing data can also be used to count professionals who are required to be licensed. However, licensing or registration is a state-level function, and there are no centralized databases that provide the numbers of professionals licensed in multiple states.

Workforce productivity also affects supply. In most cases, younger and female health professionals work fewer hours and select different kinds of work settings. This translates into a change in the productivity of a particular workforce as, for example, more women become pharmacists and more men become nurses. Also, the proportion of female physicians increased from 10% in 1975 to 26% in 2002 (see TABLE 12.4) (American Medical Association [AMA], 2004), whereas the proportion of male nurses increased from 3.3% in 1988 to 5.9% in 2000. More males nurses are in the younger age groups, and more of them are employed (88%) than female nurses (81%). Physically demanding professions such as nursing can also be difficult for older workers, who tend to move from hospital and nursing home settings and to part-time positions or other settings such as education (Sprately et al., 2001).

It is also important to have an adequate number of particular types of health care workers. For example, periodically certain medical specialists such as primary care physicians or subspecialists such as anesthesiologists will be in short supply. However, determining what is an adequate supply of types of physicians or other professionals depends heavily on how health care is financed and organized. TABLE 12.5 presents the number of allopathic physicians in selected specialties from 1975 to 2002, and TABLE 12.6

## TABLE 12.5

### Allopathic Physicians by Specialty, 1975–2002

| SPECIALTY | 1975 | 1985 | 1995 | 2000 | 2002 | PERCENTAGE OF CHANGE (1985–2002) |
|---|---|---|---|---|---|---|
| Primary Care | 131,080 | 191,939 | 242,000 | 283,773 | 299,619 | 56.1 |
| Obstetrics/Gynecology | 21,731 | 30,867 | 37,652 | 40,241 | 41,038 | 33.0 |
| Medicine Subspecialties | 9,314 | 19,141 | 28,549 | 31,652 | 33,297 | 74.0 |
| General Surgery | 31,562 | 38,169 | 37,569 | 36,716 | 37,286 | −2.3 |
| Surgery Subspecialties | 34,920 | 48,150 | 58,473 | 60,132 | 62,052 | 28.9 |
| Facility-Based Specialties | 26,791 | 48,383 | 64,782 | 71,049 | 75,280 | 55.6 |
| Psychiatry | 23,922 | 32,355 | 38,098 | 39,457 | 39,895 | 23.3 |
| Other Specialties | 21,653 | 36,379 | 52,813 | 57,723 | 60,582 | 66.5 |
| Total Physicians | 393,742 | 552,716 | 720,325 | 813,770 | 853,187 | 54.4 |

SOURCE: American Medical Association (2004). Physician Characteristics and Distribution in the U.S., 2003, p. 68.

## TABLE 12.6

### Allopathic Medical School Enrollment and Demographics

| ACADEMIC YEAR | NUMBER APPLICANTS | APPLICANT ACCEPTANCE RATIO | GRADUATES | PERCENTAGE OF WOMEN GRADUATES | PERCENTAGE OF UNDERREPRESENTED MINORITY GRADUATES |
|---|---|---|---|---|---|
| 1979–1980 | 36,141 | 2.1 | 15,113 | 23.1 | 7.1 |
| 1989–1990 | 26,915 | 1.6 | 15,398 | 33.9 | 8.2 |
| 1999–2000 | 38,529 | 2.2 | 15,824 | 42.4 | 11.7 |
| 2000–2001 | 37,092 | 2.1 | 15,901 | 43.0 | 10.5 |
| 2001–2002 | 34,859 | 2.0 | 15,810 | 44.1 | 11.0 |
| 2002–2003 | 33,625 | 1.9 | 15,640 | 45.1 | 13.4* |

SOURCEs: B. Barzansky, 2003, p. 8; Barzansky et al., 1999–2002.
NOTE: This percentage* is from the American Association of Medical Colleges Data Book, 2004, p. 113.

shows medical school enrollments. In 1975, there were more than 131,000 physicians in primary care (internal medicine, family practice, pediatrics, and general practice), and 299,619 in 2002, a 56.1% increase. The 40% of all allopathic physicians in primary care or obstetrics/gynecology (AMA, 2004) does not include the 43,910 active osteopathic physicians (American Association of Colleges of Osteopathic Medicine [AACOM], 2002). This proportion of primary care physicians has been lower than in countries such as Canada, Great Britain, and Germany, where more than 50% of physicians were in primary care specialties (PHPC, 1993). This is a result of the priorities, policies and organizations that determine the operation of the health care system in that country.

### Assuring an Adequate Supply of Physicians

One of the more hotly debated, recent health workforce policy issues has been physician workforce planning. At the core of the debate is how to encourage the production of a physician workforce that can best meet the health needs of the nation. The debate has been fueled by a lack of agreement as to whether the current and projected supply is adequate to meet the nation's needs, as well as whether the marketplace, without specific government interventions, will produce the appropriate role, number, mix and distribution of physicians. The National Council on Graduate Medical Education (COGME), by statute, advises the Department of Health and Human Services and the Congress on physician workforce issues.

The supply of physicians has been growing steadily since the 1950s. As shown in Table 12.4, the physician-to-population ratio increased from 180 nonfederal physicians per 100,000 people in 1975 to 288 physicians per 100,000 population (AMA, 2004), or by about 70%. In contrast, Weiner (2004) found that HMO staffing ranged from 134 to 144 per 100,000. There were signs, such as the drop in physician incomes (Simon & Born, 1996), that a surplus existed. Physicians and other practitioners who control the ordering of tests, procedures, and treatments, may generate their own demand by ordering tests and revisits (Rice, 1998). Because of the influence of physicians on health care costs, as well as the subsidization of their education, an oversupply of physicians is a serious concern. Supply-induced demand by physicians means that an excess supply of physicians can have a serious effect on health care costs (Rice, 1998), because these professionals generate demand for their own services. This problem is compounded by the cost of subsidized physician education.

Another reason for concern arising from our health care social context and values has been the high level of public financing for graduate medical education (GME). Medicare and Medicaid provided an estimated $10 billion in 2000 (Inglehart, 1996; Council on Graduate Medical Education, 2000). If there is a physician surplus, it is hard to justify such massive public support. In 1997, the Balanced Budget Act reduced the amount of Medicare funding for GME; however, other efforts to decrease GME financing have been blocked by concerns about the impact on teaching hospitals and care for the poor in inner cities that are served by medical school residents (Inglehart).

There is considerable debate over whether the nation may face a surplus or shortage in the next decade (Cooper, Getzen, McKee, & Laud, 2002; Blumenthal, 2004; Grumbach, 2002), particularly of specialists (Cooper et al.). This reflects several factors, including the evolution of managed care to a less restrictive form than expected, the aging of the baby boom generation, the general growth in the nation's population, the growing supply of physician extenders and female physicians, and the aging of the nation's physician workforce (Cooper et al.).

## Assuring an Adequate Supply of Nurses

Cyclical shortages and surpluses of registered nurses occurred during the 20th century (Brewer, 2005). This reflects a number of factors, including the lag in response of prospective students and the educational system to changes in health care demand (see Figure 12.1). In response to severe shortages in the late 1980s, salaries for registered nurses rose significantly; these higher salaries led to an increase in the numbers of RNs being educated in the early 1990s. In addition, in response to higher RN salaries and shortages, as well as pressures to reduce costs from managed care, health facilities increasingly sought ways to substitute lower-cost personnel for RNs (Brewer & Kovner, 2001). Throughout the late 1990s, enrollment in nursing programs fell. We are now seeing a similar economic response to a shortage, with rising wages and enrollments. In fact, more than 11,000 qualified students were turned away from baccalaureate nursing programs in 2003 due to the limited numbers of faculty, clinical sites, and classroom spaces (American Association of Colleges of Nursing, 2003a; National League for Nursing, 2003).

Both the advent of managed care and the Balanced Budget Act of 1997 that reduced Medicare payments also led hospitals to try to reduce costs. Ironically, the approaches to cost cutting due to both decreased demand and shortages of staff are similar. Both focus on redesign of services and substituting less costly personnel or in improved technology (such as computerized records, medication systems, or personal digital assistants [PDAs]) to reduce costs and improve productivity.

There is concern that as the RN workforce ages, the shortage periods will become more sustained and severe. With a full economy and the growing business aspects of health care, there have been growing opportunities for nurses not involving direct patient care. In addition, the stress and physical demands of the job may lead some of the most experienced nurses to leave health facilities (Brewer, Feeley, & Servoss, 2003).

## Geographical Distribution

Another major issue for the health care workforce is its distribution across rural and urban underserved areas. Even when numbers of professionals are high in relation to the population, as in New York State, these professionals may not be evenly distributed in proportion to need. Rural areas, for example, often do not have large employers with insurance benefits, and the reimbursement rates of Medicaid and Medicare may be too low to attract practitioners in medicine and dentistry (Wright, Andrilla, & Hart, 2001).

The distribution of the workforce results from a complex interplay of all the factors shown in Table 12.2. Scholarships are available for primary care practitioners (physicians, nurses, and physician assistants), and a loan repayment program is available for the same practitioners as well as various mental health practitioners, social workers, and dental hygienists (USDHHS, 2003). Once educated and licensed, the health care worker still has to choose a geographic area, setting, and level of work participation. Many students want to stay where they were educated, which are typically urban areas, rather than in rural or underserved areas. Medically Underserved Areas (MUAs) and Health Professions Shortage Areas (HPSAs) are federally determined designations for which a county or region can apply that confer benefits upon the areas so designated. In 2004, there were nearly 2,700 health care professionals serving in urban and rural areas that were classified by the federal government as HPSAs (USDHHS, 2003). Educational costs are a major pipeline barrier to increasing the supply of health care workers.

### Nurses

The major source of information about registered nurses is the quadrennial National Sample Survey of Registered Nurses by

Health Resources and Services Administration (HRSA), Bureau of Health Professions, which is currently being conducted for 2004. About 2.7 million people had licenses to practice as registered nurses in the United States in 2000 (Sprately et al., 2001 [HRSA]). About 2.2 million (82%) were employed in nursing (an increase of about 86,000 over 1996); 59% were working full time.

The National Council of State Boards of Nursing [NCSBN] (Crawford, Marks, Gawel, & White, 2002) reported there are about 3,100,000 licensed RNs, including duplicates. An unknown number of RNs have licenses in more than one state, reflecting the difficulty in estimating accurate ratios for any profession that allows multiple state licensures. Estimates from the NSSRN data show that there is wide variation in the number of RNs in relation to the population. California, the state with the lowest ratio, had 554 RNs per 100,000, whereas Massachusetts, the state with the highest ratio, had 1,194 RNs per 100,000 (Sprately et al., 2001).

Another aspect of adequate nurse-population ratios is whether the number of minority professionals matches that of the population served. In 2000, an estimated 25% of all Americans were of minority race or ethnicity (USCB, 2000), and this percentage is expected to continue to increase. However, as shown in FIGURE 12.2, only about 10% of RNs were minorities (defined as nonwhites) in 2000. The percentage of men, another minority group in nursing, was almost 6%, a slight increase from 1996. The percentage of minority RNs is inconsistent with their representation in the general population, and typically their distribution is also nonrepresentative in urban areas where the minority populations are higher. This has been a concern of nursing, other health professions, and the government for many years.

### Physicians

The majority of physicians are concentrated in urban areas, although the doubling of the total number of U.S. physicians over time has led to some dispersal of physicians to rural areas. While 20% of the U.S. population lives in nonmetropolitan areas, only 11% of the physicians practice there (Federal Office of Rural Health Policy [FORHP], 1995). The lower physician-to-population ratio in most rural areas reflects, in part, the need for a minimum population base required to economically support a physician specialty practice and to maintain skill levels for certain specialties. International medical graduates are more likely than U.S. graduates to set-

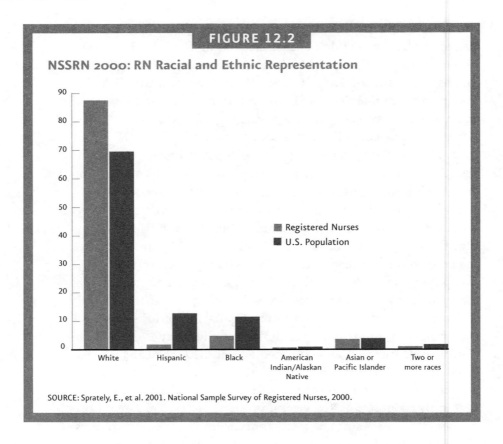

**FIGURE 12.2**

**NSSRN 2000: RN Racial and Ethnic Representation**

- ■ Registered Nurses
- ■ U.S. Population

(White, Hispanic, Black, American Indian/Alaskan Native, Asian or Pacific Islander, Two or more races)

SOURCE: Sprately, E., et al. 2001. National Sample Survey of Registered Nurses, 2000.

tle in rural areas (Croasdale, 2003), but in spite of the increase in total physician supply, serious access problems still exist in rural areas. In spite of the need, it appears that interest by U.S. medical school graduates in primary care specialties has declined (AAMC, 2002), and demand has stayed level for office based primary care physicians, except in rural areas (Guglielmo, 2003). Some of this is attributed to the much lower level and slower growth of net income for primary care physicians (Guglielmo).

## TYPES OF HEALTH CARE WORKERS

There are currently hundreds of health care professions, subspecialties, and occupations with educational requirements ranging from a high school degree to doctoral and professional degrees. Details about some of these professions can be obtained from the Web sites listed at the end of this chapter. The regulation of health professionals is a state responsibility. As such, each state has its own legal definition of the practice of the profession and its scope of responsibilities. Professions attempting to change or expand their scope of responsibilities must change the regulations in every state. States can require registration, licensure, certification, or other forms of regulation for the workforce. In addition, the state is responsible for approving educational programs and curriculums and for maintaining information about the professions and registry lists which are often used for research on the health care workforce. Multiple state licenses create difficulties in assessing the size and distribution of the workforce as well as create barriers to the interstate movement of professionals, but states are reluctant to give up their oversight function to national governing or licensing bodies.

Often the workforce structure of a discipline is based on a defined scope of practice for that discipline, and a particular professional will be licensed to practice the full the discipline (nutritionist, registered nurse, physician, dentist). However, parts of the practice may be delegated to less highly trained people with varying amounts of educational preparation, who may or may not be licensed. Examples are licensed practical nurses, radiology technicians, and dental hygienists. Unlicensed occupations have little regulation, although educational programs may be accredited. If these health workers give patient care, they generally work under the supervision of a licensed health professional.

Labor substitution means that the increase in cost (e.g., wage per hour) of one type of profession or occupation decreases the demand for it, and increases the demand for its substitute. Licensing and government regulations (particularly regarding reimbursement) can limit the substitution of less costly workers for professionals. When professionals compete on the basis of this substitution, or attempt to obtain direct insurance reimbursement for services, considerable political rivalry may occur. Examples of such competition have occurred between anesthesiologists and Certified Registered Nurse Anesthetists (CRNAs), and between dentists and dental hygienists, among others. There are many other complementary health care professions. At least in some areas, these must work together using the full scope of their practices to complete the diagnosis, treatment, and care of the patient. Demand for one creates the demand for the complement to move in the same direction. Contemporary education and practice models have focused on developing these aspects of health care practice under the rubric of interdisciplinary or collaborative care of patients.

## NURSING PRACTICE

Nurse is a generic term that is applied to a variety of practitioners from unlicensed nurses' aides and assistants to nurse researchers with PhDs. This is the largest group of health care workers.

### Registered Nurse

Each state board of nursing defines and interprets the authority and scope of practice of registered nurses, although nursing is often defined as the diagnosis and treatment of human responses to health problems. By 1923, legislation was enacted in all states for voluntary registration (Bullough, 1975).

All states require that prospective registered nurses attend an approved nursing program and take a national licensing exam developed by the NCSBN, the National Council Licensure Examination for RNs (NCLEX-RN). In 2003, of the 76,727 first-time candidates educated in the United States and its territories taking the exam, almost 87% passed, while 56% of the 16,490 foreign-educated applicants passed the exam (NCSBN, 2003, 2004). The number of first-time foreign educated RNs taking the exam has almost tripled since 1999.

### Other Nursing Personnel

Licensed practical nurses (LPNs)/licensed vocational nurses (LVNs) work under the supervision of RNs or physicians and perform caregiving tasks such as medication administration and wound dressing change. LPN/LVNs must pass a national examination to be licensed in each state. In 2003, some 56,581 people took the exam and 78.5% passed (NCSBN, 2003).

Additional nursing personnel include a variety of unlicensed assistive personnel (UAP) such as nurse aides, assistants, orderlies, and technicians. These personnel also work under the supervision of registered nurses and perform such simple tasks as taking vital signs and providing comfort measures such as bathing and linen change. These occupations are not licensed by the states, although federal regulations require that nurse aides who work in long-term care facilities that are reimbursed by Medicare and Medicaid must complete a specified educational program and pass a written and practical test. In addition, Medicare certified home health agencies have to hire certified home health aides. Some states have specific educational requirements for some of these workers. More than half of the states have regulations or guidelines for RNs who supervise UAPs (Thomas, Barter, & McLaughlin, 2000).

## The Education of Nurses

One of the most confusing aspects of the nursing profession is the variety of programs for educating nurses. Unlike medicine and most other health care professions, which have consistent educational requirements, nursing offers the student a number of options. Students can attend a 2-year college program conferring an associate's degree, a 3-year hospital-based (diploma) program, a 4-year college program, a 2-year master's degree program, or a nursing doctoral (ND) program. North Dakota is currently the only state to require a baccalaureate degree, although the American Nurses Association recommends a baccalaureate degree to become a registered nurse, and New York State's Board of Nursing passed a motion in December 2003 that all associate and diploma degree RNs should obtain a baccalaureate degree within 10 years. All other state boards of nursing accept any of these programs as appropriate preparation for the RN licensing exam.

Both the National League for Nursing (NLN) and the American Association of Colleges of Nursing (AACN) accredit nursing programs and collect data on programs, admissions, enrollments, and graduations. Neither organization has complete data, making it difficult to reliably track students in the pipeline. Accreditation standards do not specify individual course requirements, so curricula vary widely from school to school, and transfer of nursing course credits is extremely difficult. Fewer nurses are now prepared at the diploma level; about 22% of RNs had a diploma as their highest level of education; only 6% of those educated from 1995 to 2000 graduated from a diploma program and 38% graduated from a baccalaureate program (Sprately et al. 2001).

Enrollments and graduations have fluctuated over the years (see Figure 12.1). Total enrollments in baccalaureate nursing programs decreased from 1995 to 1999, the fifth year that enrollments decreased (American Association of Colleges of Nursing [AACN], 2003b). Enrollments and graduations have increased, although they have not returned to levels seen in 1996; they were sharply up in baccalaureate programs by 2003 (AACN, 2003a, 2003b).

Educational requirements for other nursing personnel, such as LPNs and nurses' aides, vary by state and employment setting. Practical nurse education, usually one year long, occurs in high schools, hospitals, junior colleges, or vocational schools. Some are educated in the setting in which they work, some in programs in high schools, and others in not-for-profit or for-profit vocational schools. Training takes from a few hours to six months or more.

### Graduate Nursing Education

Registered nurses with baccalaureate degrees can earn master's degrees in advanced clinical practice, teaching, and nursing administration/management. Most students choose to focus on advanced clinical practice. In graduate school, students usually focus on an area such as adult health, maternal-child health, psychiatric-mental health, or community health. Specific programs include everything from nursing informatics, home health care management, and geriatrics, to pediatric nurse practitioners. Clinical expertise in specialty areas can also be recognized through certification programs administered by various nursing organizations. Enrollment of nurses in master's programs did not increase until 2001, rebounding almost to the 1998 level. While the proportion of minority nurses in graduate education is better than in undergraduate education (about 17%), the lack of minority entrants in proportion to the population remains, at a minimum, of great concern (AACN, 2003b).

Three types of doctoral degrees are offered. The ND (Doctor of Nursing) is similar to the MD, that is, it is the first professional degree, building on the earlier undergraduate education and preparing the student to take the state registered nurse licensing exam. The DSN and DNSc are professional doctorates that prepare the nurse for advanced clinical practice. The PhD is a research degree, with requirements similar to the PhD in other fields; it requires extensive preparation in a narrow field and a dissertation. Enrollment of students in doctoral programs has had small but steady average increases of 31 students per year. In 2002, of the nearly 3,505 students enrolled in doctoral programs, 93.3% were female and 14.4% were minority students (AACN, 2003b).

## Employment Settings

As shown in FIGURE 12.3, in 2000, about 59.1% of RNs worked in hospitals, 18.2% worked in public health or community health care of various types, while only 6.9% worked in nursing homes. About 9.5% of RNs worked in ambulatory care settings. Staff nurses typically work in direct patient care, where they provide nursing care to individuals who may be acutely ill, as in a hospital; chronically ill or recovering from illness, as in a home setting; or well but requiring preventive care, as in a health department or HMO. About 15.6% of RNs hold more than one job (Sprately et al., 2001).

When adjusted for inflation, average salaries for RNs were relatively flat from 1992 to 2000 (Sprately et al., 2001). In 2002, the median salary for registered nurses ranged from $38,900 in Iowa to $61,700 in Maryland (*America's Career Infonet*, 2004). Because of the shortage, adjusted salaries have been rising as the market adjusts (Bauer, 2003). RN salaries vary by geographic area, setting, position, education, and experience. Detailed information about a variety of occupations (including nursing), educational requirements,

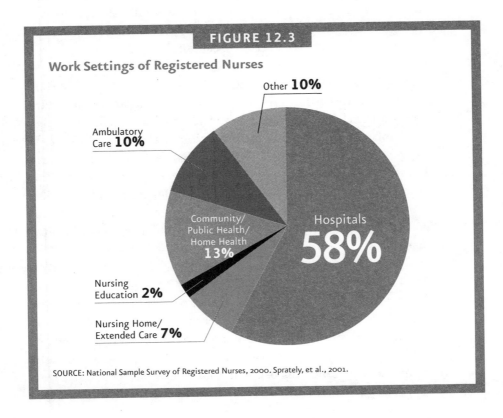

**FIGURE 12.3**

**Work Settings of Registered Nurses**

Other **10%**

Ambulatory Care **10%**

Community/ Public Health/ Home Health **13%**

Hospitals **58%**

Nursing Education **2%**

Nursing Home/ Extended Care **7%**

SOURCE: National Sample Survey of Registered Nurses, 2000. Sprately, et al., 2001.

and income is available in the *Occupational Handbook* of the Bureau of Labor Statistics (USBLS, 2004a).

## MEDICAL PRACTICE

Medical practice may be defined as the science of diagnosing, treating, or preventing disease and other damage to the body or mind (http://education;yahoo.com/reference/dictionary/entry/medicine). American medicine is undergoing a major transformation. Changes in the health care system are challenging physicians and transforming their traditional role in health care, from being the dominant, controlling force, to being one of many players. The world of solo practice and fee-for-service medicine is rapidly being replaced by group practice, integrated delivery systems, managed care, and capitation. The increased use of nurse practitioners, physician assistants, and other health care professionals is requiring greater collaboration and cooperation among health care professionals. Physicians still play a central role in determining the type of care provided, admitting patients to health facilities, ordering tests, and prescribing medicine, treatment, and referrals to therapists, but now they must generally share the responsibility and oversight with other professionals and managed care organizations.

There are two types of traditional physicians: allopathic (MD) and osteopathic (DO). Allopathic medicine is "a system of medicine based on the theory that successful therapy depends on creating a condition antagonistic to or incompatible with the condition to be treated" (Slee & Slee, 2004). Osteopathic medicine "emphasizes a theory that the body can make its own remedies, given normal structural relationships, environmental conditions, and nutrition. It differs from allopathic primarily in its greater attention to body mechanics and manipulative methods in diagnosis and therapy" (Slee & Slee, 2004).

### Undergraduate Medical Education

The majority of the 126 allopathic (Barzansky & Etzel, 2003) and 20 osteopathic medical schools (Brotherton, Rockey, & Etzel, 2003) in the United States are part of academic medical centers that include tertiary hospitals and medical complexes. Medical school usually requires 4 years following baccalaureate education. The first 2 years are usually didactic (instruction taught in the classroom), and the second 2 years are primarily clinical. Medical schools have been criticized for overemphasizing high-tech tertiary care, for emphasizing organ systems rather than the whole patient, for not encouraging primary care, for not educating more underrepresented minorities, and for not preparing physicians to work in ambulatory settings or in managed care environments.

The result of these criticisms has been a major reassessment of medical school curricula, and many schools have modified or are considering modifying the traditional curriculum. For example, many schools have added instruction on alternative/complementary medicine and many have added coursework related to cultural competence and the health care system (Barzansky & Etzel, 2003). In some schools, aspects of clinical training are presented earlier in the education process.

Once educated, allopathic and osteopathic physicians have the same scope of practice and take the same U.S. Medical Licensing Examination that tests basic sciences, clinical knowledge, and clinical skills in three parts. The final examination is after the first year of post graduate work, usually in a residency, and is required in order to be licensed by the state.

### Enrollment in Medical School

Despite high tuition and a lengthy education, medicine is still a highly sought profession and applicants exceed available slots by about 2:1 (Barzansky & Etzel, 2003). Enrollments at allopathic schools have been virtually constant since 1998. Women are 46% of enrollees in allopathic schools and 43% of osteopathic schools (Singer, 2003). Both the number of osteopathic schools (14 to 20) and enrollments (from 2035 to 3043) have increased since 1992 (Barzansky & Etzel). Allopathic medical school graduates have been relatively stable since 1980, with about 16,000 each year. As indicated in Table 12.2, however, female allopathic graduates have increased, and minority graduates have increased more slowly (Barzansky & Etzel). In 2002, 41% of osteopathic graduates were female, and 7.8% of osteopathic enrollees were minority (Singer). This has implications for the health care system, as female and minority physicians have different specialty and practice patterns than white male physicians (Forte & Salsberg, 1999).

The failure of American medical schools to enroll underrepresented minorities consistent with their representation has implications for issues of equity, access, and quality of health care. Much has been written and lamented about this fact, with little progress for changing it. Underrepresented minority physicians are more likely to serve in underserved communities; serve underserved populations, and be more sensitive to cultural and social differences of their race and ethnicity, which can be critical in diagnosis, treatment, and patient compliance (AAMC, 2002).

The medical student's average debt in 2002 was $103,855 (Barzansky & Etzel, 2003). It is a disincentive for many students to pursue medicine, although physicians can anticipate higher than average incomes once they begin practice. The lengthy period for education and training, with its relatively low salaries, combined with most loans coming due in the second year of postgraduate training, may discourage medical students from choosing primary care, a group of specialties that remains relatively low-paying (Ginsburg, Ostow, & Dutka, 1993).

### Graduate Medical Education

To be licensed as a physician and to be recognized by the profession as fully prepared, a physician must complete at least some formal, supervised, practical clinical experience through graduate medical education (GME), known as residency training. As medicine has become more complex and the number of physicians has grown, there has been greater specialization and more advanced training. After specialty training, a physician may choose to subspecialize. For example, after training for 3 years in internal medicine, a physician can choose 2 years of additional training and subspecialize in cardiology or gastroenterology.

GME, which is funded largely by Medicare ($7.8 billion in direct and indirect payments in 2000) and Medicaid ($2.3 billion in 1998), is a central determinant of the number and types of physicians available in a region (Council on Graduate Medical Education [CGME], 2000). It is a major source of funding for teaching hospitals, and in many states, it has a major impact on Medicaid costs. The expansion of managed care, growing competition in health care, and other developments have brought a series of GME issues to the foreground—nationally, in state capitals, and at teaching hospitals. Today, these hospitals are facing major challenges because the new competitive marketplace leaves little room for expenditures that are not directly related to patient care. The federal government and many states are considering legislation related to the financing of GME. In spite of the addition of physician assistants (PAs) and nurse practitioners (NPs) to the staff of hospitals, partly to replace residents whose work hours have been reduced, only a few states use GME funds for PA or NP programs. However, some funding still supports hospital based nursing schools (Aiken & Gwyther, 1995).

Historically, the vast majority of GME has taken place in large teaching hospitals. These hospitals offer residents an opportunity to see a wide range of patient conditions, and, in many cases, these academic medical centers are where medical schools and their faculty are located. As services shift to ambulatory settings, there is a growing effort to provide more training outside of hospitals to better prepare physicians for future practice and to encourage primary care. GME funding recommendations have encouraged finding methods of reimbursing GME that would broaden the location of training to more accurately reflect where physicians will actually practice (CGME, 2000).

### Residency Programs and Specialties

Allopathic residency programs are accredited by the Accreditation Council for Graduate Medical Education (ACGME) (Brotherton, Rockey, & Etzel, 2003). The ACGME is a private national body that oversees establishing standards and assesses individual residency program performance against those standards. Osteopathic internship and residency programs are accredited by the American Osteopathic Association.

U.S. residencies accept many more physicians than there are U.S. graduates; many are accepted from foreign medical schools and are called international medical graduates. Consensus on the number of residency slots and size of medical schools does not exist.

The proportion of residents who graduated from international medical schools has stayed quite constant from 1998 to 2003. The largest proportion of first-year residents, 62%, choose family practice or internal medicine and these numbers are growing (Brotherton, Rockey, & Etzel, 2003).

### Mid-Level Professionals

The term mid-level professional generally refers to physician assistants and nurse practitioners. These two practitioner levels have developed to fill the need for medical care in rural and other areas where medical practitioners are lacking as well as provide medical services that are theoretically less expensive than those provided by a physician. Cooper (2002) argues that the lessening of interest in and demand for primary care specialties is at least partially the result of increasing numbers of mid-level providers.

PAs practice under the direct supervision of the physician who remains legally responsible for the care delivered by the PA. Mid-level nurses collaborate with physicians as required by state law but practice on their own license and are legally responsible for the care they deliver. Three key issues for mid-level practitioners are the degree to which (1) they can diagnose and prescribe treatment independently of a physician's oversight, (2) the right to prescribe, and (3) the right to be directly reimbursed by insurance. Without these legal rights, it is difficult to establish an independent practice; most mid-level practitioners are salaried.

## Advanced Practice Nurses

There were about 196,275 (7.3%) advanced practice RNs in 2000 (Sprately et al., 2001). Within the generic category of advanced practice nurse (APN), those with a clinical practice focus include clinical nurse specialist (CNS), nurse practitioner (NP), nurse midwife (NMW), and certified registered nurse anesthetist (CRNA). APNs are legally responsible for their own practice. Clinical nurse specialists have advanced degrees with expert skills in a particular area, such as mental health, cancer, or women's health, and often focus their practice in acute care settings. Nurse-practitioners perform an expanded nursing role and diagnose and manage most common and many chronic health problems, often in primary care. In most states they can prescribe medicines. Their scope of practice, however, including whether or not they must have a collaborating relationship with a physician, varies from state to state. Nurse midwives are educated to provide pre-, intra-, and postpartum care, provide family planning services and routine gynecological care, as well as care for newborns. Nurse anesthetists are trained to administer anesthetics.

Legal limitations and educational requirements for advanced practice vary considerably from state to state. Most, but not all, states require a master's degree. Numerous studies support the position that nurse practitioners provide cost effective health care equal in quality to that provided by physicians (Brown & Grimes, 1995), and it costs substantially less to educate a NP than a physician.

State regulations on nurses prescribing pharmaceuticals are inconsistent. In some states advanced practice nurses (clinical nurse specialists and NPs) can prescribe without physician collaboration or authorizations, while in other states the NP must have a practice arrangement with a physician, and in some states, clinical nurse specialists do not have prescriptive privileges. Some states limit prescriptive authority to central sites, to formularies, or to specific drugs.

Reimbursement continues to be a restriction on practice. Although RNs can bill patients for services, as they have been able to do since the early part of the twentieth century, third-party reimbursement continues to be a problem. When managed care organizations do not include NPs or NMWs on their primary care panels (Mason, Cohen, O'Donnell, Baxer, & Chase, 1997), these nurses are not eligible for reimbursement for care provided. Medicare reimburses APNs for care that is within their scope of practice. In terms of NMWs, Medicaid reimbursement is available in all states; however, services covered varied from state to state (Declerq, Paine, Simmes, & DeJoseph, 1998). HCFA issued a rule in 2001 that defers to state professional practice laws and hospital bylaws to determine which licensed professionals can administer anesthesia. This would allow for more autonomy and direct reimbursement for CRNAs. Physician groups, including the American Medical Association, are opposed to this regulatory change.

## Physician Assistants

Physician assistants (PAs) work under the direct supervision of physicians, who remain legally responsible for the care delivered by the PA. While the regulation of PAs varies from state to state, supervision does not mean on-site supervision. In most states the amount of delegation to a PA is a decision between the physician and the PA.

Both the demand and supply of PAs has been increasing rapidly. PAs can expand access to primary care and improve physician productivity, both of which are promoted by the expansion of managed care. PAs can substitute for physicians in hospitals, and in some areas, PAs may replace residents in training.

In 2003, there were about 57,879 PAs eligible to practice in the United States. Of these, 59% were female, 89% were white, and 19% worked in nonmetropolitan counties. The PAs worked in a wide variety of specialties; 87% were practicing. The largest percentage,

44%, of PAs worked in primary care, and 23% worked in surgical subspecialties (American Academy of Physician Assistants [AAPA], 2004). In 2002, their median U.S. annual income was $64,700 (*America's Career Infonet*, 2004). As the effectiveness and efficacy of PAs is demonstrated in more and more specialty areas, PAs may be drawn away from primary care specialties. The PA to population ratio varies widely between states, from 43.2 per 100,000 population in Alaska, to only 2.3 per 100,000 in Mississippi (AAPA, 2003).

The physician assistant is a relatively new profession. The first PA educational program was established by Duke University Medical Center in 1965, in part to allow an opportunity for medics who had gained clinical experience in the Vietnam War to practice in the health care system. In 1971, with the passage of the Comprehensive Health Manpower Act, federal financial support became available and contributed to the rapid expansion of PA programs. These programs are located in a number of academic settings and offer a variety of credentials. Most physician assistant programs require applicants to have previous health care experience and some college education before entering a program that is about 26 months in length. Half have a bachelor's degree and 26% a master's degree as the basic PA education (AAPA, 2004).

## OTHER HEALTH CARE WORKERS

In addition to physicians, there are a variety of other health professionals educated in graduate programs beyond the baccalaureate that use the title "Doctor," as described below. Each specialty has its own body of knowledge, professional association, and educational requirements. Pharmacists have long been considered an allied health occupation, but recently changed their educational requirements to a doctoral degree. The same information is not available on all occupations because the varying sources that produce workforce data do not do so on a regular schedule or to meet standard requirements.

### Dentists

In 2002, doctors of dental surgery (DDSs) or the equivalent, doctors of dental medicine (DMDs), held approximately 153,000 dentistry jobs. The ratio of dentists to 100,000 population peaked at 59.5 in 1990 and is expected to decline to 52.7 by 2020 (Valachovic, 2001b).

Another estimate, however, is a ratio of 60.7 in 2020 (USDHHS, 2002b). They were educated in 55 schools of dentistry (American Dental Association [ADA], 2001). Females are 15.6% of the total and 33.9% of new graduates. Like nurses, dentists are an aging group of professionals. Only a 4% growth in the total number of dentists is expected by 2012, and most jobs will result from the need to replace retiring dentists. African Americans account for 12.9% of the general population but only 2.2% of active dentists and less than 5% of students enrolled in dental schools. Hispanics comprise 12.5% of the population but only 2.8% of active dentists and 5.3% of enrolled dental students in 1999–2000 (Valachovic, Weaver, Sinkford, & Haden, 2001). Dental medicine has been slow to embrace community-based training, so the distribution of dentists is problematic. Most (80%) are solo practitioners in private practice (USBLS, 2004a).

## Podiatrists

Podiatrists diagnose, treat, and prevent abnormal foot conditions. Educated at one of the seven 4-year podiatric medical schools in the U.S., they perform surgery, and prescribe and administer pharmaceuticals. In most states, a postdoctoral residency program of at least 1 year is required. Licensed by individual states, they deliver a wide range of medical and surgical services. There were about 13,000 practitioners in 1997 and about the same in 2002. Many podiatrists are solo practitioners, although more are entering partnerships with other podiatrists or other health practitioners (USBLS, 2004a).

## Chiropractors

Chiropractic medicine is a system of diagnosis and healing based on the concept that health and disease are related to nervous system function, disease is due to malfunction of the nervous system due to noxious irritants, and health can be restored by their removal (*Medical Dictionary*, 2004). These doctors treat problems of the musculo-skeletal system (particularly the spine) and neurological systems holistically and with manipulation. They do use not pharmaceuticals or surgery, but they do use diagnostic tests such as radiographs. Chiropractors are educated in 4-year programs, which follow at least 2 years of undergraduate education. There were 16 chiropractic programs and two institutions accredited by the Council on Chiropractic Education (CCE) in 2003. Their graduates are eligible for licensure in all 50 states. In 2002, chiropractors held approximately 49,000 jobs, and employment is expected to grow faster than average. Geographic imbalances exist in this profession, although many are located in small communities (USBLS, 2004a). The uncertainty of workforce planning is indicated with this profession, as the professional society claims that there are 78,000 active licenses, though the number of duplicates is uncertain (Federation of Chiropractic Licensing Boards, 2004). An estimated ratio of chiropractors to 100,000 population is 24 (USD-HHS, 2002b).

## Optometrists

Optometrists are licensed to diagnose and provide selective eye treatment. In some states, they are licensed to prescribe a limited range of pharmaceuticals. Optometrists held about 32,000 jobs in 2002 (USBLS, 2004a). There is an estimated ratio of 11.7 optometrists per 100,000 population (USDHHS, 2002b). Educated at one of the 17 accredited schools of optometry, students have 4 years of professional training following undergraduate school. Optometrists provide many of the same services as ophthalmologists, usually at a lower cost. As state government considers increasing the scope of practice of optometrists, and as managed care expands, there has been conflict about the overlapping roles of optometrists and ophthalmologists (USBLS, 2004a).

## ALLIED HEALTH PROFESSIONALS

The Committee on Allied Health Education and Accreditation of the American Medical Association, which oversees nearly 2,000 educational programs, defines allied health as " . . . a large cluster of health care related professions and personnel whose functions include assisting, facilitating, or complementing the work of physicians and other specialists in the health care system, and who choose to be identified as allied health personnel" (USDHHS, 1992, p. 177). Although this is a general definition, it allows for occupations to be added and subtracted as the health care system evolves.

Allied health occupations are among the fastest growing in health care. The number of allied health professionals is difficult to estimate and depends on the definition of allied health. The Bureau of Health Professions estimates that allied health personnel are about 50 to 60% of the total health workforce (USDHHS, 2002b).

This number includes such occupations as dental hygienists, dietetic technicians, occupational therapists, clinical laboratory workers, operating room technicians, medical transcriptionists, speech-language pathology and audiology personnel, and many others. Unlike medicine, women dominate most of the allied health professions, representing 75 to 95% of most of the occupations. Education and training can be unstandardized and variable. Many allied health occupations develop in response to the shortage or high cost of other professionals. Little is known about the implications for patient outcomes (USDHHS, 1999).

For some allied health professions (e.g., physical therapists) all states require licensure, whereas for others (e.g., occupational therapy) only some states require licensure (Posner & Jaffe, 2000). Space does not permit a thorough discussion of each of these workers, but several examples are given.

## Pharmacists

Pharmacists have traditionally prepared pharmaceutical prescriptions; however, their role has expanded to providing information to patients about pharmaceuticals and drug interactions. Pharmacists held about 230,000 jobs in 2002, with a ratio of 71.3 pharamacists per 100,000 population (USDHHS, 2002b; USBLS, 2004a, p. 51). About 62% work in community pharmacies that are either independently owned or part of a drugstore chain, grocery store, department store, or mass merchandiser. Others work in hospitals, clinics, or drug companies. All states require pharmacists to be licensed.

Pharmacy programs recently began granting the degree of doctor of pharmacy (PharmD), which requires at least 6 years of postsecondary study and the passing of the licensure examination of a board of pharmacy. In 2002, there were 85 colleges of pharmacy offering the PharmD degree. Pharmacists can specialize by obtaining advanced degrees in pharmacy and through residency programs. Pharmacy technicians assist pharmacists with activities not requiring the judgment of a pharmacist (USBLS, 2004a).

### Physical Therapists

Physical therapists (PTs) provide services that help restore function, improve mobility, relieve pain, and prevent or limit permanent physical disabilities of patients suffering from injuries or disease. They restore, maintain, and promote overall fitness and health.

Counting the number of PT jobs, of which there were 132,000 in 2002, is a little misleading. For any profession in which it is common for the professional to have more than one job, the number of jobs is more than the number of therapists. For example, some may work in a private practice but also work part time in another health care facility. Most physical therapists (about two thirds) were either in hospitals or in offices of other health practitioners. Other jobs were in home health care services, nursing care facilities, outpatient care centers, and offices of physicians.

Of the 203 accredited programs in 2003, master's degrees were offered by 113 and doctoral degrees were offered by 90. Accredited programs are required to offer degrees at the master's degree level and above, in accordance with the Commission on Accreditation in Physical Therapy Education. There are also physical therapy technicians who work under the supervision of physical therapists (USBLS, 2004a).

## Alternative Practitioners

Alternative practitioners include naturopathic physicians, homeopaths, practitioners of acupuncture and other Asian medicine, as well as traditional healers from a variety of cultures, such as the Hispanic curandero. Chiropractors are also considered alternative practitioners. Several states now license these alternative health care providers. The National Center for Complementary and Alternative Medicine (NCCAM) was established in 1998 and is dedicated to using exacting science to research healing practices and determine their effectiveness. They have categorized alternative medicine into seven types for research purposes according to the approach to treatment: mind-body medicine, alternative medical systems, lifestyle disease and prevention, biologically based therapies, manipulative and body-based systems, biofield, and bioelectromagnetics (NCCAM, 2004). Alternative therapies are well accepted by the general public and account for a significant part of health care spending. In addition, third party reimbursement is offered by some insurance programs for some types of services, primarily in response to consumer demand.

## ISSUES

The changes occurring in health care have made it clear that there are issues in workforce preparation and utilization today. Among the issues that need better solutions to prepare the health care workforce for the future are the following: (a) the scope and nature of public policy for the workforce, (b) the quality of care and accountability of the professions, and (c) interdisciplinary and collaborative education and practice.

## Public Policy and the Health Care Workforce

The health care market place has never been a free market in the economic sense of the word (Rice, 1998), and it is unclear how fast and to what degree the health care workforce markets, if left alone, would respond to imbalances. Delays caused by the educational process make it particularly difficult for the market to respond quickly to changes. Thus, legislators respond by developing federal and state programs such as the Nurse Reinvestment Act of 2002 (AACN, 2003c), which established scholarships, loan forgiveness, and training and career ladders programs. Other responses can be seen by public policy groups such as the Robert Wood Johnson Foundation that establish demonstration programs for developing and studying the workforce.

States are responsible for regulating educational programs and providing publicly funded educational programs. However, state budgetary constraints may make it difficult to respond to market opportunities. Centralized workforce policy, such as is more common in European and many other countries, has not been politically acceptable in this country. Government solutions to shortages of health care workers have generally been limited for a number of reasons. First, forecasting beyond a few years can be unreliable, due to inaccurate data or an inability to predict shocks to the health care system that may radically change how it operates. Examples are the way managed care grew so rapidly in the late 1990s, reducing the demand for acute care and consequently for some kinds of health care personnel, and the debate over the existence of a physician shortage (Blumenthal, 2004).

Another problem is the lack of agreed-upon amount and type of data collection needed across the workforce, and beyond that, the kinds of analyses of this data are needed. Workforce data collection and analyses are highly variable from state to state, and between occupations. The federal government collects Census related information that can be used for some occupations, and the Bureau of Labor Statistics collects information about jobs and wages, and makes regular forecasts. Much essential information is collected by private organizations that provide accrediting or other services to the workforce. When these private organizations discontinue, merge, or divide, the kinds of data they collect may also change in accordance with their new interests. Occupations not represented by such an organization that has the resources to collect data (such as nursing assistants or aides), no matter how essential to the system, are difficult to study or predict. Also, analyses that predict the workforce may be performed by researchers or private subcontractors, though the methods and procedures are often not transparent.

Development of workforce policy is also hindered by a lack of agreement on what is an adequate health care workforce, such well-defined standards for access and appropriate population ratios. For example, the definition of rural geographic areas is complex, complicating the assessment of the distribution of the health care workforce in rural areas (U.S. Department of Agriculture [USDA], 2003). Currently, health professions shortage areas (HPSAs) are used to define shortage areas primarily for physicians, but a comparable process has not been developed for all health professions. Medicare reimbursement regulations allow higher reimbursement in HPSA designated rural areas, and rural health clinics may receive enhanced payments as well, but in spite of these subsidies, some communities are just too small to support economically viable medical practices (Wright, Andrilla, & Hart, 2001). In contrast, perhaps because their income requirements are not as high, some midlevel practitioners have been particularly likely to settle in underserved areas. For example, CRNAs provide about 65% of the anesthesia in rural hospitals (American Association of Nurse Anesthetists, 1997).

Development of a national health care workforce policy, or even state level policy is also hindered because evaluation of the success of government workforce policies are not easily accomplished. Some government programs are designed to attract people into health care or into certain underserved areas. Area Health Education Center grants are federal workforce programs designed to address recruitment, retention, and distribution of health care workers, particularly in rural and other medically underserved areas (see the Web site listed below). The National Health Service Corps is a federal program that reduces medical student debt burden in exchange for service in underserved areas designated by the federal government. These programs are administered by the

Health and Human Resources Agency (HRSA). Some states also provide funds for these purposes. The Indian Health Service is a federal program intended to provide services to Native Americans. Educational loan repayment and scholarship programs are the primary policy tools used in these programs, and funding varies depending on the outcome of the budgetary political process outcome. However, these programs have not been able to solve the access problems of rural and some urban areas that remain chronically underserved, nor have countries with centralized workforce planning been able to solve this problem.

## Quality of Care and the Role of Systems in Health Care Practice and Accountability

Historically, the health care professions have determined the requirements for entry into their ranks, which is codified into law through state practice legislation. When legislation has been required, employers and health care systems may lobby to provide input. Further, employers have a role, especially if they receive Medicare funding, in setting internal standards for practice. The Joint Commission on Accreditation of Health Care Organizations (JCAHO), as well as Medicare and Medicaid, requires that hospitals and other facilities monitor, on an ongoing basis, health professionals who practice in their facilities, and set criteria for staff privileges. These standards are, however, often set by committees of professionals within the institution. For most professions, additional educational requirements, examinations, and/or experience are required for certification, and may be required by employers.

Problems arise when employers require employees to practice at a level not consistent with the law that governs their practice, or attempt creative solutions to workforce problems that may require new job descriptions or activities not previously included in an occupation, particularly an unlicensed one.

There is a trend toward requiring more education in some professions. Pharmacy has made a six-year doctor of pharmacy the required degree, and physical therapy now requires a master's degree to enter practice. The nursing profession so far has not been successful in requiring the baccalaureate degree to enter practice, except in North Dakota. These educational requirements have been proposed for several reasons. There is a burgeoning amount of scientific knowledge that is needed for basic practice in health care; and prestige, professional independence, and authority are enhanced by additional education, particularly (but not exclusively) in the nonphysician disciplines. Employers often do not support increased educational requirements, fearing they will reduce the supply of these professionals and drive up their costs.

Good quality of care is the result not only of adequate training and education of health care professionals but also of safe systems of care that support the reporting and correction of problems (Committee on Quality Health Care in America, 2001). (This is discussed in detail in Chapter 15.) In the health care industries that have successfully decreased errors, the approach has been to analyze systems rather than to blame individuals. Thus, there has been increased interest in evidence-based care protocols, technology, and systems of care that encourage compliance with evidence-based standards of care (such as incentives or pay for performance) and increased efficiency (such as PDA-assisted prescribing, charting, and information systems). Patient-centered and equitable care is also a goal of high quality care, and is addressed through increasing the diversity, cultural competence, and distribution of the health care workforce.

Historically, the nation has relied heavily on licensure, accreditation, and certification of health professionals to assure that health care was of high quality. The increasingly technical and sophisticated health care industry will continue to generate a need for additional training as well as new types of occupations and evolution of old ones. There may be numerous skirmishes among professionals, employers, government, and managed care organizations as to who should determine who is qualified to perform which activities, and who should be accountable for the quality of care.

Freidson (1973) argued that the autonomy of medicine is a defining characteristic of the profession, and one to which other health care workers aspire. First, the claim is that there is such an unusual degree of skill and knowledge involved in professional work that nonprofessionals are not equipped to evaluate or regulate it. Second, it is claimed that professionals are responsible—that they may be trusted to work conscientiously without supervision. Third, the claim is that the profession itself may be trusted to undertake the proper regulatory action on those rare occasions when an individual does not perform their work competently or ethically (p. 137).

The prerogative of a profession has been to monitor itself, and

states have largely allowed this practice through using professionals to conduct inspection and accreditation visits and as members
of professional licensing boards. However, the composition of the
members of licensing boards and their rates of disciplinary actions
can be a political issue. For example, physicians used to sit on nursing boards, but that is rarely the case now. In addition, certification and accreditation programs are generally controlled by the
profession. The control by professions over the conditions of practice as well as their regulation and discipline has led public advocates to complain that patients are not adequately protected from
incompetent professionals.

## Interdisciplinary and Collaborative Education and Practice

Most health care professionals today are educated in their own professional schools, health facilities, or divisions of colleges and universities. Most aspiring health professionals currently do not take
any courses together, nor do many even share the same faculty. In
many cases, students in a variety of professions receive their clinical training in the same institutions; however, there is rarely any
shared clinical teaching or learning. This pattern of education
leads to systems of care at the patient level that often are structured in "silos," which makes it very difficult for the professions
to consult or plan care with each other across boundaries, or to
deliver patient care together.

There is a growing recognition throughout the health care field
that optimal care requires extensive collaboration and interdisciplinary team work among health care personnel, including doctors, dentists, nurses, physical therapists, pharmacists, aides, and
even nontraditional caregivers, like acupuncturists and massage
therapists. In their training and education programs, an increasing number of health professions are trying to incorporate collaborative practice into the curriculum in recognition that professionals need to work together to give care (Lowry, Burns, Smith, &
Jacobson, 2000). This development in interdisciplinary models of
care reflects the complexity and multiple facets of healing, and the
belief that a team can be more effective than any profession working alone.

There is confusion in the health care literature among the terms
multidisciplinary, interdisciplinary, and transdisciplinary, and
there are large issues surrounding their implementation due to a

lack of professional guidelines, curriculum models, and controversies over core curriculums, faculty resistance, problems with faculty workload and influence on enrollments, accreditation, and licensure requirements (Lynch et al., 2003).

Despite this move toward interdisciplinary collaboration, in which professions act to complement each other, there is also likely to be greater competition between and among professions as a result of the degree to which professions can substitute for each other. Attractive professional careers, good incomes, professional autonomy, and/or an opportunity to help others have helped to fuel an increasing supply of health professionals and occupations. In some cases, less educated or trained allied health workers can be partially substituted for more highly educated professionals, sometimes in new or extended roles. These roles tend to be created by employers rather than by educators.

This growing supply of health worker substitutes, particularly in areas that are underserved, is likely to lead to conflicts, especially if an employer can save on labor costs by substituting the less costly profession. For example:

1. Psychiatrists, psychologists, social workers, and mental health nurse practitioners as well as primary care physicians have scopes of practice that overlap, and each may believe they are the best qualified to treat certain types of patients.
2. Professionals and assistive personnel will compete because of the overlap in the care they provide. Examples include physical therapists and physical therapy assistants, and registered nurses and unlicensed assistive personnel.

The competition between different professions and occupations can spill over into the legislative and/or regulatory arena, where different groups may argue for or against an expansion of the scope of practice for a particular occupation or profession. Reimbursement policies for Medicaid and/or private insurance companies can be another battleground since they can have a major impact on the economic health of an occupation or profession. Regrettably, there are few studies of the impact on outcomes of permitting different occupations to perform specific activities, or of the effects of changing how the health professions and/or occupations interact. Thus, the debates between professions are often publicity campaigns and turf issues rather than substantive policy discussions based on research into outcomes, and have a negative effect on the promotion of interdisciplinary, collaborative care.

## KEEPING CURRENT ABOUT
## THE HEALTH CARE WORKFORCE

Although we used the latest available data at the time of publication of this book, some of this data may appear to be outdated. In some cases, they are not outdated; it is the most recent information available, due to a common 1 to 2 year lag in government reports and other sources of data. Many resources in the reference list have online sources as well. We therefore include a partial list of sources and Web sites that provide recent or current data about the health workforce:

American Physical Therapy Association *www.apta.org*
U.S. Department of Health and Human Services: Health Resources Services Administration *www.hrsa.gov*
USDHHS, HRSA Bureau of Health Professions *www.bhpr.gov*
U.S. Department of Labor: Bureau of Labor Statistics *www.bls.gov*
*Occupational Outlook Handbook http://www.bls.gov/oco/home.htm*
Health Care Financing Administration *www.hcfa.gov*
U.S. Department of Commerce: U.S. Census Bureau
  *http://www.census.gov*
American Academy of Physician Assistants *www.aapa.org*
American Dental Association *www.ada.org*
American Medical Association. *www.ama-assn.org*
American Nurses Association *www.ana.org*
American Osteopathic Association *www.am-osteo-assn.org*
National Center for Health Statistics *www.cdc.gov/hchs*
National Council of State Boards of Nursing *http://www.ncsbn.org*
New York State Center for Workforce Studies *http://chws.albany.edu*
  (See also centers in Washington, California, North Carolina, and Texas.)
National Area Health Education Organization *http://www.national ahec.org/main/ahec.asp* and *www.nationalahec.org*

## CONCLUSIONS

A continuing concern for the health care workforce is in having adequate numbers of health care professionals as the demograph-

# CASE STUDY

The Executive Secretary of the New York State Board for Nursing has proposed to the Regents that to advance the profession and provide optimal patient care, regulatory change be sought that would require future graduates of associate degree and diploma programs of nursing to receive a baccalaureate degree within 10 years of graduation or have their license deemed inactive. The Board of Nursing is an advisory board to the New York State Education Department's Board of Regents, which has asked the nursing board to write a report justifying the proposal.

Associate degree or diploma-based graduates can still enter the profession, but they must earn their bachelor's degrees to continue practicing after 10 years, and would not be able to practice as RNs until they receive a bachelor's degree. Nurses would have the option to apply for waivers if extenuating circumstances kept them from meeting the 10-year deadline. Only new nurses who graduate four years after the governor signs the legislation would be affected.

Nurses need to further their education because of changing technology and advances in medicine, and to put them on par with other health professionals who are required to obtain advanced degrees to practice. Bachelor's degree nursing programs offer more research and management courses and have a liberal arts component.

Several nurses said they are concerned that the State Board's proposal to require that new nurses get their bachelor's degrees to maintain state licensure may cause some people to reconsider making nursing a career. Nurses think they have enough activity in their lives without having to worry about earning another degree to keep their job; they believe the onus of furthering one's education needs to be on the professional, not be mandated by the state. Other concerns have to do with lack of access to programs in some areas of the state, the time commitment, and the cost.

Employer concerns center on exacerbation of the shortage as nurses require time off to go to school, and expectations that they should pay part of the tuition and release-time costs when NYS hospitals are already financially strapped. AD and diploma programs are concerned about the effect on their enrollments.

ics of the workforce and population change. Lack of workers may fundamentally change how professionals' scope of practice is defined and how health care workers interact.

The rapid changes in the U.S. health care delivery system will undoubtedly lead to changes in the roles and relationships of health professionals. Managed care and managed competition will require greater collaboration among health professionals. Efforts to institute single payer insurance reform could have a profound effect on the health care workforce. It will also mean greater supervision and management of health professionals by nonhealth professionals. Some health professionals may resist this inevitable oversight as an intrusion on their professionalism. New relationships and even a new definition of professionalism may need to be developed for the health care workforce.

The provision of health care in the early 21st century will require the cooperation and coordination of the many health workers currently providing health care, and those who will be educated in these health careers in the future, and will likely include health care workers educated in newly created careers. There are large areas of overlap in the care provided by health professionals today. The focus for the twenty-first century will likely be on the issues of scope of practice, prescriptive authority, and reimbursement. If the United States moves to a system in which financial barriers to health care are removed, the use of mid-level professionals will likely expand.

It seems clear that as health care moves from the hospital to the community, even more coordination of patient care and cooperation among health providers will be required. It is also likely that any one of a variety of health professionals may be the primary, caregiver or coordinator, which will vary depending on the health problems of the clients.

## DISCUSSION QUESTIONS

*Case study:*
1. Nurses will be viewed more as a partner by physicians and others as their education is increased, attracting those who are now diverted to other disciplines by higher recognition and perceived value. Thus, retention and recruitment may be positively served. What do you think of this argument?

2. Degree programs for nursing students who are unlicensed require a 1:10 faculty ratio in New York State. When the students are already licensed nurses, there is no mandated faculty ratio. Colleges have almost unlimited capacity for students going on for baccalaureate programs. How would this help relieve the nursing shortage?

3. An additional concern is that nurses with bachelor's degrees may leave bedside nursing for management or other nonclinical roles. More numerous BSN nurses may relieve this concern. Do you agree? What might an employer's response be to this proposal? What about schools of nursing?

*General:*

1. Discuss the role the federal or state government now has in assuring an adequate supply of health professionals.

2. What role *should* the federal or state government have in assuring an adequate supply of health professionals?

3. Some people have proposed that institutions and/or organizations should be able to decide what health professionals should be able to do rather than state boards of licensure. Discuss pros and cons.

4. How should health professional education be funded?

5. What role should professional associations have in assuring that their professional members and nonmembers provide safe care?

6. Is substitution among health care workers a good or bad thing to have happen? Why? What policies could be developed to support your position?

7. What responsibility do individual practitioners have for medical errors?

8. Should the federal government set mandatory staffing levels or limit hours of work for health workers in the organizations for which the government (e.g., HCFA) pays for care? Why?

# REFERENCES

Aiken, L., & Gwyther, M. (1995). Medicare funding of nurse education: The case for policy change. *Journal of the American Medical Association, 273*, 1528–1532.

American Academy of Physician Assistants (AAPA). (2003). Information update: Projected number of people in clinical practice as PAs as of January 2004. (Available: www.aapa.org/research/03–04nom-clin-prac.pdf)

American Academy of Physician Assistants (AAPA). (2004). *2003 AAPA physician assistant census report.* American Academy of Physicians

Assistants. [Accessed December 21, 2004]. (Available: www.aapa. org/research/03census-intro.html)

American Association of Colleges of Nursing (AACN). (2003). *Thousands of students turned away from the nation's nursing schools despite sharp increases in enrollment.* American Association of Colleges of Nursing, 2003a [Accessed July 12, 2004]. Available from http://www.aacn.nche.edu/ Media/NewsReleases/enr1103.htm

American Association of Colleges of Nursing (AACN). (2003b). Enrollments and graduations in baccalaureate and graduate programs in nursing.

American Association of Colleges of Nursing (AACN). (2003c). *Nurse Reinvestment Act at a glance. American Association of Colleges of Nursing* [Accessed July 16, 2004]. Available from http://www.aacn.nche.edu/ Media/NRAataglance.htm

American Association of Colleges of Osteopathic Medicine (AACOM). (2002). Annual report on osteopathic medical education. Chevy Chase, MD: AACOM.

American Association of Nurse Anesthetists (AANA). (1997). Nurse anesthesia in rural hospitals.

American Dental Association. (2001). Distribution of dentists in the United States by region and state. Chicago: ADA.

American Medical Association (AMA). (2004). Physician characteristics and distribution in the U.S. (2003 ed.). American Medical Association, Division of Survey and Data Resources.

*America's Career Infonet.* (2004). [Accessed June 3, 2004]. Available from http://www.acinet.org/acinet/default.asp

Association of American Medical Colleges. (2002). *Minority students in medical education: Facts and figures XII*, 2002 [Accessed July 26, 2004]. Available from https://services.aamc.org/Publications/index.cfm

Barzansky, B., & Etzel, S. I. (2003). Educational programs in U.S. medical schools, 2002–2003. *JAMA*, 290(9), 1190–1196.

Bauer, J. (2004). *2003 earnings survey: The outlook is bright* [Electronic version]. RN 2003 [Accessed July 13 2004]. Available from http://www. rnmag.com/be_core/r/templates/issue/show_article

Blumenthal, D. (2004). New steam from an old cauldron: The physician-supply debate. *New England Journal of Medicine*, 350(17), 1780–1787.

Brewer, C. S. (1997). Through the looking glass: The labor market for nurses in the 21st century. *Nursing and Health Care Perspectives, 18*, 260–269.

Brewer, C. S. (in press). Health services research and the nursing workforce. Access and utilization issues. *Nursing Outlook.*

Brewer, C. S., Feeley, T. H., & Servoss, T. J. (2003). A statewide and regional analysis of New York State Nurses using the 2000 National Sample Survey of Registered Nurses. *Nursing Outlook, 51*, 220–226.

Brewer, C. S., & Kovner, C. T. (2001). Is there another nursing shortage? *Nursing Outlook, 49*(1), 20–26.

Brotherton, S. E., Rockey, P. H., & Etzel, S. I. (2003). U.S. graduate medical education, 2002–2003. *JAMA, 290*(9), 1197–1202.

Brown, S. L., & Grimes, D. (1995). A meta-analysis of nurse practitioners and nurse midwives in primary care. *Nursing Research, 44,* 332–339.

Buerhaus, P. I., Staiger, D. O., & Auerbach, D. I. (2000). Policy responses to an aging registered nurse workforce. *Nursing Economics, 18*(6), 278–284, 303.

Bullough, N. (1975). Barriers to the nurse practitioner movement: Problem of women in a women's field. *International Journal of Health Sciences, 5,* 225.

Committee on Quality Health Care in America. (2001). *Crossing the quality chasm: A new system for the 21st century.* Institute of Medicine. Washington, DC: National Academy Press.

Cooper, R. A. (2002). There's a shortage of specialists: Is anyone listening? [comment]. *Academic Medicine, 77*(8), 761–766.

Cooper, R. A., Getzen, T. E., McKee, H. J., & Laud, P. (2002). Economic and demographic trends signal an impending physician shortage [comment]. *Health Affairs, 21*(1), 140–154.

Council on Graduate Medical Education (CGME). (2000). Financing graduate medical education in a changing health care environment: U.S. Department of Health and Human Services, Health Resources and Services Administration.

Crane, M. (2001). Survey report: Earnings: Time to call a code? *Medical Economics, 18,* 74. [Accessed July 15, 2004]. Available from http://www.memag.com

Crawford, L. H., Marks, C., Gawel, S. H., & White, E. (2002). *2002 licensure and examination statistics. NCSBN Research Brief* (Vol. 13). Chicago: National Council of State Boards of Nursing.

Croasdale, M. (2003). Visa cap likely to hurt rural clinics. *AMNewsr* [Accessed July 12, 2004]. Available from http://www.ama-assn.org/amednews/2003/11/10/prsf1110.htm#relatedcontent

Declerq, E. R., Paine, L. L., Simmes, D. R., & DeJoseph, J. F. (1998). State regulation, payment policies, and nurse-midwife services. *Health Affairs, 17*(2), 190–200.

Dumpe, M. L., Herman, J., & Young, S. W. (1998). Forecasting the nursing workforce in a dynamic health care market. *Nursing Economics, 16*(4), 170–179, 188.

Farberman, H. A., Finch, S. J., Horowitz, B. P., Lurie, A., Morgan, R., & Page, J. (2003). A survey of family care giving to elders in New York State: Findings and implications. *Care Management Journals, 4*(3), 153–160.

Federal Office of Rural Health Policy. (1995). *Facts about . . . rural physicians.* U.S. Department of Health and Human Services [Accessed July 12,

2004]. Available from http://www.shepcenter.unc.edu/research_programs/rural_program/phy.html

Federation of Chiropractic Licensing Boards. (2004). *Official directory.* Federation of Chiropractic Licensing Boards 2004 [Accessed March 11, 2004]. Available from http://www.fclb.org/directory/index.htm

Forte, G. J., & Salsberg, E. S. (1999). Women in medicine in New York state: Preliminary findings from the 1997–2000 New York State Physician Licensure Re-Registration Survey. *News of New York (Newsletter of the Medical Society of the State of New York)*, 54(9), 7, 13.

Freidson, E. (1973). *Profession of medicine.* New York: Dodd, Mead.

Ginsburg, E., Ostow, M., & Dutka, A. (1993). *The economics of medical education.* New York: Josiah Macy, Jr. Foundation.

Grumbach, K. (2002). Fighting hand to hand over physician workforce policy. [comment]. *Health Affairs*, 21(5), 13–27.

Guglielmo, W. J. (2003). Physicians' earnings: Our exclusive survey [Electronic Version]. *Medical Economics* [Accessed July 15, 2004]. Available from http://www.memag.com

Inglehart, J. K. (1996). A health policy report: The struggle to reform Medicare. *New England Journal of Medicine*, 334(16), 1071–1075.

Langa, K. M., Valenstein, M. A., Fendrick, A. M., Kabeto, M. U., & Vijan, S. (2004). Extent and cost of informal caregiving for older Americans with symptoms of depression. *American Journal of Psychiatry*, 161(5), 857–863.

Lowry, L. W., Burns, C. M., Smith, A. A., & Jacobson, H. (2000). Compete or complement? An interdisciplinary approach to training health professionals. *Nursing and Health Care Perspectives*, 21(2), 76–80.

Lynch, D. C., Greer, A. G., Larson, L. C., Cummings, D. M., Harriett, B. S., Dreyfus, K. S., et al. (2003). Descriptive meta-evaluation. Case study of an interdisciplinary curriculum. *Evaluation and the Health Professions*, 26(4), 447–461.

Mason, D., Cohen, S., O'Donnell, J., Baxer, K., & Chase, A. (1997). Managed care organizations' arrangements with nurse practitioners. *Nursing Economics*, 15, 306–314.

*Medical Dictionary.* (2004). [Accessed July 29, 2004]. Available from http://medical-dictionary.com/dictionaryresults.php

National Center for Complementary and Alternative Medicine (NCCAM). (2004). *Patient information: Classification of CAM practices 2004.* Available from http://your-doctor.com/patient_info/alternative_remedies/overview_alternrx.html

National Council of State Boards of Nursing, Inc. (NCSBN). (2003). *Number of candidates taking NCLEX exam and percent passing, by type of candidate, 2003.* National Council of State Boards of Nursing, 2003 [Accessed July 12, 2004]. Available from http://www.ncsbn.org/pdfs/Table_of_Pass_Rates_2003.pdf

National League for Nursing. (2003). *NLN 2002–2003 Survey of RN nursing* programs indicate positive upward trends in the nursing workforce supply [Online]. National League for Nursing, 2003 [Accessed July 12, 2004]. Available from http://www.nln.org/newsreleases/prelimdata12.16.03.pdf

Pew Health Professions Commission (PHPC). (1995). Critical challenges: Revitalizing the health professions for the twenty-first century. San Francisco: UCSF Center for the Health Professions.

Posner, G., & Jaffe, E. A. (2000). The case for more U.S. medical students [comment]. *New England Journal of Medicine, 343*(21), 1574; [author reply] 1574–1575.

Rice, T. (1998). *The economics of health reconsidered.* Chicago: Health Administration Press.

Salsberg, E., & Forte, G. (2004). Perspective: Benefits and pitfalls in applying the experience of prepaid group practices to the U.S. physician supply. *Health Affairs,* W4–73–W4–75.

Simon, C. J., & Born, P. H. (1996). TRENDS: Physician Income in a changing environment. *Health Affairs, 15,* 124–133.

Singer, A. M. (2003). Annual report on osteopathic medicine: 2002. American Association of Colleges of Osteopathic Medicine, Ed.

Slee, V. M., & Slee, D. A. (2004). *Slee's health care terms, online 2004* [Accessed December 21, 2004]. Available from http://hctonline.net

Sprately, E., Johnson, A., Sochalski, J., Fritz, M., & Spencer, W. (2001). The registered nurse population, March 2000: Findings from the National Sample Survey of Registered Nurses. Washington, DC: U.S. Department of Health and Human Services, Bureau of Health Professions, Division of Nursing.

Thomas, S. A., Barter, M., & McLaughlin, F. E. (2000). State and territorial boards of nursing approaches to the use of unlicensed assistive personnel. *JONA's Healthcare Law, Ethics, and Regulation, 2*(1), 13–21.

U.S. Census Bureau. (2000). *Race and Hispanic or Latino: 2000.* [Accessed December 21, 2004]. Available: http://www.factfinder.census.gov/servlet/SAFFPeople

U.S. Bureau of Labor Statistics (USBLS). (2004a). *Occupational Handbook* [Electronic Version]. U.S. Department of Labor [Accessed July 11, 2004]. Available from http://bls.gov/oco/oco2003.htm

U.S. Bureau of Labor Statistics (USBLS). (2004b). *Career guide to industries* [Accessed July 15, 2004]. Available from http://stats.bls.gov/oco/cg/cgs035.htm

U.S. Census Bureau. (2003). *Statistical Abstracts of the United States, 2003.* 2003 [Accessed December 21, 2004]. Available from http://www.census.gov/prod/2004pubs/03statab/health.pdf

U.S. Department of Agriculture (USDA). (2003). *Briefing room: Measuring rurality: New definitions in 2003* [Accessed July 16, 2004]. Available from http://www.ers.usda.gov/briefing/Rurality/NewDefinitions/

U.S. Department of Health and Human Services (USDHHS). (1992). *Health* personnel in the United States. eighth report to Congress: 1991 (DHHS Pub. No. HRSPOD92–1). Washington, DC: U.S. Government Printing Office.

U.S. Department of Health and Human Services (USDHHS). (1999). Building the Future of Allied Health: Report of the Implementation Task Force of the National Commission on Allied Health. Rockville, MD: U.S. Department of Health and Human Services, Bureau of Health Professions.

U.S. Department of Health and Human Services (USDHHS). (2002). *Projected supply, demand, and shortages of registered nurses: 2000–2020* [Online]. Health Resources and Services Administration, Bureau of Health Professions [Accessed July 12, 2004]. Available from http://bhpr.hrsa.gov/healthworkforce/reports/rnproject/default.htm

U.S. Department of Health and Human Services (USDHHS). (2002b). *U.S. health workforce personnel factbook*. Health Resources and Services Administration (HRSA) [Accessed July 16, 2004]. Available from http://bhpr.hrsa.gov/healthworkforce/reports/factbook02/FB101.htm

U.S. Department of Health and Human Services (USDHHS). (2003). *NHSC Factsheet* [Online]. Health and Human Services Administration 2003 [Accessed July 28, 2004]. Available from (ftp:\\ftp.hrsa.gov/hrsa.gov/nhsc/factsheets/factsheet-RRA-2003.pdf

Valachovic, R. W. (2001). *NGA Policy Academy for state officials improving oral health care for children* [Power Point presentation]. American Dental Education Association [Accessed July 16, 2004]. Available from www.nga.org/cda/files/VALACHOVIC.ppt

Valachovic, R. W., Weaver, R. G., Sinkford, J. C., & Haden, N.K. (2001). Trends in dentistry and dental education. *Journal of Dental Education*, 65(6), 539–561.

Weiner, J. P. (2004). Prepaid group practice staffing and U.S. physician supply: Lessons for workforce policy. *Health Affairs*, 23(2), W43–W59.

Wright, G. E., Andrilla, H. A., & Hart, L. G. (2001). *How many physicians can a rural community support? A practice income potential model for Washington State*. WWAMI Rural Health Research Center [Accessed August 4, 2004]. Available from http://www.fammed.washington.edu/wwamirhrc/

# 13

# INFORMATION MANAGEMENT

Roger Kropf

## LEARNING OBJECTIVES

- Identify why collecting and using information is important to patients, clinicians, and payers.
- Illustrate how information technology can help improve the quality of medical care and prevent injury and deaths.
- Show how technology can increase patient satisfaction.
- Provide examples of how information technology can help reduce or control the increase in health care costs.
- Identify the consultants who assist providers and the vendors who sell information technology and describe their roles.
- Describe some of the issues that face providers and some of the options for dealing with them.

## TOPICAL OUTLINE

- The importance of managing information important in health care
- Improving clinical quality through information technology
- Improving health care service quality through technology
- Opportunities for controlling health care costs
- Information systems vendors and consultants
- Issues on health care and IT

## KEY WORDS

Information technology, clinical quality, service quality, wireless, computerized physician order entry (CPOE), electronic medical record (EMR), outsourcing, Enterprise Master Patient Index (EMPI), data repositories, Picture Archiving and Collections Systems (PACS), Health Insurance Portability and Accountability Act (HIPPA), decision support, Personal Digital Assistants (PDAs), Return on Investment (ROI), authorization, authentication, Virtual Private Network (VPN)

# THE IMPORTANCE OF MANAGING INFORMATION IN HEALTH CARE

Enormous advances in medical knowledge, technology, and the training of health care professionals have been made in the last 100 years. We know more and have better tools for preventing, finding, and curing disease. Yet the way in which information is managed in most health care organizations hasn't changed nearly as much. Physicians, nurses, and other clinicians still write on pieces of paper which are then filed. When information is needed, someone goes and finds that paper and brings it to the clinician. If a bank operated this way, tellers would be writing checking account balances in a book, which would have to be retrieved every time someone wanted money. In the health care industry, investment in information technology, including computer hardware, software, and services, is about $3,000 for each worker, compared with $7,000 per worker on average in private industry and nearly $15,000 per worker in banking (Lohr, 2004).

Health care organizations have fallen behind other organizations in managing information. What makes this a serious concern for all of us is that medical knowledge saves lives, and errors cost lives. We will examine why managing information is important for the patient, the provider, and the employers and insurance companies who pay for health care.

## Improving Clinical Quality

Walk into a hospital and go to one of the floors. For a particular patient there are dozens if not hundreds of pages, including reports of laboratory tests, orders for drugs, and notes written by nurses and doctors. Paper records may lead to errors, some with serious or fatal consequences for patients. Some of the handwriting is hard to read. It's left up to the nurse or physician to decide how to interpret new information that is arriving and to find the information they need. A clinician in another department who is treating the patient has no access to the entire record.

In contrast, medical records stored in a computer appear as easy-to-read text or graphics. When information arrives that requires action, the nurse or physician can be automatically alerted. The information can be searched. Clinicians in different places can all view the information they need to see.

This is only one application of information technology that offers the potential to improve the quality of health care. For the patient, this can mean a shorter hospital stay and fewer physician visits, a faster recovery and fewer complications due to errors. For the physician, the technology can save time and support better decisions. For both hospitals and physicians, it can lead to fewer lawsuits for malpractice. For the payer, both the employer and the insurance company, the result can be lower medical expenses. Despite the benefits, technologies such as the computer-stored or "electronic" medical record (EMR) exist only in a minority of U.S. hospitals and physician offices. Some of the reasons are examined

in this chapter and include both the cost of the technology and disagreement on who should pay for it.

## Improving Patient Satisfaction and Access to Care

A patient who visits a physician's office and the radiology and laboratory departments of a hospital is very likely to be asked for the
same information (name, Social Security number, etc.) three times.
Commonly, they will be asked for the same information when they
go back to that hospital a second time. It would be hard to name
another service in the U.S. that requires such redundant requests
for information.

The ways in which health care organizations fail to use information technology to serve patients grows more obvious all the
time. Individuals can track the progress of a package from FedEx or
UPS hour by hour, but have absolutely no idea where their blood
test results can be accessed once they've left a doctor's office. They
can order movie tickets on the Internet, but have to wait on hold
for a receptionist when they call to make a doctor's appointment.

Improving patient satisfaction through information technology
should be easy. We are increasingly using the technology in our
everyday lives. There's nothing to invent, yet many health care
organizations haven't adopted technology that has become commonplace for other services. Of course, there are reasons. Again,
who will pay? Shouldn't clinical technology take priority? We
explore these and other reasons in this chapter.

The problem goes beyond patient satisfaction. Technology can
make it much easier for patients to communicate with providers. A
patient who has a question about a medication may now have to
make multiple phone calls to contact a physician. This information
could be provided by email or by accessing information on a Web
site. Patients may not know whom to contact to receive a service
they need, although that information could be made available on
the Internet. Access via technology affects access to care as well as
patient satisfaction.

## Controlling Costs

Chronic conditions like asthma have to be managed. Patients must
be educated on how to monitor their conditions and to take appropriate actions. Information technology can help by facilitating the
monitoring of patients and delivering information to them. There
are devices that asthma patients can breath into and then attach to

a phone line to transmit the data to a clinician, who can provide advice on when to begin taking medication. Expensive visits to the emergency room are avoided. Personalized Web sites can provide access to tests and records that can help an emergency room physician diagnose a condition faster and avoid complications that lead to longer hospital stays. Email can be used to send messages from clinicians and health education materials that permit chronically ill patients to manage their diseases and avoid acute episodes that lead to expensive hospital stays.

Information technology can also be used to improve efficiency. Scheduling software can track the use of operating rooms and surgical equipment to assure that both are available when needed and that neither are under-utilized. Inventory management systems can control the use of drugs and other supplies.

The benefits for the patient are lower health care expenses as a result of avoiding more expensive treatment. The payer, both employer and insurance company, can avoid medical expenses normally paid through insurance. To the extent that hospitals have signed agreements to assume the financial risk of providing care, they can also benefit. Physicians can benefit from technologies that improve the efficiency of care and save them time.

While the financial impact of technologies to improve clinical quality and patient satisfaction may be hard to measure, a range of information technologies are available with the proven ability to control costs. Yet they have not been widely adopted by hospitals and physicians.

## IMPROVING CLINICAL QUALITY THROUGH INFORMATION TECHNOLOGY

### Current Issues and Problems

The Institute of Medicine's reports in 1999 and 2001 focused attention on how the quality of medical care could be improved by the adoption of information technology (Institute of Medicine (IOM) & Committee on Quality of Health Care in America, 1999, 2001). In "Using Information Technology," the Committee on Quality of Health Care in America stated that "much of the potential of IT to improve quality is predicated on the automation of at least some types of clinical data" (IOM, 2001, p. 170). They discussed four of the barriers to the automation of clinical information: privacy concerns, the need for standards, financial requirements, and human factor issues. The first two were partially addressed by the federal government as a result of the Health Insurance Portability and Accountability Act of 1996 (HIPAA), which set standards that providers must address for maintaining the security and privacy of personal health information, and for information required for transmitting insurance claims. While recognizing the efforts of a number of organizations to develop standards, they noted that "these efforts, as important as they are, amount to a patchwork of standards that address some areas and not others, and are not adhered to by all users" (p. 173). The financial requirements of information technology remain a difficult issue. They noted that reductions in Medicare payments since the 1997 Balanced Budget Act have "likely contributed to a more cautious approach to long-term investment in technology" and that "these capital decisions are also being made in an environment in which benefits are diffi-cult to qualify" and "current payment policies do not adequately reward improvements in quality" (IOM, 2001, p. 175).

The human factor issues include the highly variable IT-related knowledge and experience of the health care workforce, and vary-ing receptivity to learning and acquiring these skills. Disruptions in patient care result in lost revenues for many clinicians. IT may alter the clinician and patient relationship, which may be threat-ening to clinicians, e.g., when IT opens up new opportunities for comparing clinicians.

The Committee's response is to call for a "comprehensive national health information infrastructure," defined as "a set of technologies, standards, applications, systems, values and laws that support all facets of individual health, health care and public health" and "offer a way to connect distributed health data in the framework of a secure network" (p. 176). To do this requires the promulgation of national standards to protect data privacy and for the definition, collection, coding, and exchange of clinical data; changes in the legal and regulatory structures that impede the adoption of useful IT applications and greater effort to inform the American public of the benefits and risks of automated clinical data and electronic communication (IOM, 2001).

The creation of the office of the National Health Information Technology Coordinator (ONCHIT) in the U.S. Department of Health and Human Services in 2004 to coordinate health information activ-ities, standards development, and partnerships with the private sector is a recognition that considerable progress still needs to be made in addressing the barriers identified by the IOM (Morrissey, 2004a).

As has also been often reported, few clinicians or health care facilities have access to computer-stored clinical data. Some of the reasons for this are explored at the end of this chapter, since they cut across many other topics than the improvement of clinical quality. These include the cost of technology, who will pay, the lack of standardization, winning clinician acceptance and support, and assuring confidentiality.

There are many technologies which have been shown to improve clinical quality and outcomes. Some of them are described in the next few pages. The number of providers that have them is very small and has grown very slowly since the publication of the IOM's first report in 1999. How to accelerate adoption is a major issue for payers, including the federal government and employers. How to do that will certainly involve money, but changes in the attitude of clinicians and the priorities of providers will also be needed. Rapid adoption would also involve a larger infusion of skilled computer specialists into the health care industry, but whether they should occur by internal hiring or the use of consulting or computer firms or the vendors themselves isn't clear.

The major issue is how to accelerate the adoption of clinical information technology and electronic medical records and deal with the obstacles that have been identified by the Institute of Medicine and others. The creation of the office in HHS, headed by a single federal official reporting directing to the HHS secretary, was a recognition that leadership is needed to implement technology in health care. The formation of the Leapfrog group by major employers to press for quality improvement (www.leapfrog group.org), including the implementation of certain information technologies, is also a statement of concern that providers will not move quickly ahead. Again, many providers would say that rapid movement without new funding made this inevitable. New federal grant funds for information technology implementation and the additional payments being offered by employer members of the Leapfrog Group for the Adoption of Computerized Physician Order Entry (CPOE) suggest at least partial agreement.

## Technologies for Clinical Quality Improvement

Shortliffe and Perreault (1990) have categorized the role of computers in clinical decision support as "tools for information management," "tools for focusing attention," and "tools for patient-specific consultation." Each category offers the opportunity to improve how care is provided. Systems that manage information can gather and display relevant information about the patient; systems that focus attention can alert the clinician to conditions that should be dealt with, such as abnormal lab values; and those that provide consultation or advice use patient-specific data and the latest information or judgments about appropriate care. The advice might be what antibiotic to use, taking into account patient allergies, age, and other relevant factors. Just by moving from hand-written records to computer entry, errors resulting from legibility could be eliminated and data made available to anyone with online access.

Care can also be provided in a more timely way. Skarulis reports a reduction in average medication order turnaround time of 2 hours and 26 minutes after the introduction of Computerized Physician Order Entry (CPOE) at Rush-Presbyterian-St. Luke's Medical Center in Chicago (Skarulis, Brill, & Lehman, 2002). CPOE refers to the entering of an order for services by a clinician using a computer or PDA.

### Reducing Medication Errors

Unlike paper ordering, CPOE allows for interaction between the clinician and information stored in the computer. When a physician at the Weiler Hospital of Montefiore Medical Center in the Bronx orders a drug, the computer checks whether the patient is already taking it, is allergic to it, whether there might be a negative interaction with another drug the patient is taking, whether any lab tests indicate a danger, whether the dosage is correct given the patient's size and age, and whether there is a cheaper alternative. When orders were handwritten, "12 percent of inpatient prescriptions led to some kind of error—wrong drug, wrong timing, wrong dose—though the patient was rarely harmed" (p. C6). The error rate is now 2.5%. Montefiore has spent $100 million on its system (Perez-Pena, 2004).

A cheaper alternative would be for the physician to enter the order on paper, but use a PDA and software like ePocrates (www.epocrates.com) which stores information on drugs, including when they should be used and when not to use them. The physician can manually input patient data such as allergies, age, and weight.

The physician will then order the medication, but the order may not be legible and must be entered manually into the order entry system, if it exists. A pharmacy information system can then check (for the first time or again) for errors. This provides a second check of the appropriateness of the order.

The medication will then be dispensed and sent to the nursing unit. Danville Regional Medical Center in Virginia uses bar codes attached to the medication and to the patient's wristband to assure that the right patient is given the right medication. The nurse scans both and is given approval to give the medication. The administration of the medication is recorded automatically, providing a record of when it was given. The nurses use wireless computers and wireless bar code scanners that are brought into patient rooms. Danville has documented an average of 84 to 264 potential errors prevented each week (Sublett, 2002).

In a physicians office, the visit usually ends with the doctor giving the patient a prescription. Ambulatory CPOE could provide the physician with information, assure that the prescription is legible, and provide an automatic record in the patient's chart (McDonald, Turisco, & Drazen, 2003).

A medication error may still occur if the patient has received medications from a number of physicians and this information may not be available. A physician may order an inappropriate prescription. This is a particular problem during the transition to and from a hospital. It is rare for Americans to have a single medical record that covers all contacts with health care providers. The creation of a data repository for an entire health care system of hospital and physicians, or the sharing of information among providers in a community, would help resolve this problem (McDonald et al., 2003).

While the use of PDAs and software like ePocrates is rapidly spreading, other technologies are not being used by most hospitals. Only 125 of more than 5,000 hospital systems use bar code systems for medication administration, in part because only about 35% of hospitals' drug suppliers included bar codes on drugs in 2004. The FDA published a rule in February 2004, requiring bar codes on the labels of all drugs in hospitals within two years (ABC, 2004a).

Many medication errors can be prevented by a CPOE system (Kaushal et al., 2003). CPOE systems have been shown to reduce the incidence of serious medication errors by as much as 55% (Bates et al., 1998; Teich et al., 1996). Yet Ash and his colleagues estimate that only 10 to 15% of U.S. hospitals had a CPOE system in 2002 (Ash et al., 2004). The Leapfrog Group requires that 75% percent of physicians use an online hospital system to order prescriptions and tests to win its approval, but only 40 hospitals in the U.S. met that standard in 2004 (Freudenheim, 2004).

### Adherence to Clinical Guidelines and Protocols

Berwick (1999) has noted that since important medical journals number in the hundreds, reading and memory are the wrong processes to rely on for incorporating important changes into care practices. To use evidence-based medicine, a fact base must be created and made accessible to clinicians at any time. From that fact base, clinical guidelines and protocols can be developed. This knowledge can then be incorporated into clinical systems, merging the processes of looking for knowledge and then applying it. For example, clinical guidelines and protocols can be offered to physicians as part of a CPOE system. When an order is entered, the physician can be reminded that a particular test or procedure is suggested by a guideline. The physician can also be asked to provide a written justification for not following the guideline or even be asked to seek approval from a department head or medical director for ordering a test or drug not deemed necessary or appropriate. The absence of an order can also be noted and a reminder or alert sent to the physician or nurse. For example, if the medication order log doesn't show that aspirin has been ordered upon discharge for a patient who has suffered a heart attack, a reminder can be sent (Dexter et al., 2001).

The way in which technology is used therefore has to be consistent with the philosophy, culture and politics of a health care organization. It may simply not be acceptable to the medical leadership to require physicians to justify a decision in any way. It may not be acceptable to remind a physician of what the guideline is.

University Health Network, a three-hospital system in Toronto, has an IT clinical advisory committee that recommends which lab tests should be ordered for which patient conditions, and why. Its recommendations are sent to a medical advisory committee for the entire system that has final approval on which evidence-based rules and alerts are programmed into the Decision1 system from Per-Se technologies. The medical advisory committee measures the impact of each new automated rule six months later and often modifies the rule. The governance structure has helped assuage physician fears about evidence-based guidelines implemented through a computer-based system (Schuerenberg, 2003a).

## Availability and Accuracy of Patient Records

Storing patient records in a computer opens up a number of possibilities for improving their availability and accuracy. While a paper record is available only in one location, computerized patient records can be accessed from multiple locations in the same building or another state. Clinicians can consult with each other on the care of the patient.

Until the 1990s, access was only available to those who had special software installed on their computers. They used a telephone line to connect to the computer on which patient records were stored. If a physician wanted to consult a specialist, software had to be installed on the specialist's computer that permitted the connection. With the development of Internet tools and standards (including browsers such as Netscape and Internet Explorer), it became possible to offer access to anyone by giving them a password or other method of identification and authorization. "Web-enabled" systems are offered by health care software vendors to allow such access (Briggs, 2002). Patient records can also be made available to patients, who can then examine and verify medical information. Providing information over the Internet is being made easier by the development of "web services" software by vendors such as IBM and Microsoft. Such software allows programmers to create forms that are filled with information automatically, permitting clinicians to view information from multiple systems (e.g., lab and pharmacy) on one screen (Briggs, 2003a).

If clerks enter data from hand-written documents into a computer, the accuracy of that data could be worse than the paper record. A trained nurse will interpret a physician's handwriting or call to verify the information, but clerks are more likely to type what they believe they see. The great advance in accuracy from computerized records comes when clinicians enter the information themselves, or it is automatically sent from lab or other equipment through a connection called an interface. Equipment manufacturers now offer such interfaces. Getting clinicians to directly enter information is more difficult, since it involves a change in the location and method of data entry. The ways in which clinician acceptance and support can be achieved will be discussed later. The technologies to assist in data entry include wireless systems that connect the clinician to the computer from a patient room or hallway, and devices such as personal digital assistants (PDAs) and tablet computers.

Regardless of whether a clerk, nurse, or physician is entering data, computer systems can check whether data are missing and whether it is logical given what is known about the patient. This can be as simple as checking the date of a lab test and rejecting one that precedes the date of a hospital patient's admission. Or it could be a more complex check that rejects a procedure inconsistent with other information such as diagnosis. Such "edit checks" are also important for receiving payment from an insurance company, which will run similar checks and reject claims with illogical data, delaying payment.

Far less frequently, computer systems are used to look across the various places where patients receive care to validate the accuracy of data. A home care nurse who visits a patient after hospital discharge will carry a list of medications that doesn't match the one in a primary care physicians office records or the bottles in the patient's home. Patients usually see physicians and hospitals whose computer systems aren't linked, even if the physician is a member of the hospital's staff. Efforts are now being made within hospital systems and even communities to provide such information either through connections between computer systems or "data repositories" that can be accessed by all providers. Even when such repositories exist, determining which data are accurate is no easy task, but at least the physician would be able to see what data have been entered by all or most of the clinicians who have seen the patient, a task now done by telephone if at all.

Inland Northwest Health Services, a collaboration of 5 Washington State hospitals and 25 regional facilities, has created a unified electronic medical record for more than 2 million patients. Physicians can access the EMR from their homes, offices, and at the point of care (Drazen & Fortin, 2003).

Sentara Norfolk General Hospital in Norfolk, Virginia, monitors patients in multiple intensive care units from a remote location. When intervention becomes necessary, the virtual staff can communicate with on-site personnel though a video and audio connection. A study of Sentara's first year "showed faster intervention lead to a 25% decrease in hospital mortality rates for ICU patients" (p. 10). Use of the system also meets the Leapfrog Group's standard for around-the-clock coverage by an intensivist, making the hospital eligible for additional reimbursement (Drazen & Fortin, 2003).

Hospital patients may have multiple record numbers because each department or facility may maintain separate medical records systems. On a subsequent visit, they may be assigned additional numbers. A physician who would like to access all the information about a patient faces the time-consuming job of locating those records or even determining if they exist. An Enterprise Master Patient Index (EMPI) creates a single identifier for a patient which is then associated with all the medical records numbers a patient has been assigned. With a single request, a clinician can determine what records exist and where they are located (Joyce & Epplen, 2001).

### Access to Knowledge

Presenting information when it is needed is one type of "decision support," and information technology is available to assist the clinician. The National Library of Medicine's Medline or PubMed allow the clinician to search for and retrieve journal articles (www.ncbi.nlm.nih.gov). But it is up to the clinician to extract the information that would be useful for a particular decision.

Personal Digital Assistants (PDAs) have become popular devices for providing specific information when clinicians need it. Software such as ePocrates (www.epocrates.com) allows physicians to access drug information that is constantly updated (unlike a book on the shelf). Web sites like the *Journal of Mobile Informatics* (www.rnpalm.com/) and pdaMD.com (www.pdamd.com) offer reviews of PDA software for physicians and nurses. Updating allows such software to incorporate new medical knowledge.

Such information is not specific to the institution where the clinician practices. Guidelines or protocols can be made available using computer systems in a hospital or physician practice. The information can be downloaded to a PDA or made accessible from a computer. Such knowledge can be provided passively or actively. In passive systems, the clinician can ask for knowledge or advice. In active systems, the knowledge is presented to the clinician when a problem or diagnosis is entered or a test, procedure, or medication is ordered. This could include citations from the latest medical journals. These are sometimes referred to as "evidence-based systems" because the information comes from evidence obtained through clinical research.

Medical Center Emergency Services, which provides emergency services for the six-hospital Detroit Medical Center, purchased 160 Palm Tungsten C PDAs (www.palmone.com) for its physicians in 2003. Physicians access the Internet with their PDAs, which have built-in "Wi-Fi" wireless technology. They also have access to medical reference software and clinical guidelines (Schuerenberg, 2003b).

If the clinician is using a computer linked to the facility's system, information from the medical record can be used to tailor the information that is provided. For example, if a patient is allergic to penicillin, information on only appropriate antibiotics can be provided. Data in a clinical data repository can be analyzed and presented, such as the effectiveness of different antibiotics in treating specific types of infections seen in the hospital (Evans et al., 1998).

Computer systems can therefore greatly improve access to knowledge by presenting knowledge at the point of care and using data stored in clinical systems.

## IMPROVING HEALTH CARE SERVICE QUALITY THROUGH TECHNOLOGY

### Current Issues and Problems

A comparison of the experience of a bank customer and a patient who visits a physician's office suggests the extent to which health care providers have fallen behind in adopting information technology. Banks allow the retrieval of most information and many transactions using an automated teller. Many transactions that don't involve a physical object such as cash or checks can be carried out online using a secure Internet site. Customers can utilize interbank networks to carry out transactions at a different bank, even in foreign countries. However, most patients can do very little of their health care transactions using a computer. They cannot retrieve information, make a request for services such as the renewal of a prescription, or communicate with anyone in the physician's office. Records from a physician's office cannot be accessed even by emergency room physicians in a nearby hospital.

Berwick (1999) has predicted that by 2020, "the work of medical care will shift from the provision of a personal service to the provision of information as its core process" and that "control over care decisions will shift dramatically from professionals to patients and their families" (p. 2). The two ideas are closely related. Berwick notes that we now confuse care with encounters, offering appointments when patients need information. If we utilize the information technology now commonly available for other services (e.g., database access via the Internet), medical information would be available to consumers and providers at any time. Patients would not have to hold during a telephone call to get their blood test results, nor would physicians have to wait for a letter or fax to get the consultations they have asked for. Our current paper-based system for moving information results in delays that affect both patient satisfaction and the quality of care. If information was continually transmitted back to managers and clinicians, they would be better able to "predict demand and allocate resources through anticipation, not reaction. . . . The best hospitals of the future won't need waiting rooms" (Berwick, p. 4).

There are a number of explanations for why health care providers have not implemented technologies that are commonplace in banking, retail sales, and other consumer services. Often cited is the lack of money. The general issues concerning reimbursement and the availability of capital funds are discussed in detail later in this chapter. Technologies related to customer service raise specific issues that are discussed here. Such technologies compete with technologies for the diagnosis and treatment of illness which are both expensive and constantly emerging. Faced with the choice of acquiring an improved MRI scanner or providing patient access to medical records, the choice is often the former. Philosophical differences concerning access to information may also inhibit adoption of the means to do so. While no bank employee will deny that customers should have access to their bank records, health care providers differ in their opinions on whether full access by a patient to medical records is important, even though HIPAA makes it a patient right. There are differing opinions on whether patients can appropriately interpret the information without a physician's guidance. In the absence of a strong consensus for full and easy access, there is less incentive for the information system investments that are needed. Patient expectations may be another barrier. Patients may have no expectation of easy access to medical information and may not consider this an important factor in choosing a physician. But a bank that failed to provide 24-hour, seven-day access to cash and information would quickly lose customers. A physician's office or hospital that offers no online information can still be full of patients.

To understand what expectations patients can and should have, we describe the available technologies and address this question:

How could information technology improve both patient satisfaction and access to services?

## Technologies for Improving Service Quality

### Improving Access to Information and Services

Web sites are the most obvious way to provide online information to patients. But personalization and two-way interaction can also be provided that allow patients to customize the information they receive and actually carry out transactions such as appointment scheduling.

The University of Texas M.D. Anderson Cancer Center in Houston provides personalized web pages for patients in the Brain and Spine Center. Pages are customized with information specific to a patient's disease. Nurses select educational materials to post on a patient's myMDA site. When a patient sends a secure message to their clinical nurse, the message is automatically copied and sent to the attending physician. Patients are able to review and request appointments, request prescription refills, and review bills online (Briggs, 2003b).

Group Health Cooperative in Seattle partnered with its medical handbook vendor, Healthwise, to provide the content for its Web site for members, MyGroupHealth, for which 25,000 pages of content were reviewed by Group Health's physicians. Physicians are encouraged to cite information from the Web site in their responses to email from patients. Group Health's lab and pharmacy information systems now send lab results and medication refill approvals (with links to related information on the Web site) to patients' MyGroupHealth Web sites (Schuerenberg, 2003c).

PatientSite is another personal Web page offered by Beth Israel Deaconess Medical Center in Boston (https://patientsite.bidmc.harvard.edu/). It offers patients the ability to send and receive messages to providers; request, cancel or re-schedule an appointment; request a referral; view a current account statement; and view a personal health record that includes problems, allergies, medications, test reports and a list of visits.

Murray Hill Medical Group, a 34-physician practice in Manhattan, implemented online patient scheduling via a secure Web site (www.mhmg.net). Patients are able to view a physician's schedule for available appointments and request an appointment, which is then confirmed by email. Patients receive periodic reminders about the appointment by email. Online scheduling has reduced phone calls enough to reduce from 18 to 13 the number of staff handling calls. Other benefits to the practice include increased revenue from filling cancelled appointments and fewer patient no-shows (1% for Internet appointments versus 7% for those made over the phone) (Health Data Management, 2003).

ProviderLookup Online by GeoAccess (www.geoaccess.com) is a feature that can be added to a Web site that allows patients or health plan members to locate a physician with the characteristics they desire, such as specialty, gender, proximity to home or work, languages spoken, and hospital admitting privileges.

### Online Communication with Clinicians

Once a visit to a physician is over, most patients rely on the telephone for communication. This is at best indirect and often frustrating. Patients are put on hold or asked to leave a message for a busy physician who will call back. Calls are then returned to a patient who may not be available, leading to "telephone tag" that frustrates both parties.

Phone calls and voice mail are no longer the only options for communications between physicians and patient. (McDonald, 2003) Email applications include RelayHealth (www.relayhealth.com) and Medem (www.medem.com). Vendors of hospital and physician information systems are offering applications that allow access to medical information and the use of email to communicate with other clinicians. Examples are Elysium Clinical Messaging (www.axolotl.com) and EpicWeb (www.epicsystems.com).

Email offers the same advantages to health care as in business and personal communication. It allows each party to communicate when they are available, in legible text. It avoids inconvenient interruptions and provides better documentation. It also has disadvantages, some of which are specific to health care. Communication is not direct, so the provider can't engage in a question-and-answer conversation. The patient may leave out important information, and the patient can't follow up with additional questions without another message. Regular email is not secure, so messages could be intercepted. Physicians are concerned about a possible flood of messages which they are not paid to respond to. They also are concerned about the legal and ethical implications of email (MacDonald, Case, & Metzger, 2001).

Email systems have been developed to address some of these concerns. The assumption that email must be direct communication with the physician isn't necessarily true. As in telephone communication, a process can be developed that routes appropriate messages to the appropriate person based on physician preferences. The practice support staff play a greater role in triaging incoming requests, routing them to the appropriate staff person or physician, and tracking all messages to be sure they are attended to in a reasonable time (MacDonald et al., 2001).

RelayHealth allows for customizable message routing rules. For example, all appointment requests could be routed to a secretary. Role-based permissions enable physicians to authorize nurses and others on staff to read specific messages and respond. Customizable group coverage rules allow physicians and staff to cover for each other. Structured templates are used to assure that the desired information is transmitted and to allow for easy routing. Patients and physicians use a secure Web site to send and receive messages, which cannot be intercepted en route.

As MacDonald and his colleagues note, "The impacts of e-communication on physician productivity are not well understood because published reports of experience are rare and formal research almost non-existent" (p. 25). They quote individual physicians expressing concern that the ease of sending an email would result in increased communication; that when a practice offers email, only a minority of patients use it; that when email increases, phone calls decrease; and that email is quicker and easier to handle than a phone call. The cumulative effect is therefore difficult to measure before a practice begins allowing patients to email physicians.

A study of the use of RelayHealth was conducted at the UC Davis Primary Care Network (Liederman & Morefield, 2003). The web messaging system was preferred over telephone calls by both providers and patients for nonurgent problems. Physicians were not inundated with messages. The physician with the greatest number of enrollees and messages received only about six messages per business day in the final two weeks of the study. The average number of visits per day increased, so email did not reduce revenues, and physicians were reimbursed for answering messages. The study showed that 85% of the patients were very satisfied or satisfied with the messaging system.

The American Medical Informatics Association (www.amia.org) (Kane & Sands, 1998) and the AMA (www.ama-assn.org) have developed guidelines for email communication between physicians and patients that address ethical and legal issues. Medem is a secure messaging service created by 45 medical societies and sponsored by the American Medical Association (www.medem.com). It has developed guidelines for online communication.

Blue Shield of California has agreed to pay physicians to respond to email from patients (Chin, 2002). Blue Cross Blue Shield of Massachusetts (www.bcbsma.com) has announced a pilot program to reimburse physicians for online "webVisits." The pilot program will be conducted in conjunction with RelayHealth (www.relay health.com). Physicians can use the RelayHealth service to communicate online with patients with whom they have established relationships. BCBSMA will pay the participating physicians for each webVisit and members will pay an office visit copayment depending on their plan and the nature of the webVisit.

It might seem illogical to think of email as offering the possibility of improving the degree of compassion and empathy in physician/patient communication. Those who have developed close relationships with others as a result of frequent emails might be able to see this possibility, however. Some physicians report that emails with patients allow for more thoughtful communication at times when they are not pressured by other demands.

> Alone at night and pensive, a patient or a parent can reach out, can compose their thoughts without the pressure of sitting across from the doctor. And I, in turn, can take the time to do justice to their concerns, to take care with the nuance of my response and to know that some other lonely night, my patient can re-read those words and be consoled or informed by them again. (Fein, 1997)

Most messages will be about more mundane issues such as refilling medications and asking for clarification of information given during an office visit. Email, however, is opening up the possibility of a closer relationship than can be achieved in sporadic 15-minute office visits.

## Managing Waiting Time

St. Jude's Children's Research Hospital in Memphis implemented a centralized scheduling system that allows one scheduler to make all the appointments for a patient. St. Jude's vision was to "integrate orders with scheduling without multiple phone calls to provide patient-centered schedules" (Session 39, p. 3). The amount of time children had to wait was reduced and the number of appointments that could be made in a single day was increased, resulting in less travel (Shepherd & Dotson, 2002).

When patients at Candler Hospital in Georgia go to the ER for a minor problem, they are handed the same type of beeper as used at a busy restaurant. It allows them to go to the snack bar, and the nurse doesn't have to call out their name to find them (Hart, 2003). Candler uses PeopleAlert pagers made by Jtech Wireless Solutions (www.jtech.com), which vibrate and flash when alerted. While the pagers don't reduce waiting time, they can reduce the anxiety patients feel about missing a call when they leave the waiting room, and can reduce the boredom of waiting. It can also reduce staff frustration with patients who continually ask how long they will have to wait.

## OPPORTUNITIES FOR CONTROLLING HEALTH CARE COSTS

### Current Issues and Problems

The lack of money to invest in information technology is often cited by providers as the reason for slow adoption of the technologies for improving clinical quality and service quality. The ROI or return on investment is said to be low or nonexistent. There is evidence that some information technologies do lower costs, but those savings are not always delivered to the organization that has to incur the expense. For example, a hospital spends $500,000 on a system to reduce medication errors that uses bar codes. The result is a shorter length of stay for the patient. But if the hospital is being paid an all-inclusive per diem by the insurer, it receives no additional revenue. The savings accrues to the insurer. Nurses may spend less time administering medications, but that is likely to result in nurses spending more time on other tasks rather than on nurse staff reductions that would lower hospital expenses. The hospital may also incur lower expenses related to litigation. This estimate is difficult to make and involves speculation on what might have happened. Lower malpractice insurance rates might also represent a savings, but not all insurers offer such reductions.

This leads to a discussion in professional magazines of ROI composed of "soft" savings (uncertain or hard to estimate in dollars) versus "hard" savings (certain and in dollars). The former would include improved clinical decision-making resulting in improved patient outcomes. The latter would include a reduction in the cost of paper and film. Many of the technologies we've discussed have obvious soft savings (e.g., improvement in patient satisfaction), but the hard savings are difficult to document. The savings also may not go to the provider who bears the cost.

### Disease Management

There are three categories of disease management tools. "Predictive modeling" applies to sophisticated mathematical models and analysis to identify patients whose medical conditions or health status are most likely to lead to significant dollars spent on health care (therefore leading health care providers to more closely manage these patients to prevent serious hospitalization and thereby reducing the overall costs associated with their care). "Patient registries" are primarily database tools used to track and manage patients with certain disease states so that clinical interventions are completed as required and patients are kept healthier through preventive care. "Patient-focused disease management tools" can include a wide range of devices that patients use to help monitor and manage their own health remotely—connecting them from home to the physician office (McDonald et al., 2003).

Hospitals and physicians are not usually responsible for the care of patients over the course of a long or chronic illness. It's not surprising then that disease management programs are primarily undertaken by payers who would realize the savings in health care expenses. Harvard Pilgrim Health Plan (HPHP) in Boston selected a vendor with predictive models for identifying high-risk members, care management processes that supported the specific types of outreach, and care improvements required for the targeted members; and the technology that allowed staff to administer care plans and track performance. The first registry of 1,500 members was created, and outreach was initiated in September 2001. HPHP and its vendor identified 0.6% of the member population as appropriate for case management intervention (in line with an expected 0.5 to 1.0%). Most of these members—with few exceptions—had not been targeted for outreach and direct management. The focus of the program has been to identify members who are at high risk for future acute hospitalization. HPHP's acute hospitalization rate for both Medicare+Choice and commercial members who enrolled in the care management program has decreased from a preimplementation average rate of 16.73% to a post implementation average of 6.71% (McDonald et al., 2003).

A variety of devices are available to link patients in their homes to clinicians. One such patient-focused tool is Health Buddy, a device placed in the home and connected to a telephone line. Through this device patients can be prompted to carry out and report specific activities that are important for health maintenance and improvement (www.healthhero.com). This can include taking medications. A report is sent directly to the clinician who can evaluate the results for many patients without their having to travel. The system can also prompt the clinician to make contact with a patient who hasn't used the device or carried out a particular action.

Even simpler technology is being used. An automated messaging system using two-way pagers was used to send and receive medication reminders and confirmations to HIV-positive patients. Seventy-one percent of patients who completed exit interviews said the study improved adherence to their medication regimen (Dunbar et al., 2003). On-Cue Compliance in South Africa is sending text messages to tuberculosis patients' cell phones to improve patient compliance with treatment regimens (Advisory Board Company (ABC), 2003a).

Information technology can also help control costs in the hospital. Evanston Northwestern Healthcare, a three-hospital system in Illinois, uses software called MedMined to detect hospital-acquired infections. MedMined is an example of "data-mining" software, which can examine large amounts of data and detect relationships that would probably go undetected by people. MedMined tracks every lab test and merges the findings with details on how and where the patient is being treated. It alerts infection-control professionals to likely problems. The usual practice has been to target only certain areas of the hospital that are most likely to harbor and spread infections. This approach allows some hospital-acquired infections to go unnoticed until they become an obvious threat. Six months of surveillance by MedMined at the three hospitals detected an infection rate of 5.8% and $5 million in unreimbursed costs of treating hospital-acquired infections. In the following six months, the infection rate was cut to 5%. At Florida Hospital in the Orlando area, 956 cases of hospital-acquired infection were identified that added $10 million in costs. The source of problems can be pinpointed down to a cluster of rooms. Florida Hospital was able to trace the source of a type of mold that causes lung problems to a filter in a ventilation duct that hadn't been properly seated (Morrissey, 2004b).

While these savings might be described as "hard" because the reduction in patient days and expenses incurred can be calculated, the hospital that incurs the cost may not receive the financial benefit. A reduction in days may mean a loss of revenue. Savings may result from fewer malpractice claims, and enhanced revenue if the hospital has a lower infection rate that attracts additional patients. The cost savings and revenue enhancements may, however, be considered "soft" by hospital management, since the cost of acquiring and implementing the technology is immediate and may prevent investment in other projects that both improve quality and increase revenue or lower expenses.

### Efficient Use of Resources

There is a significant cost in not using expensive resources. An operation that is delayed because a microscope isn't available or because an instrument is broken or missing costs a hospital and physicians revenue and costs are still incurred for staff. When patients do not appear for an appointment, the result is lost revenue. All of these problems can be handled by scheduling systems which not only record the day and time of a procedure, but can check to see that the needed resources are available. They can also prompt staff to call patients in advance to remind them of the visit. Some systems will even call the patient and provide a reminder using a physician's own voice.

The centralized scheduling system at St. Jude's Children's Research Hospital in Memphis decreased reschedules and cancellations due to inappropriate sequencing or patient availability. The system schedules visits, as well as any resource whose availability may impact the patient (Shepherd & Dotson, 2002).

Computerized resource management systems can be used to track and control inventory. The Louisiana State University Health Sciences Center uses automated MedSelect drug-dispensing cabinets at nursing stations for narcotics and "as-needed" medications (drugs that are dispensed when the patients needs them rather than on a specific schedule). After entering a password and pin, the nurse enters the patient's name; a list of approved medications appears, the needed drugs are chosen, and the corresponding drawers in the cabinet open. The hospital's emergency department has saved approximately $20,000 per month due largely to better inventory control through this automated system (Stammer, 2001).

Digital acquisition and transmission of images from radiographic, MRI, and CT equipment can permit radiologists to provide services to multiple facilities without traveling. The University of California at San Francisco (UCSF) Department of Radiology provides primary interpretations and second opinions of unusual or difficult cases, as well as second opinions for difficult modalities such as cardiac magnetic resonance imaging (MRI) for images sent electronically or by courier (www.radiology.ucsf.edu/physicians). If a provider switches to digital images, the expense of film and chemicals is eliminated, as well as the cost of filing, delivering, and refiling films. Systems that collect, store, and retrieve digital images are called Picture Archiving and Collection Systems (PACS).

The filing and retrieval of films is an example of a huge cost (and potential "hard" savings) that is largely forgotten in examining the cost of information technology. Staff spend a significant amount of time handling paper and finding it when it is misplaced. Paper and film also need to be copied and delivered. While the cost of computerization is frequently discussed, the cost of paper and film is not always calculated. These savings alone may justify the purchase of a PACS system, even without calculating "soft" savings such as the impact of returning interpretations more quickly to a physician.

Transmitting images over a secure connection (teleradiology) can allow a hospital to avoid the expense of a full-time night radiologist. There may not be one available in rural areas in any case. Services such as Nighthawk Radiology Services in Australia provide preliminary interpretations for U.S. hospitals, with a final read being done in the daytime by the hospital's radiologists. The cost in 2004 was $50 to $70 per study. A small hospital with 100 cases per month would spend $60,000 to $84,000 per year, less than the cost of a full-time night radiologist (ABC, 2004b).

Wireless communications systems that allow quick communication between staff can also improve patient satisfaction while reducing the time wasted as clinicians try to locate each other. Rather than spending time finding the physician or nurse assigned to a patient, a clinician can immediately communicate and give an order or answer a question. El Camino Hospital in California has installed such a wireless communication system that uses voice recognition to call staff. A staff member simply says a person's name and is connected to that person. The system uses wireless badges from Vocera Communications (www.vocera.com) (California HealthCare Foundation, 2003).

Bon Secours Richmond (Virginia) has tagged approximately 12,000 pieces of movable equipment at its three hospitals with Radio Frequency Identification (RFID) tags like those used to allow cars to move through toll plazas without paying cash. The chips in the tags emit radio signals which are detected by a wireless "WiFi" network throughout the facility. Rather than spending time looking for an IV pole or wheelchair, a nurse can go to a computer and click on an icon to locate the equipment. The system is expected to save money by utilizing equipment more frequently and avoiding additional equipment purchases, from theft prevention, and from improved employee productivity (Becker, 2004).

Advocate Health Care in the Chicago area uses the Visicu "eICU" to monitor patients in intensive care from a central command center (www.visicu.com). Critical care specialists and ICU nurses use 24-hour audio and video to monitor patients. Advocate Lutheran General Hospital has reduced its average mortality rate from 9.7% to 8.6%. Multiple ICUs in a single hospital can be monitored from one location (ABC, 2003b).

## INFORMATION SYSTEMS VENDORS AND CONSULTANTS

Hospitals and physicians have come to rely on consultants and vendors to acquire, implement, and maintain information technologies. The consultants include health care divisions of firms such as Accenture (www.accenture.com), Bearingpoint (www.bearing point.com), Cap Gemini Ernst & Young (www.capgemini.com), and Deloitte (www.deloitte.com). Some are consulting divisions of information technology firms such as Computer Sciences Corporation (www.csc.com), EDS (www.eds.com), IBM (www.ibm.com), and Perot Systems (www.perotsystems.com). Firms such as First Consulting Group (www.fcg.com) and Superior Consulting (www.super iorconsultant.com) serve only the health care industry.

Numerous vendors of computer software sell to hospitals and physicians. A list of some of the vendors and the products they offer is maintained by the Healthcare Information and Management Systems Society (www.himss.org). In terms of 2003 revenue, the two largest were Siemens Medical Solutions (www.siemensmed ical.com) and McKesson Information Solutions (www.infosolu tions.mckesson.com) (Johnson & Associates, 2004). Both were independent companies that were bought by much larger firms.

## History

When computers were first introduced to hospitals, they were primarily used for billing and financial management. The consulting firms hired to assist in purchasing them were divisions of financial auditing firms. Other consulting firms were formed specifically to assist hospitals in acquiring computers. In either case, the role of the consulting firm was to help hospital managers make a decision on which system to purchase, not to implement or maintain the technology.

The vendors were firms that developed computer software, often in a partnership arrangement with a hospital or physicians. The products they offered changed as computer technology evolved. For example, Shared Medical Systems, now Siemens Medical Solutions (SMS), started by developing financial and clinical systems for hospitals that ran on large "mainframe" computers. It installed the computers and software, trained staff, and then provided support and upgrades when available. SMS later allowed hospitals to connect over telephone lines to SMS's mainframe computers so that the hospital could avoid buying one and hiring staff to operate it. IDX Corporation (www.idx.com) provided similar services to larger physician group practices when smaller and cheaper "minicomputers" were introduced. Some vendors focused on just a few products and relied on minicomputers that could be used to run one service or department. This included the Cerner Corporation (www.cerner.com), which began by developing laboratory information systems. After "microcomputers" or PCs and Macs were introduced, dozens of systems for small physician offices were developed by small companies and sometimes by computer-savvy physicians themselves.

The history of the companies that offer technology is important for understanding the current attitudes of hospitals and physicians toward vendors and their products. Providers have watched small companies go out of business or be absorbed by larger companies. Technology that providers had invested in and relied on was sometimes abandoned by the vendor or not supported. Some products were offered after testing in only a few locations and failed to produce the expected results or required extensive and expensive customization when installed elsewhere. Companies that acquired others or purchased software struggled to integrate and support products that were written in different programming languages and ran on different types of computers. Doubts about the performance or the survival of vendors has been one cause of the slow adoption of technology, which has left vendors with less money for research and development. Providers have then complained that products were aging and purchases should be delayed. Computer-based technology is complex and expensive, and concerns about vendor performance have made the decision to proceed with implementation more difficult.

## Roles

Since 2000, hospitals have shown a greater interest in turning over the management of information technology to outside firms (i.e., outsourcing). The impetus is a desire to control the cost of technology, acquire expertise that is not available in-house, and avoid costly mistakes in selection and implementation. A hospital can negotiate a fixed cost contract with a firm to manage some or all of its information technology. Costs are not only fixed but also lower than projected if the hospital continued alone. This has led to considerable change in the roles of consultants and vendors. Consulting firms such as First Consulting Group (FCG) will now manage all of a hospital's computer technology. The hospital can decide if it wants to retain ownership of the computers and retain any IT staff, who otherwise will work for FCG. The hospital can continue to pick which computer vendors to use, with FCG providing advice. The hospital can choose to hand over only part of its information system. IBM will sign a contract to maintain a hospital's software on IBM computers but leave the installation, customization and maintenance of the software to the hospital's staff. Vendors such as Elipsys (www.eclipsys.com) offer similar "outsourcing" agreements. Hospitals can therefore continue to use consulting firms and vendors in the traditional way or turn over all or part of the technology operations to these firms.

Some computer services have also moved overseas to take advantage of lower-cost labor and telecommunications services. Just as a telephone or computer firm might use a firm in India to answer customer questions, hospitals are using "call centers" overseas to provide assistance to users who call on the telephone or send messages from a Web site. Overseas "network operating centers" are used to monitor computers and computer networks during the night and weekend hours.

## Challenges

The economics of outsourcing suggest that the trend will continue and fewer hospitals and physicians will be operating information technology. Consultants and vendors can combine the computer centers of several hospitals and achieve significant economies of scale. They can hire specialized staff with expertise that a single hospital would find expensive or difficult to find and retain. For-profit firms can offer benefits that nonprofit hospitals would not often be able to match, and provide staff with career opportunities that don't exist in a single hospital.

Outsourcing relieves a hospital of managing computer hardware and software but leaves many other tasks to be carried out. The challenge for providers will be to develop a strategy and vision of what the organization should be doing and to manage the human dimension of change (Morrissey, 2004d). Should the organization aim to be "paperless" and how soon? How can it help physicians and staff adjust to the changes? How can it manage the outsourcing firm to assure that it delivers on the service agreements that are signed? How can it use the firm's expertise in a positive way so that it makes the right choices? Hospitals and physicians need to realize that rather than getting rid of its responsibility for technology, outsourcing requires significant effort of a different kind. Outsourcing permits them to focus on important strategic choices and leave the day-to-day tactical issues to the outsourcing firm.

## ISSUES ON HEALTH CARE AND IT

Health care organizations are far behind those in other parts of the economy in the use of information management technology. Why? There isn't just one reason. The cost of technology, disagreement on who should pay, the perceived lack of information on the benefits, a lack of standardization that makes implementation costly and difficult, resistance by clinicians, and concerns about security and patient confidentiality are all frequently mentioned as obstacles. Each of these factors and possible solutions is discussed below.

## Cost of Technology

Information technology competes with technology for diagnosis and treatment, such as Magnetic Resonance Imaging (MRI) scanners. Information technology competes with salary increases for nurses, renovation and construction of facilities, and other proposed uses of funds. These requests come at a time when many hospitals are faced with lower reimbursement, higher expenses for indigent care, and competition from other hospitals, including single specialty hospitals for cardiac and cancer care.

Estimates of the cost of CPOE have ranged from $3 to $10 million depending on hospital size and level of existing IT infrastructure (Advisory Board Company, 2001). A report prepared by FCG for the American Hospital Association estimated one-time combined capital and operating costs from $6.3 to $26 million with an average of $12 million. Annual operating costs were estimated to be $370,000 to $3 million, with an average of $1.5 million. "The factors that exhibited the greatest impact on the cost of CPOE implementation were the size and complexity—particularly the number of sites— of the implementation and the extent to which organizations had to acquire additional hardware and software beyond what they had already" (First Consulting Group, 2003, p. 25). Implementing a CPOE system requires implementation of components of an electronic medical record to achieve the benefits of providing information to the clinician. Patient allergies must be recorded as well as lab and other tests which help the clinician make a decision on what to order.

The historical low level of investment has worsened the problem for hospitals and physicians. A bank that has made recent investments in computers can consider only the cost of new software and training in deciding whether to install a new system. A hospital that doesn't have PCs at all nursing stations or computer cables connecting them will have to bear the cost of installing them before considering use of an electronic medical record (EMR). Similarly, a physician's office with one PC in the office of the business manager faces hardware costs before implementing an EMR.

However, the cost of hardware and software may not be the best estimate of the true cost of implementing information technology. Baylor Health Care System in Dallas launched a $119 million initiative to transform clinical care, using information technology in 2004. But less than half the expense of the seven-year project represents information technology investment. The majority of the expense is to buy professionals' time to complete an internal reorganization emphasizing efficiency, evidence-based medicine, and patient safety. Rather than automating overly complex and poorly organized care processes, Baylor has chosen to redesign the processes first (Morrissey, 2004c).

Poon et al. (2004) divide the possible ways of dealing with the high cost of CPOE into "hospital-centric" and "external" approaches. One hospital-centric approach is to "re-align the hospital's priorities to focus on patient safety," which could result in putting competing capital investment projects on hold. Another is to "leverage external influence" such as "public outcry against medical errors and the threat of market share loss" (p. 187). A third is to measure CPOE impact on hospital efficiency and the benefits to individual providers.

External approaches rely on outside groups. One approach is to improve system interoperability so that CPOE becomes more affordable because fewer interfaces are required. This would require the adoption of standards through private efforts or government intervention. The Health Insurance Portability and Accountability Act of 1996 (HIPAA) is an example of how government can assist in reducing costs. For example, HIPAA required the establishment of a unique identifying number for all providers. This makes it easier to exchange information and identify the source of information. Another external approach would be for payers or government to bear part of the cost of systems (Poon et al., 2004).

## Paying for Technology Improvements

If we accept the principle that those who benefit should pay, there isn't a clear answer to whether providers or payers should bear the cost of information technology. Information technologies that are likely to improve quality do not necessarily result in higher net revenues for hospitals and physicians, and they do require additional investment. For example, Computerized Physician Order Entry (CPOE) could result in fewer medication errors, lower expenses for care, and reduced patient stays. Hospitals that receive a payment per day might gain if patients need fewer services, but lose revenue from the shorter length of stay. Only if the hospital receives a lump-sum payment for the entire stay does it gain when patients' stays are shorter. While lower malpractice insurance premiums might result from fewer medication errors, those savings are hard to predict and not guaranteed.

So perhaps payers who might realize lower health care costs should be asked to pay part of the cost of CPOE. Some of the members of the Leapfrog Group (www.leapfroggroup.org), including Boeing, have offered to increase payments to hospitals that adopt specific information technologies (Freudenheim, 2004). Empire BlueCross BlueShield in New York is making bonus payments of 2% of a hospital's 2004 claims for employees of IBM, Verizon, Xerox, Pepsico, and Empire itself. All of these companies are members of the Leapfrog Group. To obtain the bonus, hospitals must have implemented or be in the process of implementing CPOE and have an intensive care unit staffed by certified intensivists (Health Data Management, 2003).

The Federal government is also a possible source of funds either through grants or incentive payments to hospitals serving Medicare and Medicaid recipients who adopt information technology such as CPOE. There is no consensus in the U.S. on whether information technology is a cost of business that should be borne by providers, regardless of whether they obtain any financial benefits, or a cost of providing health services that should be borne by payers. Increased hospital and physicians investments may therefore require either external funding, a demonstrated return on investment (ROI), or a commitment to proceed resulting from values or external pressure, including actions by competitors that threaten existing market share. The immediate problem of how to obtain capital might be lessened by providing low or no-cost revolving loans to provider organizations for the adoption of certain technologies.

## Information for IT Decision Making

Obtaining the information to make appropriate decisions on information technology (and to calculate ROI) requires clinical information systems which many providers don't have. Billing and financial systems provide a continual flow of information for management decisions, while clinical data resides in paper charts. So when clinicians and managers face opposition or skepticism about the value of technology, they are often forced to refer to studies at other, dissimilar organizations. Much of the research on the effect of information technology in improving quality and controlling costs has been done in large teaching hospitals. Vendors will provide data from hospitals that use their products, but this can be discounted as promotional. Policymakers in the federal and state governments, as well as insurers and employers, face a similar dilemma in deciding which technology to subsidize.

As Johnston and Pan (2002) point out, the value of health care IT falls under three dimensions: financial, clinical and organizational. To determine the financial benefits, any cost reductions, revenue enhancements, and productivity gains need to be measured. Clinical value would come from better adherence to clinical protocols and improvements in the stages of clinical decision-making or clinical outcomes improvement. Organizational value would come from stakeholder satisfaction improvements resulting from decreased wait times, improved access to health care information, and more positive perceptions of care quality and clinician efficacy; or from risk mitigation resulting from decreases in malpractice litigation and increased adherence to federal, state, and accreditation organization standards.

> It turns out, however, that inpatient CPOE is a rare case regarding demonstrated benefit. Few rigorous studies prove the value of other HIT implementations. And even with CPOE, the data is specific to the clinical benefits, with little attention paid to financial or organizational value. Instead, healthcare executives must rely on anecdote, inference, and opinion to make critical IT decisions. (Johnston & Pan, 2002, p. 1)

At the federal level, this is being addressed by grants offered by the Agency for Healthcare Research and Quality (AHRQ) (www.ahrq.gov) to evaluate and study the implementation of technology in a wider range of provider organizations, including rural hospitals and physician groups.

The eHealth Initiative is a nonprofit organization whose members include providers, vendors, consultants, consumer organizations, and universities. It was created to drive investment in research related to the value of IT in addressing quality, safety and efficiency challenges and to fund strategic demonstration projects that evaluate and demonstrate the impact of IT and further the development of strategies and tools for accelerating the adoption of IT and electronic connectivity (www.ehealthinitiative.org).

The evidence on the effect of technologies such as CPOE is sufficient enough for the Leapfrog Group of employers (www.leapfroggroup.org) to begin offering financial incentives to hospitals that use it. The fact that CPOE hasn't been rapidly adopted suggests that persuasive evaluation isn't the only obstacle to adoption. The absence of rigorously conducted studies of the value of information technology is, however, an obstacle to adoption and more rigorous studies are needed.

## Lack of Standardization

A U.S. bank customer can go to an ATM in Europe and get cash because standards exist for the transmittal of data between banks. Such standards have not been widely adopted for the exchange of clinical data among U.S. physicians and hospitals, however. Under HIPAA, standards have been developed for the exchange of billing data, but no such standards are required for clinical data in electronic medical records. The federal government has adopted identification numbers for each provider and a format for the transmittal of billing information. It has mandated that the pharmaceutical industry adopt bar codes for every drug to reduce medication errors. Health care industry groups have developed standards. For instance, HL7 is a standard for how data should be organized so that it can be exchanged. Many of the computer applications used by physicians and hospitals don't follow that standard either because they were acquired before the standard was written or the vendor chose not to follow the voluntary standard.

When spreadsheet (e.g., Excel or Quattro Pro) or database (e.g., Access or Paradox) users exchange files, the program knows how the data is organized and can use it. If Quattro Pro users want to send data to an Excel user, they can convert the data to the required format. But since dozens of computer programs are used by physicians and hospitals, converting the files becomes expensive. An "interface" has to be programmed or an "interface engine" purchased so convert files and pass them to other programs. This is often done by larger hospitals and health care organizations, but many other providers lack this capability. So if a patient appears in the emergency room of a hospital, it is usually not possible for the ER physician to call that patient's physician and ask for records to be transmitted electronically. Instead, information is passed by phone with the danger of misunderstanding or incomplete transmittal of information.

Progress in resolving this information-sharing problem has been made, but resolution is unlikely very soon. The HL7, provider identification and billing standards under HIPAA, and bar-code standards for drugs are a beginning. Larger organizations will continue to invest in interfaces and interface engines, but changing the individual pharmacy, laboratory, and other systems that generate the data is likely to be a much slower process. Installing up-to-date information systems in physician offices remains a major challenge. Technology to allow patients to carry their own medical records or get access to them on a secure Web site has appeared, but this usually puts the burden on the patient to collect the information from each provider and store it.

There is frequent discussion of community-wide and even state-wide medical data exchange that would facilitate and provide an incentive for the adoption of standards. A few such systems, called Community Health Information Networks (CHINs), were established in the 1980s, but often ceased operation because the problem of who could and would pay for them wasn't solved. That issue remains today. While it is certainly in the interest of patients to have their medical information available to anyone they choose to see, it is not clear that the benefits to clinicians and facilities justify the costs and what they perceive to be the risks of data exchange. Such exchanges could allow patients to move more easily between providers and expose the provider to an easy review of the care rendered.

So we can expect that, with the exception of a few communities and large health care systems, such as Kaiser-Permanente, patients and clinicians will not have easy access to clinical information. This is hardly the situation faced by customers when they enter a bank, or one they would tolerate.

## Winning Clinician Acceptance and Support for IT

Indifference or hostility on the part of physicians and nurses to clinical information systems is often attributed to age, prior training, or culture. The most experienced and powerful clinicians were trained without this technology, may be concerned about their ability to use it, and believe it may affect their ability to practice as they see fit, e.g., by advising what care to provide. Using a technology such as CPOE is said to take more time and reduce efficiency (Poon et al., 2004).

Berkowitz has categorized physicians into "resistant users," "variable users," "consistent users," and "technophile users," reminding us that the physician population isn't uniform in its attitude towards technology. He suggests that our response should also not be uniform. Resistant users could initially be left alone, while variable users are continually shown the benefits and potential of expanding their use. Consistent users need to be given a usable system and supported well. Technophile users can help in defining future plans for the use of technology (Bria, Berkowitz, Gaillour, & Wald, 1999).

Much has been written on how health care organizations should respond. Physician involvement is considered critical (Skarulis et al., 2002). New roles for clinicians have been proposed. A physician or nurse "champion" should be identified (Poon et al., 2004). This is an influential (but not necessarily the most knowledgeable) clinician who could offer support once they are educated on the benefits. They would then be included on committees involved in selection and implementation. A full or part-time paid position for a physician and nurse would provide advice to managers and a voice for clinicians within the information technology team (Schuerenberg, 2003c). They could be recruited from clinicians who have a strong interest in the technology and would be offered opportunities for learning. CareGroup in Boston has gone so far as to make a physician the CIO (Chief Information Officer) of the system. The Association of Medical Directors of Information Systems is an organization for physicians who have such a formal title and role (www.amdis.org).

Fine tuning the process of implementation is also advocated. Pilots are suggested that allow the documentation of positive results and the identification of problems. The pace of implementation needs to be monitored to assure that it is neither too fast nor too slow. Careful training is advocated, as well as constant personal support. The systems themselves need to be customized to the needs of clinicians (Poon et al., 2004).

Cedars-Sinai Medical Center in Los Angeles halted implementation of CPOE in 2003 after doctors protested. Cedars' plan called for full use of CPOE within 14 weeks. Since all of its 1,800 physicians were required to pass a test proving they could use the system, 165 who hadn't done so had their privileges suspended. Physicians also complained that the system was too complex and time-consuming (Morrissey, 2003; Freudenheim, 2004).

Bates and his colleagues at Brigham and Women's Hospital in Boston have developed a list of "ten commandments for effective clinical decision support" that focus on the process of providing information (Bates et al., 2003). They believe that "speed is everything" and "speed is the parameter that users value most" (p. 524).

Systems need to "anticipate clinician needs and bring information to clinicians at the time they need it" (p. 524). Systems need to "fit into the user's workflow" (p. 525), for example, a guideline on medication should appear at the time of ordering.

Another strategy adopted by Baylor Health Care System in Dallas is to make computers "an easy and attractive component of daily practice for physicians and their office staffs" (p. 17). Office staff were first given access to billing and demographic data on patients kept by the hospital. Physicians were then provided access to clinical information using the same secure Web site. This resulted in 40% of physicians using the web portal daily in 2004. Physician order entry will not be introduced until the later stages of the system's 7-year clinical care transformation project (Morrissey, 2004c).

Much can be done to help clinicians accept and use information technology. Success isn't guaranteed just because the technology has significant benefits for the patient, hospitals, or payers.

## Assuring the Confidentiality of Patient Information

It's not surprising that the continual flow of stories about computer viruses and hackers would make everyone concerned about the confidentiality of medical information stored in computers. Yet many people do their banking online, use their credit cards to purchase on the Internet, and are aware that their personal information is being held by a wide variety of private and government organizations. Less well known is the extent to which medical information on paper is not secure. Physicians and nurses not involved in a patient's care can look at their chart when they are in the hospital. Staff who do billing in hospitals and physician offices have access to medical information, as do workers in insurance companies.

Yet the current flow of stories about unauthorized access to computer records puts the burden of proof on those who advocate computer storage of medical records. How can that information be kept secure and private? Grady (1997) reminds us that storing medical information in a computer makes it "easier to snoop, but also easier to catch the snoopers" (p. C8). Computer systems with "audit trails" record the identity of each person who looks at a medical record. Patients can ask to see who has been reading their records, and have that right under HIPAA. Employee education and a schedule of penalties help to deter inappropriate access.

We need to recognize that the privacy and security of medical information in computers depends as much on people as on the technology. A hospital can require the use of passwords to access files, but if a medical resident is willing to give that password to another resident while taking a break, security and privacy have been compromised. This is also true when a physician working at home accesses patient records while others are in the room and are able to view the screen. Clearly stated procedures, training on these procedures, and monitoring and enforcement are critically important.

Equally important is the use of the specific technology for assuring privacy and security. This includes technology for "authorization," i.e., determining who has access. Unlike paper files, access to specific elements of the medical record in a computer can be restricted on a "need to know" basis. A clerk arranging for transportation to the radiology department needs to know the patient's room number and name but not their diagnoses. A food service worker in the cafeteria should have no access to the record at all.

Technology is also available for "authentication," i.e., verifying the identity of those who attempt to access information. A common procedure requires the user to "know something and have something." They must not only know a password and user name, but also possess a key or special card encoded with information on a magnetic strip or in a computer chip. The voluntary or involuntary sharing of passwords and user names is then no longer a threat to confidentiality. There is growing interest in devices that use fingerprints, the iris of the eye, and facial images to authenticate identity (International Biometric Group www.biometric group.com/).

Once the user has gained access, measures need to be taken to assure that others don't use the opportunity to view information inappropriately. Systems can be set to disconnect the user after a period of inactivity, preventing someone from gaining access after a user has left without logging off. Printing or transfer of data may not be permitted.

Access to the information system outside of the health care facility raises many security issues that need to be addressed. Virtual Private Networks (VPNs) allow private, protected communication on the public Internet (Gillespie, 2003). Access may be allowed only through secure Web sites to prevent unauthorized access. PDAs and laptops may be set to access information only on Web sites so that nothing is stored on the device itself.

The security regulations in HIPAA require that health care

organizations take measures to maintain the security and privacy of information that are consistent with their resources (U.S. Department of Health and Human Services, 2004; Office of the Assistant Secretary for Planning and Evaluation, 2004).

The office of a single physician is not required to purchase and implement the most advanced technology. On the other hand, an academic medical center would be held to a higher standard based on common practice in similar organizations. HIPAA puts a major emphasis on procedures and training, not just on technology. Organizations must do a risk analysis, define procedures, and decide how they intend to implement them.

Measures to secure the security and privacy of patient data would be necessary even without federal regulations. Health care organizations would be facing incidents (reported loudly in the media) where patient information was exposed. Ennis (2003) notes that HIPAA is concerned with only part of the sensitive information that must be protected. Financial, marketing, and employee information must also be protected. Avoiding "business interruption" (i.e., the inability to provide care or bill for services as a result of the failure of systems due to an internal or external attack or disaster) is a major reason for investment in security technology and backup capabilities such as an alternative computer center in another location.

So while the vulnerability of patient data is cited as a reason for caution in adopting information technology, the problem is much larger and solutions will have to be found regardless of whether or not providers implement clinical information systems. Once safeguards are put in place, obtaining the benefits of access to clinical information is an important return on the investment in securing information. Foregoing a clinical information systems doesn't obviate the need for investments in security, and the investment, once made, is one justification with proceeding to implement a clinical information system that offers significant benefits to patients and clinicians.

The ability to identify a patient is important in providing care and avoiding errors. Some hospitals have implemented Enterprise Master Patient Indexes (EMPI) so that they can locate all the records of a patient in a hospital or health care system (Joyce & Epplen, 2001). This doesn't solve the problem of locating date coming from other providers, and the methods that are used are not perfect, so some errors will still occur (Aspden, Corrigan, Wolcott,

& Erickson, 2004). A unique health identifier (UHI) would be another solution. HIPAA required the development of a UHI for patients, but Congress withheld funding for the implementation of a UHI until adequate privacy protections could be put into place. Now that HIPAA privacy and security rules have been published, a committee of the Institute of Medicine has called on Congress to authorize the Department of Health and Human Services to identify options for a UHI (Aspden et al., 2004). The issue is not a simple one to resolve, since there is concern that a single national identifier would then be used for many other purposes (e.g., driver's licenses, taxes). Access to that one number would therefore provide access to many sensitive databases, a widely-recognized problem with Social Security numbers (Goldman & Tossell, 2004). The problem is how to link information in multiple databases while protecting privacy and ensuring security, but there is no consensus at this time on how to do that.

## CONCLUSIONS

Information technology that can improve the quality of health care, increase patient satisfaction, and help control costs is available. It is used by a small minority of hospitals and physicians in the U.S. The obstacles are real but concrete ways of overcoming them are being debated by providers themselves and payers, including government. The growing gap between what consumers, government, and employers expect from the technology used by other sectors of our economy and what is delivered by health care providers will create an increasing demand for change. An important unresolved issue is who will pay as health care expenditures continue to mount.

## DISCUSSION QUESTIONS

1. Why do you think hospitals and physicians have invested less than banks in information technology?
2. Who do you think should pay for improvements in information technology: providers, patients, or payers (including government and employers)?
3. What are the causes of resistance by physicians to CPOE? What can hospitals do to reduce it?

## CASE STUDY

Paul Schaeffer, MD, is the president of a group practice of 20 internal medicine physicians. He is preparing for a monthly meeting next week of the group's physicians and reviewing a proposal to begin using a secure email system called RelayHealth (www.relay-health.com) to communicate with patients. Researchers at UC Berkeley and Stanford have published studies showing that both patients and physicians at two pilot sites were satisfied with the use of RelayHealth to allow patients to request appointments and prescription renewals, receive lab reports, and to communicate about nonurgent health problems. RelayHealth will charge $50 a month per physician for the service, but the local Blue Cross plan has begun to allow physicians to bill $20 for each email concerning a health problem, with patients paying a co-payment of $5. A number of physicians have expressed concern about RelayHealth. They are unsure if this will increase the chances of a malpractice suit, are concerned about being inundated by email messages, and feel that using email dehumanizes the practice of medicine. Dr. Schaeffer believes these are not major concerns, and also feels that email offers the possibility of significant improvement in both patient satisfaction and the quality of care provided. What information should he ask the practice administrator to gather before the meeting? What are the most important arguments in favor of the proposal?

4. Should hospitals outsource the operation of their computer hardware and software to consulting firms or vendors?
5. What can be done to insure the privacy and security of patient information?

## REFERENCES

Advisory Board Company (ABC). (2001). *Computerized physician order entry: Lessons from pioneering institutions.* Washington, DC: Advisory Board Company.

Advisory Board Company (ABC). (2003a, January 30). Firm launches text message service for TB patients. *iHealthBeat, California Healthcare Foun-*

*dation.* Retrieved January 30, 2003, from http://www.ihealthbeat. org

Advisory Board Company (ABC). (2003b, November 14). Remote ICU lowers mortality rate. *iHealthBeat, California Healthcare Foundation.* Retrieved July 28, 2004, from http://www.ihealthbeat.org

Advisory Board Company (ABC). (2004a, February 25). FDA announces final bar code rule. *iHealthBeat, California Healthcare Foundation.* Retrieved February 25, 2004, from http://www.ihealthbeat.org

Advisory Board Company (ABC). (2004b, April 8). Teleradiology services help meet demand, shortages. *iHealthBeat, California Healthcare Foundation.* Retrieved July 14, 2004, from http://www.ihealthbeat.org

Ash, J., et al. (2004). Computerized physician order entry in U.S. hospitals: Results of a 2002 survey. *Journal of the American Medical Informatics Association, 2,* 95–99.

Aspden, P., Corrigan, J., Wolcott, J., & Erickson, S. (2004). *Patient safety: Achieving a new standard for care.* Washington, DC: Institute of Medicine, National Academies Press.

Bates, D., et al. (1998). Effect of computerized physician order entry and a team intervention on prevention of serious medication errors. *Journal of the American Medical Association, 280*(15), 1311–1316.

Bates, D., et al. (2003, November/December). Ten commandments for effective decision support: Making the practice of evidence-based medicine a reality. *Journal of the American Medical Informatics Association, 10*(6), 523–530.

Becker, C. (2004, July 12). A new case of leapfrog. *Modern Healthcare.*

Berwick, D. (1999, September 27). Knowledge always on call. *Modern Healthcare,* 2–4.

Bria, W., Berkowitz, L., Gaillour, F., & Wald, J. (1999). Physician adoption strategies for CPR systems. In *Proceedings of the 1999 Annual HIMSS Conference* (Vol. 3, pp. 11–20). Chicago: HIMSS.

Briggs, B. (2002, October). Web-based technology closing gap with physicians. *Health Data Management.*

Briggs, B. (2003a, August). Patient data online and on time. *Health Data Management.*

Briggs, B. (2003b, March). Provider's web pages get personal. *Health Data Management.*

California HealthCare Foundation. (2003, November 11). California hospital's wireless system improves response time. *iHealthBeat* (http://www.ihealthbeat.org).

Chin, T. (2002, 25 November). Some California physicians will be paid for online advice. amednews.com

Dexter, P., et al. (2001, September 27). A computerized reminder system to increase the use of preventive care for hospitalized patients. *New England Journal of Medicine, 345*(13), 965–970.

Drazen, E., & Fortin, J. (2003). *Digital hospitals move off the drawing board.* California HealthCare Foundation.

Dunbar, P. J., et al. (2003, January/February). A two-way messaging system to enhance antiretroviral adherence. *Journal of the American Medical Informatics Association, 10*(1), 11–15.

Ennis, J. B. (2003, Summer). Information security strategy: Questions you wish the CEO would ask. *Journal of Healthcare Information Management, 17*(3), 5–8.

Evans, R. S., et al. (1998, January 22). A computer-assisted management program for antibiotics and other infective agents. *New England Journal of Medicine, 338*(4), 232–238.

Fein, E. (1997, November 20). For many physicians, e-mail is the high-tech house call. *New York Times,* A1, B8.

First Consulting Group. (2003). *Computerized physician order entry: Cost, benefits and challenges* (First Consulting Group). Long Beach, CA: Author.

Freudenheim, M. (2004, April 6). Many hospitals resist computerized patient care. *New York Times,* C1.

Gillespie, G. (2003, September). Are VPNs safe for the wild wild web? *Health Data Management.*

Goldman, J., & Tossell, B. (2004, February 26). Linking patient records: Protecting privacy, promoting care. *iHealthBeat.* Retrieved August 5, 2004, from http://www.ihealthbeat.org

Grady, D. (1997, March 12). Hospital files as open book. *New York Times,* C8.

Hart, A. (2003, November 1). Patience lost, patients gained. *Savannah Morning News.*

*Health Data Management.* (2003a, September). Doc: Web scheduling yields benefits.

*Health Data Management.* (2003, April 9). Payer still shelling out for CPOE.

Institute of Medicine & Committee on Quality of Health Care in America. (1999). *To err is human: Building a safer health system.* Washington, DC: National Academy Press.

Institute of Medicine & Committee on Quality of Health Care in America. (2001). *Crossing the Quality Chasm: A new health system for the 21st century.* Washington, DC: National Academy Press.

Johnson, R. L., & Associates. (2004, May 17). Top healthcare software application providers: Ranked by 2003 health care revenue. *Modern Healthcare, 34.*

Johnston, D., & Pan, E. M., Blackford. (2002). *Finding the value in health care information technologies.* Retrieved July 28, 2004, from Center for IT Leadership, Partners Health care: http://www.citl.org/finding TheValue.pdf

Joyce, P., & Epplen, M. (2001). Integration, indexing and EMPI: Powerful foundation tools for enterprise architecture. *Proceedings of the 2001 Annual HIMSS Conference.* Chicago: HIMSS.

Kane, B., & Sands, D. (1998, January/February). Guidelines for the clinical use of electronic mail with patients. *Journal of the American Medical Informatics Association, 5*(1), 104–111.

Kaushal, R., et al. (2003). Effects of computerized physician order entry and clinical decision support systems on medication safety: A systematic review. *Archives of Internal Medicine, 163*(12), 1409–1416.

Liederman, E., & Morefield, C. (2003, May/June). Web messaging: A new tool for patient-physician communication. *Journal of the American Medical Informatics Association, 10*(3), 260–270.

Lohr, S. (2004, July 21). Government wants to bring health records into computer age. *New York Times,* C1, C3.

MacDonald, K., Case, J., & Metzger, J. (2001, November). E-encounters. Oakland, CA: California HealthCare Foundation. Available: http://www.chcf.org

McDonald, K. (2003). *Online patient-provider communication tools: An overview.* California HealthCare Foundation.

McDonald, K., Turisco, F., & Drazen, E. (2003). *Advanced technologies to lower health care costs and improve quality.* Massachusetts Technology Collaborative.

Morrissey, J. (2003, February 10). An info-tech disconnect. *Modern Healthcare,* 6–7, 36–48.

Morrissey, J. (2004a, May 17). Adding voltage to e-records. *Modern Healthcare,* 28, 29, 31.

Morrissey, J. (2004b, April 26). Debugging hospitals. *Modern Healthcare,* 30, 32.

Morrissey, J. (2004c, January 12). Information transformation. *Modern Healthcare,* 17.

Morrissey, J. (2004d, July 12). The process comes first. *Modern Healthcare.*

Office of the Assistant Secretary for Planning and Evaluation. (2004). *Administrative simplification in the health care industry.* Retrieved July 29, 2004, from U.S. Department of Health and Human Services: http://aspe.hhs.gov/admnsimp/index.shtml

Perez-Pena, R. (2004, April 6). Bronx Hospital embraces online technology that others avoid. *New York Times.*

Poon, E., Blumenthal, D., Jaggi, T., Honour, M., Bates, D., & Kaushal, R. (2004, July/August). Overcoming barriers to adopting and implementing computerized physician order entry systems in U.S. hospitals. *Health Affairs, 23*(4), 184–190.

Schuerenberg, B. K. (2003a, May). Clearing the hurdles to decision support. *Health Data Management.*

Schuerenberg, B. K. (2003b, December 10). Docs get PDAs—Stat. *Health Data Management.*

Schuerenberg, B. K. (2003c, April). Is there a doctor in the I.T. department? *Health Data Management,* 42, 44, 46.

Shepherd, G., & Dotson, P. (2002). The design and implementation of an integrated scheduling application. In *Proceedings of the 2002 Annual HIMSS Conference*. Chicago: HIMSS.

Shortliffe, E. H., & Perreault, L. E. (Eds.). (1990). *Medical informatics: Computer applications in health care* (pp. 469, 475–480). Reading, MA: Addison-Wesley.

Skarulis, P., Brill, J., & Lehman, M. (2002). Rush physician order entry: From physician resistors to physician champions. In *Proceedings of the 2002 Annual HIMSS Conference*. Chicago: HIMSS.

Stammer, L. (2001, March). Dispense account. *Healthcare Informatics*.

Sublett, P. (2002, November). Technology's impact on reducing medication errors. *Health Management Technology*.

Teich, J., et al. (1996). Toward cost effective, quality care: The Brigham Integrated Computing System. In Computer-Based Records Institute Staff (Ed.), *Proceedings of the CPR Recognition Symposium: 2* (pp. 19–56). New York: McGraw-Hill.

U.S. Department of Health and Human Services (USDHHS). (2004). Retrieved July 26, 2004, from Office of Civil Rights: http://www.hhs.gov/ocr/hipaa

# PART III
## SYSTEM PERFORMANCE

# 14

# GOVERNANCE, MANAGEMENT, AND ACCOUNTABILITY

Anthony R. Kovner

- Specify how governance and management contribute to health care organization (HCO) performance.
- Identify the pros and cons of for-profit, not-for-profit, and public ownership.
- Describe how performance is measured in health care organizations.
- Apply concepts of accountability to health care organizations
- Identify ways to improve HCO governance, management, and accountability.

KEY WORDS

Accountability, benchmarking, board composition, structure and function, chief executive officer, competencies, environmental scanning, governance, governing boards, integrated delivery system, mission, organizational autonomy and performance, managerial skills and performance, not-for-profit, for-profit and governmental ownership, political terrain, position description, product line management.

---

PUT SIMPLY, GOVERNANCE is the system for making important decisions, such as about mission, goals, budget, capital financing, and quality improvement. Management is responsible for implementing these decisions. And, accountability means being answerable for the decisions that an organization (or individuals and governments) make. Increasingly, in large organizations governance is differentiated from management. In smaller organizations, the owner-managers often govern as well as manage, and they may also arrange for patient care. Organizations are constrained by the accountability mandates of government, and by the autonomy of customers (to include physicians) who decide whether or not to use services. The mechanisms of accountability are also opportunities for these organizations to manage the expectations and commitment of major stakeholders.

This chapter has three parts. The first, on governance, defines what governance is, describes the contribution of owners to measuring performance, reviews the advantages and disadvantages of different patterns of ownership, and discusses current governance issues. The second part, on management, describes what managers do and how managerial work is carried out in health care organizations, and discusses current management issues. The third part, on accountability, describes how organizations are accountable to stakeholders and how their behavior is limited and focused by customers.

## GOVERNANCE AS A PROCESS FOR DECISION MAKING

The governance system is how decisions are made in organizations, such as what services are provided to whom at what price. Those who govern or own the organization exercise ultimate direction, control, and authority. They are accountable to payers and users for the use of resources by the organization to provide care. The governance process in any organization may be dominated by a few individuals or by many; governance may be exercised in an authoritarian or participatory way.

Every organization has a set of stakeholders who have interests in organizational performance. For health care organizations (HCOs), the list of stakeholders includes payers, users, clinicians and other employees, accreditors, and regulators. Stakeholders often want the organization to perform in different ways—as to what services are provided by whom, or what employees are to be compensated. HCOs are dependent on the resources required to achieve their purposes and survive. Such resources include patients, clinicians, facilities, and legitimacy. Governance influences the supply of resources as well as their allocation.

### Governance as Contrasted with Management

Although those who govern should make policy and those who manage should implement policy, it is well known that there is no clear cut boundary between governance and management. In practice, those who manage at the top are often key participants in governance, as they have the necessary time and information to define an issue or limit consideration among policy alternatives. In large part, this is what managers are paid to do. On the other hand, because they at least potentially have the power and will to do so, trustees or directors may carry out policy or manage as well. A more useful distinction between governance and management therefore concerns the nature of the decisions and their relative importance. Decisions about who governs, the mission of the organization, and major capital investment decisions are governance and not management decisions. Hiring, scheduling, and coordinating front-line providers of care are typically day-to-day management decisions.

Griffith, Sahney, and Mohr (1995) specify four types of organizational decisions: what the mission/vision is, how resources are to be allocated, how the organization is designed, and how its programs are to be implemented. They point out that these processes may be considered at a strategic (policy) or at a programmatic (operations) level. For example, at the strategic level, mission/vision can be considered as assessing the environment and developing a strategic plan; at the programmatic level, as developing and carrying out a marketing plan or a joint venture with another organization. These decisions involve governance, as they concern the scope of service and the generation of resources; or they involve management, as to generating information and motivating workers to carry out policy decisions. Governance includes decisions about what services the organization provides to whom at what price. Management involves implementing those governance decisions through specification of priority objectives and strategies, and reconsideration of objectives and strategies as circumstances change. (See Griffith & White, 2002, for the contrast between functions of the governing board and the executive office in HCOs.)

## MEASURING ORGANIZATIONAL PERFORMANCE

One reason for attempting to specify effective or acceptable organizational performance is to focus attention on who controls organizational decision-making. If performance is acceptable to trustees, managers, and clinicians, does it matter what anyone else thinks? If it does matter, what are other stakeholders going to do if they find performance unacceptable?

A second reason for developing measures of performance concerns the distribution of organizational resources. To adjudicate claims on resources, questions may be raised about the scope of the organization's mission, if performance goals are not clearly specified. (Or, if they are clearly specified but not being achieved, questions may also be asked.) For example, "How is our HMO doing? How does what we do compare with what our physicians and nurses, accreditors and regulators, customers and potential customers think we ought to be doing?"

Prior agreement about standards of performance helps to facilitate agreement on performance evaluation and compensation. Statements such as "The hospital made a $100,000 surplus this year, 1% of patients made formal complaints, and our turnover rate in nursing was 15%," are ambiguous indicators of performance unless they can be related to agreed-upon standards and purposes. The standards of performance for which the organization and its managers are to be held accountable must be made clear in measurable terms and in advance. Of course, as circumstances change, targets can be adjusted for fully explained reasons.

Individuals or institutions that own HCOs are typically concerned with organizational performance. This includes defining standards, specifying measures of acceptable and superior performance, and hiring, retaining, or firing the key managers who are responsible for achieving organizational objectives. Superior organizational performance is defined differently by different stakeholders. Employees want higher salaries, clinicians want the latest equipment, patients want more convenient and higher quality services, and payers want better cost containment. A common way to evaluate HCO performance is in terms of market share or financial profitability. Those governing the organization must decide what is acceptable performance and how it is to be measured. If they do not formally decide this, the judgments on performance outcomes will be based on the behavior of individuals and groups at lower organizational levels. Further, different parts of the same HCO obviously may operate at different levels of success relative to each other or to the organization as a whole.

## OWNERSHIP OF HEALTH CARE ORGANIZATIONS

Different sponsors or owners of HCOs have different goals. HCO owners include physicians and nurses, cooperatives, government, churches, investors, employers, unions, and philanthropists. Different categories of owners establish an HCO for different reasons, although their motives are often mixed. A classification of some main reasons and goals by type of sponsor is shown in TABLE 14.1.

### TABLE 14.1

**Governance by Group and by Some Key Goals**

| GROUP | GOALS |
|---|---|
| Physicians and nurses | Autonomy for providers |
| Cooperatives | Service to membership |
| Government | Votes for politicians |
| Church | Service for coreligionists |
| Employer | Lower costs |
| Investors | Profit |
| Union | Jobs for union members |
| Philanthropists | Prestige, advancing social goals |

For example, a politician's goal in securing funding for a new public hospital may be to gain votes and create jobs as well as to improve health services. An archdiocese may seek to maintain ownership of a hospital in part to assure that Catholic doctrines are followed in the community, for example, with regard to policies about abortions.

HCOs are commonly grouped as to whether they are for-profit, not-for-profit, or public. What kind of ownership makes the most sense varies according to what population is being served, the nature of the local competitor providers, and the interests of sponsoring stakeholders, such as trustees, and of the attending physician staff. Ownership may change from one form to another. For example, a church may sell a nonprofit hospital to a for-profit corporation because the church officials decide that the monies gained from the sale can be used elsewhere to better serve the poor, while the for-profit corporation can better attract the capital required to upgrade and expand hospital facilities.

## Boards of Directors (Trustees)

Most organizations have a governing body with legal responsibility for control of the organization. Corporations are required to designate membership of the governing body as a condition of incorporation by the state in which home offices are located.

Bylaws outline the purposes of the organization, the composition, and duties of the governing board, the requirements for periodic meetings of the board and notice of meetings, the duties and nature of corporate officers and the method of their selection, the nature and purpose of board committees, and how the bylaws can be amended. A physician partnership agreement, for example, may typically specify the responsibilities of the partners, how net income is shared and losses borne, disability provisions, termination of a partner's agreement, and the composition of the executive committee or board and its functions.

The legal powers of the governing board, as suggested in a model constitution and bylaws for nonprofit hospitals published by the American Hospital Association (1981), are specified as follows:

> The general powers of the corporation shall be vested in the governing board which shall have charge, control and management of the property, affairs, and funds of the corporation; shall fill vacancies among the officers for unexpired terms; and shall have the power and authority to do and perform all acts and functions not inconsistent with these bylaws or with any action taken by the corporation. (p. 11)

Although in theory the governing board has the responsibility for making policy, in practice the power and function of governing boards vary widely, depending on population served, resource dependence, and local power structure. Policy for the HCO may be decided by different internal subgroups and by external organizations. For example, while hospital capital funding allocation may be decided by the board of a multi-unit health system of which it is a part, the scope of hospital services is decided by the local governing board, the nature of clinical education program, by the professional staff and accrediting organizations, and initiatives in marketing and community relations by management.

Board members of nonprofits are often less clear than those of their for-profit counterparts as to their responsibilities and functions. In the nonprofit, board members may not even be aware that they are (technically) the HCO owners. Board members serve for a variety of reasons: community service, contacts, compensation, status, access for their own medical care, or belief that their skills and experience add value to the HCO mission attainment.

## Selection of Board Members

The functions and powers of a governing board are strongly influenced by its composition and its method of selecting members. At first, a governing board consists of the HCO's founders, who may be contributing the key resources to begin the enterprise. Officers are elected by members of the governing board. For investor-owned organizations, owners of shares elect the governing board. In non-profits, board members usually elect themselves. Or board members may be chosen from superordinate nonprofit corporate bodies that, in effect, own the HCO. For example, an archdiocese may own several hospitals and appoint board members for each hospital. Or a hospital may be owned by members in a community who pay a fee to join the hospital corporation.

Large HCOs typically have boards dominated by businessmen, bankers, and lawyers, white males between 50 and 70 years of age. Board composition varies widely by type of control. Unsurprisingly, government and religious hospitals have greater proportions of government officials and religious leaders on their respective boards. For-profit and osteopathic hospitals have a greater proportion of physicians on their boards.

Board members may be "insiders" (managers or clinicians) or "outsiders" chosen for some special expertise, status, or access to resources. The type of person selected often depends on the functions and role of the board. If the primary purpose of the board is to raise money or give advice and counsel to the chief executive officer (CEO), then outsiders will be selected. If the primary function is policy making, then the directors will have detailed knowledge of the business; in which case, insiders may be preferred. For example, nonprofit hospital boards have been dominated by outsider community influentials and for-profit group practices by insider physicians.

According to Bowen (1994), the principal functions of a board of directors or trustees are as follows:

- To select, encourage, advise, evaluate, and if need be, replace the CEO.
- To review and adopt long-term strategic directions and to approve specific objectives, financial and other.
- To insure, to the extent possible, that the necessary resources, including human resources, will be available to pursue the strategies and achieve the objectives.
- To monitor the performance of management.
- To ensure that the organization operates responsibly as well as effectively.
- To nominate suitable candidates for election to the board and to

establish and carry out an effective system of governance at the board level, including evaluation of board performance.

Most board members, certainly of nonprofits, are not paid for their participation. The vast majority of nonprofits do not pay board members. Board service can require a great deal of time. Board members could be spending that time earning money. Payment to board members for their time might improve accountability or provide a more realistic opportunity for lower income persons to serve.

## Board Composition, Structure, and Function

Governing boards vary in their make-up, structure, and function. According to an Ernst and Young study (1997), the average hospital board had 13 members, although some boards had fewer than 7 or more than 16 members. Boards usually meet on a monthly basis; some boards meet quarterly. Most boards have committees of two types: standing committees and special committees, which are discharged on completion of a task. Typical standing committees are: long range planning, finance, and nominating. Some boards will appoint nonboard members to serve on their committees.

Appropriate composition, structure and function depend on organizational circumstances. The boards of a national for-profit nursing home corporation with facilities in 40 states, and that of a nonprofit academic medical center with one site, will in all likelihood not have the same composition, structure, or function. What makes the most sense for a health care organization depends on mission, strategy, resources, and expected board contribution to results.

## The Changing Role of the Board

Views differ and are changing regarding the role of the board of directors. More than 45 years ago, Burling, Lentz, and Wilson (1956) argued that a not-for-profit hospital governing board has a responsibility to provide and maintain the hospital to serve a community need according the wishes of the donor(s). To Umbdenstock (1987), the board must be the "organization's conscience, constantly assessing proposed directions . . . in light of what these steps mean for the implementation of a mission to serve and care for all" (p. 47).

According to Griffith and White (2004), the managerial functions of HCO governing boards include: appoint the chief executive, establish mission and vision, approve long range plans and the annual budget, ensure quality of care, and monitor performance against plans and budget.

It is easy to say that the board should be concerned with policy and oversight functions and that the staff should be responsible for management and administration (Bowen, 1994). But how best this is worked out in any organization depends upon, among other factors, the skills, experience, and trust of the board chair and the CEO, the particular challenges the organization is facing at any particular time, and the expectations of major stakeholders.

### Board Relationship to Independent Medical Staff

According to Griffith et al. (1995), in the nonprofit HCO, the governing board "owns" the organization but obviously cannot practice medicine. The independently practicing physicians are appointed to the medical staff—given privileges in the hospital by the board and practice medicine. The CEO is the board's designate on site. The privileges agreement between attending physicians and the HCO grants these physicians permission to practice medicine and to collect private fees from patients in return for their commitment to the hospital to abide by the requisite bylaws, rules, and regulations. Especially important are those pertaining to the quality of medical care. The board (and there may be some physicians on the board) participates in implementing and revising the medical staff bylaws. The medical staff organization develops and enforces the rules so long as the board agrees that these are beneficial (in nonprofits, to the community; in for-profits, to the shareholders). Griffith specifies that the compact breaks down if the board does not act vigorously as trustees for community (or shareholder) interests.

## CURRENT GOVERNANCE ISSUES

Two current governance issues are as follows: What are preferable HCO ownership patterns, and how can nonprofit governance be improved?

### Preferable Ownership Patterns

Does it make any difference whether HCOs are owned by government or by for-profit or by nonprofit organizations? (For a review of the arguments for and against these three types of ownership for all organizations, see Hansmann, 1996.) Does it make enough of a difference to justify tax exemption for nonprofits? Currently, government is the primary owner of facilities that provide long-term mental health care and those that serve veterans. For-profits dominate in the HMO, nursing home, and physician practice sectors. Nonprofits are the form of ownership for most short-term community hospitals, particularly in the northeastern United States, principally for historical reasons. The first nonprofit hospitals were founded over 200 years ago by local community leaders as institutions to care for the "deserving" poor (The well-to-do were treated in their homes and the "undeserving" poor were treated in almshouses.).

There is insufficient evidence to make scientific conclusions regarding the effect of the type of ownership per se on the cost and quality of medical care, or as to whether the performance of nonprofit HCOs justifies continued preferential tax treatment. Tax exemption applies to income, state, and local taxes. Exempt status makes gifts to the organization tax deductible for donors and allows the organization access to tax-free bonds. A related issue concerns conversions from nonprofit to for-profit status and their valuations.

Arguments against for-profit ownership follow: first, for-profits concentrate on providing only those services that are profitable, leaving the nonprofit and public HCOs to provide services to those who lack adequate insurance. Second, for-profits build facilities only in expanding high-income communities, leaving nonprofits and governmental HCOs to provide services to the poor. Third, the monies allocated to the shareholders of for-profits can better be reinvested in the delivery of care to those lacking access, and that care is of lower quality in for-profits than in other HCOs.

Arguments in favor of for-profit ownership counter that: first, even allowing for profit, these HCOs are more efficient, and they pay taxes. Second, consumers should be charged for the costs of the services that they use, rather than overcharged (in most cases, have their third party payers overcharged), as in the nonprofits, to subsidize the payment of costs for others who cannot pay. Third, for-profits respond more quickly and more flexibly in meeting market demand, and the quality of care most of them provide is adequate and sometimes higher than that of competing nonprofits and public HCOs.

Arguments in favor of public ownership follow: first, nonprofits' total costs and unit costs are lower, signifying greater efficiency. Yet every user gets treated similarly, based on health needs and regardless of income or disease status. Second, the quality of care is not lower than that provided by other HCOs. Arguments against public ownership are as follows: first, primary emphasis in public HCOs is on keeping costs low, especially in this area of continual tax-cutting for the better-off, rather than on providing adequate health care. Second, government operations are bureaucratic and inflexible. Third, the quality of care in public HCOs is lower.

Arguments in favor of nonprofit ownership follow: first, nonprofits provide a higher quality of care and more service to the community. Arguments against the non-profit form are: first, their higher cost, and second, in some or in many cases, the quality of care is low and the community services nonexistent.

In order to reach informed conclusions as to preferred auspices, further research relating ownership to performance must be carried out. To properly do this, conditions other than ownership, such as organizational size, must be held constant. And evaluators must agree as to what is adequate and effective HCO performance.

## Improving Nonprofit Governing Board Performance

What is the value added of the nonprofit governing board, and how can this value added be increased? Answering this question cogently assumes some agreement on the criteria for evaluating board performance. Boards represent an ownership interest that is different from management's. Different owners choose to maximize different values. Such values may include improving health care in a community at acceptable levels of cost and quality. In any case, nonprofit boards add value by holding management accountable for results and by helping plan the future to fulfill organizational mission and to meet certain objectives and expectations of stakeholders.

Boards can certainly add more value, relative to the expectations of stakeholders regarding HCO performance. (For excellent recommendations as to how to improve HCO governance, see Pointer & Orlikoff, 2002). Government HCOs are usually not run by boards but rather by executives, with oversight from the legislative branch. The goals of for-profits are usually clear cut—to make more money now and in the future. Some of the critics of nonprofit boards point to the lack of agreement among board members as to mission and their roles as board members (Kovner, 2001), the length of time it takes for these boards to make policy decisions, the lack of relevance/utility of decisions when board members don't understand the business, and the time and effort it takes for management to educate boards and provide staff support.

An important issue is what stakeholders should do when non-profit boards do not perform well. Obviously where there is healthy competition, the market forces accountability, and how boards add value may be of less stakeholder concern. Although top management should assist the board in carrying out its responsibilities, obviously management should be accountable to the board, as owners, rather than the other way around. Government should at least set rules for governance and disclose the performance of health care organizations. Organizations that accredit HCOs have similar responsibilities. Setting the rules includes establishing personal liability for board members when they have committed a breach of fiduciary duty, as when they pursue self-interest for firms for whom they work, which sell to the institution on whose board they sit. Disclosing performance includes that of measures related to board performance, such as limitation, if any, on terms of office, the presence or absence of measurable objectives for the board, and the numbers and types and value added of board committees.

An argument can be made that government should set requirements for boards, such as who can serve, for how long, whether meetings should be open to the public, and establishing committees to review quality of care in HCOs. A common suggestion is to extend the Sarbanes-Oxley legislation enacted by the federal government to combat corruption in corporate boards to non-profit boards as well.

## MANAGEMENT

Now we focus on managers in HCOs—what they do, and how their work is organized. We shall also consider certain management issues, such as how management performance can be improved, how managers should be compensated, and how managers should be trained.

### What Managers Do

Managerial work can be viewed as occupying positions, carrying out functions, requiring competencies, and performing roles. Managers do, invariably, what they are supposed to do, what they are asked to do, what they want to do, and what they can do. Managerial work is characterized by choice or discretion after constraints are obeyed and demands are complied with.

## Positions and Functions

A job or position description is one way of looking at the work that managers do. (See TABLE 14.2 for the position description of an HCO operations coordinator.) Implicit in this job description are managerial functions, each of which comprises a group of activities. Longest (1980) views the basic managerial functions as:

- Planning, which involves the determination of goals and objectives.
- Organizing, which is the structuring of people and things to accomplish the work required to meet the objectives.
- Directing, which is the stimulation of members of the organization to meet the objectives.
- Coordinating, which is the conscious effort of assembling and synchronizing diverse activities and participants so that they work toward the attainment of objectives.
- Controlling, in which the manager compares actual results with objectives to provide a measure of success or failure.

## Competencies

Boyatzis (1995) has developed a model that includes three groups of managerial competencies. These include, first, the primarily "people skills" of efficiency orientation, planning, initiative, attention to detail, self-control and flexibility (goals and action management), empathy, persuasiveness, networking, negotiating, self-confidence, group management, developing others, and oral communication; second, use of concepts, systems thinking, pattern recognition, theory building, technology, quantitative analysis, and social objectivity; and, third, written communication (analytic reasoning).

Goleman (1998) has found that most effective leaders have a high degree of what he calls emotional intelligence, which is twice as important as are technical skills and IQ for managerial jobs at all levels. The five components of emotional intelligence in managerial work are self-awareness, self-regulation (e.g., the ability to think before acting), motivation, empathy (e.g., the ability to understand the emotional make-up of other people), and social skills.

## Managerial Roles

Roles are aspects of behavior that can be isolated for analytical purposes, such as leading, or handling disturbances. Positions can be

## TABLE 14.2

### Position Description of Operations Coordinator

**REASON POSITION EXISTS**

To assist in all operational aspects of the physician hospital organization (PHO).

To provide analytical support, maintain PC systems and coordinate various implementation projects.

**REPORTS TO**

Executive director, PHO.

**DUTIES AND RESPONSIBILITIES**

Schedule, coordinate, and maintain minutes for all IPA and PHO board meetings and board committee meetings.

Prepare written correspondence, including, but not limited to, position papers and research, education and information pieces, and memos and letters.

Maintain PC files on database, spreadsheet, and word processing programs.

Possible desktop publishing responsibilities.

Maintain financial income and expense spreadsheets for preparation of financial statements; maintain bank accounts and perform banking functions; maintain files for budget preparation and presentation.

Design and produce reports for distribution on IPA and PHO activity.

Maintain and assist in the analysis of reports from utilization management, HMOs, hospital systems, and IDX to produce data, as needed to analyze PHO performance.

Maintain, update, and assist in the preparation of reports on IPA membership demographics, finances, and utilization performance.

Assist in other projects as needed.

**KNOWLEDGE, SKILLS, AND ABILITIES**

Knowledge of managed care reimbursement and operations, working knowledge of physician and hospital reimbursement.

Proficiency in spreadsheet and database applications.

Excellent writing, organization, and presentation skills.

Motivation to initiate/recommended action or research options for problem solving or program enhancement. Ability to follow up appropriately and effectively to affect action.

Superior interpersonal skills and judgment.

Comfort level with financial issues and accuracy in financial work.

**EDUCATION AND EXPERIENCE**

Bachelor's degree in public administration, health care administration, or finance/accounting with health care course work or experience; master's degree preferred.

Managed care experience in finance, analysis, utilization management, contracting, or a combination of the above; experience may be in a hospital, physician group, HMO, or regulatory setting.

Proven organizational or project management experience.

viewed as combinations of roles. Kovner (1984) has conceptualized managerial roles into four sets of activities: motivating others, scanning the environment, negotiating the political terrain, and generating and allocating resources.

*Motivating Others.* Managers spend a great deal of time recruiting and retaining their managerial and supervisory staff, and in making decisions about rewards and promotions, work procedures, and development and training. To carry out these activities, they use communications and analytical skills. Managers facilitate the work of subordinates in doing what is required and in doing what subordinates want to do, within organizational limits.

Managers motivate others through development, pay level, and training. And managers must be developed, appropriately rewarded, and trained themselves. Motivation is affected by a worker's self image of her job performance in any particular job. Managers can help improve performance by starting from where the worker is and using whichever strategies the worker will buy into to attain organizational goals and objectives. Worker performance can be enhanced through improvement of systems and processes, rather than by workers working harder and smarter. Also important in improving quality and productivity is the organizational culture. For example, workers can be rewarded for treating patients as customers, with high expectations for quality and service, or paid as necessary complements to the physician's work.

*Scanning the Environment.* Effective managers scan or search the environment for potential problems and targets of opportunity. Scanning activities include market and product research, long-range planning, and quality bench marking. The development of management information systems may be essential for effective scanning. In large HCOs, scanning activities are usually performed by special units for marketing, quality improvement, fund-raising, and planning. In smaller HCOs, managers scan the environment themselves and are assisted by colleagues. Information about how similar organizations and managers perform is available from journals, books, the Internet, newsletters, and advertisements. Managers attend continuing education and trade association meetings, and are part of online networks where colleagues and experts communicate. Managers visit similar organizations to learn firsthand about ways to improve effectiveness and efficiency. Openness to such visits has been a hallmark of public and nonprofit HCOs.

*Negotiating the Political Terrain.* Effective managers maintain trust and build alliances with groups and individuals. A positive political climate contributes to effective decision-making and implementation. New managers must find out "who is doing what to whom" across a wide variety of organizational issues and problems. Or put another way, managers must learn "what is the ballpark in which I am really playing, who are the players and what are the rules?" Managers learn the informal power structure by looking and listening. The operative rules are not always easy to discover. Organizational cultures vary, and within organizations, subcultures impact differently according to the issue. Stakeholders involved in overhauling a management information system are different from those establishing a new renal dialysis unit.

Activities that managers carry out when negotiating the political terrain include public relations, lobbying, labor relations, negotiating with governing boards and medical staffs, arbitrating among units and departments, and making alliances with other organizations.

*Generating and Allocating Resources.* Effective managers spend a great deal of time looking for ways to increase revenues and decrease expenses. In this analysis, managers consider past performance, performance in best practice organizations, and industry standards. For example, managers streamline buying procedures, secure long-term and working capital at low rates of interest, maintain effectively buildings and equipment, set optimal prices, and sequence appropriately new construction and renovations. In managing stakeholder expectations, managers listen closely to what subordinates, clinicians, and customers say.

Effective managers make decisions about generating and using resources. This occurs as part of the budgetary process and in response to emergency or extraordinary requests. Less tangible resources, such as staff time, must also be allocated, as must resources that may be less amenable to negotiation, such as use of space.

## MANAGERIAL WORK IN HEALTH CARE ORGANIZATIONS

Hilsenrath and others (1993) have reviewed Bureau of Labor Statistics data estimating a total of 362,500 health care managers in 1990, with projections showing an increase to 517,800 in 2,005. Organizations that employ health services managers include hospitals and health systems, nursing homes, health maintenance organizations and other insurance companies, group practices, neighborhood health centers, home care agencies, ambulatory surgery centers, medical day care programs, durable equipment companies, home infusion agencies, and hospices.

In simple organizations such as the physician's office, clinicians themselves may perform managerial functions, such as billing patients or contracting with vendors to bill patients (see FIGURE 14.1). In a group practice, the hiring, paying, and firing of physicians is done either by the whole group, or generally in the larger groups, by a subset of physicians who also practice medicine, while the billing function is supervised by nonphysician managers. In the large hospital or health maintenance organization (HMO), specialized functional managers support clinician and nonclinician general managers. Such functions include human resources (personnel), finance, information services, and marketing, among others. In multiunit organizations (also called integrated delivery systems), which include hospitals, nursing homes, group practices and HMOs, managers of these units report to divisional managers for a geographic area, such as the northeastern United States. Divisional managers, in turn, report to managers in corporate headquarters who are accountable to the board of directors. In these large organizations, certain management functions are allocated among headquarters, divisions, and local HCOs. Headquarters functions commonly include legal affairs, construction, capital financing, and corporate public relations. Other functions, such as quality improvement and production standards, may be divided among the three organizational levels.

A newer development in the organization of managerial work in HCOs is product line management (see FIGURE 14.2). The health system, large hospital, or group practice is reorganized into several divisions, such as women's' health services, emergency care, cancer care, and rehabilitation services, each product line with its own manager and budget (see Herzlinger, 1997). The logic behind such reorganization is that these services can be more effectively managed as separate "businesses" than as part of a large HCO. Whether or not this is so, is yet unproven.

Accountability of health care organizations is uncertain unless there are measurable objectives set in advance and negotiated with stakeholders. Managerial contribution to organizational performance in health care has been criticized, as managerial costs are high per dollar of expenditures, and managerial salaries are often high.

## FIGURE 14.1

Average Health Care Expenditures among Medicare Beneficiaries

### A. Doctor's office

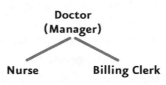

### B. Group Practice

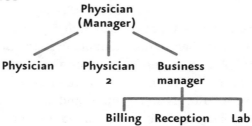

### C. Hospital

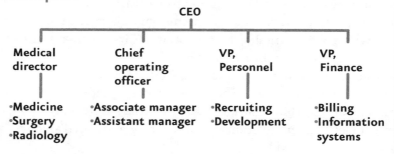

### D. Mulitunit hospital corporation

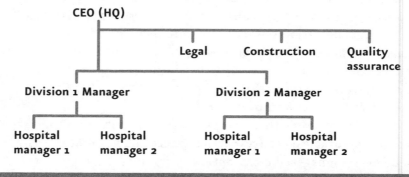

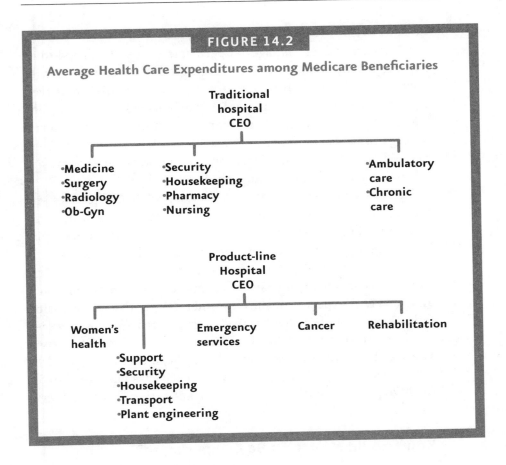

**FIGURE 14.2**

**Average Health Care Expenditures among Medicare Beneficiaries**

Traditional
hospital
CEO

- •Medicine
- •Surgery
- •Radiology
- •Ob-Gyn

- •Security
- •Housekeeping
- •Pharmacy
- •Nursing

- •Ambulatory
  care
- •Chronic
  care

Product-line
Hospital
CEO

Women's
health

Emergency
services

Cancer

Rehabilitation

- •Support
- •Security
- •Housekeeping
- •Transport
- •Plant engineering

It has been difficult to isolate managerial contribution to organizational performance. For example, despite substantial managerial contributions, an HCO may be floundering because of a hostile environment or poor decisions by previous managers. Or the reverse situation may be occurring; despite little or ineffective managerial contribution, an HCO may be growing rapidly and even improving the quality of service rendered due to lack of competitors, excellent performance by previous managers, and because of the performance of dedicated clinicians.

## CURRENT MANAGEMENT ISSUES

Some current issues in HCO management are: How can performance be improved, how should managers be compensated, and how should managers be trained?

## Improving Managerial Performance

To what extent does managerial performance in HCOs need to be improved? Why don't more HCOs have a greater capacity to change? Why do they invest so little in training? Why is quality so uneven and service to customers not sufficiently user-friendly in some organizations, while in others, management has been transforming organizational performance? Costs per unit of service have been reduced, quality has been improved, and market share has grown, in part because service has improved.

Disclosure to customers and stakeholders of HCO objectives and the degree of their attainment relative to best practice is an excellent way to hold managers accountable for improving service, monitoring quality, cutting waste, and improving health status. It is the responsibility of stakeholders—government, owners, clinicians, and customers and payers, to expect improved performance and to act, if expectations are not met. When the organization fails, the customers either try to change performance or they seek services elsewhere, and the managers are fired or forced to resign. This has been the American way. It has been highly regarded by other developed nations, even as we are criticized as a society for the high preference given to organizational performance relative to community solidarity.

## How Should Managers Be Compensated?

The median total compensation in 1999 for hospital administrators and chief executive officers, according to a survey by Hewitt Associates (Moore, 1999), was $210,000, and some health system CEOs make more than $1,00,000 per year. And of course, managers get fringe benefits on top of that. Some CEOs have bonus arrangements keyed to organizational performance, which allows them to make more money in any particular year. Is that too much, or too little, relative to managerial contribution and relative to what comparable managers make in other sectors of the economy? Or relative to what physicians make? Once again, different stakeholders come up with different answers to these questions.

Part of the answer on compensation relates to the contribution top managers make to organizational performance, and part relates to determinations of what are acceptable profits in a just society. Proponents of paying managers more money argue that health care is increasingly a competitive sector of the economy as patients are choosing lower cost and higher quality HCOs that are managed better. The management function contributes to keeping costs down and quality and revenues up, and the best managers must be attracted to work in health care rather than in other sectors of the economy.

Opponents of higher managerial compensation argue that the money paid to highly paid managers could be better spent on, for example, improving access of the uninsured to health care. Of course, this would not go very far as there are few highly paid managers relative to the many uninsured. Opponents argue that since health care is a right and not a privilege, HCOs should be competing not against each other for market share, but rather working cooperatively to improve population health. And they argue that health care managers should be paid like managers in other public service organizations such as education, welfare, and religion.

## How Should Managers Be Trained?

How do people learn to be health care managers? Can health care management be taught? Is it a science, an art, a craft, or some of all three? What can best be learned at school and on the job?

Learning health care management is done on the job, through continuing nondegree education, in undergraduate programs, and in graduate programs leading to a degree. But despite the existence of large numbers of formal educational programs in management, much of what managers learn about what works in an organization and about how they can best work with clinicians and customers must be learned on the job. Most large HCOs have formal orientation programs and offer special training courses on site, as well. Managers can learn from others at work how to write what they mean, how not to always say what they are thinking, and how to more effectively influence others. Superiors, subordinates, and peers can assist managers in developing agendas, and in forming and energizing networks through which to accomplish goals and objectives.

Continuing nondegree educational programs are of various lengths and cover various subjects, such as developing an efficient and sustainable physician compensation system or developing an integrated information system for an HCO. These programs are offered by universities, by free standing centers, sometimes sponsored by professional associations, or by vendors, and by large HCOs, themselves.

Undergraduate programs train managers for intermediate level positions in large HCOs, and for higher level positions in smaller organizations. The curriculum is often similar in subject matter to that of graduate programs. Courses that are generally required include introduction to the health care field, economics, law, management, human resources, financial management, information, and quantitative methods.

There are over 250 graduate programs in health care management in the United States today.[1] Programs are housed in various schools, such as business, public health, public administration, allied health, and medicine. Curricula commonly cover the following areas:

- Structuring, marketing, positioning, and governing health organizations
- Financial management
- Leadership, interpersonal relations, and written and oral communications skills
- Managing human resources and health professionals in diverse organizational environments
- Managing information
- Economic and financial analysis to support decision-making
- Governmental health policy formation, regulation, and impact
- Assessment and understanding of the health status of populations, determinants of health and illness, and managing health risks and behaviors in diverse organizations
- The management of change in health care organizations
- Quality improvement. (Accrediting Commission on Education for Health Services Administration [ACEHSA], 2003)

Questions remain as to where and how managers should be trained at various phases of their managerial careers, and as to what managerial competencies are required for which managerial positions. And as to what responsibility employers should take for management development, and how important clinical training is to management performance.

## ACCOUNTABILITY

Governance can be analyzed at various levels of the organization or with regard to an organization's accountability to various stakeholders. Decisions are also made outside the HCO by government that affect governance. For example, the Medicare and Medicaid legislation of 1965 provided its beneficiaries with better health benefits

1 For information about specific undergraduate and graduate programs, contact the Association of University Programs in Health Administration, 730 11th St., NW, 4th Floor, Washington, DC, 20001; http://www.acehsa.org

coverage than many of them had prior to this enactment. This redesign of the entitlement programs was not made by individual HCOs but by the elected representatives of the American people, who decided to have government collect and reimburse more uniformly for services provided to the populations to be covered. Decisions are also made which affect HCO governance by front-line clinicians and by patients and consumers. For example, registered nurses may choose to work in a home care agency or a nursing home, rather than in a hospital. Patients may choose to enroll in one or another of competing health plans, such as United Health Care or Aetna.

Government and consumers have to be accountable, too, for their behavior, which affects the performance of HCOs. Legislation is often passed, particularly at the state level, without funding adequate to pay for mandated benefits. And many consumers lack basic health education; many graduate from high school without understanding much about health and health practices.

## The Extent of Organizational Autonomy

To what extent should an HCO determine what services to provide to whom at what price? The autonomy of HCO governing boards has been shrinking since 1960. Federal and state governments have passed legislation, for example, forbidding discrimination against patients who seek admission or persons seeking employment, and invalidating a requirement that staff physicians of a nonprofit hospital be graduates of a medical school approved by the Liaison Committee on Medical Education and be members of the county medical society. Government has removed the exemption of hospitals from state labor laws, specified standards to be met by HCOs in order to be licensed by a state or reimbursed by Medicare, and forbidden construction of hospitals, nursing homes, and related facilities in some states without prior approval by state planning authorities. Medicare and Medicaid limit payment for new technology; some states require community service for hospitals to retain nonprofit status; in West Virginia, community representation is required on hospital boards; some states cap hospital revenue; and Medicare limits hospital reimbursement to average length of stay regardless of cost. Some states require that all Medicaid beneficiaries enroll in managed care plans. Some states require managed care plans to pay for hospital stays of 48 hours for normal deliveries, and that physicians be allowed to discuss with patients treatments for which the HMO will not pay.

Different stakeholders in health care delivery have different responses to questions about the degree of HCO autonomy that are useful in deciding what services they offer, what prices they charge, and what populations they serve. The same stakeholders may answer questions differently, depending on whether they are sick or well at the time. HCOs should have enough leeway to decide issues regarding when they have better information than government, so long as there are ways to change HCO behavior when it falls unaccountably short of stakeholder expectations.

Too little autonomy for the HCO will result in the withdrawal from leadership positions of highly qualified individuals who have helped HCOs adapt appropriately in their local communities. Excessive standardization and centralization of decision-making in governmental bureaucracies will result in decreased HCO innovation and ultimately in lower productivity. On the other hand, too much HCO autonomy may have been responsible, at least in large part, for the present unevenness in age-adjusted mortality and morbidity rates by race and by income, in over-utilization of acute care, and in underutilization of long-term care, uneven productivity across HCOs, uneven service to customers, and high cost of health care.

## Accountability to Those Served

How should HCOs be accountable and to whom? Some advocate more formal accountability mechanisms than presently exist, for example, insisting that HCO governing boards be controlled by consumer representatives. Opponents argue that such control will result in ineffective decision-making by boards and eventual withdrawal from the organization of community resources formerly donated. They ask what evidence there is that the newly chosen representatives will be any more accountable to users and payers.

At the same time, most stakeholders will agree that on major decisions directly affecting their interests, appeal mechanisms should be available in HCOs for consumer surveys and manager hotlines. As with most solutions, there are reasons, if not excuses, why health care providers do not meet patient and taxpayer expectations. For the consumer, to whom does he or she appeal if dissatisfied with the response of a patient advocate, who reports, after all, to HCO management? Appeal mechanisms may be costly in relation to benefits obtained by the consumer from following through on them. And there are many aspects of care that consumers (and providers) find objectionable but about which little can be done by the HCO, such as obtaining acceptable payment for services provided to the uninsured. Finally, appeal mechanisms may serve only as buffers that satisfy the occasional vocal complainant but do little to change the system of care that may be a cause of much unreported dissatisfaction.

An important issue here is the extent to which health care organizations appropriately manage the expectations of customers, whether these are patients or physicians. To what extent are health care organizations ethical in their marketing and employment practices, not taking unfair advantage of either customers or employees. Of course, reasonable people will differ regarding fair

## CASE STUDY

What follows is the mission statement, vision and values and behavior statement of the Henry Ford Health System of Detroit, Michigan in 2004.

**Mission**
To improve human life through excellence in the science and art of healing.

**Vision**
To put patients first by providing each patient the quality of care and comfort we want for our families and for ourselves.

**Values and Behaviors**
We serve our patients and our community through our actions, which always demonstrate:

- respect for people
- high performance
- learning and continuous improvement
- social conscience

Please answer the following questions regarding this case:

1. How should organizational performance at Henry Ford be measured?
2. Why don't all HCOs have statements of purpose similar to Henry Ford's?
3. What contribution should the board of Henry Ford make to accomplish the statement of purpose?
4. What contribution should the management team of Henry Ford make to the attainment of the statement of purpose?

---

advertising and employment practices, as in other industries. And to what extent do health care organizations allow physicians to responsibly provide services in the way that they were trained (we assume that such training is evidence-based).

## CONCLUSIONS

Governance and management are vitally important to the success of health care organizations, and to the provision of accessible, efficient health care of high quality. Governance and management of HCOs have a cost and produce a benefit. Governance is a mechanism to focus accountability of HCOs to the stakeholders who provide these organizations with resources. And managers are the means through which the mission of health care organizations is articulated and accomplished. It is vitally important that patients, taxpayers, and the health care workforce understand better how and why HCOs are governed and managed. It is only through understanding current governance and management behaviors and processes, and the reasons for current functioning, that advocates can reasonably drive for changes in governance and management to improve HCO performance.

## DISCUSSION QUESTIONS

1. What are the advantages and disadvantages of the different forms of ownership of HCOs?
2. What mechanisms of accountability are most effective for not-for-profit HCOs?
3. What are some of the ways to measure the performance of HCOs?
4. What are some of the ways to measure managerial performance in HCOs?
5. What skills and experience are required to own and manage HCOs?
6. Who should be in charge of HCOs and how should they be trained?

## REFERENCES

Accrediting Commission on Education for Health Services Administration (ACEHSA). (2003). *Criteria for accreditation* (3rd rev. ed.). Arlington, VA: Author.

Alexander, J. A. (2001). Hospital trusteeship in an era of institutional transition: What we can learn from governance research. In B. Jennings, B. H. Gray, V. A. Sharpe, & A. R. Fleischman (Eds.), *The ethics of hospital trustees* (pp 58–76). Washington, DC: Georgetown University Press.

American Hospital Association. (1981). *Guide for preparation of constitution and bylaws for general hospitals.* Chicago, IL: Author.

Bowen, W. G. (1994). *Inside the boardroom: Governance by directors and trustees.* New York: John Wiley.

Boyatzis, R. E. (1995). Cornerstones of change: Building the path to self-directed learning. In R. E. Boyatzis, S. S. Cowen, D. A. Kolb, & Associates (Eds.), *Innovation in professional education* (pp. 50–94). San Francisco: Jossey-Bass.

Bureau of Labor Statistics. (1998–1999). *Occupational outlook handbook.* http://www.stats.bls.gov/oco/

Burling, T., Lentz, E., & Wilson, R. (1956). *The give and take in hospitals.* New York: Putnam.

Ernst & Young. (1997). *Shining light on your board's passage to the future.* Cleveland, OH: Author.

Goleman, D. (1998). What makes a leader. *Harvard Business Review, 76*(6), 93–102.

Griffith, J. R., Sahney, V. K., & Mohr, R. A. (1995). *Reengineering health care: Building on CQI.* Ann Arbor, MI: Health Administration Press.

Griffith, J. R., & White, K. R. (2002). *The well managed health care organization* (5th ed., pp. 65–144). Ann Arbor, MI: Health Administration Press.

Hansmann, H. (1996). *The ownership of enterprise.* Cambridge, MA: Belknap Press of Harvard University Press.

Herzlinger, R. (1997). *Market-driven health care.* Reading, MA: Addison-Wesley.

Hilsenrath, P. E., Levey, S., Weil, T. P., & Ludke, R. (1993). Health services management manpower and education. Outlook for the future. *Journal of Health Administration Education, 11,* 407–419.

Kovner, A. R. (2001, Jan/Feb). Better information for the board. *Journal of Healthcare Management, 46*(1), 53–66.

Kovner, A. R. (1984). *Really trying: A career guide for the health services manager.* Ann Arbor, MI: Health Administration Press.

Longest, B. B. (1980). *Management practices for the health professional.* Reston, VA: Reston.

Moore, J. D., Jr. (1999, July 12). Holding the line (for you down there). *Modern Healthcare,* 43–48.

Pointer, D., & Orlikoff, J. (2000). *Getting to great.* San Francisco, CA: Jossey-Bass.

Seay, J. D. (2004). The legal responsibilities of voluntary hospital trustees. In B. Jennings, B. H. Gray, V. A. Sharpe, & A. R. Fleischman (Eds.), *The ethics of hospital trustees* (pp. 41–57). Washington, DC: Georgetown University Press.

Umbdenstock, R. J. (1987). Refinement of board's role required. *Health Progress, 68*(1), 47.

# 15

# THE COMPLEXITY OF HEALTH CARE QUALITY

Douglas S. Wakefield and
Bonnie J. Wakefield

- Describe and apply the concept of complex adaptive systems to health care quality.
- Describe how differing definitions of quality health care are influenced by the perspectives of different stakeholders.
- Describe and analyze alternative approaches for health care purchasers to implement pay for performance (P4P) quality improvement initiatives.
- Describe the importance of risk adjusting health care outcomes.
- Describe basic strategies for managing quality within the inherent complexity of health care organizations.

- Health care
- Complexity and the health care quality challenge
- Defining quality of health care
- Pay for Performance (P4P): Helping to make the business case for quality
- Risk-adjusted quality outcomes
- Strategies for managing quality in the health care zone of complexity

Complexity, quality, structure, process, outcome, risk adjustment, outcome attribution, pay-for-performance (P4P)

ALTHOUGH THERE HAS been a longstanding interest in measuring and improving the quality and safety of health care, two recent Institute of Medicine (IOM)/Committee on the Quality of Health Care in America reports have galvanized interest nationally. The first, *To Err Is Human: Building a Safer Health System* (2000a), with its estimate that between 44,000 and 98,000 Americans die each year as a result of medical mistakes, captured the attention of policy makers, providers, payers, patients, and importantly, the popular press about the need to reduce the tremendous gaps in patient safety. Arguably less sensational but of greater importance was the second report, *Crossing the Quality Chasm: A New Health System for the*

*21st Century* (IOM, 2001b). This report concluded, "Quality problems are everywhere, affecting many patients. Between the healthcare we have and the care we could have lies not just a gap, but a chasm" (p. 1). The Quality Chasm report continues,

> The dominant finding of our review is that there are large gaps between the care people should receive and the care they do receive. This is true for preventive, acute, and chronic care, whether one goes for a checkup, a sore throat, or diabetic care. It is true whether one looks at overuse, underuse, or misuse. It is true in different types of healthcare facilities and for different types of health insurance. It is true for all age groups, from children to the elderly. And it is true whether one is looking at the whole country or a single city. (p. 236)

In its call for major system change, this latter groundbreaking report identified six common sense aims for improvement, asserting that patient care should be:

1. *Safe:* patients should not be injured from the very care processes designed to help.
2. *Effective:* scientific knowledge and evidence should be used to determine both what to and what not to do to meet a patient's care needs.
3. *Patient-Centered:* care should be provided in a respectful manner while honoring the patient's values, beliefs, and preferences.
4. *Timely:* better care will come from reducing waits and untimely delays.
5. *Efficient:* it is essential to avoid wasting time, equipment, supplies, ideas, and people's energy because of poorly designed health care processes.
6. *Equitable:* care quality should not vary as a function of geography, gender, ethnicity, or socioeconomic status.

One cannot readily disagree with the face value or intuitively appealing nature of these six aims. Thus, these six assertions have been transformed into demands for improved patient care quality and safety. Throughout America, health care providers, organizations, and systems have been put on notice that the quality and patient safety status quo is no longer acceptable. With increasing frequency, health care providers, organizations, and systems are being required to demonstrate, and are being held accountable for, the level of patient care quality and safety achieved.

What does health care quality mean? Would technically perfect health care quality guarantee great outcomes? How does the concept of risk-adjusted outcomes relate to health care quality? How can patients and third-party payers purchase quality health care? How can providers improve quality and safety? These are but a few of the intriguing questions facing patients, providers, payers, purchasers, and policymakers today. In this chapter, we explore these and other questions by beginning with discussions of health care and complexity, followed by consideration of the challenges and approaches in defining quality, and measuring and purchasing quality health care.

## HEALTH CARE

In framing this chapter's discussion of health care quality, it is useful to begin with a consideration of what we mean by health care. Health care is defined as "care provided to individuals or communities by agents of the health services or professions for the purpose of promoting, maintaining, monitoring, or restoring health" (Lexicon, p. 345). An historically important body of research by Donabedian framed the concept of quality assurance in terms of three types of quality measures: structure, process, and outcomes (1980, see FIGURE 15.1). Donabedian noted that any efforts to improve quality needed to account for the fact that health care is embedded in, and greatly influenced by, the larger external environment. His model posits that health care providers and organizations draw both patients being served as well as the resources necessary to care for these patients (e.g., funding, personnel, equipment, and supplies) from the external environment. These resources are combined in a variety of ways to create structures from which specific patient care processes can be developed through which specific patient care services are ultimately provided to patients. Patient outcomes are the direct results or outcomes of the patient care processes. Feedback about patient outcomes influences subsequent changes in the external environment, as well as the providers' patient care structures and processes.

In applying this model to a hospital, Donabedian would argue that structural aspects of the hospital (e.g., its physical plant, equipment, staffing levels and personnel mix, licensure and accreditation status, organizational culture) reflect both patient

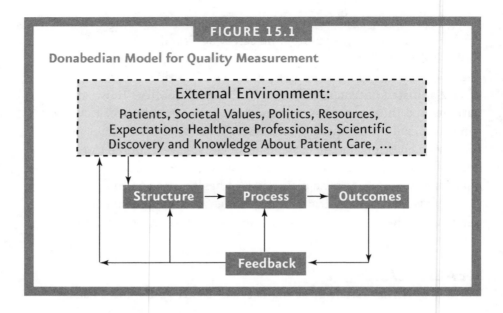

**FIGURE 15.1**

Donabedian Model for Quality Measurement

needs and the fiscal and other resources available to meet these needs. It is a hospital's structural elements or characteristics (e.g., staff types and mix, plant, equipment and organizational structures) when combined with the patient population or market being served that directly influence the complex range and mix of specific diagnostic and treatment services that are ultimately used to meet a patient's care needs. It is through the combined influence of structures and processes as well as patient characteristics that patient outcomes result. Outcomes (e.g., physiological status, mortality, morbidity, disability, functional status, satisfaction, quality of life, lost work days, costs) can be assessed for individuals and groups and used for feedback to influence subsequent changes in the external market (e.g., market share, payment levels), patient care structures and processes, as well as to assess the external environment from which patients and resources come.

A 1993 Life magazine collage highlights the complexity inherent in providing health care services though its depiction of the wide range of clinical and support staff, expertise, and equipment involved in a patient's double coronary artery bypass graft and aortic valve replacement operation (Duncan, 1993). The underlying patient-care process is actually composed of a large number of sequential and parallel patient-care services and actions carried out buy a large number of individuals, representing dozens of dif-

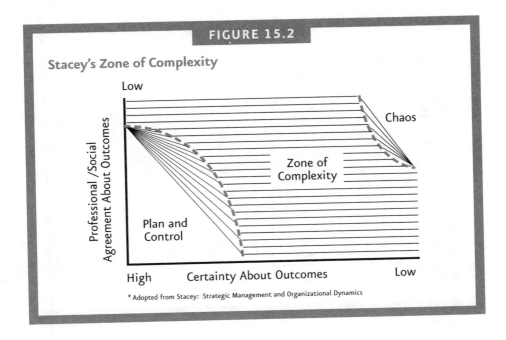

**FIGURE 15.2**

Stacey's Zone of Complexity

Low

Professional /Social Agreement About Outcomes

Chaos

Zone of Complexity

Plan and Control

High          Certainty About Outcomes          Low

* Adopted from Stacey: Strategic Management and Organizational Dynamics

ferent job titles. **FIGURE 15.2** provides a partial listing of the different job titles. Adding to the complexity of coordinating the efforts of many different individuals is the fact that services received by this patient were carried out over several days, requiring extensive communication among all those involved. It is also important to note that both the original picture and the list of personnel included in **TABLE 15.1** reflect the unique blend of services required to care for only one type of patient. In reality hospitals care for a complex range of different types of patients, each with their unique needs, and each requiring individualized treatments. Because of the inherently complex nature of and interaction among structures, processes, and outcomes in health care it is useful to consider how such complexity can affect quality.

## COMPLEXITY AND THE HEALTH CARE QUALITY CHALLENGE

Complicating any consideration of health care quality is the fact that neither need nor demand for health care services, nor what might possibly be provided as treatments for a given disease or condition, are static. If the Life magazine collage were recreated today one would expect to see major changes in equipment and specific

---

**TABLE 15.1**

**Partial Listing of Different Personnel Involved in a Double Bypass and Aortic Valve Replacement**

| CLINICAL PERSONNEL | CLINICAL SUPPORT SERVICES | ADMINISTRATIVE SUPPORT SERVICES |
| --- | --- | --- |
| Physicians: Heart Surgeon, Cardiovascular Surgeon, Anesthesiologist, Intensivist, Cardiologists, Radiologist, Trainees (i.e., Fellows, Residents, Medical Students) <br><br> OR and Nursing: Registered Nurses (e.g., Pre-Op, OR, Post-Op, ICU), Perfusionist, Phlebotomist | Pharmacy (e.g., Pharmacists, Pharmacologist, Pharmacy Technologists), Laboratory (Medical Technologists, Specimen Technologists, Chemistry, Immunology, Microbiology), Radiology (Radiology Technologists), Blood Bank Technologists, Respiratory Therapists, Sterile Processing Tech, Social Work | Housekeeping, Food Service, Plant (e.g., Security, Engineer, Plumber, Maintenance, Electrician), Patient Transport, Materials (e.g., Purchasing, Receiving, Distribution), Billing and Insurance, Administration (Hospital CEO, VP Patient Services, Department Managers, Unit Managers, Shift Supervisors) |

SOURCE: Adapted from D. D. Duncan (1993), The Big Picture: Anatomy of a $64,589 Medical Bill. *Life*, December, pp. 15–19.

---

patient care pre and postsurgical care processes. This is due to the constant bombardment of forces driving continual change. Zimmerman, Lindberg, and Plsek (1998) and Plsek (2001) draw many useful insights from complexity science in their discussion of health care organizations as complex adaptive systems. Critical to thinking about health care organizations as complex adaptive systems is Stacey's Zone of Complexity (1996). Stacey argues that when there is a high degree of certainty about how specific actions can lead to specific outcomes, and if there is a high degree of agreement among those who carry out the actions, an organization can rely on mechanical systems (i.e., plan and control) design principles (see Figure 15.2). In contrast, where there is little agreement about which actions in isolation or in combination automatically lead to specific outcomes, and little agreement among those acting, an organization is faced with the daunting prospect of managing what Stacey calls "Chaos." Between "Plan and Control" and "Chaos" is what Stacey calls the "Zone of Complexity."

Stacey's model can be very useful in understanding some of the challenges associated with ensuring the delivery of high-quality health care services, and the ensuing assessment. The Zone of Complexity varies greatly depending on what is known about the etiology and relative effectiveness of available treatment options for a particular disease or condition. Coming out of the "Chaos Zone" is an unending stream of factors that can directly and indirectly affect how one might view health care quality (see **FIGURE 15.3**). Factors that require health care providers and organizations to be complex adaptive systems include the changing knowledge base, new and refined diagnostic and treatment technologies, changing health care financing and regulatory environments, and the emergence of new diseases or health/bioterrorism threats.

Take for example patients undergoing balloon angioplasties for the treatment of coronary artery disease. With the angioplasty procedure, narrowed portions of a patient's coronary arteries are widened by inserting and inflating a small balloon-like device. Medicare alone paid for about 500,000 angioplasty procedures in 2002. Unfortunately, approximately 30 to 50% of patients who receive this procedure subsequently experience restenosis, or a narrowing of the artery. Restenosis, while most frequently occurring within a 6 to 9-month period, can also occur after a few years. When the restenosis becomes serious enough, the patient must undergo a repeat angioplasty or, in some cases, a coronary artery bypass graft. Research subsequently found that by placing a metal

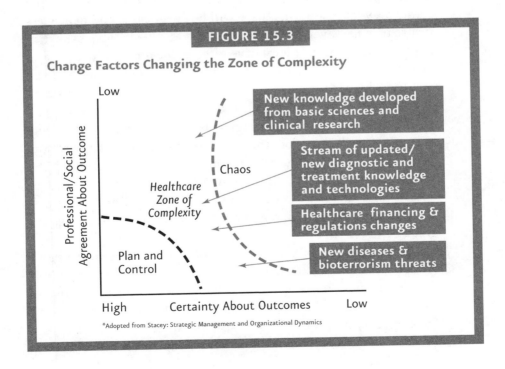

**FIGURE 15.3**

**Change Factors Changing the Zone of Complexity**

Low

Professional/Social Agreement About Outcome

New knowledge developed from basic sciences and clinical research

Stream of updated/ new diagnostic and treatment knowledge and technologies

Chaos

Healthcare Zone of Complexity

Healthcare financing & regulations changes

Plan and Control

New diseases & bioterrorism threats

High          Certainty About Outcomes          Low

*Adopted from Stacey: Strategic Management and Organizational Dynamics

stent at the site of the angioplasty, the estimated incidence of restenosis was reduced to between 17 and 30% of cases. Stents are a metal, spring-like device that helps hold the artery open while allowing the blood to flow through. Subsequent research yielded the development of a new type of restenosis-inhibiting, drug-impregnated stent that further reduced the incidence of restenosis by another 14%. These drug-eluting stents, approved by the FDA in 2003, have been rapidly accepted in the marketplace despite the fact that they cost nearly $3,000, or about three times that of the traditional stent.

From a quality of care standpoint, the question arises if everyone who receives an angioplasty should also receive a drug eluting stent? There are rather broad ranges of estimates of non-stented patients (30% to 50%) and traditionally stented angioplasty patients (17% to 30%) who will experience restenonsis. The new, and much more expensive, drug-eluting stents claim to achieve an additional 14% reduction in restenosis over the traditional stents. Complicating the issues further, third-party payers such as Medicare are unwilling to pay the full cost of using the drug-eluting stent. Hospitals electing to use the drug-eluting stents are financially penalized in two ways. First is the cost of subsidizing the cost of the stents. Second, to the extent that the drug-eluting stents prevent restenosis, there will be fewer cases and hence less future income. Given the current state of knowledge about the incidence of restenosis, the relative effectiveness of traditional and drug-eluting stents in preventing restenosis, stent costs, and the fact that there is little ability to accurately predict which patients will experience restenosis, it is problematic to conclude that good quality demands that every angioplasty patient receive the drug-eluting stents. So how does the absence or presence of the use of the new stents influence the assessment of patient care quality? The best answer is probably, "It depends." Unfortunately, this answer applies to much of health care, and reflects the reality that the definition, measurement, and management of health care quality are greatly influenced by the realities of the "Zone of Complexity."

The applicability of Stacey's work to health care quality is readily apparent when one thinks about the predictability of patient outcomes, given the uncertainty about the relationship between specific actions and outcomes (see FIGURE 15.4). In the Plan and Control Zone, the probability of a specific patient care process yielding a given outcome is very high. For example the clinical labora-

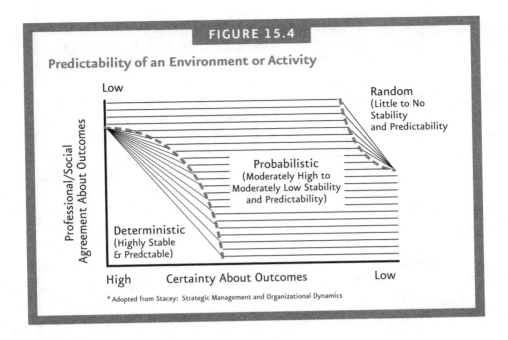

**FIGURE 15.4**

**Predictability of an Environment or Activity**

Low

Random
(Little to No
Stability
and Predictability

Professional/Social
Agreement About Outcomes

Probabilistic
(Moderately High to
Moderately Low Stability
and Predictability)

Deterministic
(Highly Stable
& Predctable)

High          Certainty About Outcomes          Low

\* Adopted from Stacey: Strategic Management and Organizational Dynamics

tory uses well-designed and highly standardized testing protocols when testing for a specific antibiotic resistant organism. Examples of deterministic approaches include the use of process/flow engineering techniques, automated diagnostic testing, and robotic medication dispensing. High degrees of agreement reflect high levels of predictability and standardization, and low variability in the resulting outcomes. Additional Plan and Control examples in which a deterministic approach can be taken include routine elective surgeries for noncomplex patients, and use of appropriate antibiotics to treat known bacterial organisms.

In contrast, low degrees of agreement between the desired outcomes and actions that will yield specific outcomes reflect situations in which there is little or no predictability and standardization, and great variability in outcomes. The resulting uncertainty prohibits the use of probabilistic and mechanical approaches. Examples of clinical randomness coming out of the Chaos Zone include the early stages following discovery of new diseases (e.g., HIV-AIDS, SARS), emergence of new scientific discoveries and/or health care knowledge, and the introduction of new technologies or new but unapproved uses for existing technology. At these times there is great confusion among patients, providers, payers/purchasers, and policymakers as to what could and should be done. Hence, there is also great confusion over what is good quality care.

In the Zone of Complexity, the probability that a given action will yield a specific outcome can vary greatly as seen in the previous angioplasty example. Depending on the specific disease or condition, the probability that a specific health care intervention or service will by itself yield a given level of outcome varies greatly. The Zone of Complexity is where significant portions of health care occur. In this zone there are moderately low to moderately high degrees of variation in the levels of certainty and agreement among the different stakeholders as to what could and should be done to achieve a desired outcome. Therefore, a probabilistic approach, based on the current state of the underlying science, must be taken because of the low to moderately high predictability, standardization, and variability in outcomes. A number of different strategies to improve quality used in this zone include evidence-based clinical guidelines and algorithms; computerized clinical data capture; reporting and real-time decision support systems; and continued investment in the education and development of the clinical workforce. Despite all theses strategies, the resulting variability in outcomes reflects the complexity of defining, measuring, and improving an inherently complex service—health care!

## DEFINING QUALITY OF HEALTH CARE

A central challenge when discussing health care quality is that it has no universally accepted definition. Quality has many dimensions and each can be emphasized or de-emphasized by the range of actors affected by quality (see Figure 15.5). Providers, who are accountable for quality and safety, tend to emphasize "technical quality," which emphasizes performing procedures correctly and providing the correct care needed. Patient care, while caring about technical quality, also emphasizes "touch quality," which implies the interactions between the patient and providers. Payers add a concern for efficiency, value, and appropriateness to the quality construct. And, finally, policymakers—who also are often payers—add the dimensions of access, equity, disparities, and legal responsibilities to quality considerations.

The definition of quality of care used in the 2001 IOM *Crossing the Quality Chasm Report*, originally from the JCAHO *Lexicon* is, "the degree to which health services for individuals and populations increase the likelihood of desired health outcomes and are consistent with current professional knowledge" (Joint Commission on Accreditation of Healthcare Organizations [JCAHO] *Lexicon*, p. 664). Patient health outcome is then defined as

> The result that happens to a patient from performance (or nonperformance) of one or more processes, services, or activities carried out by healthcare providers. A patient health outcome represents the cumulative effect of one or more processes at a defined time, as in survival to discharge following a gunshot wound to the chest or an acute myocardial infarction. (p. 594)

Intuitively appealing and consistent with the Donabedian model, this definition has as its primary focus of quality health care the "result" or "outcome" of the care process. It is important to note, however, that there is a wide range of potential patient care outcomes. For example, the Dartmouth Clinical Value Compass lists four primary outcome categories including clinical outcomes, functional status, risk status, and well-being, satisfaction with care and the perceived benefit, and cost (Nelson, Mohr, Batalden, & Plume, 1996). Each dimension has quality indicators specific to the disease or condition of interest.

---

**FIGURE 15.5**

**Stakeholders' Differing Perspectives on Health Care Quality**

■ Providers: "Technical Quality"
  - "5 Rights": Providing the Technically Right Care, to the Right Patient in the Right Time, Right Way and Right Amount

■ Patients: "Touch Quality"
  - How Well the Patient Feels Treated (Satisfaction, Access to Care)
  - Communication, Coordination, Compassion, Respect, Personalization, and Time Spent with Patient are Key

■ Payers: "Technical and Touch Quality"
  - The Appropriateness, Timeliness, Cost, Effectiveness, and Resulting Patient Satisfaction are Key

■ Policy Makers: "Technical and Touch Quality"
  - Some Elements Shared with Payers include Appropriateness, Timeliness, Cost, Cost Effectiveness, and Resulting Patient Satisfaction
  - Care Also Should be Accessible and Meet the Needs of the Larger Population and Societal Needs

While a focus on outcomes in defining and measuring quality is reasonable, to what extent is it also reasonable to assume that a specific combination of health care services used to care for a patient actually lead to the outcome? That is, to what extent will a provider's specific actions dictate the patient's outcomes? In reality, patient care outcomes may be influenced by two categories of factors that reside outside the control of health care providers and organizations. The first category relates to the fact that patients may receive patient care services simultaneously from several, frequently independent, sources including themselves. For example, patients with multiple chronic diseases may be seen by a number of different specialists (who may not share a common medical record or information about the same patient), obtain prescribed medications from different pharmacies, and use self-prescribed, over-the-counter medications, herbal, and dietary supplements without informing their physicians. The end result may be that, while in isolation each provider gave the patient technically perfect treatment, the combination of different prescribed medications and patient self-treatments may be canceling out potentially positive effects, and perhaps creating treatment combinations that increase morbidity, mortality, reduced functional status, and ultimately an ineffective use of health care resources.

The second set of factors that potentially affects patient care outcomes relates directly to differences in patients' individual characteristics. Patient characteristics that potentially influence an outcome include health status, genetic make-up, personal health habits and behaviors (e.g., diet, exercise, smoking, excessive alcohol consumption, and drug abuse), personal wealth and/or health insurance coverage, social support systems, and personal attitudes towards and beliefs about the health care system. Take for example two patients undergoing the same surgical procedure. Let's assume Patient A was in very poor physical and nutritional health, with a long history of smoking, alcohol, and drug abuse, and too poor to buy prescribed medications, whereas Patient B was in excellent physical and nutritional health, did not have a history of smoking, alcohol, and drug abuse and could afford to purchase prescribed medications. Assuming that the technical aspects of the surgery were performed in a technically perfect manner and were provided in exactly the same manner to each patient, it would not be realistic to expect identical outcomes in nonidentical patients.

In nonhealth care industries, quality has been improved and controlled by reducing the variability in the quality of the "raw material" being used in the production processes. In contrast, health care providers generally do not have the luxury of selectively caring for just the healthiest and wealthiest patients. In fact, evidence of "patient dumping" can have serious financial and legal repercussions for health care providers and organizations. Thus, the inherent variability in patient characteristics (i.e., the clinical process's "raw material") adds significantly to the complexity of assessing the quality of care received, particularly in terms of patient outcomes.

This problem of how and to what extent to attribute a patient's outcome to the patient care services actually received can be seen in cases of both good and poor clinical outcomes. Taking the case in which the patient care services that were provided were technically perfect, timely, and appropriate to the patient's clinical needs, the patient may have a poor outcome (e.g., death, disability, reduced functional status) because of poor general health status, genetic predisposition for early organ failure, significant history of excessive smoking, drinking, and poor nutrition and exercise practices, or the lack of financial resources or health insurance to purchase needed drugs or supplies needed to comply with the prescribed treatment. Ironically, the reverse is also true. A generally healthy patient with good personal health habits and behaviors, and adequate financial resources to purchase needed drugs and supplies may receive technically inferior care, but ultimately may experience a good clinical outcome despite poor quality care because she is physically, socially, and economically better prepared to handle the insults of both the disease and poor quality technical care. Therefore, if one were to focus on patient care outcomes as the measure of quality there is a clear need to adjust for important differences in patients' characteristics (risk adjustment is discussed below).

If there is a limited ability to use patient care outcomes as a definition of quality, perhaps a greater emphasis on process should be considered. Chin and Muramatsu (2004) provide a useful definition of health care quality that links outcomes to process: "Quality of care is that portion of a patient's outcome over which healthcare providers, whether individuals or organization, have control" (p. 7). That is, the focus should be on outcomes for which there are reasonably well-known process-outcome relationships. With available resources (e.g., equipment, staff, supplies) providers have the most control over process, that is, what is or is not done to and for the patient. Thus, when thinking about the quality of patient care processes we would suggest that health care quality be further defined and assessed within the concept of the Five Rights of Patient Care.

- *Right Care.* Quality health care requires that physicians, nurses, and other health care providers be held responsible for accurately assessing and providing appropriate patient care interventions given their knowledge about the underlying disease(s) or condition(s) being treated, and within the constraints of available resources.
- *Right Patient.* Quality health care requires that patients should only receive the care (e.g., diagnostic tests, medical, or surgical treatments) that was specifically planned for them. Just as replacing a radiator in a car that needs a new water pump represents poor quality, so does giving one patient the wrong treatment.
- *Right Way.* Quality health care requires that health care providers be held responsible for using the appropriate equipment and patient care protocols in the appropriate way, that patients be informed of and participate in decisions regarding treatment options, and be treated in a respectful and considerate manner.
- *Right Time.* Quality health care requires that it be provided in a timely manner with no inappropriate/avoidable delays in care (e.g., surgery cancellations, failure to perform required tests, excessive clinical or E.R. wait times). As noted earlier, complex surgeries such as a CABG are actually comprised of a series of different processes of care that must be appropriately synchronized for good quality to occur. Thus failing to complete the appropriate pre-op assessments prior to the scheduled elective surgery time result in avoidable delays and poor quality.
- *Right Amount.* Quality health care requires that both under- and over-utilization of health care services represent be avoided. In the first instance, quality is affected because patients do not receive the needed services. In the latter instance, quality is affected because of the potential for iatrogenic harm resulting from receiving too much care, and costs. Fisher (2003) has highlighted the wide variation in use of health services in different health care markets. The variation is not due to differences in patient need but rather difference in practice patterns. Fisher's work clearly documents that in fact more care is not better care.

Given the realities of health care complexity, disagreement about what quality means, health care payment practices that sometimes mitigate against quality, and limited resources with which to purchase health care services, is there anything that can be done to improve the quality of care being given? In response, third-party payers have begun to experiment with alternative ways to create an incentive for higher health care quality through "pay-for-performance" initiatives.

## PAY FOR PERFORMANCE (P4P): HELPING TO MAKE THE BUSINESS CASE FOR QUALITY

Crossing the "Quality Chasm" requires a fundamental change in the way that health care services are organized, provided, evaluated, and financed. Needed is a change in the incentives to stimulate innovations that result in higher quality health care. The difficulty of specifying a clear and compelling "business case" for high quality health care has been clearly defined as a barrier to quality improvement (Leatherman et al., 2003; Porter & Teisberg, 2004). Shine (2001) highlights the current disconnect between quality improvement and third-party payer practices.

> . . . A hospital in the Midwest implemented a program to improve choices of initial antibiotics to treat pneumonia. Mortality rates went down, hospital days went down, and costs went down, but it cost the hospital money because these patients were less sick, their DRG categories were less serious, and the hospital received less money. The system itself is bizarre. If the system makes a mistake and produces kidney failure, this will put the patient into a higher-paying RG. That is not aligning incentives with regard to quality. (p. 8)

Leatherman et al. (2003), in their discussion of the lack of a business case for quality, note:

> . . . the misalignment of financial incentives creates a formidable obstacle to the adoption of quality interventions. . . . a healthcare organization may be reluctant to implement improvements if better quality is not accompanied by better payment or improved margins, or al least equal compensation. Without a business case for quality, we think it unlikely that the private sector will move

quickly and reliably to widely adopt proven quality improvements. (pp. 17–18)

As a result of the growing recognition that healthcare payment practices have focused on paying for services without specific linkage to their quality, the U.S. health care system is in the very early stages of attempts by third party payers to more explicitly link payment to quality (Bailit Health Purchasing, 2001, 2002; Baker, 2003; TrendWatch, 2003; Strunk & Hurley, 2004; Endsley, Kirkegaard, Baker, & Murcko, 2004; DeWitt, 2004). These so-called "Pay for Performance" or "P4P" quality improvement initiatives are experimenting with a variety of direct and indirect financial incentives targeted to different categories of providers, i.e., making a business case for quality.

Because of the inherent complexity of health care services and patient-specific factors influencing outcomes, there are a number of factors to consider in implementing a P4P approach to quality improvement. **FIGURE 15.6** provides a framework highlighting three core issues to address in implementing a P4P strategy to improve quality: Whom to target with incentives, which incentive

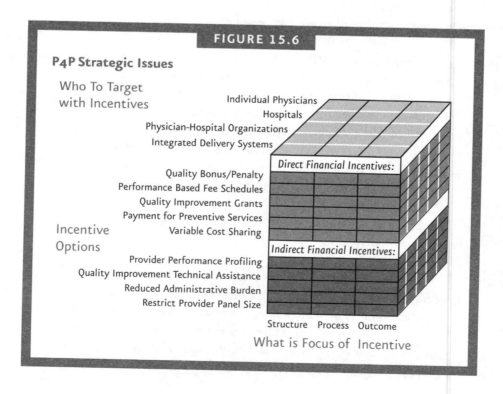

**FIGURE 15.6**

**P4P Strategic Issues**

Who To Target with Incentives
- Individual Physicians
- Hospitals
- Physician-Hospital Organizations
- Integrated Delivery Systems

Incentive Options

Direct Financial Incentives:
- Quality Bonus/Penalty
- Performance Based Fee Schedules
- Quality Improvement Grants
- Payment for Preventive Services
- Variable Cost Sharing

Indirect Financial Incentives:
- Provider Performance Profiling
- Quality Improvement Technical Assistance
- Reduced Administrative Burden
- Restrict Provider Panel Size

Structure   Process   Outcome

What is Focus of Incentive

options to use, and what to focus the incentives on. Determining the appropriate approach to incenting quality improvement requires consideration of these three interconnected questions.

### Whom to Target with Incentives

The choice of whom to target for P4P quality improvement incentives has significant implications for what to target and the types of incentives that will be used. Choice options range from individual physicians, medical groups, hospitals, physician-hospital organizations, and integrated delivery systems (Bailit, 2001, 2002). For a variety of reasons, focusing quality improvement incentives on individual physicians will have only a very limited effect on broad efforts to improve quality. Because of the extensive specialization within medical practice, it is increasingly rare, especially for the Medicare population, that patients will be cared for by only one physician. Although patients may have a primary care physician, they may also be cared for by a number of specialists depending on medical need. Given this, and the fact that the different health care treatments may interact or otherwise affect each other, it may be very difficult to have meaningful P4P quality improvement initiatives targeted to individual physicians unless the focus is on specific interventional procedures (e.g., CABG, angioplasty, or hip replacements) or on disease-specific patient care processes (e.g., HbA1c and blood pressure control, annual eye exams for diabetic patients). Even with such a specific focus, the issue may arise as to whether an individual physician will care for a sufficient number of patients for which meaningful risk adjustments can be made in order to have statistically valid and reliable results. While aggregating a P4P quality improvement focus at the medical group level may help to address some of the limitations in focusing on individual physicians, the issue of whether patients receive all their care from the same medical group remains. Because many medical groups are still relatively small and tend to be single specialty or contain a limited number of specialists, many of the problems in targeting individual physicians still remain. Regardless of whether an individual physician or medical group focus is taken, a basic problem remains as to whether quality improvement incentives should focus on a specific disease or procedure or whether it would be more effective to focus on a cluster of diseases or procedures. For example, in the case of primary care, if a physician or medical group is found to provide excellent care to heart failure patients, is excellent care also being provided for pulmonary disease, diabetes, or depression?

Alternatively, a P4P quality improvement approach could focus on hospitals as is the case with the CMS's Voluntary Hospital Reporting Initiative and Premier Hospital Quality Demonstration Project (http://www.cms.hhs.gov/quality). The approach in both is to focus on common conditions for which there are generally agreed upon process of care measures (i.e., what should be done for the typical patient). For example, the Voluntary Hospital Reporting Initiative was begun with a focus on three conditions including acute myocardial infarction, heart failure, and pneumonia for which 10 specific process of care indicators have been identified. Quality is then assessed in terms of the percentage of all patients receiving these process of care indicators for whom they are not contraindicated. In addition to the several limitations associated with focusing on process of care measures (discussed below), other potential limitations of the hospital focus include insufficient number of cases in small hospitals, absence of risk-adjusted patient groupings, wide variation in physician staffing patterns in different hospitals, and patients receiving care in different hospitals depending on care needs and service availability.

Further aggregations to the physician–hospital organization (PHO) and to the integrated delivery system (IDS) levels can be beneficial because of the ability to aggregate patients into larger groups and to the extent that individual patients receive all or the majority of care from these organizations. Because these are much larger organizations typically caring for populations of patients, P4P quality improvement incentives can be targeted to create system-wide changes. Unfortunately, only a portion of the U.S. population receives care within a single PHO or IDS.

### Incentive Options

A second major issue to consider in implementing a P4P quality improvement incentive plan is to consider what types of incentives might be used. A recent report provides a useful comparison of direct and indirect financial incentives (Bailit, 2002). Direct financial incentives are intended to flow directly to the provider and to be explicitly linked to specified actions or performance. As shown in Figure 15.6 direct financial incentives include quality bonuses/incentives, pay for performance, performance fee-based scales, quality improvement grants, payment for preventive services and variable cost-sharing arrangements. In contrast, indirect financial incentives try to create change in provider performance through the provision of comparative information and/or by influencing the actions of the patient. Examples of indirect financial incentives include provider performance profiling, publicizing provider performance, providing technical assistance for quality improvement, reducing administrative burdens imposed by third-party payers, and reducing the size of a physician's patient panel.

To the extent that specific provider behaviors and incentives can be linked, there is great potential to improve health care quality. With all incentive schemes, a key challenge is to anticipate and mitigate the effect of any unintended consequences. The recently published Leapfrog Incentive and Reward Compendium (http://www.leapfroggroup.org/ircompendium.htm) documents the growing use of specific incentives for P4P quality and patient safety initiatives. In reviewing 15 P4P initiatives (Web site accessed June 12, 2004) targeting quality improvement in hospitals, direct financial incentives were used exclusively in 7 initiatives while the remaining 8 P4P initiatives reported using both direct and indirect incentives. Among direct financial incentives, quality bonuses were used most frequently ($n = 10$), followed by compensation being at risk ($n = 3$) and performance fee schedules and tiering ($n = 2$ respectively) of the P4P initiatives. The most frequently used indirect financial incentives included the use of provider profiling ($n = 4$) and publicizing hospitals' performance in 2 of the initiatives. In 18 P4P initiatives targeting physicians, a combination of direct and indirect financial incentives was used in about 14. Quality bonuses were used in 14 of these physician-targeted initiatives versus the use of compensation at-risk approaches in approximately 4 of the initiatives. The use of indirect financial incentives is more pronounced in the physician P4P initiatives, with 10 of the initiatives using provider profiling, and 9 publicizing provider performance.

## What to Target for Quality Improvement

As shown in Figure 15.6, potential quality improvement targets can be grouped into the three Donabedian categories of Structure, Process and Outcome. Examples of potential P4P Structure Targets currently being pursued include investment in information technologies, staffing patterns, and volume-based referral practices

(Leapfrog Group, Blue Cross Blue Shield of Mass, Bridges to Excellence, Integrated Healthcare Association). Specific P4P information technology targets include investment in and use of computerized physician order entry systems with real-time decision support, bedside bar-coding systems, patient data warehouse creation, and enhanced clinical decision support systems. The best example of a P4P staffing pattern target would be the Leapfrog Group's patient safety standard of full-time, intensivist-only staffing in intensive care units (http://www.leapfroggroup.org). Such staffing coverage could potentially be provided both on-site and through the use of electronic-ICUs (e-ICU ref). For many conditions, there is a lack of valid and reliable evidence of differences in quality among competing providers. With growing support from the literature, the Leapfrog Group has endorsed the use of volume-based referral. The underlying assumption is that, all things being equal, providers (e.g., hospitals and physicians) having higher volumes are able to develop higher quality care and better outcomes.

P4P Process Targets focus on the ways in which care is delivered. The primary goal of this approach to improving quality is to standardize patient care processes whenever possible based on the best available science. Examples of potential P4P Process Targets currently being pursued include the Center for Medicare & Medicaid Services (CMS) initiatives targeting hospitals, nursing homes, and home health agencies (http://www.cms.hhs.gov/quality). There are two CMS hospital quality initiatives. In the National Voluntary Hospital Reporting Initiative, the focus is on three conditions and 10 specific processes of care measures. The conditions (and processes of care measures) include acute myocardial infarction (aspirin at arrival, aspirin at discharge, beta blocker at arrival, beta blocker at discharge, ACE inhibitor for left ventricular systolic dysfunction), heart failure (left ventricular function assessment, ACE inhibitor for left ventricular systolic dysfunction), and pneumonia (initial antibiotic timing, pneumococcal vaccination, oxygenation assessment). Quality is then measured by the extent to which patients for whom these specific care processes are appropriate actually receive them. All acute care hospitals receiving Medicare payments will be required to regularly submit these data.

P4P Outcome Targets, as the name implies, is focused on the outcomes of patient care. An excellent example of an outcome approach can be seen in the Project Bridges to Excellence: Rewarding Quality Across the Healthcare System funded by the Robert Wood Johnson Foundation (http://www.bridgestoexcellence.org/bte/index.html). In addition to an IT-focused physician office linkage project, the Bridges to Excellence (BTE) initiative is comprised of two condition-specific programs focused on diabetes and cardiac care. Examples of the diabetes outcome measures for adult patients include HbAıc, blood pressure and cholesterol control as measured by specific laboratory values. The Integrated Healthcare Association initiative also includes patient satisfaction outcome measures related to items such as timely access to care, patient-physician communications and overall care ratings (http://www.iha.org).

In returning to the Leapfrog Group's Incentive and Reward Compendium (http://www.leapfroggroup.org/ircompendium.htm), our analysis of the 15 P4P quality and patient safety improvement initiatives targeted on hospitals reveals that only 2 of the initiatives focused exclusively on Structures, 4 focused exclusively on Processes, and the remaining 9 focused on some combination of Structures, Processes and Outcomes. For the 18 P4P initiatives targeted on physicians, 6 focused exclusively on Processes, one focused exclusively on Outcomes, and the remaining 11 focused on some combination of Structures, Processes, and Outcomes.

In deciding whether to focus on structures, processes, and/or outcomes as quality improvement targets, it is important to recognize their respective strengths and limitations. Without the appropriate structures, such as the required physical plant, staff, equipment, and supplies, the ability to provide high quality care is limited. Given the relatively unadvanced status of clinical information technology systems in many hospitals, P4P incentives to support investment in information technology is not surprising. However, there is no guarantee that simply having access to state-of-the-art equipment will guarantee that the best or most appropriate patient care will actually be provided. Having access to the "perfect" clinical information technology system will not in and of itself guarantee the provision of high quality care. Thus, health care structures can be thought of as being necessary, but not sufficient, to guarantee high quality care.

A P4P quality improvement focus on patient care processes is useful only to the extent that there is good scientific evidence supporting the provision of that type of care. Because of its many serious clinical complications, high quality diabetes care requires routine monitoring of HbA1c, blood pressure, and cholesterol levels. In addition is the need for periodic eye, foot, and neuropathy assessments as well as smoking cessation advice and treatment. As discussed earlier, because of patient-specific factors, such as personal health habits, behaviors, and beliefs, genetic predispositions, and poverty and lack of health insurance, there still may not be good clinical outcomes, even with the appropriate, ongoing monitoring and treatment. A second potential limitation of a process-only approach is the relative state of knowledge regarding exactly what and when specific care processes should be provided for a wide number of conditions. Finally, as Porter and Teisberg (2004) note, targeting incentives on compliance with specific processes rather than on improved health may in the long run inhibit significant improvements in quality.

Ideally P4P initiatives should be focused on outcomes. Unfortunately outcomes-focused quality improvement initiatives are relatively rare at this point due to several factors. First, the specific outcome or outcomes of interest must be determined. Four outcomes categories contained in the Dartmouth Quality Compass (Nelson, Mohr, Batalden, & Plume, 1996) are useful to highlight range of potential outcomes of interest. These outcome categories include Clinical, Patient Care Experience, Functional Status, and Financial Outcomes. In selecting clinical outcomes, consideration needs to be given to focusing on single diseases, a subset of diseases, or all acute and chronic diseases or conditions being cared for. Patient Care Experience outcomes might include patient satisfaction with specific aspects of the care process, assessment of the quality of patient-provider communications, or an overall assessment of the patients' perspective of the care experience. Functional Status outcomes might include changes in patients' abilities to perform activities of daily living, instrumental activities of daily living, or ability to perform successfully in a work role. Financial Outcomes may focus potentially on the costs of care, including both the direct and indirect costs (e.g., waiting time, travel costs) associated with care.

A second challenge associated with focusing on patient care outcomes is the question of whose perspective the outcome should reflect. For the individual patient, the desired outcome may be being symptom free and able to return to work. From the third-party payer's perspective, the outcome may be defined in terms of the cost effectiveness of the intervention. For the public policy-maker, undifferentiated access to care may be of greatest interest.

A third issue to consider is whether an outcome focus should be service or disease specific. For example, should the outcome reflect the specific services or interventions (e.g., hospitalization, surgical procedure, office visit) versus the overall combination of related inpatient and outpatient services provided over a longer period of time? Likewise, should the outcome have a disease specific focus such as diabetes or heart failure versus focusing on an individual's entire set of health care conditions? Focusing on individual diseases ignores the growing reality of an aging population typically experiencing multiple chronic diseases.

Finally, and perhaps of greatest importance in being able to "purchase" quality care, one needs to be able to compare outcome quality for similar types of patients cared for by different providers. To do this requires the presence of valid, reliable and meaningful risk adjusted outcomes, yet one more layer of complexity in "Crossing the Quality Chasm."

## RISK-ADJUSTED QUALITY OUTCOMES

The central issue is how to assess the quality of care provided given the complexity and variability of patient factors over which providers and health care organizations have no control. The answer in part is to risk adjust the outcomes. Risk adjustment attempts to account for the differences that patients bring to the health care encounter so that outcomes can be compared across different patient groups, treatments, providers, health plans, or populations (Iezzoni, 2003). These techniques recognize that patient outcomes are a function of care provided (including consideration of both structure and process variables) and patient factors (demographics, comorbid conditions, social factors, preferences). Because risk adjustment techniques help account for differences in patient-related factors affecting outcomes of care, they increase health care providers and organizations' ability to assess and manage quality in the health care zone of complexity.

Several different risk adjustment methodologies have been developed (Iezzoni, 2003). Two examples of these include the Acute Physiology and Chronic Health Evaluation (APACHE) and Diagnosis Related Groups (DRG). Each of these methods defines risks in relation to outcomes differently and uses different populations. For example, APACHE has three versions, two of which focus on in-hospital mortality in adult patients in intensive care units. DRGs focus on total hospital charges of all hospitalized patients. If using an established risk adjustment model, the patient population and outcome of interest must be congruent with the chosen methodology.

## Basic Risk Adjustment Strategies

Devising appropriate risk adjustment strategies requires answers to four major questions (Iezzoni, 2003) discussed below:

- What outcomes require risk adjustment?
- Over what time frames should risk adjustment methodologies be applied?
- For which patient populations will the risk adjustment methodology be applied?
- For which purpose(s) will the risk-adjusted outcomes be used?

### What Outcomes Require Risk Adjustment?

Historically, the outcome of interest, i.e., "risk of what?" has been mortality. However, outcomes may also include resource use (including charges and length of hospital stay), clinical outcomes, patient satisfaction, functional status, complications, and quality of life. As noted earlier, the Dartmouth Clinical Value Compass lists four primary outcomes categories including Clinical Outcomes, Functional Status, Patient Care Experiences, and Financial (Nelson et al., 1996). Issues surrounding the choice of outcome were discussed earlier in the P4P section, and include a focus on single versus multiple disease states, the question of whose perspective the outcome should reflect, and whether the outcome focus should be service or disease specific. The specific outcome of interest must be appropriate to the purpose of risk adjustment.

### Over What Time Frames Should
### Risk Adjustment Methodologies Be Applied?

Selection of the timeframe for risk adjustment is important as different timeframes provide different perspectives on risk adjustment. For example, is there a need to assess lifetime risks, such as the development of complications of diabetes (e.g., retinopathy, amputations) or heart disease (e.g., prolonged hypertension leading to stroke)? Or is there a need to risk-adjust for short-term outcomes such as post-operative mortality, measured as in-hospital or within 30 days of the procedure? It is important to note that the timeframe selected can be used to reflect individual patient care interventions such as a single surgical procedure, or larger episodes of care as reflected in the combination of inpatient and outpatient care received prior to the surgical procedure. Because patient characteristics can and do change over time (e.g., income, health status) it is essential to specify the timeframe of interest when adjusting for risk factors.

### For What Patient Populations Will the Risk Adjustment Methodology Be Applied?

The patient population characteristics must be specified. Risk adjustment approaches designed for children will not be appropriate for elderly individuals. Patient populations might also be defined in terms of the type of care previously received. For example, there is a growing literature highlighting the importance of patients' transfer status as a predictor of referral hospitals (Clough et al., 1993; Gordon & Rosenthal, 1995; Wyatt et al., 1997; Riggs et al., 2002; Jencks & Boboula, 1988) and referral hospital ICU (Dragsted et al., 1989; Rosenberg et al., 2003; Durairaj et al., 2003) resource use and mortality. In these studies both overall and ICU resource use were significantly higher for transfer patients. Thus, for hospitals, particularly academic medical centers (AMCs), that receive large numbers of referral patients, the need to risk-adjust resource use and mortality for transfer status has been recognized in several studies (Gordon & Rosenthal, 1995; Dragsted et al., 1989; Rosenberg et al., 2003). Additional population characteristics used in risk-adjusted outcomes are discussed below.

### For What Purpose(s) Will the Risk Adjusted Outcomes Be Used?

Finally, the purpose of risk adjustment must be identified. The purpose can be comparison across providers or health plans, for setting payment levels or encouraging health plans to accept and treat high-risk, high-cost patients (Iezzoni, 2003).

### Sources of Data for Risk Adjustment

Risk adjustment methods can use administrative (claims) data, clinical data (patient record abstraction), and patient surveys. Each of these data sources has distinct advantages and disadvantages.

Risk adjustment is most often accomplished using administrative data, usually claims data. These data offer a number of advantages (Iezzoni, 2003), such as including large numbers of individuals, being representative of the community, providing the ability to track people over time, having relatively standardized content, and being inexpensive for researchers to acquire. A significant disadvantage of using administrative data is that these data are primarily collected for financial purposes (e.g., paying claims and tracking utilization) and are not intended to examine or track changes in health and health status. Thus, many important variables needed for risk adjustment are not available in administrative databases, e.g., functional status and health literacy. Furthermore, most administrative databases do not include uninsured individuals or noncovered services (Iezzoni).

A second source of data is clinical abstraction of patient medical records. While clinical data offer more detailed information about patients compared to administrative data, data on key risk adjustment variables may be absent for a variety of reasons. These include, among others, documentation practices that focus on documenting only the presence of abnormalities. Inconsistent documentation across clinicians may result in reliability issues. Documentation systems vary across health care facilities and settings. Clinical abstraction is also a labor-intensive method of data collection. Records may be missing or unavailable. Privacy regulations may limit access to individual medical records. The increasing use of electronic medical records may improve the availability, standardization, and cost-effective use of medical records.

A third source of data is surveys of patients. Surveys are probably the best way to assess patient preferences and self-report of health (self-reported health status is a good predictor of outcomes), but low response rates will bias the data and sicker people may be less likely to respond to surveys. Patients may give socially acceptable answers, resulting in biased results. Surveys also incur costs for postage, copying, and data entry. With mailed surveys, one cannot be sure whether the intended individual answered the survey. If answered by another individual, responses may not accurately reflect those that would have been given by the survey target. For example, methods to measure functional status are not interchangeable. Patients tend to overstate their functional abilities, whereas significant others tend to understate the patient's ability, relative to the nurse's ratings (Rubenstein, Schairer, Wieland, &

Kane, 1984). Nurses tend to rate patients as significantly less independent as either occupational or physical therapists and patients would, the latter more likely to rate themselves as improved during therapy (Malzer, 1988).

## STRATEGIES FOR MANAGING QUALITY IN THE HEALTH CARE ZONE OF COMPLEXITY

As depicted earlier in Figure 15.3, the health care zone of complexity is constantly being influenced by new basic science and clinical discoveries, updated and new diagnostic and treatment technologies, new and emerging diseases, and even bioterrorism threats. Over time, as additional information is gained about such intrusions, and the effectiveness of different interventions used to address them, information is gradually developed to support the use of probabilistic-based approaches in general practice (see Figure 15.4). Because a great deal of health care resides within the zone of complexity, strategies for managing and improving quality should center on ways of increasing the probability of achieving the desired outcomes. Five fundamental strategies, each building on the previous, are presented in **FIGURE 15.7**, which are discussed below.

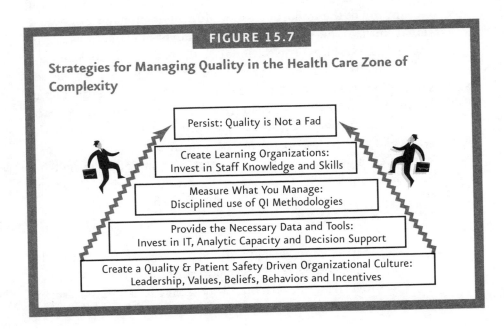

**FIGURE 15.7**

**Strategies for Managing Quality in the Health Care Zone of Complexity**

Persist: Quality is Not a Fad

Create Learning Organizations: Invest in Staff Knowledge and Skills

Measure What You Manage: Disciplined use of QI Methodologies

Provide the Necessary Data and Tools: Invest in IT, Analytic Capacity and Decision Support

Create a Quality & Patient Safety Driven Organizational Culture: Leadership, Values, Beliefs, Behaviors and Incentives

## Create a Quality & Patient Safety-Driven Organizational Culture: Leadership, Values, Beliefs, Behaviors and Incentives

Health care is all about people . . . those receiving, paying for, and providing services. Every organization is comprised of people, who through their shared experiences, values, and combined efforts create a product or service. The glue holding everything together and serving as the "invisible hand" of internal control is the organizational culture in which people work. There are a number of terms used to discuss organizational culture including group norms, espoused values, formal philosophy, climate, and shared meanings (Schein, 1992). Schein provides a useful framework clarifying the linkage between organizational culture and leadership.

> Culture and leadership are two sides of the same coin in that leaders first create cultures when they create groups and organizations . . . if cultures become dysfunctional, it is the unique function of leadership to perceive the functional and dysfunctional elements of the existing culture and to manage culture evolution and change. . . . The bottom line for leaders is that if they do not become conscious of the culture in which they are embedded, those cultures will manage them. (p. 15)

There are many recent examples in health care of the growing recognition of the importance of building and managing organizational cultures that facilitate the provision of high quality and safe patient care services. The National Quality Forum, in its Safe Practices for Better Healthcare (2003), published a list of 30 endorsed safety practices (see APPENDIX 15A). While the first safety practice is explicitly to create an overall health care culture of safety, many of the remaining practices are either directly related to or the result of a health care organization's culture of safety. Three papers in the December 2003 issue of *Quality & Safety in Health Care* journal provide examples of this growing recognition. Berwick (2003) considers the relationships among improvement, trust, and health care workers:

> Accelerating improvement will require large shifts in attitudes toward and strategies for developing the healthcare workforce . . . (required is) a workforce capable of setting bold aims, measuring

## APPENDIX 15A

### The National Quality Forum Safe Practices For Better Healthcare, 2003[*]

1. Create a healthcare culture of safety.
2. For designated high-risk, elective surgical procedures or other specified care, patients should be clearly informed of the likely reduced risk of an adverse outcome at treatment facilities that have demonstrated superior outcomes and should be referred to such facilities in accordance with the patient's stated preference.
3. Specify an explicit protocol to be used to ensure an adequate level of nursing based on the institution's usual patient mix and the experience and training of its nursing staff.
4. All patients in general intensive care units (both adult and pediatric) should be managed by physicians having specific training and certification in critical care medicine ("critical care certified").
5. Pharmacists should actively participate in the medication-use process, including, at a minimum, being available for consultation with prescribers on medication ordering, interpretation and review of medication orders, preparation of medications, dispensing of medications, and administration and monitoring of medications.
6. Verbal orders should be recorded whenever possible and immediately read back to the prescriber—i.e., a healthcare provider receiving a verbal order should read or repeat back the information that the prescriber conveys in order to verify the accuracy of what was heard.
7. Use only standardized abbreviations and dose designations.
8. Patient care summaries or other similar records should not be prepared from memory.
9. Ensure that care information, especially changes in orders and new diagnostic information, is transmitted in a timely and clearly understandable form to all of the patient's current healthcare providers who need that information to provide care.
10. Ask each patient or legal surrogate to recount what he or she has been told during the informed consent discussion.
11. Ensure that written documentation of the patient's preference for life-sustaining treatments is prominently displayed in his or her chart.
12. Implement a computerized prescriber order entry system.
13. Implement a standardized protocol to prevent the mislabeling of radiographs.
14. Implement standardized protocols to prevent the occurrence of wrong-site procedures or wrong-patient procedures.
15. Evaluate each patient undergoing elective surgery for risk of an acute ischemic cardiac event during surgery, and provide prophylactic treatment of high-risk patients with beta blockers.

[*]NQF-Endorsed Set of Safe Practices

**(Continued)**

## APPENDIX 15A (Continued)

16. Evaluate each patient upon admission, and regularly thereafter, for the risk of developing pressure ulcers. This evaluation should be repeated at regular intervals during care. Clinically appropriate preventive methods should be implemented consequent to the evaluation.

17. Evaluate each patient upon admission, and regularly thereafter, for the risk of developing deep vein thrombosis (DVT)/venous thromboembolism (VTE). Utilize clinically appropriate methods to prevent DVT/VTE.

18. Utilize dedicated anti-thrombotic (anti-coagulation) services that facilitate coordinated care management.

19. Upon admission, and regularly thereafter, evaluate each patient for the risk of aspiration.

20. Adhere to effective methods of preventing central venous catheter-associated blood stream infections.

21. Evaluate each pre-operative patient in light of his or her planned surgical procedure for the risk of surgical site infection, and implement appropriate antibiotic prophylaxis and other preventive measures based on that evaluation.

22. Utilize validated protocols to evaluate patients who are at risk for contrast media-induced renal failure, and utilize a clinically appropriate method for reducing risk of renal injury based on the patient's kidney function evaluation.

23. Evaluate each patient upon admission, and regularly thereafter, for risk of malnutrition. Employ clinically appropriate strategies to prevent malnutrition.

24. Whenever a pneumatic tourniquet is used, evaluate the patient for the risk of an ischemic and/or thrombotic complication, and utilize appropriate prophylactic measures.

25. Decontaminate hands with either a hygienic hand rub or by washing with a disinfectant soap prior to and after direct contact with the patient or objects immediately around the patient.

26. Vaccinate healthcare workers against influenza to protect both them and patients from influenza.

27. Keep workspaces where medications are prepared clean, orderly, well lit, and free of clutter, distraction, and noise.

28. Standardize the methods for labeling, packaging, and storing medications.

29. Identify all "high alert" drugs (e.g., intravenous adrenergic agonists and antagonists, chemotherapy agents, anticoagulants and anti-thrombotics, concentrated parenteral electrolytes, general anesthetics, neuromuscular blockers, insulin and oral hypoglycemics, narcotics and opiates).

30. Dispense medications in unit-dose or, when appropriate, unit-of-use form, whenever possible.

progress, finding alternative designs for the work itself, and testing changes rapidly and informatively. It also requires a high
degree of trust in many forms, a bias toward teamwork, and a
predilection toward shouldering the burden of improvement,
rather than blaming external factors. (p. 12)

In Hudson's (2003) discussion of the safety practices of organizations in high-risk industries, he describes their organizational cultures as being characterized by being informed, wary, just, flexible, and learning. He also presents an evolutional model of the
development of patient and safety cultural maturity that pro-
gresses through five stages:

- Pathological (Who cares as long as we're not caught.)
- Reactive (Safety is important, we do a lot every time we have an accident.)
- Calculative (We have systems in place to manage all hazards.)
- Proactive (We work on the problems that we still find.)
- Generative (Safety is how we do business round here.) (p. 19)

Barber, Rawlins, and Franklin (2003), in their paper examining
ways to reduce prescribing error, argue for changes in organizational cultures " . . . which do not support the belief that prescribing is a complex, technical, act, and that it is important to get it
right" (p. 129).

Finally, in our work examining medication administration error
(MAE) reporting by nursing staff, we found markedly different perceptions of the percentages of MAE being reported. We have consistently found four organizational cultural categories of reasons
for not reporting: disagreement over what constitutes an error;
amount of effort it takes to report an error; fear of being perceived
by peers, physicians or patients as being incompetent; and the
nature of the administration's response when errors are reported
(Wakefield et al., 1996, 1998, 1999a, 1999b, 2000, 2001). Each of the
categories has strong implications for organizational and professional cultures.

Making things more complex, many health care organizations
(particularly hospitals) are composed of several different cultures.
These include the culture of the overall organization, as well as cultures of the major subunits (e.g., clinical and support service
departments, nursing units, clinics) and specific patient care

teams. In addition, there are also specific cultures reflecting the values, beliefs, and priorities of a host of different health care professions (e.g., medicine, nursing, pharmacy, allied health) and managers. In the best of all worlds, these cultures work in concert to define, assess, and make necessary adjustments as quickly as possible to ensure the provision of high quality and safe patient care. At worst, these organizational cultures are in conflict over defining what is high quality and safe patient care, how to assess quality and safety, and making appropriate and timely changes. Both IOM reports, *To Err is Human* and *Crossing the Quality Chasm*, indicate that much remains to be done to align all of the many cultures to ensure the provision of high quality and safe patient care. Hiam (1992) has noted, "The culture of an organization is not always apparent . . . until it becomes an obstacle to progress"(p. 157) (AHRQ, http://grants.nih.gov/grants/rfa-files/RFA-HS-01-0003.html). Without understanding and managing the many organizational and professional cultures at play in health care organizations, the ability to move from the status quo to make major improvements in quality and patient safety is limited. Put another way, "An organization is a system, with a logic of its own, and all the weight of tradition and inertia. The deck is stacked in favor of the tried and proven way of doing things and against the taking of risks and striking out in new directions" (John D. Rockefeller, *The Second American Revolution*, 1973).

## Provide the Necessary Data and Tools: Invest in IT, Analytic Capacity and Decision Support

Improving health care quality is not just about collecting more data. Rather it requires the ability to convert that data into something useful. Davis and Meyer (1998) provide a framework that can enhance our understanding of the relationships between quality improvement and the concepts of data, information, and knowledge. They argue that data become useful information only after they have been processed or analyzed in some way to derive meaning. In our case, data from several difference sources (e.g., lab values, patient history, and physical examination) are combined and processed to generate useful information, the diagnosis. The diagnosis is then used to develop and guide a specific treatment plan for a particular patient. A challenge faced by all health care providers and organizations is how to convert individual patient information into more generalized knowledge that could be used for similar patients or throughout the organization.

To successfully achieve the transformation of data into information, and information into knowledge requires significant investment in health care organizations' information technologies (IT) and the analytic and decision support capabilities. Today, several health care organizations and systems have made great progress in developing computer-based comprehensive electronic medical records which gather intensive amounts of data including not only the specific services provided (e.g., diagnostic and therapeutic procedures, nursing care, pharmaceutical use), but also detailed clinical data (e.g., specific lab values, vital signs, risk factors).

Because of the tremendous increase in the amount of specific clinical data being collected and the ability to automatically analyze it, it is now possible to have automated, real-time clinical care monitoring and decision support services. A prime example currently receiving considerable attention in hospitals are Computerized Physician Order Entry (CPOE) systems. CPOE has been widely touted as a potential solution to medication prescribing errors. True CPOE systems are more than simply enabling a physician to use a computer to order a patient's medication. True CPOE systems simultaneously analyze a patient's discrete data elements from several different sources (e.g., laboratory, physician notes, pharmacy, and nursing notes, including the medication administration record) to evaluate the potential appropriateness of a physician's medication order *at the time the order is initially made.* That is, it provides computerized decision support by applying specified decision algorithms to the available data in order to determine if there are any potential contraindications.

The logic behind using computers as a way of addressing the complexity of medication ordering is compelling. While CPOE has been enthusiastically endorsed by purchaser groups such as the Leapfrog Group, relatively few hospitals currently have true CPOE systems. The primary reason is that most hospitals currently have a mix of IT systems from different vendors that use software packages that do not communicate with each, and thus are unable to create a single computer file containing all the needed data. Retooling a hospital's existing IT systems is extremely expensive, and third-party payers typically do not provide additional payments for IT investments. However, among the emerging P4P initiatives, four hospital-targeted and two physician-targeted initiatives noted above (http://ir.leapfroggroup.org/compendiumselect.cfm, accessed July 6, 2004) are conducting early experiments in providing quality bonuses for IT infrastructure investments such as CPOE and electronic health records.

## Measure What You Manage: Disciplined Use of QI Methodology

With an organizational culture centered on providing high quality and safe patient care supported by an IT and analytic infrastructure, the stage is set to sharpen the focus of quality care and patient assessment and improvement efforts. Such a sharpened focus requires two things: prioritization of what is important to monitor and manage, and the disciplined use of quality improvement approaches.

### What to Measure

If one assumes that what is measured gets managed, then the choice of measurement indicators and metrics is critical. For example, one could focus on specific processes of care for selected types of patients such as found with the CMS Voluntary Hospital Reporting Initiative. Likewise, an outcomes orientation could be used in which specific outcome indicators such as mortality, functional status, patient satisfaction, and/or resource use for specific diseases or conditions could be monitored on an ongoing basis. One could also focus on error-related indicators that could be used to monitor a hospital's total patient population or subcategorized to track specific patient care service lines or patient care units. Sentinel events, "unexpected [occurrences] involving death or serious physical or psychological injury, or the risk thereof" (JCAHO, 2004), could also be used as a primary focus. Examples of sentinel events include patient suicides, wrong-site surgery, medication errors, and transfusion errors.

In leading the national quality improvement and safety research agenda, the Agency for Healthcare Research and Quality has identified and defined three primary categories of error-related indicators that might be used for ongoing monitoring (http//:www.ahrq.gov). The first, *Medical Errors*, are defined as: "The failure[s] of a planned action to be completed as intended or the use of a wrong action to achieve an aim. . . . Errors can include problems in practice, products, procedures, and systems" (http://

grants.nih.gov/grants/rfa-files/RFA-HS-01-0003.html). Note, that medical errors may include both acts of *commission and omission*. Next are *Adverse Events*, defined as: "*Undesirable and unintended incidents in care that may result in adverse outcomes, or may require additional care efforts to thwart an adverse outcome*" (http://grants.nih.gov/grants/rfa-files/RFA-HS-01-0003.html). Because adverse events do not always result in harm to the patient, organizations must make the strategic decision as whether they will collect, analyze, and act in the absence of harm. Focusing only on adverse events causing harm will result in ignoring critical information about potential weaknesses in the way care is currently being provided. Finally, *Near Misses* are defined as: "*Events in which the unwanted consequences were prevented because there was a recovery by identification and correction of the failure. Such a recovery could be by a planned or unplanned barrier*" (p.677) (AHRQ, http://grants.nih.gov/grants/guide/rfa-files/RFA-HS-01–00003.html, accessed July 8, 2004).

Near miss data raise the interesting question of whether, and to what extent, it is useful to track things that almost happened. The potential value of near miss data has been dramatically demonstrated in the aviation and nuclear power industries, and potentially other industries such as health care, requiring high reliability production processes. Several potential advantages of supplementing adverse event and error reporting with near miss reporting have been identified: (a) Near misses are thought to occur much more often than actual adverse events or errors and thus enhance the use of quantitative analytic strategies; (b) near misses have fewer barriers to reporting because of a shift in focus *from the occurrence of an adverse event or error to how the occurrence of an adverse event or error was prevented*; (c) a focus on prevention allowing for systematic learning about how recovery from the potential error was achieved; and (d) a reduction in hindsight bias (Van der Schaaf et al., 1991).

There are a growing but limited number of near miss health care applications. These include a focus on blood transfusions (Callum et al., 2001; Ibojie & Urbaniak, 2000; Kaplan et al., 1998; Linden & Wagner, 2000; Battles et al., 1998), anesthesia (Runciman et al., 1993), and medication safety (Schmidt & Bottoni, 2003). Examples of near misses in health care might include a patient *nearly* getting the wrong medication, defective equipment *nearly* being used to provide patient treatment, and clarification of communications among patient care team members that prevented an error. At issue is to what extent near miss data and information enhance a health care organization's ability to improve quality and enhance the safety of its patient care processes.

Regardless of which categories of indicators are selected, the question arises as to the extent to which the organizational culture and data collection systems capture all the indicators of interest. There are a number of limitations associated with most existing adverse event and error reporting systems. Most of these systems were designed to emphasize accountability at the expense of learning. This emphasis includes (a) risk management orientation emphasizing the reporting of known major adverse events and errors rather than minor adverse events and near misses; (b) participation in comparative reporting systems motivated primarily by external groups' (i.e., JCAHO, purchaser groups, and state facility licensure agencies) requirement that health care organizations obtain comparison information; (c) organizations failing to systematically assess the quality of their internal "reporting cultures" as a means of gauging how well the adverse event and error reporting systems are working; and (d) use of adverse event and error data as part of individual performance appraisals rather than as opportunities to learn about reducing systems-related adverse events and errors.

Although unintended, the design of many organizational policies, practices, and cultures has incorporated adverse event and error reporting primarily within risk management programs at the expense of quality and performance improvement. The result has been a major barrier to adverse event and error reporting, and greatly reduced opportunities for open and positive learning experiences.

In summary, some basic questions to consider when evaluating the validity, reliability, and usefulness of the health care quality and patient safety related indicators actually being used to improve practice include the following.

- To what extent does your organization rely on automated systems to measure quality or detect and report patient safety problems?
- To what extent do the processes used to measure quality or report patient safety problems rely on individual physician, nurse, or other health care provider's decisions and actions?

- To what extent does the combination of organizational and professional cultures present enhance or reduce the validity, reliability, and usability of the care quality and patient safety indicators?
- What percent of errors, adverse events, or near misses do you want to be reported?
- To what extent will quality and patient safety indicator information be used for accountability versus organizational learning purposes?

### Quality Improvement Methodologies

In conjunction with the decision about what to measure, it is also critical for health care organizations to adopt a consistent quality improvement methodology. These methodologies typically provide an iterative framework and tools for analyzing existing processes or problems, developing and testing interventions, and continued monitoring and evaluation for potential subsequent revisions. Examples of such methodologies range from the process-specific focused PDCA (Plan-Do-Check-Act) cycle developed by Shewhart and endorsed for widespread use by Deming (http://www.dartmouth.edu/~ogehome/CQI/PDCA.html), to the more organization-wide Six Sigma (http://www.isixsigma.com/), ISO-9000 (http://www.iso.ch/iso/en/ISOOnline.frontpage), and Baldridge National Quality Program (http://www.quality.nist.gov/).

Regardless of the QI method or approach taken, each shares several commonalities. Each approach was widely used in nonhealth-care organizations prior to their adoption in health care settings. Each approach also relies on the use of similar types of data collection and analytic tools to evaluate production or patient care processes of interest. Among the most common tools for collecting and displaying data are focus groups, surveys, check sheets, logs, histograms, Pareto charts, trend charts, and run charts (Leebov & Ersoz, 1991). Tools commonly used to making improvement include flowcharts, brainstorming, affinity charts, relationships diagrams, cause-and-effect diagrams, force-field analysis, decision matrices, and tree diagrams (Leebov & Ersoz). Finally, each approach emphasizes the need for ongoing monitoring and intensified study if performance problems emerge. While it is beyond the scope of this chapter to discuss in detail the variety of specific quality improvement approaches or methodologies that might be used, APPENDIX 15B offers the reader a number references containing more detailed discussion and applications of QI.

## APPENDIX 15B

### Selected References For Additional study

#### Quality Improvement Tools and Methods

Al-Assaf, A. F., & Schmele, J. A. (1993). *The textbook of total quality in health care*. Delray Beach, FL: St. Lucie Press.

Boonan, K. J. (1995). *The Juran Prescription*. San Francisco, Jossey-Bass.

Donnell, A., & Dellinger, M. (1990). *Analyzing business process data: The looking glass*. Indianapolis: AT&T Quality Steering Committee.

Gaucher, E. J., & Coffey, R. J. (2000). *Breakthrough performance: Accelerating the transformation of health care organizations*. San Francisco: Jossey-Bass.

Kelly, D. L. (2003). *Applying quality management in healthcare: A process for improvement*. Chicago: Health Administration Press.

Langley, G. J., Nolan, N. M., Nolan, T. W., Norman, C. L., & Provost, L. P. (1996). *The improvement guide: A practical approach to enhancing organizational performance*.

Leebov, W., & Ersoz, C. J. (1991). *The health care manager's guide to continuous quality improvement*. Chicago: American Hospital.

Lighter, D. E., & Fair, D. C. (Eds.). (2004). *Quality management in health care: Principles and methods* (2nd ed.). Boston: Jones & Bartlett.

Longo, D. R., & Bohr, D. (1990). *Quantitive methods in quality management*. Chicago: American Hospital.

Moen, R. D., Nolan, T. W., & Provost, L. P. (1999). *Quality improvement through planned experimentation* (2nd ed.). New York: McGraw Hill.

#### Change Management

Ashkansay, N. M., Wilderom, C., & Peterson, M. F. (Eds.). (2000). *Handbook of organizational culture and climate*. Thousand Oaks, CA: Sage.

Blumenthal, D., & Scheck, A. C. (Eds.). (1995). *Improving clinical practice: Total quality management and the physician*. San Francisco: Jossey-Bass.

Dlugacz, Y. D., Restifo, A., & Greenwood, A. (2004). *The quality handbook for health care organizations: A manager's guide to tools and programs*. San Francisco: Jossey-Bass.

Jick. T. D., & Peiperl, M. A. (2003). *Managing change: Cases and concepts* (2nd ed.). Boston: McGraw Hill.

Weick, K. E., & Sutcliffe, K. M. (2001). *Managing the unexpected: Assuring performance in an age of complexity*. San Francisco: Jossey-Bass.

## Create Learning Organizations: Invest in Staff Knowledge and Skills

Health care organizations have a unique opportunity to improve patient safety and the quality of care by tapping into the knowledge of its workers and by studying near miss data. In nonhealth care organizations, organizational development and learning strategies have helped sharpen the focus on ways to more effectively and efficiently extract and share what is already known or might be learned about the HCO. Examples from other literature include Davenport and Prusak's framework for understanding the differences among data, information, and knowledge in the context of knowledge management within organizations, Senge's (1994) *Fifth Discipline*; deGeus's (1997) *The Living Company*; Pfeffer and Sutton's (2000) *The Knowing-Doing Gap*; and O'Dell and Grayson's (1998) *If Only We Knew What We Know*.

Central to this rapidly expanding body of literature is the basic question of how organizational productivity, including the value, quality, and safety of health care services and products can be enhanced through the creation of learning organizations. Potential answers to this question include the first three strategies discussed earlier in this section: understanding the organizational culture; having the necessary data and analytic tools; and systematically measuring what we hope to manage. Beyond these three are additional strategies that can be helpful in building health care organizations that learn: making quality and safety the core competencies; focusing professional educational on what matters; and considering quality improvement as fundamental to every organizational initiative.

## Quality and Safety As Core Competencies

Whose job is it to ensure that the patient care services being provided are high quality and safe? Everyone for whom the answer is yes must have the specific relevant quality and safety competencies explicitly specified as part of their position descriptions and roles within the organization. At a minimum we would encourage that, in addition to the specific technical competencies associated with a particular position, additional competencies include the ability to interpret and use specific types of quality and patient safety related information being generated in their particular part of the organization. Depending on the level of supervisory or managerial responsibility, additional competencies might include conducting basic process analyses, leading quality/safety improvement teams, and designing, implementing, and testing interventions. For every manager, specific competencies related to change management skills are essential. After all, inherent in any effort to improve quality or patient safety is the desire to create meaningful and appropriate change in the way things are done. While beyond the scope of this chapter to discuss change management issues and tactics, Appendix B provides some suggested references for those desiring to learn more about this topic.

### Organizational and Professional Educational as an Opportunity for Quality Improvement

Each year health care providers and organizations invest significant amounts of resources in ongoing education. Most state licensure laws require that licensed health care professionals complete a minimum amount of professional education each year. This continuing education is generally offered by outside organizations and is frequently paid for by health care organizations. In addition, these same organizations also provide a variety of in-house educational programs designed to improve their staff's knowledge of specific legal, administrative, and patient care related processes and skills. Continuing education costs include not only the direct expenses of attending external educational programs (e.g., registration fees, travel, hotel) and of internal educational programs (e.g., program preparation and delivery), but also paid time away (e.g., participant salary and benefits, and replacement worker salary and benefits). Depending on the size and nature of the health care organization, the combined investments in external and internal continuing education programming can range from several thousands to millions of dollars each year. Ironically, few if any hospitals have ever calculated their annual educational expenditures or the return on investment.

To date, many health care organizations have not maximized the educational investments being made in their personnel. Take for example external continuing education programs used to meet state professional licensure requirements. There is generally wide latitude in the educational programming content that qualifies for credit towards meeting the licensing requirement. Even if the choice of types of educational programs the staff might attend is restricted to educational content related to the type of unit in which they work, the specific educational content may not have much to do with the specific types of services being offered, or the types of care for which the unit is have difficulty providing in a high quality or safe manner. Few hospitals have developed comprehensive plans for targeting both external and internal continuing education investments on what matters most to improve quality and safety. Implicit in creating effective learning organizations is aligning educational investments and strategies with patient care quality and safety priorities. That is, focusing learning on what matters.

### Quality Improvement as Fundamental to Every Organizational Initiative

An additional strategy to consider when creating learning organizations is to view every organizational initiative as an opportunity to improve quality. This is true regardless of whether the initiative is focused on improving service excellence, reducing nosocomial infections, making new IT investments, or carrying out revenue and supply chain management initiatives. Consider the recent development of supply chain management initiatives.

### Persist: Quality Is Not a Fad

There are no quick quality improvement fixes in healthcare. The challenge of providing high quality, individualized, appropriate, and effective health care services within the dynamic internal and external environments is daunting. Daily minor and true crises stemming from uncertainty in dealing with changing financial, regulatory, and legal requirements can and do distract clinical and nonclinical leaders' focus on improving quality. Without fully integrating a commitment to quality into the organization's culture, organization-wide efforts to improve quality run many of the same risks of failure as management fads.

It is no longer sufficient for a provider or health care organization to simply proclaim that only the best quality care is given. Rather, there is an increasing demand for proof. The P4P quality improvement initiatives is but one of the markers of this change. Accompanying P4P is the rapid growth of consumer driven health care initiatives that by shifting an increasing share of the economic costs of health care to the patient will further stimulate the demand for valid, reliable, and meaningful information differentiating quality among providers. Therefore, persistence in integrating quality concerns and implications into every decision is essential if quality gains are to be maintained.

Persistence in improving the quality of health care must become everyone's job.

## CASE STUDY

You are the CEO of a large academic medical center located in a highly competitive health care market. Recently there have been major changes in the membership and leadership of your Board of Trustees. Among others on the Board, the new Board Chairwoman, who is also president of a Fortune 500 company, is very insistent that your academic medical center publish its quality data for all product lines as a way of improving patients' and third-party payers' ability to assess whether they are receiving/paying for high quality care. As such, you have been instructed to prepare a plan for publicly reporting and publishing your institution's quality data.

As you prepare the plan what are your options in addressing the following issues and questions?

1. Who is the intended audience for these data, and how might that change the kinds of quality related data that you will publish?
2. Should both hospital and physician quality related data be reported?
3. To what extent will the publicly reported quality data reflect structure, process, and outcome indicators?
4. Will quality data be presented just for your facility, or in comparison with other providers? If in comparison with other providers, which providers represent the most appropriate comparisons?
5. In what ways will you account for comparisons to dissimilar organizations?

## DISCUSSION QUESTIONS

1. Third-party payers such as Medicare, Medicaid, and commercial insurance traditionally pay for hospitals and physicians separately for the patient care services being provided. To what extent, and how, does paying hospitals and physicians separately either facilitate or inhibit the provision of care that is safe, effective, patient-centered, timely, efficient, and equitable?
2. As a member of the Board of Trustees of a 500-bed community hos-

pital, you have been given the chairmanship of the newly created
Quality and Safety Board of Trustee's Subcommittee. The subcommittee is charged with the responsibility to monitor and make recommendations to the full board regarding quality of care and safety
issues.

- What are the key questions that you must address in determining
  what to monitor?
- In what ways will the specific indicators that you select to monitor as a Board subcommittee be similar to, and different from,
  the quality and safety indicators already being used at the individual physician, clinic or unit, department, and hospital-wide
  levels?

3. Frequently, new patient care technologies, such as the drug-eluting
   stents, are very costly and third-party payers are not willing to pay
   hospitals for the full incremental costs associated with their use.

   - Would you conclude that the quality of care in your hospital is
     lower if you decide to not use the new technology because the
     reimbursement is inadequate?
   - Is it ethical to use the new technology for only some, but not all,
     patients who might benefit from the new technology because of
     third-party reimbursement practices?

4. Pay-for-Performance (P4P) as a strategy for improving quality is an
   appealing concept. As a self-insured employer providing health care
   benefits for over 100,000 covered lives, you are very interested in
   implementing a P4P system.

   - What are the potential advantages and disadvantages of develop-
     ing your P4P incentives targeted on structures, processes, and
     outcomes?
   - What portion of hospital or physician total payments should be
     based on specific P4P incentives?

## REFERENCES

Agency for Healthcare Research. (2004). Accessed July 8, 2004 at
http://grants.NIH.gov/grants/guide/RFA-files/RFA-HS-04–012.html

Bailit Health Purchasing. (2001). The growing case for using physician
incentives to improve health care quality. National Health Care
Purchasing Institute. Accessed July 12, 2004 at http://www.bailit-
health.com/articles/index.shtml

Bailit Health Purchasing. (2002). Ensuring quality providers: A purchaser's toolkit for using incentives. National Health Care Purchas-

ing Institute. Accessed July 12, 2004 at http://www.bailit-health.com/articles/index.shtml

Baker, G. (2003). Pay for performance incentive programs in healthcare: Market dynamics and business process. Accessed July 12, 2004 at http://www.medvantageinc.com/documents/MVP4PWP_TOC2.pdf

Barber, N., Rawlins, M., & Franklin, B. D. (2003). Reducing prescribing error: Competence, control, and culture. *Quality & Safety in Health Care, 12*(Suppl. 1), i29–i31.

Battles, J. B., Kaplan, H. S., Van der Schaaf, T. W., et al. (1998). The attributes of medical event reporting systems: Experience with a prototype medical event reporting system for transfusion medicine. *Arch Pathology Laboratory Medicine, 122,* 231–238.

Berwick, D. M. (2003). Improvement, trust, and the health care workforce. *Quality & Safety in Health Care, 12*(Suppl. 1), i2–i6.

Callum, J. L., Kaplan, H. S., Merkley, L. L., Pinkerton, P. H., Fastman, B. R., Romans, R., et al. (2001). Reporting of near-miss events for transfusion medicine: Improving transfusion safety. *Transfusion, 41,* 1204–1211.

Chin, M. H., & Muramatsu, N. (2004). What is the quality of quality of medical care measures. *Rashomon-Like Relativism and Real-World Applications, 1*(1), 5–20.

Davenport, T. H., & Prusak, L. (1998). *Working knowledge: How organizations manage what they know.* Boston: Harvard Business School Press.

Davis, S. M., & Meyer, C. (1998). *Blur: The speed of change in the connected economy.* New York: Warner Books.

Donabedian, A. (1980). *Explorations in quality assessment and monitoring: The definition of quality and approaches to its assessment* (Vol. I). Ann Arbor, MI: Health Administration Press.

de Geus, A. (1997). *The living company: Habits for survival in a turbulent business environment.* Boston: Harvard Business School Press.

Duncan, D. D. (1993, December). The big picture: Anatomy of a $64,589 medical bill. *Life,* 15–19.

Endsley, S., Kirkegaard, M., Baker, G., & Murcko, A. C. (2004). Getting rewards for your results: Pay for performance programs. American Academy of Family Physicians. Accessed July 12, 2004 at http://www.aafp.org/20040300/45gett.html

Ferguson, J. A., Tierney, W. M., Westmoreland, G. R., Mamlin, L. A., Segar, D. S., Eckert, G. J., et al. (1997). Examination of racial differences in management of cardiovascular disease. *Journal of the American College of Cardiology, 30,* 1707–1713.

Fisher, E. S. (2003). Medical care—Is more always better? *New England Journal of Medicine, 349*(17), 1665–1667.

Gordon, H. S., & Rosenthal, G. E. (1995). Impact of marital status on outcomes in hospitalized patients. *Archives of Internal Medicine, 155,* 2465–2471.

Hiam, A. (1992). *Closing the quality gap: Lessons from America's leading companies.* Englewood Cliffs. NJ: Prentice Hall.

Hudson, P. (2003). Applying the lessons of high risk industries to health care. *Quality & Safety in Health Care,* 12(Suppl. 1), i7–i12.

Ibojie, J., & Urbaniak, S. J. (2000). Comparing near misses with actual mistransfusion events: A more accurate reflection of transfusion errors. *British Journal of Haematology,* 108, 458–460.

Iezzoni, L. I. (2003). *Risk adjustment for measuring healthcare outcomes* (3rd ed.). Chicago: Health Administration Press.

Institute of Medicine (IOM) & Committee on Quality Health Care in America. (2000a). *To err is human: Building a safer health system.* L. T. Kohn et al., Eds. Washington, DC: National Academy Press.

Institute of Medicine (IOM) & Committee on Quality Health Care in America. (2001b). *Crossing the quality chasm: A new health system for the 21st century.* Washington, DC: National Academy Press.

Jha, A. K., Varosy, P. D., Kanaya, A. M., Hunninghake, D. B., Hlatky, M. A., Waters, D. D., et al. (2003). Differences in medical care and disease outcomes among black and white women with heart disease. *Circulation,* 108, 1089–1094.

Joint Commission on Accreditation of Healthcare Organizations (JCAHO). (2004). Sentinel events. Accessed July 6, 2004 at http://www.jcaho. org/accredited+organizations/ambulatory+care/sentinel+events/ glossary.htm

Kaplan, H. S., Battles, J. B., Van Der Schaff, T. W., & Mercer, S. (1998). Identification and classification of the causes of events in transfusion medicine. *Transfusion,* 38(1), 1071–1081.

Leatherman, S., et al. (2003). Making the business case for quality. *Health Affairs,* 22(2), 17–30.

Leebov, W., & Ersoz, C. J. (1991). *The health care manager's guide to continuous quality improvement.* Chicago: American Hospital.

*Lexicon: Dictionary of health care terms, organizations, and acronyms for the era of reform.* (1994). Oak Brook Terrace, IL: Joint Commission on Accreditation of Healthcare Organizations.

Linden, J. V., & Wagner, K. (2000). Transfusion errors in New York State: An analysis of 10 years' experience. *Transfusion,* 40(10), 1207–1213.

Malzer, R. L. (1988). Patient performance level during inpatient physical rehabilitation: Therapist, nurse, and patient perspective. *Archives of Physical Medicine and Rehabilitation,* 69, 363–365.

National Quality Forum. (2005). Safe practices for better health care. Accessed Jan. 6, 2004 at http://www.qualityforum.org/TXSAFEEX ECSUMM+ORDER6–8-03public.pdf

Nelson, G., Mohr, J., Batalden, P., & Plume, S. (1996). Improving health care, part 1: The clinical value compass. *The Joint Commission Journal on Quality Improvement,* 22(4).

O'Dell, C., & Grayson, Jr., C. (1998). *If only we knew what we know: The transfer of internal knowledge and best practice.* New York: Free Press.

Pfeffer, J., & Sutton, R. I. (2000). *The knowing-doing gap: How smart companies turn knowledge into action.* Boston: Harvard Business School Press.

Plsek, P. (2001). Redesigning health care with insights from the science of complex adaptive systems. In Institute of Medicine (Ed.), *Crossing the quality chasm: A new health system for the 21st century* (Appendix B, pp. 322–355). Washington, DC: National Academy Press.

Porter, M. E., & Teisberg, E. O. (2004). Redefining competition in health care. *Harvard Business Review, 82*(6), 64–77.

Riggs, J. E., Lithell, D. P., & Hobbs, G. R. (2002). In-hospital stroke mortality, hospital transfers, and referral beds at a rural academic medical center. *Journal of Rural Health, 18,* 294–297.

Rockefeller, J. D. (1973). *The second American revolution: Some personal observations.* New York: Harper & Row.

Rosenberg, A. L., Hofer, T. T., Strachan, C. J., Watts, M., & Hayward, R. A. (2003). Accepting critically ill transfer patients: Adverse effect on a referral center's outcome and benchmark measures. *Annals of Internal Medicine, 438,* 882–890.

Rosenthal, G. E., Harper, D. L., Quinn, L. M., & Cooper, G. S. (1997). Severity-adjusted mortality and length of stay in teaching and non-teaching hospitals. *Journal of the American Medical Association, 278,* 485–490.

Rubenstein, L. Z., Schairer, C., Wieland, G. D., & Kane, R. (1984). Systematic biases in functional status assessment of elderly adults: Effects of different data sources. *Journal of Gerontology, 39*(6), 686–691.

Runciman, W. B., Sellen, A., Webb, R. K., et al. (1993). Errors, incidents and accidents in anesthetic practice. *Anesthesia Intensive Care, 21,* 506–519.

Senge, P. M. (1994). *The fifth discipline: The art and practice of the learning organization.* New York: Doubleday/Currency.

Schein, E. H. (1992). *Organizational culture and leadership* (2nd ed.). San Francisco: Jossey-Bass.

Shine, K. (2001). 2001 Robert H. Ebert Memorial Lecture: Health care quality and how to achieve it. Milbank Memorial Fund. Accessed July 12, 2004 at http://www.milbank.org/reports/020130Ebert/020130Ebert.html

Stacey, R. D. (1996). *Complexity and creativity in organizations.* San Francisco: Berrett-Koehler.

Strunk, B. C., & Hurley, R. E. (2004). Paying for quality: Health plans try carrots instead of sticks. Accessed July 12, 2004 at http://www.hschange.com/CONTENT/675/675.pdf

TrendWatch. (2003). Paying for performance: Creating incentives for quality improvement. Accessed July 12, 2004 at http://www.lewin.com/NR/rdonlyres/eyzniiua4jsqz6v7patsjmd54vlkjol

4ifb64ilsanyeiphentkgkwchchwlm4shfvhojnxwo554be/Vo15No3.pdf

Van der Schaaf, T. W., Lucas, D. A., & Hale, A. R. (Eds.). (1991). *Near miss reporting as a safety tool.* Oxford: Butterworth-Heinemann, Elsevier.

Wakefield, D. S., Wakefield, B. J., Uden-Holman, T., & Blegan, M. A. (1996). Perceived barriers in reporting medication administration errors. *Best Practices and Benchmarking in Healthcare,* 1(4), 191–197.

Wakefield, B. J., Wakefield, D. S., Uden-Holman, T., & Blegan, M. A. (1998). Nurses' perception of why medication administration errors occur. *MEDSURG Nursing* 7(1), 39–44.

Wakefield, D. S., Wakefield, B. J., Borders, T., Uden-Holman, T., Blegen, M., & Vaughn, T. (1999a). Understanding and comparing differences in reported medication administration error rates. *American Journal of Medical Quality,* 14(2), 73–80.

Wakefield, D. S., Wakefield, B. J., Uden-Holman, T., Borders, T., Blegen, M., & Vaughn, T. (1999b). Understanding why medication administration errors may not be reported. *American Journal of Medical Quality,* 14(2), 81–88.

Wakefield, B., Wakefield, D. S., & Uden-Holman T. (2000). Improving medication administration error reporting systems. *Ambulatory Outreach* (Spring), 16–20.

Wakefield, B., Blegen, M., Uden-Holman, T., Vaughn, T., Chrischilles, E., & Wakefield, D. S. (2001). Organizational culture, continuous quality improvement, and medication administration error reporting. *American Journal of Medical Quality,* 16(4), 128–134.

Wyatt, S. M., Moy, E., Levin, R. J., Lawton, K. B., Witter, D. M., Valente, E., et al. (1997). Patients transferred to academic medical centers and other hospitals. *Academic Medicine,* 72, 922–930.

Zimmerman, B. Lindberg, C., & Plsek, P. (1998). *Edgeware: Insights from complexity science for health care leaders.* Irving, TX: VHA.

# 16

## ACCESS TO CARE

John Billings and
Joel C. Cantor

SINCE THE EARLY twentieth century, the U.S. health care system has struggled to assure access to health care services for all Americans. There have been major steps forward: the growth of private, employer-based health insurance following World War II, the passage of the Medicare and Medicaid programs in 1965, and the growth of federal programs in the 1970s to expand direct service programs (such as community health centers) for low-income patients helped improve access for many. But the debate surrounding the proposed Clinton Health Reform Plan of 1993 and its subsequent failure illustrate the difficulties that are entailed in making further progress.

Access is often viewed as a one-dimensional problem: too many Americans lack health insurance coverage. By this measure, approximately 44 million persons were estimated to be uninsured in 2002—more than 15% of the U.S. population (U.S. Census Bureau

[USCB], 2003). That number is closer to 45 million in 2005. More-over, the situation has actually deteriorated over the past 25 years, with the rates of the uninsured growing.

The potential impact of lack of insurance on patients is obvious and well documented—delaying or forgoing needed care can lead to adverse health outcomes, and the costs of obtaining necessary care can be financially ruinous (Hadley, 2003). The impact that large numbers of uninsured patients have on the health care delivery system is also serious, as providers of uncompensated care struggle to have other payers subsidize the expense incurred by patients without coverage. These efforts by providers can create structural distortions in the health care delivery system, steering uninsured patients toward "safety-net" providers, further increasing the costs of care for these patients, undermining the financial integrity of many institutions, and reinforcing the development of a two-tiered health care delivery system in many communities. With the expansion of managed care and the emergence of stronger market forces, the situation is expected to get worse.

The problem of access itself, however, is enormously more complex than insurance coverage. An insurance card alone does not eliminate barriers to access. First, there are issues of the extent and adequacy of coverage. Are outpatient services covered as well as inpatient care? Are prescription drugs included? Mental health and substance abuse services? What about long-term care? And what about the levels of copayments and deductibles? As many as 29 million Americans are estimated to be "underinsured," with levels of coverage inadequate to assure financial access to care (Short & Banthin, 1995). Another important factor is the adequacy of payments to providers made by third-party payers. For example, low payment levels to physicians have historically plagued the Medicaid program, discouraging participation of many private physicians and limiting where Medicaid patients can receive care.

In addition, patients with an insurance card can also face serious noneconomic barriers to care that can have a dramatic effect on access, utilization patterns, and health outcomes. The delivery of care remains largely disconnected, creating substantial barriers for many users. Moreover, to the extent that the health care delivery system fails to respond to differences in language, culture, health care beliefs, care-seeking behavior, or educational levels, additional impediments to access can be created. These nonfinancial barriers are often aggravated for low-income patients by quasi-economic barriers. Obtaining timely care for a child may require that a parent get off work, forgo wages, arrange child care for siblings, or get transportation—all of which may be difficult for families with limited resources or who are socially isolated.

In this chapter, the nature and extent of all of these barriers to care are examined. In the next section, economic barriers to care are explored, including an overview of the characteristics of the uninsured, a discussion of problems associated with extent and adequacy of coverage, and an examination of the consequences that lack of adequate insurance has on patients and providers. In the following section, barriers other than economic are described, and their impact documented. In the final section, reforms are examined, their potential impact and limitations are discussed, and future issues related to access are explored.

## ECONOMIC BARRIERS TO CARE

### Identifying the Uninsured

It is important to note that the level of uninsurance among the elderly is very low (0.8%), reflecting the impact of the Medicare program that provides almost universal coverage for Americans age 65 and over (see TABLE 16.1). Although there are important limitations in coverage for the elderly and some noneconomic barriers for this population, the Medicare program has done much to reduce barriers to access for the elderly. Among the nonelderly, the highest rates of uninsurance are among the young adult population (ages 18 to 34). The higher rates among these age groups reflect two important factors: a dependence on employer-based coverage for private insurance, and the impact of the federal/state Medicaid program. When employers in the U.S. fail to provide or offer insurance to their workers, or when an individual becomes unemployed, the risk of becoming uninsured increases enormously. The cost of individual coverage is prohibitive for most persons without coverage, especially low-income workers or the unemployed. Young adults have higher rates of unemployment, are often recent entrants to the workforce (often with lower wage/part-time jobs).

Young adults also often have difficulty establishing eligibility for Medicaid coverage, which varies among states. Medicaid eligibility is limited to low-income persons who fall into one of the following eligibility categories: child, elderly, blind/disabled, preg-

## TABLE 16.1

### Persons Without Health Insurance Coverage by Demographic Characteristics

| CHARACTERISTIC | PERCENTAGE OF TOTAL UNINSURED | PERCENTAGE WHO ARE UNINSURED |
|---|---|---|
| Total | 100.0 | 15.2 |
| Male | 53.5 | 16.7 |
| Female | 46.4 | 13.9 |
| < 18 | 19.6 | 11.6 |
| 18–24 | 18.7 | 29.6 |
| 25–34 | 22.4 | 24.9 |
| 35–44 | 17.9 | 17.7 |
| 45–64 | 20.9 | 13.5 |
| 65+ | 0.6 | 0.8 |
| Non-Hispanic White | 47.7 | 10.7 |
| Black alone | 16.6 | 20.2 |
| Asian alone | 4.9 | 18.4 |
| Hispanic (of any race) | 29.2 | 32.4 |
| Native US | 74.3 | 12.8 |
| Foreign Born | 25.7 | 33.4 |
|    Citizen | 5.2 | 17.5 |
|    Noncitizen | 20.5 | 43.3 |
| < $25,000 annual income | 33.9 | 23.5 |
| $25,000–$49,999 | 33.6 | 19.3 |
| $50,000–74,999 | 15.8 | 11.8 |
| $75,000+ | 16.7 | 8.2 |
| Northeast | 16.2 | 13.0 |
| Midwest | 17.3 | 11.7 |
| South | 40.8 | 17.6 |
| West | 25.7 | 17.1 |
| < High School | 22.4 | 28.0 |
| High School | 29.1 | 18.8 |
| Some College (no degree) | 14.3 | 15.0 |
| Associate Degree | 4.5 | 12.1 |
| Bachelor's or Higher | 10.1 | 8.4 |

SOURCE: U.S. Census Bureau (2003). *Health Insurance Coverage in the United States: 2002.*

nant woman, single parent, or unemployed parent (in some states). Employed parents or childless adults simply cannot become eligible for Medicaid, regardless of income (unless they become blind, disabled, or pregnant), although some states provide coverage through state-financed programs (home relief, medically indigent, etc.) for some of these noncategorically eligible individuals. The targeted nature of the Medicaid program is also reflected in the lower rates of uninsurance for children (categorically eligible) and women (more likely to be single parents or to become eligible through pregnancy).

Most uninsured persons work at least part-time. About 85% of the uninsured live in households where the family head has been employed during the past year. Accordingly, the problem of uninsurance is typically due to the failure of an employer to offer insurance or to the refusal of coverage by an employee. The highest rates of uninsurance are among nonprofessional or managerial occupations in the retail, service, construction, and agricultural sectors, with much higher rates of uninsurance among small employers (and the self-employed). Low-wage earners (incomes less than 200% of the federal poverty level) represent more than half of the working uninsured and have rates of uninsurance (37.8% uninsured) more than 6 times greater than higher income workers (6.0%) (see **TABLE 16.2**).

Rates of uninsurance also differ significantly among states. For example, less than 9% of the population is uninsured in Iowa, Rhode Island, Minnesota, and Wisconsin, while rates of uninsurance are above 20% in Texas and New Mexico (USCB, 2003). In addition to the categorical requirements noted above for Medicaid coverage (children, aged, blind/disabled, etc.), there are also minimum income standards for eligibility. These standards are set by the states and have been historically tied to welfare payment levels,[1] again with considerable differences among states.

The profile of the typical uninsured person might be a young adult in a low-wage job working for a small employer in the retail/services sector. Accordingly, any realistic solution to the problem of uninsurance cannot be dependent on the uninsured themselves—more than half of the uninsured earn less than 200% of the federal poverty level (USCB, 2003). The uninsured tend to be in the weakest sectors of the economy, among smaller employers, with very low wage levels. Adding insurance coverage would represent a large percentage increase in labor expense for these employers, and resistance to "reform" among these groups. The situation

---

1 Recent federal reforms have broken this link and given states more flexibility in setting eligibility standards.

## TABLE 16.2

### Nonelderly Workers Age 18–64 without Insurance Coverage Employment Characteristics—2002

| CHARACTERISTIC | PERCENTAGE OF TOTAL UNINSURED | PERCENTAGE WHO ARE UNINSURED |
|---|---|---|
| Total | 100.0 | 18.1 |
| Full time/Full Year | 56.4 | 14.8 |
| Full time/Part Year | 21.1 | 27.0 |
| Part-time/Full Year | 11.6 | 23.7 |
| Part-time/Part Year | 10.9 | 23.4 |
| Professionals/Managers | 19.0 | 9.3 |
| Agriculture | 0.7 | 20.5 |
| Construction | 1.6 | 16.7 |
| Finance | 1.2 | 6.4 |
| Health and Social Services | 1.9 | 7.1 |
| Information, Communication & Education | 2.4 | 6.4 |
| Mining/Manufacturing | 1.2 | 5.3 |
| Professions | 2.8 | 9.8 |
| Public Administration | 0.4 | 3.6 |
| Services | 3.3 | 18.8 |
| Utilities/Transportation | 0.4 | 6.9 |
| Retail/Wholesale Trade | 3.2 | 13.2 |
| Other Occupations | 81.0 | 23.2 |
| Agriculture | 1.9 | 42.7 |
| Construction | 12.4 | 37.8 |
| Finance | 2.8 | 14.0 |
| Health and Social Services | 6.5 | 16.8 |
| Information, Communication, & Education | 3.3 | 12.9 |
| Mining/Manufacturing | 8.3 | 17.0 |
| Professions | 8.6 | 28.9 |
| Public Administration | 0.9 | 7.2 |
| Services | 19.6 | 34.6 |
| Utilities/Transportation | 4.2 | 19.1 |
| Retail/Wholesale Trade | 12.4 | 21.5 |
| Self-Employed | 13.7 | 26.3 |
| < 25 Workers in Private Firms | 35.0 | 31.2 |
| 25–99 | 13.8 | 20.7 |
| 100–499 | 9.6 | 14.6 |
| 500–999 | 2.9 | 11.7 |
| 1000+ | 19.3 | 12.6 |
| Public Sector Workers | 5.9 | 7.3 |
| < 100% Poverty | 22.8 | 48.9 |
| 100–199% | 32.0 | 37.8 |
| 200–399% | 30.3 | 17.3 |
| 400%+ | 14.9 | 6.0 |

SOURCE: The Kaiser Commission on Medicaid and the Uninsured. (2003). *Health Insurance Coverage in America—2002 Data Update.*

is likely to worsen—small employers in the services and retail sectors are where much of recent job growth has occurred.

The profile of the uninsured at a point in time is informative but insufficient for developing strategies to expand coverage. For example, would providing coverage to seasonal workers between jobs or unemployed significantly reduce the percentage of the population without coverage? Or would providing an extra 6 or 12 months of coverage for Medicaid or SCHIP coverage for individuals entering the workforce reach many of the uninsured? To answer these and related questions, analysts have used longitudinal studies to characterize individuals' transitions in and out of health coverage. Longitudinal surveys of the uninsured are revealing on several counts. First, many more individuals go without coverage over a period of time than show up in the annual statistics. One estimate from a four-year study showed that nearly 85 million are without coverage for at lease one month, more than double the number identified in studies taken at a single point in time (Short & Graefe, 2003). That same study showed that only about 12% of those uninsured during the 1996–1999 study period were without coverage throughout the four-year study. This suggests that for many, uninsurance is transitory while for others it is a long-term proposition. More than half of this study cohort was uninsured for a year or less, and about one in four of those ever uninsured during the period lacked coverage for four months or less. These data show that the uninsured are a heterogeneous lot, and no single policy (short of universal government insurance) is likely to address all of their coverage needs.

## Underinsurance and Other Limitations of Coverage

An insurance card does not always assure financial access to care, as private insurance often excludes mental health services, preventive care, and long-term care. Most plans have exclusions or waiting periods for preexisting conditions that were present at the time of enrollment. These limits affect those most in need of coverage and subject them to substantial financial risk if workers change jobs. Many plans also lack adequate coverage for catastrophic illnesses, with maximum lifetime benefit limits too low to cover the costs of serious illness or accident. Moreover, virtually all private insurance plans, even most managed care plans, have some form of copayment or deductible, which can have the effect of discouraging patients from seeking needed preventive care, especially lower income patients most sensitive to out-of-pocket costs.

While almost 97% of Americans over age 65 have Medicare coverage, the program has substantial patient cost-sharing provisions and serious gaps in coverage. The deductible is more than $850 for hospital care and $110 for outpatient care, with substantial co-payments (20%) also required in many cases. Moreover, until 2006 Medicare will provide virtually no coverage for outpatient prescription drugs. Medicare also has substantial restrictions on long-term care (only 2% of nursing home costs of the elderly are paid by Medicare). As a result of these limitations in coverage, Medicare is estimated to pay less than 50% of the total costs of health care for the elderly. Many elderly have supplemental coverage for some of these expenses (Medi-Gap plans), either through their employer/retirement plan or by purchasing such coverage directly. More than 20% of the elderly (35% of low-income elderly) have no supplemental coverage, however, exposing them to serious financial risks, and potentially creating substantial barriers to access.

Low-income elderly qualify for coverage by Medicaid. Medicaid coverage is generally very comprehensive, covering most services (including drugs and long-term care) and having few restrictions or copayments. However, Medicaid suffers from serious problems of provider nonparticipation. While hospitals historically have been guaranteed payment levels that were reasonably related to costs, physician payments are set by state administrative agencies facing staggering increases in program costs. Not surprisingly, payment levels for physicians and other noninstitutional providers have often been set below market rates. For example, in New York, the office-based physician payment rate for an "intermediate office visit" was set at $11, a level unchanged since 1985.

The most significant federal health coverage expansion since the enactment of the State Children's Health Insurance Program (SCHIP) addresses the problem of underinsurance for the elderly and disabled, rather than the problem of uninsurance in the nonelderly population. The Medicare Prescription Drug, Improvement, and Modernization Act of 2003 contained a broad range of provisions, at the center of which is drug coverage under a new Part D of Medicare beginning in 2006. Under this law, coverage is provided for prescription drugs through competing pharmacy benefit managers. The new benefit is "means tested," with substantially more generous benefits for low-income beneficiaries. Very low income beneficiaries (with incomes less that 135% of the federal poverty level) have no premium payments or deductibles, with modest co-payments depending on the level of annual prescription expenses. For non-low income beneficiaries, the level of coverage is substantially less generous. For persons with incomes above 150% of poverty, there will be a $35/month premium and an annual deductible of $250. The level of copayment is dependent on the amount of drug expenses incurred during the year. For the first $2,250, the copayment level is 25%. Between $2,250 and $5,100, the copayment is 100%—the so-called "donut hole." Above $5,100, Medicare pays 95% of drug expenditures. Accordingly, beneficiaries must have drug costs in excess of $810 before benefits exceed out-of-pocket expenses for premiums, the deductible, and copayments. The effective level of copayment (including premium, deductible, and copayments) exceeds 20% until drug expenditures reach $25,000. The median annual prescription expense of Medicare beneficiaries is about $2,000 (Cooper & How, 2004), where out-of-pocket expenses for patients who elect to enroll in the program will be 55% (http://www.kff.org/medicare/rxdrugscalculator.cfm; accessed July 12, 2004).

## The Impact of Economic Barriers to Care

For patients, the impact of the lack of insurance can be profound (Hadley, 2003). Uninsured patients are less likely than those who are privately insured to have a usual source of care (24% vs. 8%). Among patients with health problems, uninsured patients are more likely to have had no physician visits during a 12-month period than those with private insurance (22% vs. 9%) and to have had fewer average number of physician contacts (9.1 vs. 14.8)—and these differences persist, even after adjusting for socioeconomic status among the insured and uninsured (Millman, 1993).

The impact of coinsurance on utilization is also significant, especially among lower income patients. While one goal of coinsurance is to discourage frivolous utilization, lower rates for preventive services (such as immunizations for children or screening tests for cervical cancer for adult women), suggest that these barriers to care affect other utilization as well.

The lack of insurance can also affect hospital utilization. Uninsured patients are more likely to be admitted for preventable/avoidable conditions, such as asthma, diabetes, cellulitis, or other infections (Billings & Teicholz, 1990). In one study, hospitalized uninsured patients were found to have substantially lower rates for common diagnostic tests (colonoscopy, endoscopy, coronary arteriography, etc.) and for costly surgical procedures (bypass surgery, joint replacement, eye surgery, etc.), even after controlling for sociodemographic and diagnostic case-mix factors (Hadley, Steinberg, & Feder, 1991).

Although it is difficult to document the effect of insurance status on health status and health outcomes, since the lack of insurance tends to be somewhat episodic (with individuals going on and off of insurance periodically), substantial differences for the uninsured have been observed. Uninsured mothers have been found to begin prenatal care later and to have fewer total visits than privately insured mothers (Braveman, Egerter, Bennett, & Showstack, 1991), and uninsured newborns have been shown to have more adverse outcomes than babies with insurance (Braveman, Oliva, & Miller, 1989). Uninsured women have also been found to present with later stage breast cancer than privately insured patients and have lower survival rates (a 49% higher risk of death among uninsured patients) (Ayanian, Kohlker, & Toshi, 1993).

Most dramatically, overall mortality rates for uninsured patients have also been shown to be higher than for those with insurance. In a study of a national cohort of patients between 1971 and 1987, uninsured patients were found to have a 25% increased risk of dying during the study period, even after adjusting for differences in sociodemographic characteristics, general health status, and health habits (Franks, Clancy, & Gold, 1993).

Although the cost of uninsurance and underinsurance is high in human terms, there is also a serious impact on the health care delivery system that can affect all patients. First, distortions in utilization patterns can increase total costs. While uninsurance promotes underutilization, it also has the effect of steering uninsured patients to providers who are willing to provide care regardless of ability to pay. These providers tend to be institution-based providers, such as hospital outpatient departments, emergency rooms, and community-based clinics. Costs in these institution-based settings are often higher, therefore increasing total costs for the health care delivery system.

Potentially worse are the financial disequilibriums these utilization patterns can create for providers. Providers serving large numbers of uninsured patients must cover the costs of unreimbursed care. These same providers usually serve substantial numbers of Medicaid patients for whom costs of care often exceed reimbursement rates, which may subject them to arbitrary payment limits and restrictions. These expenses can either be "cost-shifted" to other payers (by raising charge levels for these payers sufficiently above actual costs to raise enough revenue to cover unreimbursed expenses), or providers can seek government or private subsidies. Although some states have established elaborate pooling systems to offset some of these costs and many publicly operated providers receive direct subsidies, in most jurisdictions providers are dependent on the cost-shift. Today, market forces make cost-shifting less viable. Managed care plans steer their patients to facilities with lower charges, making cost-shifting even more difficult, as the base of paying patients shrinks and even larger increases in charges are required to shift costs. The wholesale movement of Medicaid patients into managed care plans that has begun in most states will further worsen this situation for many providers.

The impact of hospital closures and provider failures on access to care for low-income patients may be serious. The providers most at risk are those with the highest levels of care to vulnerable populations. With the loss of these traditional safety-net providers, it is not clear that these patients will be assured access to needed care from the remaining providers, who may be located further away and who have previously avoided provision of care to these patients.

# NONECONOMIC AND QUASI-ECONOMIC BARRIERS TO CARE

## Comparing Medicaid Coverage

The impact of uninsurance on health outcomes and utilization has been previously documented—though, in many of these studies it was not possible to analyze Medicaid patients separately. Rates of preventable hospitalizations for Medicaid patients were below those of uninsured patients, but were still found to be almost 75% higher than the rate for insured patients (Billings & Teicholz, 1990). Incidence of late detection of breast cancer and survival rates for cancer among the uninsured and Medicaid patients were found to be comparable (Ayanian et al., 1993), and pregnant women on Medicaid had rates of late initiation of prenatal care and average total prenatal care visit rates similar to those of uninsured mothers (Braveman et al., 1991). For these patients, Medicaid coverage failed to eliminate all barriers to needed care. Vulnerable populations face special problems in dealing with the complexities of our fragmented health care delivery system, creating impediments to timely and effective care for many.

## Race/Ethnicity

Large and persistent differences in health status, utilization, and outcomes among racial and ethnic groups are well documented. Black and Hispanic/Latino populations have been shown to be less likely to have a usual source of primary care, to have fewer physician visits, higher rates of no/late prenatal care, lower rates of immunizations and screening tests, and worse self-reported health status. Large racial differences have also been documented in rates for infant mortality, low-birthweight infants, late-stage diagnosis of cancer, and mortality from all causes (Council on Ethical and Judicial Affairs, 1990; Fiscella, Franks, Gold, & Clancy, 2000; Millman, 1993).In American society, socioeconomic status and race/ethnicity are intertwined, and research has attributed a part, but not all, of racial/ethnic disparities in health to socioeconomic conditions. A growing body of research that attempts to control for socioeconomic and other factors, suggests that minority status itself is an important determinant of utilization and health outcomes. For example, after adjusting for differences in insurance coverage, minority adolescents were found to be less likely to have a usual source of primary care, to have fewer annual physician contacts, and lower levels of continuity of care (Lieu, Newacheck, & McManus, 1993). Among children enrolled in managed care plans, minority status was linked to lower rates of utilization, even after controlling for differences in health status (Riley, Finney, & Mellits, 1993).

In other research that could adjust for insurance coverage differences, African Americans with end-stage renal disease have been found to be 50% less likely to receive kidney transplants, and those ultimately receiving surgery had been on waiting lists significantly longer than nonminority patients (Gaston, Ayres, Dooley, & Diethelm, 1993). Similarly, among patients with coronary artery disease, Black patients have been found to receive fewer angiographies and to have lower rates of coronary artery bypass surgery controlling for insurance status and disease severity (Johnson, Lee, & Cook, 1993).

Similar differences in rates for invasive cardiac procedures have also been observed for Hispanic/Latino populations (Carlisle, Leake, Brook, & Shapiro, 1996). A study of patients visiting a trauma center emergency room with bone fractures found that nonHispanic Whites were more than twice as likely to receive pain medication as Hispanic patients, even after accounting for patient differences in injury severity, pain assessment, insurance status, gender, and language (Todd, Lee, & Hoffman, 1994; Todd, Samaroo, & Hoffman, 1993). Other studies have documented additional differences among Hispanic/Latino subgroups, with Mexican American, Puerto Rican, and Cuban American populations experiencing different rates of no usual source of care, no preventive care, and no physician visits (Council on Scientific Affairs, 1991).

Large racial/ethnic disparities in utilization have also been observed within the Medicare program. African American beneficiaries have fewer physician visits and lower rates of preventive care, such as influenza immunizations. African Americans with Medicare coverage also have lower rates for many diagnostic procedures (such as CT scans, barium enema x-rays, mammography, etc.), surgical procedures (coronary bypass, prostatectomy, hysterectomy, orthopedic surgery, etc.), and other services (Friedman, 1994; Gornick et al., 1996). Even within the Veterans Administration hospital system, White veterans have been shown to be significantly more likely to receive coronary surgery than Black veterans (Whittle, Conigliaro, & Good, 1993).

Of course, there are many potential explanations for these differences in utilization, outcomes, and health status associated with race/ethnicity. In research, controlling for factors such as socioeconomic status, education, disease incidence/prevalence, illness severity, resource availability, and even insurance coverage can be extraordinarily difficult, and interpretation of these research findings must be tempered by recognition of these methodologic limits. However, these differences by race/ethnicity are substantial and persistent across numerous studies that use a variety of research designs. But even isolating race as the determining factor in these differences leaves many unknowns. The impact of overt or latent racial/cultural bias at all levels of the health care delivery system cannot be discounted, however. A landmark study in which a large sample of physicians were presented with computerized patient scenarios in which actors were interviewed about their hypothetical chest pain showed that race and sex were important independent determinants of physicians' decisions to refer patients for advanced diagnostic procedures. That study showed that referral rates for cardiac catheterization were lower for women and Blacks (84.7% of each group) compared to White men (90.6%) (Schulman et al., 1999). However, further research is required to understand more about the factors that contribute to or mediate any bias, and to identify how patient preferences (e.g., in weighing risks and benefits of medical intervention), care-seeking behavior, and attitudes toward the health care delivery system affect utilization and outcomes.

Managed care offers the hope of establishing a "medical home" for all enrollees, but it may erect other barriers to appropriate care. In one national survey, African American, Asian, and Hispanic respondents with private coverage were 25 to 100% more likely than their White counterparts to lack a usual source of care, but these differences were much smaller between minority and White members of managed care plans. In contrast, minority managed care members were much more likely to report dissatisfaction with their usual source of care compared to minority members of traditional (nonmanaged care) health plans, while dissatisfaction among Whites was low whether they were in managed care or not (Phillips, Mayer, & Aday, 2000).

## Culture/Acculturation/Language

The effect of culture and acculturation on health care use and outcomes is not well understood. It is often hypothesized that cultural barriers may contribute to lower or less optimal utilization patterns by Hispanic/Latino and Asian immigrant populations in the U.S. These barriers can involve a broad range of potential problems, including social isolation, distrust of Western medicine, unfamiliarity with the U.S. delivery system, differences in concepts of disease/illness, alternative care-seeking behaviors, perceptions of provider disrespect, fears about immigration status, or language difficulties.

Several studies have attempted to evaluate how increased acculturation tends to ameliorate these impediments to access. This research is limited by the difficulty of assessing levels of acculturation. One of the better designed studies suggests that language proficiency may be either the best indicator of acculturation or the most important component of these cultural factors in facilitating access. In that study, better language skills resulted in more use of preventive services such as physical exams, cancer screening, and dental checkups (Solis, Marks, Garcia, & Shelton, 1990).

Of course, acculturation itself may create new problems and new barriers. For example, many immigrant families have stable family structures, including strong intergenerational ties. To the extent that these relationships become more attenuated in urban America, the ability to cope with the requirements of managing a health condition or chronic disease may be impaired.

## Gender

Less research has been conducted on gender-related barriers to health care. Similar differences in rates of procedures have been documented, however, with female end-stage renal disease patients less likely to receive a kidney transplant than male patients (Held, Pauly, & Bovberg, 1988; Kjellstrand, 1988). Women have also been shown to have lower rates of cardiac surgery than men (Udvarhelyi, Gatsonis, & Epstein, 1992), although these differences were not associated with higher mortality rates for women (raising an important issue about whether access to more surgical care is always beneficial).

Again, the impact of patient preferences and attitudes toward risk/benefit when considering surgical and diagnostic procedures requires further study to understand their influence on utilization rates. However, there are three emerging lines of research that underscore the potential seriousness of gender-related impediments to health care for women. First, it is well established that women have historically been systematically excluded from clinical trials for new drugs and procedures (Cotton, 1990a, b). The impact of bias in medical research is not yet fully established, but the potential is obvious. To the extent that medical practice is based on findings of medical research, many practitioners may be reluctant to prescribe medications or recommend surgical/diagnostic procedures that have not been fully tested for women. Accordingly, access to newly emerging drugs and technologies may be delayed for women, and resource utilization patterns significantly altered. But the corollary also raises serious concerns: when care provided to women is based on research that has been generalized from gender-biased studies, it may be inappropriate, creating impediments to optimal medical care for women.

A second body of research has begun to document how physician gender can affect practice patterns and utilization rates of care for women. For example, in one study of preventive care, it was documented that patients of female physicians were more than twice as likely to receive cervical cancer screening tests (Pap smears) and 40% more likely to receive mammograms than women whose physicians were male (Lurie, Slater, & McGovern, 1993). Again, the full impact of how differences in physician gender can influence the care provided to female patients has not yet been determined. While the number of female physicians is growing, the potential for serious barriers to needed health care services for female patients is large.

Finally, many women do not have access to family planning, abortion counseling, or abortion services. There are explicit restrictions on use of Medicaid funds for these services, and many religiously affiliated providers simply do not offer such services. Moreover, the aggressive tactics of many antiabortion groups has deterred many providers from offering these services and discouraged many women from seeking care. Medicaid and provider restrictions tend to affect low-income patients disproportionately since they are likely to have fewer alternatives, but the chilling effect of politicization of abortion-related care affects access for all women (Henshaw, 1995; Mathews, Ribar, & Wilhelm, 1997; Rosenblatt, Mattis, & Hart, 1995).

## Education

As with other indirect barriers to health care, it is difficult to isolate and quantify the effect of education on health care utilization and outcomes. Parental education deficits, however, have been shown to be associated with lower levels of well-baby and other preventive services (Short & Lefkowitz, 1992), and lower overall use by their children (Newacheck, 1992). Differences in education have also been linked to lower rates of breast cancer screening, even after adjusting for a broad range of economic and sociodemographic factors (Lantz, Weigers, & House, 1997). In another study, Medicaid patients with limited education were found to be less likely to use preventive services, have greater difficulties following medical regimens, miss more appointments, and seek care later in the course of an illness (Weiss, 1994).

A growing body of research has begun to document the impact of "functional health literacy," or the ability to use reading, writing, and computational skills in typical, everyday patient situations, such as reading prescription labels, following diagnostic test instructions, or understanding treatment directions. Because 40 million Americans are estimated to be illiterate and another 50 million marginally literate (Kirsch, Jungeblut, Jenkins, & Kolstad, 1993), the potential impediments to timely and effective care are serious. In a study conducted in two public hospitals, 42% of patients could not understand directions for taking medication on an empty stomach, 26% could not comprehend information on an appointment slip describing the scheduled follow-up visit, and more than 25% could not follow instructions for preparing for a gastrointestinal radiological exam. Overall, almost 30% of patients using the facilities were determined to have inadequate functional health literacy, and another 14% to have only marginal levels (Williams, Parker, & Baker, 1995).

## Resource Availability/Performance

The supply of health care resources has obvious implications for access. In remote rural areas, the absence of a primary care practitioner, an obstetrician/gynecologist, or even a hospital can have a serious impact on the ability of area residents to obtain timely care (Kindig & Ricketts, 1991; Nesbitt, Connell, & Hart, 1990). In urban areas, supply issues are often more complex. There are huge differences in physician supply across and within communities that have been well documented (Cooper, 1995; Grumbach, 1995; Politzer, Harris, & Gaston, 1991), with some central city areas having serious shortages of practitioners.

The issue for access is availability of providers, however, not supply. Many large urban hospitals (and their associated medical office buildings) are located in or nearby lower income neighborhoods—but this proximity does not assure access. While many hospital outpatient departments accept patients without restrictions on ability to pay (or charge on a sliding-fee schedule), this is certainly not necessarily the case for the privately practicing physicians clustered nearby. Moreover, the low Medicaid reimbursement rates for physician visits noted previously discourage many of these physicians from participating in the Medicaid program, creating potential barriers even for Medicaid cardholders. Therefore, while a simple physician-to-population ratio for the areas surrounding these hospitals would suggest a sufficient supply, a substantial portion of the supply is simply not available to low-income residents.

There is little known about the performance of the primary care delivery system and access to care. Clearly a more efficient provider that can serve more patients has the potential to reduce barriers in its service area. But more important, providers can create care delivery approaches that reduce many of the indirect barriers to care discussed previously (e.g., eliminating language barriers, reducing wait times, developing a culturally sensitive environment, using telephone consultations more effectively, and developing more effective compliance techniques for chronic disease patients with literacy problems).

Recently, for middle-class medicine, patient satisfaction has become the focus of many health care delivery systems as they struggle to attract and maintain their patient base. These developments have spawned a mini-industry of researchers and consultants attempting to assist providers in becoming more responsive to this new world. A parallel effort needs to be targeted at understanding the indirect barriers to care for low-income patients and helping safety-net providers better adapt their care delivery approach to these needs. This is not yet on the horizon.

## NONECONOMIC AND QUASI-ECONOMIC BARRIERS/PREVENTABLE HOSPITALIZATIONS

As illustrated in many of the studies described previously, the impact of noneconomic and quasi-economic barriers on utilization patterns and health status can be substantial. A growing body of analysis has also begun to explore how barriers to primary care services can result in increased utilization of other health care services, such as more costly hospital care (Billings, Anderson, & Newman, 1996; Billings, Zeitel, & Lukomnik, 1993; Bindman et al., 1995; Weissman, Gatsonis, & Epstein, 1992).

This research is based on the simple premise that timely and effective primary care can often (a) prevent the onset of an illness (e.g., congenital syphilis, pertussis, tetanus, etc.), (b) control a condition before it becomes more acute (e.g., ear infections in children, urinary tract infections, dehydration, etc.), or (c) manage a chronic disease or condition to help reduce the chances of a serious flare-up (e.g., asthma, diabetes, congestive heart disease, hypertension etc.). To the extent that barriers exist for ambulatory care services, and that a patient may delay or be unable to obtain care, an illness or condition may deteriorate beyond control in an outpatient setting, resulting in the need for hospitalization for its effective management.

By analyzing hospital admission rates for diagnoses related to these conditions, referred to as ambulatory care sensitive (ACS) conditions, researchers have documented huge differences in rates among areas (see TABLE 16.3). Areas with high ACS rates have been found to have higher levels of self-reported barriers to access than low ACS rate areas (Bindman et al., 1995). Moreover, these differ-

| TABLE 16.3 | | | |
|---|---|---|---|
| **Preventable/Avoidable Hospitalizations, Ambulatory Care Sensitive (ACS) Admissions/1,000, Age < 65, 1990** | | | |
| | ALL ZIP/FSA AREAS | | |
| MSA | ACS ADMS PER 1,000 | ASSOCIATION WITH INCOME (RSQ) | RATIO LOW-INCOME/ HIGH-INCOME |
| Boston | 11.84 | 0.581 | 2.58 |
| Buffalo | 8.90 | 0.840 | 2.92 |
| Jersey City/Bergen/Passaic, NJ | 13.20 | 0.675 | 3.21 |
| Los Angeles | 10.34 | 0.518 | 2.09 |
| Miami | 10.90 | 0.371 | 1.58 |
| New York City | 15.16 | 0.663 | 3.13 |
| Newark | 14.48 | 0.827 | 3.51 |
| Oakland | 8.90 | 0.674 | 2.55 |
| Orlando | 10.29 | 0.557 | 2.36 |
| Portland | 6.85 | 0.586 | 2.59 |
| Rochester, NJ | 8.21 | 0.734 | 2.95 |
| San Diego | 7.15 | 0.756 | 2.64 |
| San Francisco | 8.55 | 0.633 | 3.70 |
| Seattle | 6.92 | 0.606 | 2.32 |
| Tampa/St. Petersburg | 9.63 | 0.513 | 2.05 |
| Hamilton | 7.25 | 0.409 | 1.58 |
| Ottawa | 7.43 | 0.672 | 1.79 |
| Toronto | 7.38 | 0.103 | 1.39 |

*More than 40% households with income < $15,000
**$20,000 Canadian $
AU: What is MSA? Also, no asterisks in table body; please add.

ences have been found to be strongly associated with area income, with more than 80% of the variation in admission rates among zip codes in some communities being explained by the percentage of low-income persons living in an area. Admission rates for ACS conditions in low-income areas have been found on average to be 2.5–3.5 times higher than more affluent areas, those associated with individual zip code in some low-income neighborhoods being as much as 20 times higher than rates in high-income zip code areas of the same community. (See **FIGURES 16.1** and **16.2** illustrating these differences.)

Of course, not all admissions for these ACS conditions are preventable. However, the extraordinarily high rates among low-income areas and the strong association between area rates and the level of poverty suggest that significant barriers to primary care exist in most low-income areas. Insurance coverage is undoubtedly an important factor—differences in rates among Canadian urban areas (with universal insurance coverage) have been found to be significantly lower than U.S. urban areas (Billings et al., 1996; see Table

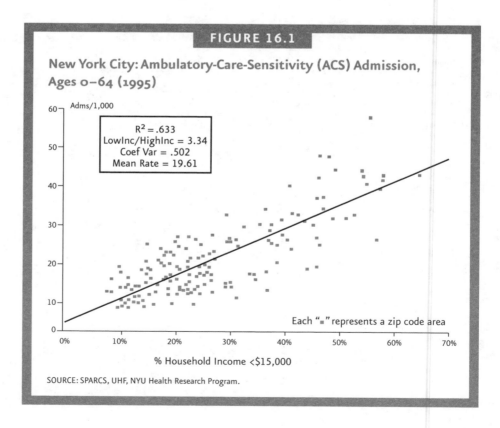

**FIGURE 16.1**

New York City: Ambulatory-Care-Sensitivity (ACS) Admission, Ages 0–64 (1995)

$R^2 = .633$
LowInc/HighInc = 3.34
Coef Var = .502
Mean Rate = 19.61

Adms/1,000

Each "■" represents a zip code area

% Household Income <$15,000

SOURCE: SPARCS, UHF, NYU Health Research Program.

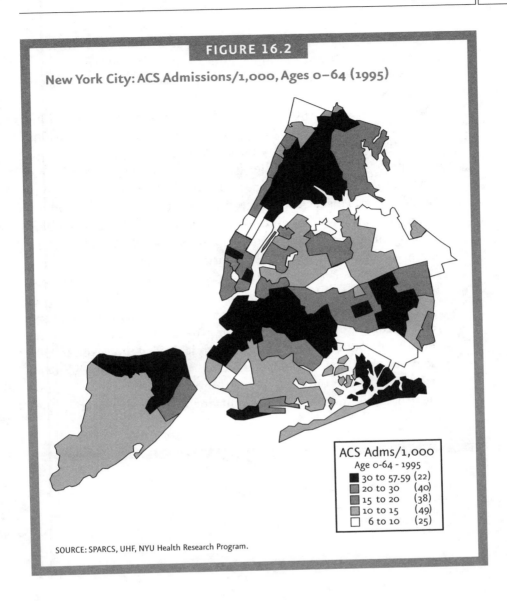

**FIGURE 16.2**

New York City: ACS Admissions/1,000, Ages 0–64 (1995)

ACS Adms/1,000
Age 0-64 - 1995
- ■ 30 to 57.59 (22)
- ▨ 20 to 30     (40)
- ▨ 15 to 20     (38)
- ▢ 10 to 15     (49)
- ☐ 6 to 10      (25)

SOURCE: SPARCS, UHF, NYU Health Research Program.

16.3). Nevertheless, lack of insurance coverage is unlikely to be the sole or even predominant cause for the disparities documented in most U.S. urban areas, since the overwhelming majority of low-income patients admitted had Medicaid coverage. The impact of the noneconomic and quasi-economic barriers discussed above is undoubtedly substantial. A low-income patient who has no regular source of care, who is dissatisfied with available providers (because of long wait times, language difficulties, or lack of cultural sensitivity), or who has difficulties arranging child care, getting off work, or simply coping with problems associated with illness, is clearly at significant risk of delaying or not getting needed care.

The potential relationship between these noneconomic factors and access is illustrated by the findings for ACS admission rates in Miami, Florida. Although like most U.S. urban areas, Miami has significant concentrations of poverty and minority populations, the difference in ACS admissions rates between low- and high-income areas is much smaller (only about 1.6 times higher in low-income areas), and the association between area rates and income is also lower. This lack of a large difference between hospital admission rates in low- and high-income areas is particularly evident among Cuban American persons' zip codes (see FIGURE 16.3), where admission rates were virtually identical, regardless of area income. In fact, in the other non-Latino persons' zip code areas, the association was comparable to other U.S. metropolitan areas (Billings et al., 1996). These data offer some promise that the noneconomic and quasi-economic barriers to care for other low-income persons are not insurmountable. Further research is needed, however, to help sort out the impact of various factors, such as the family/social structure of the Cuban American immigrant population, their health status and care-seeking behavior, and the organization/per-

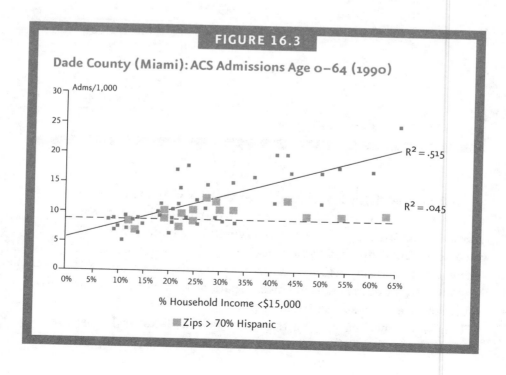

**FIGURE 16.3**

Dade County (Miami): ACS Admissions Age 0–64 (1990)

$R^2 = .515$

$R^2 = .045$

% Household Income <$15,000

■ Zips > 70% Hispanic

formance of the primary care delivery system servicing this population (including a substantial cadre of Cuban American physicians who also left Cuba).

The extent and nature of some of these indirect barriers to care are illustrated in a study of patients hospitalized for ACS conditions in New York City (Billings, Mijanovich, & Blank, 1997). In interviews after hospital admission and medical stabilization, 60.9% of low-income patients reported that they had received no care prior to the admission, and another 17.4% had received care only in the emergency room (compared with 31.4% of higher income patients receiving no care and 5.8% with only emergency room care). More than half of low-income patients reported that they had delayed or not obtained needed care (compared with about one fourth of higher income patients). The leading explanations for delay or the failure to obtain care among low-income patients were not directly related to the costs of care (the overwhelming majority had Medicaid coverage) but rather to a range of social and quasi-economic problems reflecting the difficulties encountered by low-income patients and their families in their daily lives and in negotiating the complexities of the health care delivery system. Over 25% of adult patients indicated they were "too nervous or afraid," "too busy with other things," or simply "not up to going," reflecting their serious ambivalence about the health care delivery system. Substantial numbers also reported difficulties arranging child care, problems with transportation, concern about having to wait too long, uncertainty about where to go, or apprehensions that providers wouldn't understand their needs (see TABLE 16.4).

These nonfinancial barriers to timely and effective care are substantial and serious. It is clear that successful interventions go beyond simply providing an insurance card to the uninsured. Part of the solution will require development of a health care delivery system that recognizes that low-income patients are struggling with many other aspects of their lives (as well as their health care problems)—these patients are "busy with other things" and do have difficulty getting off work or arranging child care. Longer clinic hours, home visits, and special outreach may be required to better serve them. Many of these problems necessarily will require that social service, education, and other programs become more responsive to the needs of these populations.

## TABLE 16.4

Type of "Access" Problems Reported by Low-Income Patients
Hospitalized for Preventable/Avoidable Conditions

| ACCESS PROBLEM | PERCENTAGE OF LOW-INCOME PATIENTS WITH "ACCESS" PROBLEM WHO REPORTED TYPE OF REASON* | | |
| --- | --- | --- | --- |
| | 6 MOS–17 YRS. | 18–64 YRS. | ALL AGES |
| Not up to going | 5.1 | 36.1 | 29.2 |
| Too nervous or afraid | 10.2 | 33.8 | 28.6 |
| Unable to get free time to get care | 8.1 | 27.2 | 22.9 |
| Had to wait too long to get appointment | 20.3 | 20.4 | 20.4 |
| Problems with child care | 32.8 | 14.3 | 18.2 |
| Costs too much | 13.8 | 18.1 | 17.2 |
| Unable to keep medical appointment | 7.4 | 20.2 | 17.1 |
| Couldn't fill prescription | 16.4 | 16.9 | 16.8 |
| Transportation difficulties | 19.3 | 15.8 | 16.5 |
| Didn't know where to go to get care | 8.6 | 13.8 | 12.7 |
| Not sure provider would understand needs | 22.4 | 9.1 | 12.2 |
| Care not available when needed it | 11.3 | 12.1 | 12.0 |
| Denied care | 13.4 | 9.7 | 10.6 |
| Didn't like usual place to get care | 17.2 | 7.9 | 9.9 |
| Lose pay/trouble getting off work | 12.1 | 6.0 | 7.3 |
| Language problem | 1.8 | 4.7 | 4.3 |

*NOTE: Percentages total more than 100% because some patients indicated multiple reasons.
SOURCE: Hospitalized Patient Interview Study, United Hospital Fund.

# HEALTH CARE REFORM: IMPROVING ACCESS

## At the Federal Level: Failure of Comprehensive Reform

In 1992 public support for some form of national health insurance
reached a 40-year high of 66%. During the presidential election of
that year, voters ranked health care as the third most important
issue facing the nation after the economy and the federal budget
deficit. By the time President Clinton took office in 1993, the issue
had risen to second place, with 90% of Americans indicating they

believed there was a crisis in health care (Blendon, Brodie, & Benson, 1995).

Clinton responded by appointing a task force that developed a proposal for a "Health Security Act" in the fall of 1993. The plan assured coverage for a comprehensive benefits package for almost all Americans. The elderly would continue to be covered by Medicare. The plan excluded undocumented immigrants and prisoners. However, coverage for everyone else would be provided through competing plans that would administer enrollment, collect premiums, and pay participating health plans. The cost of coverage would be made affordable for low-income and high-cost individuals through a system of mandatory subsidies. Large employers (5,000+ employees) could opt out, but would be required to offer comparable coverage from an array of competing plans and would be assessed a 1% payroll tax to support medical education and care for low-income/high-cost individuals insured in regional health alliances.

The restructuring of the health care marketplace by inducing competition among competing health plans was expected to help control health costs, but there was also a mechanism to impose caps on premiums if costs began to rise more than expected. The proposal also included other provisions to help reduce barriers to access. Expanded funding was to be provided for public health services and for programs to support "essential" community providers. This latter group included so-called safety-net providers, which have traditionally provided care to uninsured and Medicaid patients. The support for these entities was intended to assure continuation of patient outreach programs, and to ease the transition to a more competitive health care environment. The Clinton Health Plan avoided any new broad-based taxes to support the coverage expansions and premium subsidies, but rather relied on a combination of funding sources such as mandated employer contributions, Medicaid/Medicare savings (lower provider payments), assessments of large employers who opted out of alliances, and an increase in the tobacco tax. The expected costs of the program ($300+ billion by 2002) would be offset by these program savings and new revenues, making the proposed plan budget-neutral.

Of course, the plan failed. Large employers never supported the proposal, even though they were exempted from many of its requirements and the approach had promise of eliminating their financing of the cost-shift for uninsured patients embedded in their current premiums. Small employers were strongly opposed to the mandated coverage, although many would have been insulated from some of its effects by premium subsidies. Insurance companies strongly resisted the proposal, perhaps concerned that not all would survive in the competitive managed care environment contemplated by the approach of the alliances. Conservatives saw further encroachment of government into health care, with the complex system of quasi-governmental alliances and premium caps. Many liberals were concerned that the plan did not go far enough, or had discomfort with the concept of managed competition. Virtually everyone had reservations about the numbers: Was it really possible to create such a huge expansion of coverage and restructuring of the system without large amounts of new revenue?

The net effect of the failure of the Clinton Health Plan has been to virtually extinguish comprehensive health reform from the national public policy debates. Only 5% of voters in the 1996 elections indicated that reforming health care was a top issue for the new administration (Blendon, Benson, & Brodie, 1997). Since the 1996 elections, the percentage of Americans who rank health care (including Medicare) as one of the two most important issues for the government to address has fluctuated between about 10% and 20% (Blendon, Benson, Brodie, Altman, & James, 2000). Not surprisingly, the focus at the federal level has largely returned to consideration of incremental reforms and cost control. In 1996, the Kennedy-Kassebaum proposal was enacted to assure greater portability of insurance coverage when an employee changes jobs (an important issue for many middle-class workers, but having only a small effect on the 40+ million uninsured). The 1995–1997 budget battles focused primarily on how much savings can be extracted from Medicare and Medicaid. In fact, the Balanced Budget Act of 1997 included Medicare/Medicaid reductions of almost $140 billion (mostly from reduced payments to providers), an amount comparable to the $190 billion savings contemplated by the Clinton Health Plan. Of course, these savings were targeted for budget deficit reduction, whereas in 1993 the monies were intended to expand coverage for the uninsured and to broaden Medicare benefits.

However, two important features of the Balanced Budget Act of 1997 address access issues more directly and also provide a strong indication of the probable locus of near- and medium-term health reform activity. First, states obtained greater flexibility in the administration of Medicaid programs. Many states have begun to examine strategies to use managed care more effectively for Medicaid patients and/or to expand coverage to populations who are ineligible for Medicaid (because of the "categorical" requirements noted previously). These initiatives have historically required a discretionary federal "waiver," an uncertain process that usually caused substantial delay and inevitably entailed limitations on state initiatives. Under the new law, states are not required to obtain waivers for many of these reforms. While there are concerns that states may abuse this new flexibility, it will also undoubtedly encourage even greater state-level activity and innovation.

The Balanced Budget Act also included $24 billion to provide coverage for some of the estimated 10 million uninsured children in the U.S. through the State Children's Health Insurance Program (SCHIP). Again the action is at the state level, with funding distributed to states based on the number of low-income, uninsured children in the state, adjusting for differences in wages and the cost of health care. States can use the funding, which must be matched with local support (up to 35%, depending on current Medicaid match rates), to expand Medicaid coverage for children up to 200% of the poverty level or to create new programs targeted at providing coverage for low-income, uninsured children. Up to 15% of the funding can be used for direct service programs and outreach services. After a slow start, the SCHIP program has become a major new source of coverage in many states, extending health care coverage to over 4.3 million children (http://www.cms.hhs.gov/schip/enrollment/2004ever1qt.pdf; accessed July 18, 2004).

As SCHIP has matured, states have encountered challenges sustaining their progress. Recent budgetary constraints have led several states to freeze enrollment in their SCHIP programs. As of November 2003, Alabama, Colorado, Florida, Maryland, Montana, and Utah have all stopped enrolling eligible children in their respective programs (Cohen & Cox, 2004). One other state, New Jersey, has continued to enroll children in their program, but stopped enrollment of parents and other adults in SCHIP (www.statecoverage.net/schip-1115.htm; accessed July 21, 2004).

Since enactment of SCHIP, there has been little federal policy-making addressing health insurance coverage for the nonelderly uninsured. Nevertheless, the debate about how to address the still growing uninsured gap is active. Each of the presidential candidates in the 2004 election cycle proffered a proposal. The campaign of Democrat John Kerry proposed a coverage expansion over 10 years with new federal costs estimated between $653.1 billion and $1.3 trillion blending new tax subsidies and public program eligibility expansions. His opponent, Republican incumbent George W. Bush, proposed spending between $90.5 and $195.4 billion over the same period (Collins, Davis, & Lambrew, 2004). One analysis showed that the Kerry proposal would cover most of the uninsured, whereas the Bush proposal would lead to a reduction in the uninsured of about one third (Collins, Davis, & Lambrew, 2004).

Rather than emphasizing coverage expansions during the Bush Administration, Congress and the Administration promoted a policy of expanding direct funding for "safety net" providers. Congress established the Healthier Community Access Program (HCAP) within the Health Resources and Services Administration (HRSA), with an annual funding level of over $100 million, to provide grants to help safety net providers develop integrated, community-wide systems that serve the uninsured and underinsured. HCAP grants are typically intended to increase access to health care by eliminating fragmented service delivery, improving efficiencies among safety net providers, and by encouraging greater private sector involvement. Many HCAP models provide for integration of substance abuse and mental health treatment into the primary care model and have made social and human services organizations as well as the faith community their collaborative members (http://bphc.hrsa.gov/cap; accessed July 12, 2004). The Bush Administration has also promoted funding for HRSA's Community Health Center (CHC) Program, increasing appropriations from $1.3 billion in federal fiscal year 2002 to $1.63 billion in fiscal year 2004, with an proposed increase of $219 million (13.5%) for fiscal year 2005. These increases have funded the creation of more than 600 new or expanded community health centers across the country.

Tax policy options for promoting extending private coverage to the uninsured have long been supported by the Administration and conservatives in Congress. Tax policies have received renewed emphasis recently. President Bush and some of the Democratic candidates for President (including John Kerry and John Edwards) offered proposals to offer tax credits for health insurance for individuals or employers. Proponents of tax-subsidy strategies for promoting health coverage argue that they would avoid government mandates and limit the growth of public entitlement programs, which are very costly. Opponents counter that tax subsidies are not "target efficient" because much of the revenue lost to government as a result of tax breaks would go to individuals or businesses that already purchase coverage; they also cite studies that show that very large subsidies would be needed to induce voluntary purchase of coverage among the uninsured (Jackson & Trude, 2001).

## State Initiatives to Improve Access: Innovations and Limitations

Most state activities or proposed approaches fit into one of the following major categories: (a) initiatives to stimulate/facilitate voluntary action by employers or individuals to purchase insurance, (b) efforts to coerce employers to provide coverage ("pay or play" approaches), (c) support of direct services for uninsured (e.g., community-based clinics), and (d) purchase of coverage for targeted uninsured populations (with or without federal assistance).

Many of the initial efforts in the 1980s focused on coping with the apparent failure of the insurance market for small employers where rates of uninsurance were observed to be high (see Table 16.2). Because of the inherently high marketing costs for small employers and the difficulties of spreading risks for small groups, it was believed that new products needed to be developed that could lower premiums for small employers. Attempts were made to stimulate development of larger groups or cooperative purchasing pools that could centralize marketing and spread risks, giving small employers some of the advantages of larger employers and reducing premiums by 10 to 20%. While some of these initiatives have had some successes (Jacobson, Merritt, & Bartlett, 1994), most faced the difficult problem that for many small employers any premium was perceived as too much, and a relatively small number of small employers previously not providing coverage opted to purchase care from the pools.

Many states also established pools for high-risk individuals who could not get coverage in the private market because of their health status or history of high utilization. These programs have historically tended to reach only a small number of individuals. Without significant subsidies, the premiums for individuals using these pools is typically very high and beyond the means of many who are most in need. Second, the overwhelming majority of uninsured individuals lack coverage not because it has been denied for health reasons, but because their employer simply does not offer coverage and the individual insurance market is beyond their means.

While these voluntary efforts have met with only limited success, more coercive approaches have not fared well either. The approach considered by many states has been a "pay or play" strategy, where employers who do not offer coverage to their employees ("play") are assessed a tax ("pay") sufficient to support state-sponsored plans for uninsured workers. The goal is either to induce employers to offer insurance plans to their employees or to raise enough revenue to finance state-subsidized plans for employees of firms not offering coverage.

These approaches have faced two major obstacles: legal challenge and political feasibility. The legal challenge relates to the federal Employee Retirement Income Security Act of 1974 (ERISA), which has been interpreted to preempt state law in regulation of state employee benefit plans. To the extent that the "pay or play" requirement is interpreted as a mandate to provide coverage, it may be subject to legal challenge. The political obstacle is obvious—small employers strongly oppose the approach, even when subsidies or exemptions for new and very small employers are included. Of the several states that have considered or even initially legislated some variant of "pay or play," none has actually fully implemented the approach.

Initiatives to support direct services for the uninsured, such as community-based clinics, have generally fared better. The financial support typically goes to publicly operated facilities or, in some cases, to not-for-profit entities. Financing can come from general tax revenue, earmarked taxes (e.g., sales tax add-ons, tobacco/alcohol taxes, etc.) or from assessments on providers (usually hospitals). The smaller scale of these initiatives makes them more politically feasible, but also limits their reach. The federal government shares the cost of direct service support programs, particularly for hospitals, through Medicare and Medicaid disproportionate share (DSH) funding. Federal policy decisions in the late 1990s (most significantly through the Balanced Budget Act of 1997), however, have limited the availability of DSH payments, further limiting the reach of state direct provider subsidy programs.

The area that has generated the most interest at the state level is the last category, efforts to purchase coverage for targeted groups of the uninsured. In the 1990s, several states used the Section 1115 waiver process to expand Medicaid coverage to those groups that would otherwise not be "categorically" eligible or who are above income eligibility thresholds. These Section 1115 waiver coverage expansion initiatives attempt to avoid increasing total costs of the

Medicaid program (a requirement of the waiver) by use of managed care/provider payment limits (e.g., Tennessee) or by cutting the services covered by the program (e.g., Oregon). Through the late 1990s, state initiatives in health coverage reform held significant promise, but also had serious limitations. First, most were narrow in scope, typically reaching a relatively small portion of the uninsured. Of the 14 states with the most developed initiatives in 1995, only 5% of the total uninsured had been reached. Because of the targeted nature of these initiatives (children, pregnant women, etc.), even if they reached their enrollment goals, only about 20% of the uninsured would receive coverage, assuming current levels of uninsurance and no dropping of coverage to take advantage of the new programs (Lipson & Schrodel, 1996).

Moreover, the focus on children and pregnant women, although important and politically understandable, tends to overlook the more serious problems of uninsurance among the adult population, which often experiences the most serious barriers to access.

State initiatives were also often hindered by limits on revenue sources. General tax revenues are seldom a viable or reliable source, and initiatives are often dependent on a more limited potential revenue base of "sin taxes" (tobacco and alcohol excise taxes), earmarked sales taxes, or complicated provider "assessments." The undependability of state revenue shortfalls became evident in the early 2000s. In fiscal 2003, the cumulative shortfall in state budgets amounted to nearly $80 billion, and with nearly one in six dollars of state spending going to Medicaid and related programs, these programs were prime targets for savings. During that year, for instance, every state froze or reduced Medicaid provider payments and half reduce eligibility thresholds or froze enrollment (Kaiser, 2004). As well, as noted above, seven states stopped enrolling new, otherwise eligible children or adults in their SCHIP program (www.statecoverage.net/schip-1115.htm; accessed July 21, 2004). In addition, as recent federal budget reductions for welfare and Medicaid have begun to be felt at the state level, state budget problems have been exacerbated.

The Balanced Budget Act of 1997, despite a legislative intent to reduce federal financial liabilities, sparked renewed interest among the states in expanding coverage. Beginning in the late 1990s, states focused on implementing their SCHIP programs, part of the Balanced Budget Act. Following delays in program implementation, most states have fully operational SCHIP initiatives, and the federal government has offered increased flexibility to states to use SCHIP as a platform for expanding coverage beyond children under 200% of poverty. As of early 2004, as many as 39 states had extended SCHIP coverage to children to 200% or more of the federal poverty level (FPL). Six states extended eligibility to 300% of poverty or more, with New Jersey offering the most generous SCHIP eligibility limit at 350% FPL.

SCHIP addressed two major barriers to state policy to address the problem of the uninsured: lack of fiscal capacity and lack of technical competencies. SCHIP presented a new, long-term source of federal revenue to states for coverage expansions, with matching rates more favorable than Medicaid. Moreover, SCHIP pushed states to expand the capacity of their bureaucracies to implement broad new coverage mechanisms. For instance, many states focused for the first time on actively reaching out to nonwelfare populations and marketing state-subsidized coverage options. Many states also expanded their capacity to solicit and procure managed care contracts.

Some states have begun to use SCHIP as a platform for extending coverage to adults as well. Minnesota, New Jersey, Rhode Island, and Wisconsin have received federal approval to offer coverage to uninsured parents of some SCHIP recipients through Section 1115 waivers (www.statecoverage.net/schip-1115.htm; accessed July 21, 2004). In the face of state fiscal constraints, discussions of new coverage expansions have come largely to a halt, yet states are still viewed as a laboratory for health insurance coverage reforms. The State of Maine offers the best recent example of continuing discussions about new state-based approaches to expanding coverage. Maine's Dirigo Health Reform Act of 2003 phases in coverage for nearly all Maine residents by 2009 through a combination of Medicaid expansion and a voluntary, subsidized state insurance program. After the first year, the plan would not require state general revenue funding. Rather, the plan would be financed by a combination of savings from cost control measures, fees paid by insurers and insurance administers, and new federal Medicaid matching funds received by the state. The new federal funds would be raised by submitting employer health insurance contributions for Medicaid-eligible workers for federal Medicaid match. Obtaining federal approval will be a critical step toward full implementation of Dirigo, but even if the federal government rejects Maine's financing approach, the state will have advanced its health reform agenda (Nalli, 2004; Rosenthal & Pernice, 2004).

# THE FUTURE: CONTINUING AND EMERGING ISSUES

Broad fundamental issues related to access are likely to continue in the short and medium term. Even with the SCHIP-sparked renewal of state action to cover the uninsured, large numbers of Americans remain without coverage, and patients and providers continue to struggle to cope with the consequences of this reality. As of 2001, three new sets of access issues are emerging that will become increasingly important.

First, within the next few years, virtually all Medicaid patients (except the elderly in long-term care and some special needs populations) will be enrolled in managed care, and state SCHIP expansions will deliver coverage almost exclusively on managed care. Passage of the Balanced Budget Act of 1997 removes most restrictions on mandatory Medicaid managed care enrollment. While this transformation has the potential to help reduce some of the indirect barriers to care for public coverage program recipients, it also raises many new concerns and issues.

On the positive side, capitated payments create strong financial incentives for managed care plans to solve some noneconomic or quasi-economic barriers to care, for example, to the extent that preventable hospital admissions for conditions, such as asthma, can be reduced by more timely and effective outpatient management (better patient education on the use of inhalers, improved medication regimens, and nurse hotlines for care management advice during acute flare-ups) or by development of a more accessible health care delivery system (longer clinic hours, shorter waits in clinics, child care services on site, and in-home visits). Managed care plans have an interest in solving these problems that have historically eluded the fee-for-service world. Research is needed to monitor how plans respond in order to develop new strategies to improve access as Medicaid and SCHIP managed care matures.

Publicly funded managed care also creates new enforcement mechanisms and opportunities for government agencies to assure better access for enrolled patients. For example, some states have instituted policies that plans must assure that patients with urgent care needs can obtain an appointment with their primary care provider within a specified period (e.g., 48 hours). Medicaid patients have historically adapted to long wait times for appointments at some clinics and outpatient departments (60 days or more in many cases) by using emergency rooms for routine care or by turning to Medicaid mills for much of their care. Medicaid agencies often had no effective means to compel providers to be more responsive because of the logistical problems of monitoring a huge number of care sites and the difficulties inherent in penalizing providers who were often already in financial distress and who were critical to assuring some access in low-income communities. Moreover, since patients often used multiple providers, it was not possible to hold any single provider responsible for patient care, for example, when a newborn failed to receive the requisite schedule of well-baby care visits or appropriate immunizations, as it was not always clear who should be held accountable.

In a managed care environment, a single health plan is responsible for each patient. Regulators can more effectively monitor the performance of the smaller number of plans (e.g., using mock patients attempting to schedule appointments with the plan's providers by telephone; monitoring disenrollment rates; tracking performance indicators for immunizations, well-baby visits, or follow-up after hospitalization) and have a realistic enforcement mechanism to assure accountability: closing enrollment for new patients or denying reenrollment of current patients. Noncomplying plans can be forced to expand capacity or improve performance of their primary care providers, or face serious loss of revenue. Again the potential may exceed the reality. Accordingly, a critical issue for the future certainly concerns the extent and effectiveness of government oversight of Medicaid managed care. The explosion of Medicaid managed care is happening at a time of overall government cutbacks, and it will be critical to examine whether and how public agencies will adapt to this new environment.

Medicaid managed care also presents a serious risk of creating a whole new set of barriers to care for low-income patients. The confusion associated with the enrollment process undoubtedly has negative consequences. For example, many patients may enroll in plans not realizing that they will be required to change providers, perhaps requiring unrealistic travel times to new care sites and certainly disrupting continuity of current utilization patterns. Other problems are likely to emerge, as well. Aggressive, entrepreneurial plans may enroll more patients than their primary care network can adequately serve. New providers brought in by managed care plans may underestimate the special needs of Medicaid populations. Requirements that patients use a gatekeeping primary care practitioner may discourage needed care among patients who have difficulty adapting to the new rules. And, of course, the most serious concern relates to the new set of incentives for providers: provision of less care can mean higher profits or a bigger margin. While barriers to care may ultimately lead to increased morbidity and costly hospitalization for some patients, in the short run, low or no utilization of primary care services may be highly profitable. As patients jump on and off Medicaid and from one plan to another, some plans may find no financial advantage in improving access for many of their patients. Therefore, it is critical that policymakers have a capacity to monitor these developments carefully and to learn more about how these new incentives are affecting utilization and outcomes.

There are new risks as states gain more flexibility to structure public coverage programs through managed care plans. Until the Balanced Budget Act, states were required to apply for waivers to mandate managed care enrollment of Medicaid beneficiaries. Waivers brought extra layers of scrutiny from the federal government through mandated program evaluations. But today, states may employ managed care plans to deliver care under Medicaid and SCHIP without waivers, and less scrutiny may put program beneficiaries at greater risk.

The second set of emerging issues relates to the consequences of the changing health care marketplace. With the growth of managed care (in commercial, Medicare, and Medicaid markets) and the strengthening of market forces in the health care sector, the ability of traditional safety-net providers to survive, as discussed previously, remains in some doubt. The consequences of their failure are likely to be most dire for the uninsured, especially among immigrant populations who will find it increasingly difficult to take advantage of public programs to provide health insurance coverage. Although the market-clearing effect of competition may help reduce system-wide overcapacity, the impact on patients dependent on these vulnerable providers may be serious. A critical issue in the next decade will be how well the imperative to reduce unneeded beds and services is balanced by efforts to assure the availability of resources to these vulnerable populations. Will we allow these safety-net providers to fail? What will be the consequences of such failures for other providers who begin to see more uninsured patients in their emergency rooms and outpatient departments?

Finally, as efforts to cope with access problems continue to devolve to states and localities, it will be become critical to more fully understand the impact and limits of incremental reforms at these levels. What are the most effective means of expanding coverage for children? How should insurance coverage be balanced with support/subsidies to providers for direct services to the uninsured? What about uninsured adults (who use substantially more health resources than children)? Will children, and adults, in similar economic circumstances but living in different states be treated equitably?

As other innovations are attempted at the state and local levels, sorting out the balance between what is politically feasible (programs for children and pregnant women) and where limited funds might be invested most effectively (adult immigrant populations, substance abuse programs, safety-net providers) will undoubtedly be a major challenge. Disparities among states and localities will also emerge as some move forward while others remain intransigent, and it will be important to monitor the extent and effect of these differences.

Clearly, serious access problems will remain for many millions of Americans for the foreseeable future. The ultimate issue is when these problems will reemerge as a major national policy concern, at least regarding economic access, and whether national policymakers will yet again fail to find a politically viable and financially affordable strategy to assure universal access to needed care.

## CASE STUDY

You are the governor of a midsize industrial state. You have just read this chapter and have decided you want to take on the "health reform/health care access" issue. How would your proceed? How would you staff the effort? Who are the stakeholders? How would you obtain input from stakeholders? How would you limit inappropriate influence by stakeholders? What is the likely nature of the problem in your state? What are the realistic range of solutions/reforms that might be considered? What is the likelihood of meaningful reform?

## DISCUSSION QUESTIONS

1. Who are the uninsured and what does this tell us about the nature of the problem?
2. What are the implications of characteristics of the uninsured on efforts to expand coverage?
3. Who is responsible for reducing noneconomic and quasi-economic barriers to timely and effective health care?
4. What are the costs of barriers to access and how are these costs financed in the current health care delivery system?
5. What were the critical factors in the failure of the Clinton Health Plan? What are the prospects for meaningful reform in the immediate future?

## REFERENCES

Ayanian, J. Z., Kohlker, B. B., & Toshi, A. (1993). The relationship between health insurance coverage and clinical outcomes among women with breast cancer. *New England Journal of Medicine, 329*(5), 326.

Billings, J., Anderson, G., & Newman, L. (1996). Recent findings on preventable hospitalizations. *Health Affairs,* 239.

Billings, J., Mijanovich, T., & Blank, A. (1997). *Barriers to care for patients with preventable hospital admissions.* New York: United Hospital Fund.

Billings, J., & Teicholz, N. (1990). Uninsured patients in the District of Columbia. *Health Affairs,* 158.

Billings, J., Zeitel, L., & Lukomnik, J. (1993). Impact of socioeconomic status on hospital use in New York City. *Health Affairs,* 162.

Bindman, A., Grumbach, K., Osmond, D., Komaromy, M., Vranizan, K., Lurie, N., et al. (1995). Preventable hospitalizations and access to health care. *Journal of the American Medical Association, 274*(4), 305.

Blendon, R. J., Benson, J. M., & Brodie, M. (1997). Voters and health care in the 1996 election. *Journal of the American Medical Association, 277*(15), 1253.

Blendon, R. J., Benson, J. M., Brodie, M., Altman, D. E., & James, M. (2000). Health care in the upcoming 2000 election. *Health Affairs,* 210.

Blendon, R. J., Brodie, M., & Benson, J. (1995). What happened to Americans' support for the Clinton health plan. *Health Affairs,* 7.

Braveman, P. A., Egerter, S., Bennett, T., & Showstack, J. (1991). Differences in hospital resource allocation among sick newborns according to insurance coverage. *Journal of the American Medical Association, 266*(23), 3300.

Braveman, P. A., Oliva, G., & Miller, M. G. (1989). Adverse outcomes and lack of health insurance among newborns in an eight-county area of California, 1982–1986. *New England Journal of Medicine, 321*(8), 508.

Carlisle, D. M., Leake, B. D., Brook, R. H., & Shapiro, M. F. (1996). The effect of race and ethnicity on the use of selected health care procedures: A comparison of south central Los Angeles and the remainder of Los Angeles County. *Journal of Health Care for the Poor and Underserved, 7*(4), 308.

Cohen, D. R., & Cox, L. (2004). *Out in the cold: Enrollment freezes in six State Children's Health Insurance Programs withhold coverage from eligible children.* Washington, DC: Kaiser Commission on Medicaid and the Uninsured.

Collins, S. R., Davis, K., & Lambrew, J. M. (2004). *Health care reform returns to the national agenda: 2004 presidential candidates' proposals.* New York: The Commonwealth Fund.

Cooper, R. A. (1995). Perspectives on the physician workforce to the year 2020. *Journal of the American Medical Association, 274*(19), 1534.

Cooper, B., & How, S. (2004). *Medicare's future: Current picture, trends, and Medicare Prescription Drug Improvement and Modernization Act of 2003.* New York: Commonwealth Fund.

Cotton, P. (1990a). Is there still too much extrapolation from data on middle-aged White men? *Journal of the American Medical Association, 263*(8), 1049.

Cotton, P. (1990b). Examples abound of gaps in medical knowledge because of groups excluded from scientific study. *Journal of the American Medical Association, 263*(8), 1051.

Council on Ethical and Judicial Affairs, American Medical Association. (1990). Black-White disparities in health care. *Journal of the American Medical Association, 263*(17), 2344.

Council on Scientific Affairs, American Medical Association. (1991). Hispanic health in the United States. *Journal of the American Medical Association, 265*(2), 248.

Fiscella, K., Franks, P., Gold, M. R., & Clancy, C. M. (2000). Inequality in quality, addressing socioeconomic, racial, and ethnic disparities in health care. *Journal of the American Medical Association, 283*, 2579.

Franks, P., Clancy, C. M., & Gold, M. R. (1993). Health insurance and mortality: Evidence from a national cohort. *Journal of the American Medical Association, 270*(6), 737.

Friedman, E. (1994). Money isn't everything: Nonfinancial barriers to access. *Journal of the American Medical Association, 271*(19), 1535.

Gaston, R. S., Ayres, I., Dooley, L. G., & Diethelm, A. G. (1993). Racial equity in renal transplantation: The disparate impact of HLA-based allocation. *Journal of the American Medical Association, 270*(11), 1352.

Gornick, M. E., Eggers, P. W., Reilly, T. W., Mentnech, R. M., Fitterman, L. K., Kucken, L. E., et al. (1996). Effects of race and income on mortality and use of services among Medicare beneficiaries. *New England Journal of Medicine, 335,* 791.

Grumbach, K. (1995). *The problems of shortages of physicians and other health professionals in urban areas.* Report prepared for the Council on Graduate Medical Education. San Francisco: University of California, San Francisco, Center for the Health Professions.

Hadley, J. (2003). Sicker and poorer—the consequences of being uninsured: A review of the research on the relationship between health insurance, medical care use, work, income and education. *Medical Care Research and Review, 60*(2), 3S.

Hadley, J., Steinberg, E. P., & Feder, J. (1991). Comparison of uninsured and privately insured hospital patients: Conditions on admission, resource use, and outcome. *Journal of the American Medical Association, 265*(3), 374.

Held, P. J., Pauly, M. V., & Bovberg, R. R. (1988). Access to kidney transplantation. *Archives of Internal Medicine, 148,* 2594.

Henshaw, S. K. (1995). Factors hindering access to abortion services. *Family Planning Perspectives, 27*(2), 54.

Jackson, L. A., & Trude, S. (2001). Stand-alone health insurance tax credits aren't enough. (Issue Brief No. 41). Washington, DC: Center for Studying Health System Change.

Jacobson, P. D., Merritt, R., & Bartlett, L. (1994). *California health care delivery: A competitive model? In state health reform initiatives: Progress and promise.* Baltimore, MD: Health Care Financing Administration.

Johnson, P. A., Lee, T. H., & Cook, E. F. (1993). Effect of race on the presentation and management of patients with acute chest pain. *Annals of Internal Medicine, 118*(8), 593.

Kaiser Commission on Medicaid and the Uninsured. (2003). *Health insurance coverage in America—2002 data update.* Washington, DC: Author.

Kindig, D. A., & Ricketts, T. C. (1991). Determining adequacy of physicians and nurses for rural populations: Background and strategy. *Journal of Rural Health, 7*(Suppl.), 313.

Kirsch, I., Jungeblut, A., Jenkins, L., & Kolstad, A. (1993). *Adult literacy in America: A first look at the results of the National Adult Literacy Survey.* Washington, DC: National Center for Education Statistics, U.S. Department of Education.

Kjellstrand, C. M. (1988). Age, sex, and race inequality in renal transplantation. *Archives of Internal Medicine, 148,* 1305.

Lantz, P. M., Weigers, M. E., & House, J. S. (1997). Education and income differentials in breast cancer and cervical cancer screening. *Medical Care, 35*(3), 219.

Lieu, T. A., Newacheck, P. W., & McManus, M. A. (1993). Race, ethnicity, and access to ambulatory care among U.S. adolescents. *American Journal of Public Health, 83*(7), 960.

Lipson, D. J., & Schrodel, S. P. (1996). *State initiatives in health care reform:*

*State-subsidized insurance programs for low-income people.* Washington, DC: Alpha Center.

Lurie, N., Slater, J., & McGovern, P. (1993). Preventive care for women: Does the sex of the physician matter? *New England Journal of Medicine, 329*(7), 478.

Mathews, S., Ribar, D., & Wilhelm, M. (1997). The effects of economic conditions and access to reproductive health services on state abortion rates and birthrates. *Family Planning Perspectives, 29*(2), 52.

Millman, M. (Ed.). (1993). *Access to health care in America.* Washington, DC: National Academy Press, Institute of Medicine.

Nalli, G. (2004, April). *Health care reform in Maine: A work in progress.* Seminar presented at the Rutgers University Center for State Health Policy, New Brunswick, New Jersey. Retrieved from http://www.cshp.rutgers.edu/presentations/GinoNallySpeakerSeminar04_05_04.pdf July 21, 2004.

Nesbitt, T., Connell, F. A., & Hart, L. G. (1990). Access to obstetric care in rural areas: Effect on birth outcomes. *American Journal of Public Health, 80*(7), 814.

Newacheck, P. W. (1992). Characteristics of children with high and low usage of physician services. *Medical Care, 30*(1), 30.

Phillips, K. A., Mayer, M. L., & Aday, L. (2000). Barriers to care among racial/ethnic groups under managed care. *Health Affairs,* 65.

Politzer, R. M, Harris, D. L., & Gaston, M. H. (1991). Primary care physician supply and the medically underserved. *Journal of the American Medical Association, 266*(1), 104.

Riley, A. W., Finney, J. W., & Mellits, E. D. (1993). Determinants of children's health care use. *Medical Care, 31*(9), 767.

Rosenblatt, R. A., Mattis, R., & Hart, L. G. (1995). Abortions in rural Idaho: Physicians' attitudes and practices. *American Journal of Public Health, 85*(10), 1423.

Rosenthal, J., & Pernice, C. (2004). *Dirigo Health Reform Act: Addressing health care costs, quality, and access in Maine.* Portland, ME: National Academy for State Health Policy.

Schulman, K. A., Berlin, J. A., Harless, W., Kerner, J. F., Sistrunk, S., Gersh, B. J., et al. (1999). The effect of race and sex on physicians' recommendations for cardiac catheterization. *New England Journal of Medicine, 340,* 618.

Short, P. F., & Banthin, J. S. (1995). New estimates of the underinsured younger than 65 years. *Journal of the American Medical Association, 274*(16), 1302.

Short P. F., & Graefe, D. R. (2003). Battery-powered health insurance? Stability in coverage of the uninsured. *Health Affairs, 22*(6), 244.

Short, P. F., & Lefkowitz, D. C. (1992). Encouraging preventive services for low-income children: The effect of expanding Medicaid. *Medical Care, 30*(9), 766.

Solis, J. M., Marks, G., Garcia, M., & Shelton, D. (1990). Acculturation, access to care, and use of preventive services by Hispanics: Findings from HHANES 1982–1984. *American Journal of Public Health, 80*(Suppl.), 11.

Todd, K. H., Lee, T., & Hoffman, J. R. (1994). The effect of ethnicity of physician estimates of pain severity in patients with isolated extremity trauma. *Journal of the American Medical Association, 271*(12), 925.

Todd, K. H., Samaroo, N., & Hoffman, J. R. (1993). Ethnicity as a risk factor for inadequate emergency department analgesia. *Journal of the American Medical Association, 269*(12), 1537.

Udvarhelyi, I. S., Gatsonis, C., & Epstein, A. M. (1992). Acute myocardial infarction in the Medicare population. *Journal of the American Medical Association, 268*(18), 2530.

U.S. Census Bureau (USCB). (2003). Health insurance coverage: 2002.

Weiss, B. D. (1994). Illiteracy among Medicaid recipients and its relation to health care costs. *Journal of Health Care for the Poor and Underserved, 5*(2), 99.

Weissman, J., Gatsonis, C., & Epstein, A. (1992). Rates of avoidable hospitalizations by insurance status in Massachusetts and Maryland. *Journal of the American Medical Association, 268,* 2388–2394.

Whittle, J., Conigliaro, J., & Good, C. (1993). Racial differences in the use of cardiovascular procedures in the department of Veterans Affairs Medical System. *New England Journal of Medicine, 329,* 627.

Williams, M. V., Parker, R. M., & Baker, D. W. (1995). Inadequate functional health literacy among patients at two public hospitals. *Journal of the American Medical Association, 274*(21), 1677.

# 17

# COST CONTAINMENT

Steven A. Finkler

- Discuss the growth in health care costs over the last several decades.
- Explain some of the reasons for the rapid rise in health care costs.
- Describe some potential policy solutions to constrain the growth in health care costs.
- Describe some potential management solutions to constrain the growth in health care costs.
- Analyze whether available solutions are likely to be effective, and if not, explain why not.

KEY WORDS

Health, hospital, cost, nursing shortage, aging, pharmaceuticals, malpractice, tort, management, antitrust, Medicaid, Medicare, universal, one-payer, technology, evidence-based management, cost-analysis, cost-effective

FOR DECADES HEALTH services policymakers and managers have struggled with rapidly rising health care costs. This chapter provides an introduction to the problem and potential solutions. It begins by assessing the magnitude of this problem. It next moves on to an examination of some of the causes of the problem, before moving on to potential solutions. The discussion of solutions is divided into a section on policy approaches, and one on management initiatives. The chapter concludes with a brief discussion of some of the dilemmas that still face us.

## THE PROBLEM OF COST CONTAINMENT

This chapter is concerned with the problem of cost containment in the United States health care system. Inherent in that statement is the assumption that there is a problem. If the problem is cost containment, what do we know about the growth of health care costs over time? (see TABLE 17.1)

From 1960 to 2002, national health care spending rose from $27 billion to $1.6 trillion. Over that time period the population of the United States rose from 186 million to 285 million, and the Gross Domestic Product (GDP) rose from $527 billion to $10.4 trillion. One thing that stands out from these numbers is the fact that health care spending rose at a much faster rate than the population growth. This is confirmed by the fact that per capita spending on health care rose from $143 per person to $5,440 per person over that time period.

Throughout the period from 1960 to 2002, the annual percentage increase in the gross domestic product was always less than the percentage of increase in health care expenditures. One might ask, "Didn't the cost of almost everything rise during those years as a result of inflation?" Yes, but not nearly as fast as health care costs. This can best be seen by considering health care spending as a percentage of the GDP. In 1960, health care spending was 5.1% of the GDP, and by 2002 had risen to 14.9%. This means that while the GDP

### TABLE 17.1

**National Health Expenditures and GDP, 1960–2002**

| CALENDAR YEAR | 2002 | 2000 | 1990 | 1980 | 1970 | 1960 |
|---|---|---|---|---|---|---|
| National health expenditures | | | | | | |
| Amount in $ billions | 1553 | 1310 | 696 | 245.8 | 73.1 | 26.7 |
| Per capita amount in dollars | 5440 | 4672 | 2738 | 1067 | 348 | 143 |
| Annual percent change | | | | | | |
| Gross Domestic Product (GDP) | 3.6 | 5.9 | 5.7 | 8.9 | 5.5 | |
| National health expenditures | 9.3 | 7.4 | 11.8 | 14.9 | 13.1 | |
| U.S. population in millions1 | 285 | 280.4 | 254.2 | 230.4 | 210.2 | 186.2 |
| GDP in billions of dollars | 10446 | 9825 | 5803 | 2796 | 1040 | 527 |
| National health expenditures as a percentage of GDP | 14.9 | 13.3 | 12 | 8.8 | 7 | 5.1 |

1 Census resident-based population less armed forces overseas and less the population of outlying areas. Source: U.S. Census Bureau, June 2003.
SOURCE: Centers for Medicare & Medicaid Services, Office of the Actuary: Data from the National Health Statistics Group: http://www.cms.hhs.gov/statistics/nhe/historical/tables.pdf
Abstracted from: Table 1 National Health Expenditures Aggregate, Per Capita, Percent Distribution and Annual Percent Change by Source of Funds: Calendar Years 1960–2001, and from Table 2 National Health Expenditures Aggregate and Per Capita Amounts, Percent Distribution, and Average Annual Percent Growth, by Source of Funds: Selected Calendar Years 1980–2002.

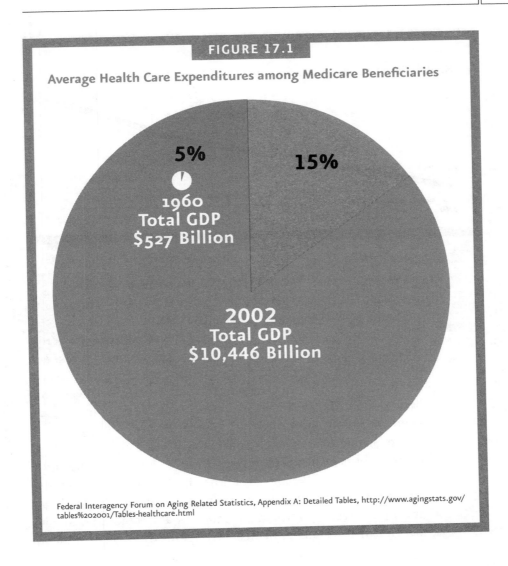

## FIGURE 17.1

### Average Health Care Expenditures among Medicare Beneficiaries

5%

15%

1960
Total GDP
$527 Billion

2002
Total GDP
$10,446 Billion

Federal Interagency Forum on Aging Related Statistics, Appendix A: Detailed Tables, http://www.agingstats.gov/
tables%202001/Tables-healthcare.html

was rising, creating a much bigger pie, health care spending was rising more rapidly, consuming an ever larger slice of that pie (see FIGURE 17.1). This means that less of the pie is available for spending on all other things.

In FIGURE 17.2, we can see the trend in health care spending over time, as a percentage of all resources available to American society. It becomes clear from this figure that if this trend were to continue indefinitely, eventually health care would squeeze out all other spending. Is the trend likely to continue? Federal estimates show that health care spending is expected to more than double

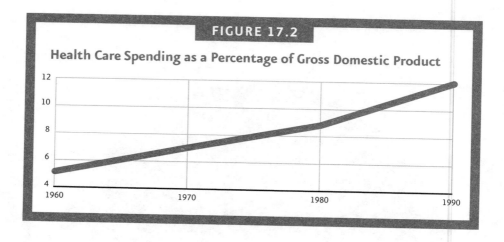

**FIGURE 17.2**

**Health Care Spending as a Percentage of Gross Domestic Product**

from 2001 to 2011 (see **TABLE 17.2**). And the problem seems to be getting worse. The federal government estimates that by 2013, health care spending will consume 18.4% of the GDP.[1]

There is substantial variation in the rate of cost increase across different parts of the health care sector. The overall increase in health care costs during 2002 was 9.3%. That year's increase in hospital spending of 9.5% and the physician increase of 7.7% were not substantially different from the overall rate. Nursing home costs rose only 4.1%, but prescription drugs rose at a rate of 15.3%.[2]

So, let's start to answer the question, What do we know about the growth of health care costs over time? We know that they have grown substantially. We know that they have grown at a rate faster than the growth rate of either the population or the GDP. We know that they are projected to continue to grow at a rapid rate. And we know that if unchecked, health care spending will consume an ever-growing percentage of the GDP, squeezing out spending on other things. Since that is generally viewed as being an undesirable outcome, health care cost containment has been and continues to be an important national concern.

1 Heffler, S., Smith, S., et. al. Health Spending Projections Through 2013, Health Affairs, February 11, 2004, Exhibit 1.
2 Source: Table 2: National Health Expenditures Aggregate Amounts and Average Annual Percent Change, by Type of Expenditure: Selected Calendar Years 1980-2002. Centers for Medicate & Medicaid Services, Baltimore.http://www.cms.hhs.gov/statistics/nhe.historical/t2.asp

| TABLE 17.2 |
| --- |

## Total Projected National Health Expenditures, 2002–2010

| YEAR | TOTAL EXPENDITURES IN MILLIONS |
| --- | --- |
| 2001 | $1,424,541 |
| 2002* | 1,547,636 |
| 2003 | 1,660,542 |
| 2004 | 1,778,798 |
| 2005 | 1,907,268 |
| 2006 | 2,044,223 |
| 2007 | 2,194,021 |
| 2008 | 2,354,599 |
| 2009 | 2,524,958 |
| 2010 | 2,702,235 |
| 2011 | 2,886,616 |
| 2012 | 3,079,836 |

NOTES: Federal, state, and local Medicaid expenditures include Medicaid SCHIP Expansion. Federal, state, and local "Other" funds include SCHIP.
*The first projected year is 2002
SOURCE: Centers for Medicare & Medicaid Services, 7500 Security Boulevard, Baltimore, MD. http://www.cms.hhs.gov/statistics/nhe/
Abstracted from: Table 1: National Health Expenditure (NHE) Aggregate Amounts and Average Annual Percentage Change by Type of Expenditure and Source of Funds: Selected Calendar Years 1965–2012. The health spending projections were based on the 2001 version of the NHE released in January 2003.

## WHY THIS PROBLEM EXISTS

The rising costs of health care have long concerned managers and policymakers alike. There are many possible causes, a few of which are discussed here. A recent study indicated that the most significant causes for increased hospital spending were volume and increasing costs of goods and services. Volume-induced cost increases result from both population growth and increased utilization per person. The most significant portion of the increase in the costs of goods and services was labor. Utilization per capita (34%), population growth (21%), and wages and benefits (39%) combined to account for 94% of the increase in hospital spending from 1997 to 2001 (PricewaterhouseCoopers, 2003, p. 1).

Why are we spending more in these hospital areas? What other areas, outside of hospitals, are driving up health care costs? There are many factors that come into play. Part of the utilization increase is due to advances in health care treatments available. Such advances are expected to continue. Utilization rates are also rising, at least partly because of the aging of America. That will likely continue. Others argue, however, that a big share of utilization results from a payment system that is less generous in paying for prevention, nonphysician care, and nonhospital care, and more generous in paying for procedures, hospitalizations, and physician care. Labor costs are on the rise due to a national nursing shortage. There is little relief in sight for that shortage. Other areas of growing concern are the cost of pharmaceuticals, skyrocketing malpractice insurance costs, and a reversal of the cost constraining impact of managed care. These various cost drivers are discussed in this section. However, this discussion is not all-inclusive. There are many elements that together account for health care cost increases. It is a mistake to try to find one culprit, e.g., physicians, technology, administrative costs, or insurers, and blame that one group for "the" cause of rising health care costs.

One might ask, just why are we concerned about the issue of cost containment in health care? Do we worry about cost containment in car production or banking services? Health care is a fairly unique commodity. In some cases, acquiring health care services is an issue of life or death. As a result, people are not always as price sensitive as they are about other products. Recall that two key elements in rising costs are volume and increasing costs of goods and services. People tend to get saturated with products like cars. If the prices of cars rise, people tend to buy fewer cars, in accord with the normal laws of supply and demand. Even if the price doesn't rise, most individuals will buy only 1 or 2 cars (although there are exceptions) before deciding that the marginal benefit of other purchases exceeds the marginal benefit of buying more cars. However, people seem to get less saturated with health care services.

Part of the problem is that consumers do not know if they have a serious illness. This lack of knowledge makes it hard to gauge how much health care service is needed. Also, consumers lack information about quality. Often they are willing to pay more for higher perceived quality, whether that perception is correct or not. This tends to drive up prices (Thorpe, 2002).

## Health Insurance

Even with the problem of lack of knowledge, which might lead to over or under-consumption,[3] why should we worry about health care costs? It's a free market. If people want to spend their money on health care, aren't they making a choice they should be allowed to make? A problem with this line of reasoning is that most Americans have health care insurance. Furthermore, employers get a tax deduction for the premiums they pay for insurance for their employees. This effectively provides a government subsidy for the insurance (Thorpe, 2002). The subsidy means that people have more insurance then they would otherwise have. And insurance leads to greater consumption of health care services because of what is referred to as "moral hazard." Since consumers do not directly bear the full cost of the services they consume, they are likely to consume more of those services than they would if they paid for them directly.

## The Dynamic Nature of Health Care Services

One argument is that health care costs are rising partly because the health care products are changing. Medical care offered today and medical care of yesterday are two different products or services. Physicians apply new techniques, new technology, and new pharmaceuticals. Yes, we are paying more, but we are buying something different, so the cause of expanding health care costs per patient is not just price increase, but rather product or service changes (Cutler, McClellan, & Newhouse, 1998).

Health care product change can be viewed in several ways. One is that there are better but more costly products, so some patients receive more expensive products in place of obsolete, less expensive ones. Another is that these new products and services can be sold to individuals who might not have even been candidates for them in prior years. For example, with respect to treatment for heart attacks and ischemia, it has been noted that "the cost per surgical procedure has actually declined. Nevertheless, surgery is now deemed appropriate for an ever-larger percentage of patients . . ."

---

3 Although we tend to think that part of the cost problem is over-consumption of care, a recent study indicated that Americans receive too little care for many medical conditions. See McGlynn, E., Asch, S., et. al., "The Quality of Health Care Delivered to Adults in the United States," New England Journal of Medicine, 348(26), June 26, 2003, pp. 2635-2645. Efforts to improve quality of care by providing appropriate care might increase health costs even further.

(Lee & Skinner, 1999, p. 131). We can save more people now, but that increases the amount we spend.

Another element is that technology creates a potential for unlimited spending. Recent innovations such as total body magnetic resonance imaging (MRI) serve as a case in point (Queenan, 2002). As facilities start marketing this service directly to symptomless consumers, we open a pandora's box. The potential cost of medical care services to rule out possibilities created by false positive findings from the scan is enormous. Is society willing and able to handle the potential explosion in health care costs that these "direct-to-consumer" marketing campaigns for new technologies and drugs can generate?

## The Aging Population

However, even if the product were the same, one cause of the problem is that we are buying more medical care, if for no other reason, than because our population is aging. This trend toward an older population will likely create increasing pressure on total health care spending as time goes by. It has been estimated that in the time it will take the U.S. population to grow by two thirds, the population over age 65 will have tripled and the population over age 85 will have increased eight fold (Lee & Tuljapurkar, 1994). In general, the elderly consume more health care services than younger individuals:

> The retirement of baby boomers during the next few decades will lead to a very large increase in the number of Medicare enrollees. In addition, enrollees are increasingly likely to live to advanced ages. Older Medicare enrollees typically use more health care than younger enrollees and are more expensive; therefore increasing longevity is viewed as causing an increase in Medicare costs. (Miller, 2001, p. 215)

Medicare is a federal program that pays for health care services, primarily for individuals age 65 and older. Not only will such growth in the number of elderly create pressure for health care spending to increase, but it also creates pressure on those who will have to pay those increasing costs. This is the case because the ratio of the population over 65 to the working age population has been growing steadily, and will rise steeply from 2010 to 2030, the years during which the baby boom population retires (Lee & Skinner, 1999).

## Labor Issues

From time to time labor shortages create pressure for salaries to rise, thus increasing health care costs. One of the most serious issues confronting us today is the nursing shortage. An aging population will naturally need more nurses. Elderly people have more acute illnesses, which are more likely to need the skilled care that nurses provide. However, it is not only growing demand but also declining supply that has created a nursing shortage. For six consecutive years (from 1995 through 2000), enrollments at undergraduate nursing schools declined (PricewaterhouseCoopers, 2003). Furthermore, hospitals are high stress environments for nurses, and many skilled nurses are shifting to careers in physician practices, or working as school nurses, or elsewhere. Also, a significant portion of the nursing labor force is nearing retirement age. Government projections indicate that between the growth in demand for nurses and the need for replacements due to retirements, by 2010 there will be more than *one million* vacant positions for registered nurses (Hecker, 2001).

These factors combine to cause hospitals to have to pay increasing wages to attract nurses. Even with higher wage rates, hospitals often fail to attract sufficient nursing staff and have to pay high hourly amounts for either overtime or per diem nurses from temporary employment agencies. Exacerbating this entire issue are recent legislative efforts to make mandatory overtime for nurses illegal. At least in the short run, such laws will inevitably drive up wages (and therefore health care costs) substantially, as hospitals try to hire more nurses than are available.

At times, employment also becomes a political issue. A city may desire to close a public hospital in a poor neighborhood. However, the hospital may be one of the few employers in the community that pays high wages. Closure of the hospital would not only affect access to care, it would also mean layoffs of individuals whose wages pump money into the local community economy. Thus, at times, politics comes into play, keeping the hospital open, even if it is a high cost provider of care. This would tend to cause health care costs to be higher than they otherwise would be.

## The Cost of Prescription Drugs

Pharmaceutical costs have been a rapidly rising component of the overall costs of health care. For example, note that in 1998 spending on nursing homes was $89 billion and spending on prescription drugs was $87 billion. By 2002, spending on nursing homes had risen to $103 billion, while spending on prescription drugs had risen to $162 billion.[4] In 2003, a law was passed providing an outpatient prescription drug benefit to Medicare enrollees.[5] While the government contends the law will restrain the growth of prescription drug costs, others argue it will actually increase overall pharmaceutical costs.

## Malpractice Insurance Costs

Medical liability insurance costs have long been a concern to those interested in controlling overall health care spending. Recently, however, there has been an increasing focus on this issue, as malpractice insurance costs, for both hospitals and physicians, have undergone a rapid increase, and in some cases, physicians are having trouble obtaining insurance regardless of price (Mello, Studdert, & Brennan, 2003). This in turn leads to a cycle of even higher health care costs as physicians and other health providers practice defensive medicine, preferring to err on the side of extra caution (and extra cost) of providing care, rather than risking enormous malpractice settlements or legal awards which would in turn lead to even higher malpractice insurance rates.

Insurers contend that increased premiums are required to deal with increases in their administrative costs, in the average payout for malpractice claims, and in the increasing size of extremely large, high-end outliers awards. Physicians tend to blame the legal profession for having convinced the public that they are entitled to a payment if there is a bad outcome in health care, regardless of whether there was medical negligence, and trial attorneys contend that the problem is that there are too many medical errors (Mello et al., 2003). Others argue that insurers are trying to make up for large losses in their investment portfolios. Regardless of the underlying cause, there is no question that the rapid, large increases in insurance premiums will be passed on, and are being reflected in the overall costs of health care. Many argue that fundamental tort reform is needed to reign in the growth of malpractice awards by the court system, and in turn, malpractice insurance rates.

---

4 Heffler, S., Smith, S., et al., Health Spending Projections Through 2013, Health Affairs, February 11, 2004, Exhibit 1.
5 The Medicare Prescription Drug, Improvement and Modernization Act of 2003 (P.L. 108-173).

## Current Issues Related to Managed Care

Managed care has been one major attempt by society to control rising health care costs. One way health plans do this is through *disease management*, defined as

> a population-based, pro-active, and preventive strategy that identifies individuals at risk of developing costly diseases (e.g., hypertension, diabetes, cancer, or heart disease) *before* the disease appears and provides preventive, educational, and early detection and treatment services, thus minimizing or averting future health costs associated with disease consequences and complications. (Cohen, 1999, pp. 701–702)

That sounds pretty good. At their best, managed care organizations improve health and lower costs. But at their worst, managed care organizations are perceived as inappropriately preventing patients from getting necessary care, in order to maximize profits (Thorpe, 1999). So costs may be constrained by managed care companies that prevent unnecessary (and in some cases, necessary) care. But they also create another costly layer of marketing, administration, and profits.

Regardless of which view is more accurate, recent years have definitely seen a consumer backlash to perceived limits on appropriate care by managed care organizations. In response to both this backlash and the enactment of "any-willing-provider" laws, health plans have relaxed their restrictions on care in recent years, resulting in the currently observed growth in the rate of increase in health care costs (Lesser & Ginsburg, 2003). Any-willing-provider laws require managed care plans to contract with any health care providers who are willing to conform to the plan's normal terms and rates. While one study has shown that such laws don't affect HMO profits (Carroll & Ambrose, 2002), there is definitely the potential for them to drive up the costs of managed care organizations by forcing them to contract with providers who are not committed to their organization's philosophy of how to practice medicine. In other words, HMOs believe that they are being required to contract with physicians they feel prescribe unnecessary services for their patients.

# THE POTENTIAL SOLUTIONS TO COST CONTAINMENT

Many authors approach the issue of cost containment from a policy perspective. What can government policymakers do to constrain the overall societal spending on health care, while still making progress in the areas of access and quality? Equally important, however, is the management perspective. What can managers do in their institutions to control their costs? It is contended here that either perspective is incomplete without the other. Government must assure that managers have appropriate incentives to constrain costs. But managers must proactively determine approaches that will minimize the costs of providing care without compromising outcomes. One physician argues,

> With our high standard of living, the public expects that we have skilled personnel, sophisticated new equipment, the latest pharmaceuticals, and modern technological advances. So medical costs will always be on the high side in developed countries. (Queenan, 2002, p. 629)

There is certainly some truth to this statement. But it doesn't mean that we must simply allow health care costs to rise unchecked. The remainder of this chapter focuses on some of the efforts that both policymakers and managers can undertake to constrain the growth of health care costs, while still providing a high level of access to and quality of care.

## Policy Focused Solutions

In recent years policy efforts to constrain health care spending have focused on several key areas. These include prescription drug costs, tort reform, antitrust, medicaid reform, and universal health care.

### Prescription Drug Reform

Of particular concern to policymakers in the last few years has been the spiraling costs of pharmaceuticals. Historically, the role of federal policy in the United States has been limited in the area of prescription drugs. As Kane (1997) notes,

> there are no national price controls, no national drug formularies, no universal policies regarding consumer cost-sharing. Rather, the main role undertaken by the national government has been regula-

tory control over entry into the market. . . . While high regulatory barriers to entry discouraged the introduction of marginal drugs into the US market, stringent regulations also discouraged the entry of lower-priced generic substitutes as well. (p. S72)

Individual states have been more active in their efforts to control costs, but this has not constrained the overall rapid growth in spending on prescription drugs.

There is evidence that indicates that drugs are a substantial economic burden on the elderly, and without coverage, they are less likely to take appropriate medications (Blustein, 2000a, 2000b). Failure to take medications could conceivably lead to even greater treatment costs. In 2003, the Medicare Prescription Drug, Improvement and Modernization Act was passed into law, providing an outpatient prescription drug benefit for Medicare enrollees. The government contends that this new expanded coverage will not only reduce the direct costs for pharmaceuticals paid by Medicare members, but will also restrain the overall growth in drug costs. The Congressional Budget Office has estimated that provisions in the Act, which allow comparison shopping and health plan negotiations with pharmaceutical manufacturers, will result in 25% initial reductions in the prices of prescription drugs. The government also contends that the law encourages assessment of the comparative effectiveness of alternative drugs, to ensure that Medicare gets the best value for its money.[6] Further, there is the argument that appropriate drug use will reduce other health care costs, saving money overall. However, some fear that this broader drug coverage will lead to a new explosion in health costs.

There has been some research that indicates that since there are many individuals who are eligible for both Medicare and Medicaid, part of the increased cost of this drug coverage by the Medicare system would be offset by decreased Medicaid costs (Dale & Verdier, 2003). Medicaid systems have instituted drug utilization review programs (Moore, Gutermuth, & Pracht, 2000; Gencarelli, 2003), but their success at stemming the increasing costs of drugs has been limited. Will Medicare have more success? Policymakers will likely spend a number of years evaluating the impacts of the Medicare prescription drug program, after it is implemented in

---

6 Frist, W. H. (2003, December 15). "The Medicare Prescription Drug, Improvement and Modernization Act: Controlling Rising Prescription Drug Costs," Office of the Majority Leader.

2006, and proposing modifications aimed at getting the maximum clinical benefit from such a program at the lowest possible cost to society. In the meantime, a debate rages over whether individuals should be allowed to buy drugs by mail order from Canada, where some drugs are sold at substantially lower prices.

Policymakers will likely continue to debate the issue of price controls on drugs. However drug research is both costly and risky, with many hundreds of millions of dollars of research never panning out. Price controls might inhibit research into new drugs. Trying to balance the societal benefit of reasonably priced drugs, with the desire to have continued drug research creates a difficult dilemma for policymakers.

### Tort Reform

Another hot topic for policymakers right now is tort reform. One study has found that

> medical liability premiums increased between 30% and more than 100% in 2002. . . . The situation is so critical that nearly 30 states are considering tort reform, including caps on non-economic damages and limits on contingency fees. (PricewaterhouseCoopers, 2003, p. 12)

Physicians have staged walk outs where they have ceased seeing patients for several days, and marched on state capitals to protest high malpractice rates. Some states have enacted tort-reform legislation.

There is no doubt that legislation can rein in the cost increases in malpractice premiums. The open question is whether laws can be crafted that don't unjustly remove the right to sue from those seriously injured by blatant malpractice. Instances in which surgeons remove the wrong limb, operate on the wrong patient causing serious injury, etc., abound. How can frivolous suits be eliminated, outlandish jury awards be tempered, while still allowing the victim of gross negligence to receive a fair settlement?

### Antitrust

Policymakers are sometimes concerned with merger activity in the health care industry. In theory, as organizations merge, it is possible that they might gain enough market power to be price makers rather than the price takers of the free-market economic model. As a result, if there are too few providers in a geographic area, they may raise prices higher than they would be in a more competitive situation. Some research has in fact lent support to the belief that hospital mergers in this country have in fact resulted in concentrated markets and higher prices (Young, Desai, & Hellinger, 2000). As a result, one way to constrain costs would be for policymakers to assure that antitrust legislation exists that is appropriate, and enforced.

### Medicaid Reform

Medicaid is a program in which the federal and state governments share the cost of medical care for certain individuals (primarily low-income mothers, children, the elderly, blind, and disabled). Each state has latitude in determining the benefits provided in that state. Medicaid is a large and growing cost for many states. As a result, states often examine their Medicaid program looking for ways to control costs. One approach is to simply cut payments. An alternative reform effort during the 1990s was a shift of Medicaid eligibles into managed care programs.

How can states simply cut Medicaid payments? There are several approaches they can take. Eligibility requirements can be changed, making it harder to qualify for Medicaid benefits. Or benefits themselves can be restructured, eliminating payments completely for certain services. Or states can simply mandate lower payment rates for the services that they do cover. Do such actions really constrain total health care costs? Perhaps to some extent. Some individuals may simply no longer consume health care services because they are no longer eligible for treatment. Some providers, under financial pressure may find less expensive ways to provide care. However, it is possible that these approaches simply shift the burden of health care costs rather than constrain them. If Medicaid doesn't pay enough to cover the cost of a patient, the rates charged to other payers may rise to cover those costs. If patients don't seek routine care because they are not covered, their illnesses may worsen and require more costly emergency or long-term care. Ultimately providers incur the costs of that more expensive emergency or lengthy care, regardless of who is actually paying for it. We must be quite careful when we consider the impact of "simple solutions" to controlling health care spending. Approaches such as cutting Medicaid payments may have little if any beneficial impact on overall costs.

The 1990s saw a dramatic shift in Medicaid towards managed care, in an effort to constrain cost increases. The percent of Medicaid recipients enrolled in managed care grew from 14.4% in 1993 to 53.6% in 1998, a rapid rate of growth (Hackey, 2000). The Medicaid managed care enrollment had reached 57.6% by 2002.[7] Yet, by the end of that period the variations were dramatic as:

> Managed care penetration in state Medicaid programs ranged from a low of 0 percent (Alaska, Wyoming) to a high of 100 percent (Tennessee). Although eleven states had enrolled more than 80 percent of their Medicaid caseload in managed care, seven other states reported managed care enrollments of less than 20 percent. (Hackey, 2000, p. 757)

While the wide variation is certainly curious, it also presents policymakers with a golden opportunity. Further research might be able to inform society as to the success of greater levels of managed care in state Medicaid programs in terms of both outcomes and cost.

### Universal Coverage

It is well known that many millions of Americans do not have health insurance. A discussion of policy issues related to cost containment would not be complete, therefore, without at least some discussion of universal health care. One argument against national health insurance is that it would simply cost too much. Consider how much health care costs rose after the introduction of Medicare, which covered just a subset of the population. What would happen if the government tried to provide insurance for all of the currently uninsured? Or, at the extreme, what if we did away with most private insurance and enrolled all Americans in Medicare? Although that may seem like an extreme solution, likely to have an extremely high cost, that is not necessarily the case.

For one thing, there are tremendous cost savings that would be realized by a one-payer system. Hospitals and physicians employ large numbers of individuals to negotiate contracts with various insurers, to process bills, and to monitor collections. A substantial

---

7 Centers for Medicare & Medicaid Services, 2002 Medicaid Managed Care Enrollment Report, http://cms.hhs.gov/medicaid/managedcare/mcsten02.pdf

part of this fixed cost incurred by each hospital could possibly be eliminated in a one-payer system. Similarly, society would save all of the costs expended by insurers negotiating contracts with providers, and processing payments, not to mention their marketing costs and profits.

For another thing, many of the people who have no insurance currently, but who would be covered under a one-payer system, now get care but don't pay for it. For these individuals, more care would not necessarily be provided. There would just be less need for cost-shifting from the person getting care to other payers who ultimately subsidize that care.

We certainly have examples of countries that have provided nationalized health insurance (NHI) and have not gone bankrupt in the process (e.g. England, Canada, Germany). A recent study in one such system (Taiwan) found that the

> single-payer NHI system enabled Taiwan to manage health spending inflation and that the resulting savings largely offset the incremental cost of covering the previously uninsured. Under the NHI, the Taiwanese have more equal access to health care, greater financial risk protection, and equity in health care financing. The NHI consistently received a 70 percent public satisfaction rate. (Lu & Hsiao, 2003)

The issue of managing health spending inflation is a critical one. It has been found in this country that Medicare actually has done a better job of constraining costs than private insurers because of its ability to set prices (Boccuti & Moon, 2003), and researchers continue to press the argument that the advantages of a single-payer system for providing universal coverage will keep costs low (DeGrazia, 1996).

### Other Approaches

This section has attempted to highlight some of the major policy efforts to control costs. Other approaches include better health education before high school graduation, better incentives for people to lead healthier lives, and capitation payment—a fixed amount for a broad range of services. The concept behind capitation is that capitated providers are likely to try to restrain costs because they receive no additional revenue if they provide additional services.

*Ineffective Policy*

Policymakers have worked long and hard to rein in the growth of health care costs. The introduction of DRGs for hospitals, physician payment systems, and certificate of need laws to restrain facilities investment are just a few examples of the many efforts over the years, by both state and federal governments, to at least slow, if not stop, the increase in health care spending. Yet the evidence is not great that policymakers really have had much impact at all on slowing the growth of health care costs. A 1995 study of several decades worth of hospital regulation aimed at controlling costs found that "hospital costs appear unresponsive to most regulatory programs" (Antel, Ohsfeldt, & Becker, 1995, p. 416).

Some have described health spending as being like a balloon (Schroeder & Cantor, 1991). When you squeeze the balloon on one side, attempting to push down health care spending, the balloon simply bulges out on the other side. For example, if DRGs are aimed at reducing health care costs by causing hospitals to decrease lengths of stay and spend less, the result is substantial increases in the volume and cost of outpatient care. It has been argued,

> The balloon metaphor seems to hold as long as we fail to get our hands entirely around its circumference. In other words, without an appropriately targeted, comprehensive, and coordinated policy strategy, the nation is unlikely to rein in systemwide health care costs. . . . It is not by accident that industrialized nations, such as Germany, Canada, France, and Japan, have gravitated toward the "high socialization, high coordinated payment" quadrant of the matrix. And it should be evident from their ability to deal effectively with cost pressures in their respective systems of care, while assuring universal coverage for their populations, that cost control and universal access are not only *compatible* goals but that a high degree of both pooled finance and coordinated payment may actually represent a means of "squeezing the balloon" from all sides. However, because many Americans—and private stakeholders in the health care system—find the concept of pooled finance either unfathomable or unpalatable, the United States is not likely to move in that direction in the near future. (Cohen, 1999, p. 701)

So, is cost control a hopeless objective? If policy efforts have been ineffective, and if Americans are unwilling to accept the types of socialized, rationed systems that exist in Europe and elsewhere, are we doomed to ever rising costs? While policymakers continue to grapple with this problem, which has not proven amenable to policy solutions, another direction is that of greater efforts by managers of health care provider organizations to find solutions that can restrain cost increases, while still improving outcomes. The discussion now shifts to such management efforts.

## Management Focused Solutions

Although society clearly has a role to play in trying to assure wide access to high quality health care services at a reasonable cost, health care organizations also play a critical role in constraining the growth of health care costs. Many of the same issues that concern policymakers also confront managers. For example, pharmaceutical costs are a macro problem but also become an organization-level problem for managed care organizations, hospitals, and nursing homes. Other areas where managers have worked and are working to constrain cost increases include controlling technology, evidence-based management, cost-effectiveness analysis, and other management approaches.

### Controlling Prescription and Over-the-Counter Drug Costs

While the national debate over pharmaceutical costs often winds up as a discussion of government price controls, health care organizations have taken a different track. Managers of insurers have taken the lead in this area, although hospital and nursing home managers also carefully scrutinize their spending on drugs to assure that they are using the least costly efficacious drug. Insurers (traditional insurance companies, managed care organizations, or employer-sponsored plans) have been pro-active in attempting to negotiate the best prices they can obtain. Beyond that, however, a good deal of their focus is on providing incentives to patients to make choices the insurer believes will help constrain costs.

Insurers can require patients to make a flat copay payment (e.g., $10) per prescription filled. The incentive is simply to dissuade the patient from filling unneeded prescriptions. Or the insurer can require a lower copay for a generic (e.g., $6) and a higher copay for a brand name drug (e.g., $12). Clearly, the latter approach gives patients an added incentive to acquire the less expensive generic version of the drug. Alternatively, insurers can require coinsurance, in which case the consumer pays a percentage of the price paid for the drug. For example, if there was a 20% coinsurance arrangement, then a prescription with a retail cost of $100, and a negotiated price to the insurer of $70, would result in a patient payment of $14 (20% x $70 = $14).

A newer approach is the use of reference pricing (Kanavos & Reinhardt, 2003).[8] In this approach, the insurer might pay 80% of the negotiated price for a particular drug. The negotiated price is referred to as the reference price. The patient pays 20% of that price if they accept that drug, but if they choose an alternate drug, they pay the entire difference between 80% of the reference price and the retail price of the drug selected. For example, if a generic drug retails for $20, the insurer might negotiate a price of $14. They will pay 80% of $14, or $11.20. The patient can accept that drug and pay 20% of $14, or $2.80. However, if they prefer a brand name drug that has a retail price of $100, they must pay the entire difference between $11.20 and $100. This $88.80 cost to the consumer provides a much stronger incentive than copays or coinsurance alone.

Another more common approach is the use of a formulary—a list of approved drugs. Formularies may be "open" or "closed." With an open formulary, there is no penalty for selecting other drugs. It is primarily an educational device showing the relative cost of drugs, and making the case for the use of a particular drug for any given condition. In closed formularies, the patient is charged higher copayments or perhaps even the full cost of drugs not included in the formulary list (Kane, 1997).

### Using Information Technology to Constrain Costs

Technology is another major part of the problem, but it also holds promise to be part of the solution that managers employ. Technology creates expensive new clinical equipment, but it also has the potential to move health care toward a paperless industry (Mahoney, 2002). Yet, while the potential is there, health care organizations have spent millions of dollars on technology, which has never fulfilled its promise, either on the clinical order-entry and clinical records side, or on the management and financial management side of health care organizations. A challenge for managers is to harness the potential management and clinical benefits, including potential cost savings, of information systems.

---

8 While relatively new in this country, reference pricing has been used for a number of years in Europe.

Managers are also starting to look at health care technology as a way to save costs in many other areas. For example, we are starting to see the use of in-home monitoring devices, which allow for shorter hospital stays (Taylor, 2003); we are seeing broader use of nursing resource management information systems (Ruland & Ravn, 2003); physician order-entry, with its potential for both clinical benefits and cost savings continues to move forward in spurts, with stops and starts as managers address concerns such as physician compliance problems (Foster & Antonelli, 2002). And we have really just scratched the surface. The Internet provides a real potential for managers to innovate and save costs (*Health Data Management*, 2003). Consider the potential benefit of having patients preregister over the Internet several days before hospital admission, allowing insurance to be confirmed, and saving time for the clerical staff and patient.

### Evidence-Based Management

Recently a movement has started that is encouraging health services managers to increase their reliance on evidence as they make decisions related to the operation of health care provider organizations. The use of such information by managers is referred to as evidence-based management (Axelsson, 1998; Kovner, Elton, & Billings, 2000; Finkler & Ward, 2003). Currently, health care organizations do not know enough about what things cost, and until they get evidence on costs, their ability to constrain costs is inhibited (Finkler, Henley, & Ward, 2003). Part of the problem is that managers do not seek out available evidence, and part of the problem is a lack of sufficient research efforts to generate evidence for managers to use. However, if managers and researchers work together to generate and use evidence as a basis for management decisions, it is possible that progress will be made in finding solutions to the problems of increasing health care costs.

For example, some might argue that we buy and pay for services that don't provide predictable value for patients. If we conduct rigorous evidence-based medicine clinical research and provide specific clinical evidence on which services do or do not add value, then insurers would be able to make more cost-effective decisions about covered services.

Of course, we need to realize that one of the difficulties in controlling health costs is that whenever insurers have tried to limit health care services because they are not cost-effective (the benefit to the patient doesn't justify the cost), consumer groups raise strong objections. Individual patients want insurance to pay for anything and everything that might possibly benefit them, even if the chances are so low that a neutral individual would say that it doesn't make sense to provide that service to everyone who might conceivably benefit.

For example, should we spend $1,000 for a test that could save someone's life? Sounds good. What if the test will save one life out of a million people tested? The cost is now one billion dollars to save one life ($1,000 per test x 1,000,000 people tested = $1,000,000,000). Society probably has many ways that one billion dollars can be spent (e.g., on roads, housing, food, and so on) that could save many more lives than one. Both insurance companies and policymakers would probably argue against paying for the test. But if that one person dies because coverage of the test was denied, the media will have a field day about how the ruthless, profit-mongering insurer allowed one of their insured members to die to save a lousy thousand dollars. Logically insurers may decide the bad press isn't worth it. They'll cover the test, and just pass the cost along in the form of higher premiums, driving up health care costs even further. Even logic and evidence cannot always prevail in the unique market for health care services.

## Use of Cost-Effectiveness Analysis

An important tool for the control of costs in health care is cost-effectiveness analysis (CEA) (Eddy, 1992; Gold, Siegel, Russell, & Weinstein, 1996). Although often thought of as a tool of policymakers, the method is extremely valuable in its role of informing managers about the implications of alternatives. Cost-effectiveness analysis assesses the resource use tradeoffs and other pros and cons of a specific intervention (Berger & Teutsch, 2000). The method is widely used to assess the impacts of clinical interventions. For example, it has been used to assess when it would be appropriate to use drug eluting stents, a new but costly medical device (Gunn et al., 2003).

CEA assesses benefits and costs. If one can find a more effective approach for achieving some end, and that approach is less costly, then it is clearly cost effective. However, CEA can also be used in situations in which a more effective result is more costly. Using the technique, one can assess the extra cost, relative to the improved effectiveness, and assess whether the extra cost of the alternative is justified.

> In assessing alternatives, CEA uses a ratio where the denominator is the gain in health (such as adverse reactions avoided) and the numerator is the incremental cost of obtaining the benefits. The denominator may be expressed in years of lives saved or undesirable outcomes averted. The primary advantage of CEA is the ability to compare two interventions aimed at the same outcome. (Jacobson & Kanna, 2001)

Information about which alternative approach aimed at achieving a clinical result provides the best outcome at the lowest cost is essential for health care organizations to be able to provide high quality care, while constraining cost increases. Further, the technique of CEA can be used by managers as they attempt to employ an evidence-based management approach to improving various management techniques employed. For example, does it make more sense for a hospital to have its own billing clerks, or to employ a billing service? Should it have an in-house laundry, or outsource that function? Careful assessment of the advantages and disadvantages of alternative approaches to achieve a desired result, including assessment of cost, allows managers to determine which alternative makes the most sense for their organization.

### Other Managerial Initiatives to Constrain Cost Increases

There are an almost unlimited number of other management-related initiatives that can be used to help constrain cost increases in health care organizations. These are a few examples:

- *Outsourcing*—As noted in the CEA section above, there are many activities carried out by health care organizations that might be less expensive if performed by outside contractors. For example, it has been suggested that it makes sense to outsource the information technology function (Joslyn, 2003).
- *The revenue cycle*—The last few years have seen a growing focus on containing costs throughout the revenue cycle. The revenue cycle is the process of collecting patient revenues. However, managers have started to focus their attention on the entire cycle, which runs from patient scheduling, to registration, treatment, discharge, and collec-

tion. To a greater degree than ever before, managers are focusing on assuring that they have the information to collect all revenues appropriately due, rather than simply thinking of this as a process of collecting accounts receivable (LaForge & Tureaud, 2003).

- *Physician buy-in*—One critical element is physician cooperation (*OR Manager*, 2002). Physicians hold an unusual role in health care organizations. They are responsible for ordering the consumption of resources in hospitals, even though they are not hospital employees. In order to effect cost controls on the consumption of tests, procedures, and drugs, the hospital manager must find ways to get the cooperation of the physician staff.

- *Nurse recruitment, retention, and substitution*—As noted earlier, the nursing shortage is likely to result in pressure on health care labor costs. One approach for managers to constrain costs is to develop effective recruitment and retention programs. However, such programs are more likely to help individual organizations than they are to constrain overall societal costs, unless their focus is on recruiting nurses from other countries, thus increasing the overall supply of nurses available in the U.S. market. Alternatively, we are likely to see at least some efforts by managers to continue searching for ways to substitute less costly labor for nurses, while still maintaining high quality of care.

- *Marginal cost analysis*—In the short-run, if an organization has excess capacity, it may make sense to offer incremental services at prices below long-run average cost, but above marginal cost (i.e., the additional cost incurred when providing service to an additional patient—often this would exclude fixed costs). Efforts by health care managers to maximize short-term profits by employing marginal cost pricing are likely to help constrain overall health care costs.

- *Product-line management*—One way for organizations to save money is to specialize in high volume services. High volumes allow fixed costs to be shared among many patients, lowering the cost per patient. To achieve this, managers can work to cull out from the services they offer those that are low volume, and therefore high cost per patient. Historically it has been politically difficult to eliminate services. However, as cost pressures mount, this is one area that managers need to focus greater attention on.

One important point to consider is that managers have been struggling with cost control for a long time. It is likely that without management efforts, health care spending would have been increasing even more rapidly than it has. Future management efforts are likely to be vigorous, and in many cases, effective at constraining cost increases, but it is not likely that management initiatives by themselves will be sufficient to slow the growth in health costs to the rate of growth of the GDP.

## THE REMAINING DILEMMAS

As policymakers and managers move forward in their efforts to control health care costs, society will need to grapple with difficult issues. As noted above, managers alone do not seem able to completely restrain the growth of health care costs, nor has policy shown itself up to the task. There is no question that managers and policymakers will both have to attack this problem as fiercely as possible. Even then, we appear to be in a holding action—trying to restrain the rise in health care costs, but never getting them fully under control.

Ultimately we will probably employ policy approaches that will lead to limits on access to care, such as increased reliance on rationing care. We must learn which approaches best balance cost, quality, and access (Dombovy, 2002). Our current dilemma largely stems from the fact that when we consider large populations we are quick to laud cost-effective care. Rationing care to the population as a whole makes good sense. But when we consider a specific individual, a person with a face and a name, we have difficulty arguing that there should be any financial limitation on care that might save that person's their life. Until we can resolve that dilemma, the fight to constrain health care costs will always be a difficult one.

If I could dictate an approach to cost control, what would it be? First of all, it would not be a perfect solution, since I don't believe that any perfect solutions are possible. The situation is much too complex. Given that caveat, my approach would be universal health care with everyone in the country covered by the Medicare system. Why? Several reasons. First, Medicare is one of the most efficient payers in the country. Second, a one-payer system would eliminate vast amounts currently spent on administrative activities. Third, a Medicare rather than Medicaid-based system, would eliminate sizeable variations in covered services that currently exist among the states.

By far, the majority of Medicare dollars are paid to providers rather than going to administrative costs. Other insurers spend huge amounts of money on marketing to consumers, negotiating contracts with employers and with providers, paying sales commissions, and earning profits. Medicare would eliminate the high percentage of total costs that are spent by insurers on administration and profits.

Furthermore, providers currently spend huge amounts negotiating contracts, billing different providers, and collecting receivables. Going to a one-payer system creates tremendous potential savings in nonmedical spending on the part of both the insurer and the provider.

Currently, there are tremendously wide variations in coverage among both different private insurers and the Medicaid program in different states. Moving to a one-payer system would create a common floor of benefits for everyone. I say floor because I believe that in a free society we should not prohibit individuals from privately paying additional funds to purchase additional or alternative services. Although we would like to believe in a classless society, that does not really exist here, and too many restrictions would just result in a flourishing illegal black market.

If we were to move in the direction of a universal Medicare system, it would need to be fairly encompassing, including not only in-patient and ambulatory hospital care and physicians, but also home health care, long-term care (nursing homes), prescription medications and so on. Furthermore, if we were to examine such a one-payer system closely, there probably would be negative aspects of such a system that would have to be overcome. Removal of free market competition often has unintended negative consequences.

In any case, do I believe there is much chance for this to become a reality? No. I agree with Cohen (1999), who notes that,

> because many Americans—and private stakeholders in the health care system—find the concept of pooled finance either unfathomable or unpalatable, the United States is not likely to move in that direction in the near future. (p. 701)

Cohen is being polite. The way I would put it is that there are many vested interests groups that profit from the current system. These include insurance companies, technology companies, and others.

These vested interest groups are likely to conduct an intense lobbying campaign that would make it politically impossible to ever move to a one-payer system.

However, even if society were able to overcome the vested interest groups and move to a system of Medicare for everyone, universal health coverage would still not solve the problems of cost containment. It would remove substantial amounts of current spending on profits, marketing, and administration. But from that point on, it would not constrain the growth of costs due to the various factors discussed in this chapter. So we need to place our hopes for cost control in piecemeal policy and management solutions that would more directly address the areas that are causing much of the increase in health care spending.

## SUMMARY

For decades, health services policymakers and managers have struggled with rapidly rising health care costs. There are many possible causes for the rapid rise of health care costs. Cost increases are due in part to the existence of health insurance, the lack of complete information on the part of patients, technological advances, the aging of America (elderly tend to consume more health care services), shortages of critical trained labor, increasing costs for pharmaceuticals, increasing health insurance profits, skyrocketing malpractice insurance costs, and a reversal of the cost constraining impact of managed care.

In recent years, policy efforts to constrain health care spending have focused on prescription drug costs, tort reform, antitrust, medicaid reform, and universal health care coverage. Additionally, the introduction of DRGs, physician payment systems, and certificate-of-need laws to restrain facilities investment are just a few examples of the many efforts to at least slow the increase in health care spending. Health care organizations also play a critical role in constraining the growth of health care costs. For example, health care managers work to constrain cost increases by controlling drug costs, and employing technology, evidence-based management, and cost-effectiveness analysis.

Even with both policymakers and managers addressing this issue, it remains a difficult problem. New solutions will need to be added to current efforts, if we are to successfully rein in the rapid rate of growth of health care costs, over the long-term.

## CASE STUDY

Suppose that obstetricians charge $5,000 for prenatal care and delivery of a baby. This is 20% higher than the previous year. No wonder health care costs are rising rapidly. The obstetrician's professional society say that obstetricians are leaving medical practice because they can't make a living. However, it turns out that on average, for each baby delivered, the obstetrician spends only 10 hours in total for all prenatal office visits and time in the hospital for the delivery. Is the $5,000 charge excessive? It would seem to translate into $1,040,000 per year if the obstetrician worked 40 hours a week for 52 weeks a year (40 hours per week x 52 weeks = 2,080 hours ÷ 10 hours per patient = 208 patients x $5,000 = $1,040,000). Consider further that obstetricians spend 200 hours a year in transit between their office and the hospital. They take 4 weeks of vacation, 10 days of holidays, and 1 week of continuing education. Due to cancellations of scheduled appointments by patients, rescheduling appointments when the doctor has to leave for the hospital suddenly to deliver a baby, and other scheduling difficulties, only 35 work hours are available each week. Costs of maintaining an office (rent, heat, etc.) run $50,000 per year. The office nurse, receptionist, and bookkeeper earn a total of $160,000 per year, including benefits. Because of bad debts from self-pay patients, and aggressive managed care negotiations for discounts, the average amount collected per patient is only $4,000. In the last two years, medical liability insurance has risen from $1,000 per patient to $2,000 per patient. Are obstetricians charging an excessive amount? Is there a cost control problem? What solutions would you suggest?

## DISCUSSION QUESTIONS

1. Why is cost containment a problem in health care? How is it different from cost containment for canned soda?
2. Health care employs 1 out of every 7 workers in America. Does this create political and economic problems that are likely to impede efforts to control health care costs?
3. Shouldn't health insurers stop paying for "health services" that don't provide predictable added value for patients? How can we balance

the desires of the individual patient with cost-effective solutions for society?

4. Which Medicaid approaches to cost control make sense? Which don't?

## REFERENCES

Antel, J. J., Ohsfeldt, R. L., & Becker, E. R. (1995). State regulation and hospital costs. *The Review of Economics and Statistics, 77*(3), 416–422.

Axelsson, R. (1998). Toward an evidence-based health care management. *International Journal of Health Planning and Management, 13*(4), 307–317.

Berger, M. L., & Teutsch, S. M. (2000). Understanding cost-effectiveness analysis. *Preventive Medicine in Managed Care, 1,* 51–58.

Blustein, J. (2000a). Drug coverage and drug purchases by medicare beneficiaries with hypertension. *Health Affairs, 19*(2), 219–230.

Blustein, J. (2000b). Medicare and drug coverage: A women's health issue. *Women's Health Issues, 10*(2), 47–53.

Boccuti, C., & Moon, M. (2003). Comparing medicare and private insurers: Growth rates in spending over three decades. *Health Affairs, 22*(2), 230–237.

Carroll, A., & Ambrose, J. M. (2002). Any-willing-provider laws: Their financial effect on HMOs. *Journal of Health Politics, Policy and Law, 27*(6), 927–945.

Cohen, A. B. (1999). Hitting the "target" in health care cost control. *Journal of Health Politics, Policy and Law, 24*(4), 697–703.

Cutler, D. M., McClellan, M., & Newhouse, J. P. (1998, May). What has increased medical-care spending bought? *AEA Papers and Proceedings, 88*(2), 132–136.

Dale, S. B., & Verdier, J. M. (2003, April). State Medicaid prescription drug expenditures for Medicare-Medicaid dual eligibles: Estimates of Medicaid savings and federal expenditures resulting from expanded Medicare prescription coverage. *Commonwealth Fund Issue Brief, 627,* 1–12.

DeGrazia, D. (1996). Why the United States should adopt a single-payer system of health care finance. *Kennedy Institute of Ethics Journal, 6*(2), 145–160.

Dombovy, M. L. (2002). U.S. health care in conflict—Part II: The challenges of balancing cost quality and access. *Physician Executive, 28*(5), 37–43.

Eddy, D. M. (1992). Applying cost-effectiveness analysis: The inside story. *Journal of the American Medical Association, 268,* 2575–2582.

Finkler, S. A., Henley, R. J., & Ward, D. M. (2003). Evidence-based financial management. *Healthcare Financial Management, 57,* 64–68.

Finkler, S. A., & Ward, D. M. (2003). The case for the use of evidence-based management research for the control of hospital costs. *Health Care Management Review, 28,* 348–365.

Foster, R. A., & Antonelli, P. J. (2002). Computerized physician-ordered entry: Are we there yet? *Otolaryngology Clinics of North America, 35,* 1237–1243.

Gencarelli, D. M. (2003, May 10). Medicaid prescription drug coverage: State efforts to control costs. *NHPF Issue Brief, 790,* 1–17.

Gold, M. R., Siegel, J. E., Russell, L. B., & Weinstein, M. C. (Eds.). (1996). *Cost-effectiveness in health and medicine.* New York: Oxford University Press.

Gunn, J., et. al. (2003). Drug eluting stents: Maximising benefit and minimizing cost. *Heart, 89*(2), 127–131.

Hackey, R. B. (2000). Review essay: Making sense of Medicaid reform. *Journal of Health Politics, Policy and Law, 25*(4), 751–759.

*Health Data Management.* (2003). Reader's perspectives: The internet has proven to be a useful tool to cut health care costs and boost revenue. *Health Data Management, 11*(3), 72.

Hecker, D. E. (2001). Occupational employment projections to 2010. *Monthly Labor Review, 124*(11), 57–84. Available from: http://stats.bls.gov/opub/mlr/2001/11/art4abs.htm

Jacobson, P. D., & Kanna, M. L. (2001). Cost-effectiveness analysis in the courts: Recent trends and future prospects. *Journal of Health Politics, Policy and Law, 25*(4), 751–759.

Joslyn, J. S. (2003). What works. An inside look at outsourcing. *Health Management Technology, 24*(1), 62–64.

Kane, N. M. (1997). Pharmaceutical cost containment and innovation in the United States. *Health Policy, 41*(Suppl.), S71–S89.

Kanavos, P., & Reinhardt, U. (2003). Reference pricing for drugs: Is it compatible with U.S. health care? *Health Affairs, 22*(3), 16–27.

Kovner, A. R., Elton, J. J., & Billings, J. D. (2000). Evidence-based management. *Frontiers of Health Services Management, Summer, 16*(4), 3–24.

LaForge, R. W., & Tureaud, J. S. (2003). Revenue-cycle design: Honing the details. *Healthcare Financial Management, 57*(1), 64–71.

Lee, R. D., & Tuljapurkar, S. (1994). Stochastic population forecasts for the U.S.: Beyond high, medium, and low. *Journal of the American Statistical Association, 89*(428), 1175–1189.

Lee, R. D., & Skinner, J. (1999). Will aging baby boomers bust the federal budget? *The Journal of Economic Perspectives, 13*(1), 117–140.

Lesser, C. S., & Ginsburg, P. B. (2003, May). Health care cost and access problems intensify. Issue Brief No. 63. Center for Studying Health System Change.

Lu, J. R., & Hsiao, W. C. (2003). Does universal health insurance make health care unaffordable? Lessons from Taiwan. *Health Affairs, 22*(3), 77–86.

Mahoney, M. E. (2002). Transforming health information management through technology. *Topics in Health Information Management, 23*(1), 52–61.

Mello, M. M., Studdert, D. M., & Brennan, T. A. (2003). The new medical malpractice crisis. *The New England Journal of Medicine, 348*(23), 2281–2284.

Miller, T. (2001). Increasing longevity and medicare expenditures. *Demography, 38*(2), 215–226.

Moore, W. J., Gutermuth, K., & Pracht, E. E. (2000). Systemwide effects of Medicaid retrospective utilization review programs. *Journal of Health Politics, Policy and Law, 25*(4), 653–688.

OR Manager. (2002). Getting MD buy-in on cost management. OR Manager, 18(6), 20–22.

PricewaterhouseCoopers. (2003, February 19). *Cost of caring: Key drivers of growth in spending on hospital care.*

Queenan, J. T. (2002). The increasing cost of medical care. *Obstetrics & Gynecology, 100*(4), 629–630.

Ruland, C. M., & Ravn, I. H. (2003). Usefulness and effects on costs and staff management of a nursing resource management information system. *Journal of Nursing Management, 11*, 208–215.

Schroeder, S. A., & Cantor, J. C. (1991). On squeezing balloons: Cost containment fails again. *The New England Journal of Medicine, 325*, 15.

Taylor, C. W. (2003). What works. Bridging the gap. In-home monitoring device reduces cost of treating underserved populations in rural Alabama. *Health Management Technology, 24*(4), 36–38.

Thorpe, K. E. (2002). Cost containment. In A. Kovner & S. Jonas (Eds.), *Health care delivery in the united states* (7th ed., pp. 427–451). New York: Springer.

Thorpe, K. E. (1999). Managed care as victim or villain? *Journal of Health Politics, Policy and Law, 24*(5), 949–956.

Young, G. J., Desai, K. R., & Hellinger, F. J. (2000). Community control and pricing patterns of nonprofit hospitals: An antitrust analysis. *Journal of Health Politics, Policy and Law, 25*(6), 1051–1081.

# PART IV
## FUTURES

# 18

# FUTURES
# IN HEALTH
# CARE

John R. Lumpkin

- Explain the importance of thinking about the future for managers in health care.
- Describe different approaches to forecasting the future.
- Identify categories of factors that will affect the future of health care.
- Predict the impact of major change factors on the health care system.

- Strategic planning and forecasting the future
- Social, governmental, and health care system drivers of change
- The impact of health trends on the future of health care in America

Forecasting, futures work, quantitative methods, qualitative methods, financial incentives, aging of the population, population diversity, Medicare, Medicaid, public health beliefs, health insurance coverage, information technology, genomics

ALL OF THE preceding chapters describe key aspects of the American health care system as they exist in the present. Many of the discussions traced historical factors that help explain why we have the health care system we have today. And, many of the discussions included analyses of the challenges that health system leaders will face in the future.

But, what are the "macro" forces that will shape our health system in the future? And, how can health leaders "manage the future" as they work to improve organizations in our health system? These questions frame this last chapter which focuses both on the issue of how to think about the future and on the issue of what will be the "drivers" shaping the future of health care delivery in the United States.

# STRATEGIC PLANNING AND FORECASTING THE FUTURE

## Change and the Need for Strategic Planning

The health care system in the United States is in a constant state of flux and seeming crisis. As health policy analysts have looked into the future, they have predicted its collapse, barring major structural changes. Yet, change over time has not been dramatic; it has been incremental. The IOM Committee on Monitoring Access to Personal Health Care Services described the challenges that exist in the system in their report, *Access to Health Care in America*:

> We hear that government agencies, physicians, and public and private hospitals are straining to keep pace with requests for services amid budget constraints. Not only are some people losing their insurance coverage, but the size of vulnerable populations is growing. Progress against several health problems is blocked because of poor access to care. . . . When the focus shifts to whether we are making headway against specific diseases, the disparity in health status between vulnerable groups and the general populace becomes apparent. . . . In addition to concerns over the less fortunate in our society, there is a growing uneasiness that the delivery system and insurance infrastructure are not meeting the needs of middle- and upper-income Americans as well as they once were. Many besides the poor may have difficulty getting access to health care. . . . Middle income people fear that shrinking insurance benefits will force them to pay more and more of the costs of health care, increasing their reluctance to seek care when they need it. (Millman, 1993, pp. 19–20)

This description of significant system stressors and the impetus for change is consistent with the views of the authors of the preceding chapters in this book. However, the IOM committee made that assessment in 1993! In that year, health care leaders had to make decisions on how to address the current and future challenges that their organizations faced. Those decisions, right or wrong were based on a vision of where the health care system was going and what it would be like in the short and long term. While few people would have predicted with any accuracy the way the system as a whole looks today, many were able to identify the important trends and to plan accordingly.

Every health care organization has a reason for existing, which is expressed in its mission statement. Generally that mission is associated with providing some form of health care to people in need of it. For-profit organizations provide health care services to meet social needs but also act in ways that meet the interests of investors and shareholders. Charitable and not-for-profit organizations also provide health care services to meet social needs and sometimes to address higher-level, community-oriented missions.

In order to assure their future viability, all health care organizations have to respond to their environments. Some institutions and organizations have endowments or other sources of funds to help them through down cycles in income. Governmentally operated organizations such as county and state-run hospitals and outpatient clinics can operate at a deficit when it is covered by tax dollars. Yet, all health care institutions and organizations are affected by the dynamics of the marketplace and the changes in the health delivery system. Each organization's vision is driven by the institution's mission and values, and serves to give direction for future decisions. Well-run organizations have a strategic plan that sets the road map to achieve that vision. It is the role of the leadership of the health care organization to develop and share the vision and to guide the development of the strategic plan.

A strategic plan is based on an assessment of the current environment and projections of a likely future. Some approaches to strategic planning involve the development of multiple futures. The leadership of the health care organization tries to develop a strategic plan that would be successful in different alternative futures. An environmental assessment involves a determination of local, regional, and national trends that potentially impact the health care organization's viability and growth. Careful synthesis of the impacts of these trends into threats and opportunities for the future, sets the boundaries of the planning process. The strategies that address the threats and take advantage of the opportunities form the basis of the strategic plan. The development and assessment of possible futures is a crucial part of the strategic planning process and is called futures work.

The Pan-European Informan 2000+ Project incorporated one approach to futures work, identifying four objectives: (a) illuminate the future and issues impacting the future; (b) use strategic future work to influence policy, either directly or indirectly; (c) formulate policy using strategic futures insight; and (d) implement policy, using strategic futures work to enact policy change (Inforrman, 2001). In the health care field, all four of the objectives are appropriate. The goal of strategic planning is to manage the future. The goal of forecasting is to understand the future well enough to take steps in the present to manage potential futures to achieve the organization's mission and goals. There are many approaches to forecasting, though they fall into three broad categories: quantitative, qualitative, and quantitative and qualitative mixed. The qualitative approach and mixed approach are often described as judgmental.

## Quantitative and Qualitative Approaches to Forecasting

Quantitative forecasting uses a mathematical model to analyze historical data to identify trends and infer the future. The model can be a simple univariate extrapolation of future expenditures based on past spending. For example, state governments have used this approach to model the impact of changing drug regimens on the cost of the Ryan White AIDS drug assistance programs. In that program, the addition of a single, newly-approved anti-retroviral drug can dramatically increase the cost of the program. The budgeting model takes the number of enrollees multiplied times the cost of an average drug package to determine the cost of the regimen. When a new drug enters the market, the cost of the average drug package is recalculated. Using the new average drug cost, it is then a simple matter to project the future costs of the program.

More complex models use multivariate analysis to determine likely changes in factors such as population, cost, and resource utilization. Many of the statistical estimates that are used in health planning are derived by using the quantitative method. These include estimates of current population, population projections, the numbers of people without health care insurance and projections of future expenditures for health care. Since exact data on the population of the United States is only collected during the decennial census, estimates of the character of the population are made using survey data, economic trend data, birth and death certificate data, and other relevant measurable statistics.

Quantitative analysis can only go so far. Methodologically, quantitative analyses are bound to the availability of good data, both historical and current. Many organizations collect and analyze extensive databases of operational data to develop their projections. These data include variables such as bed utilization rates, admissions, cost per admission, staffing levels, supply utilization, and more. In most instances, these operational data are available in real-time or with minimal delay. Other data from inside and outside the organization are plagued with problems of timeliness, data quality, and accessibility.

In addition, often there are important conceptual flaws with quantitative models. The underlying assumption with the quantitative method is that the systems being modeled respond to known inputs in constant and consistent ways. The basic assumption is that the health care system being modeled responds to changes much as an airplane does to wind and weather stresses. An airplane is a complicated mechanical system, but the function of each part and its response to input and stress is knowable. Therefore the sums of the interactions are knowable and the responses are predictable. Human and organizational systems, including the health care system, are more than just complicated; they are complex. Inputs and stressors generate responses and interactions that cannot be readily predicted. In complex systems, the cause and effect relationships between the actors are obscured due to the large number of interacting players and forces. In this type of system, strategic planning is best done using projections of alternative futures.

Since quantitative methods can only go so far in the complex health care environment, qualitative methods must be employed. Qualitative methods involve judgmental forecasting using consensus methods including guessing and hoping to get lucky, panels of experts, the Delphi technique, and surveys (Walonick, 2004). Trying to get lucky by guessing or its corollary—using the guesses of a guru, are the most common approaches used in most industries. It has the advantages of being relatively inexpensive and emotionally rewarding to the guru, but is only as good as the guru's crystal ball. Another approach for development of a vision of the future is through the use of a panel of experts. Impaneling a group of 5 to 20 experts in the field gives a broader range of ideas from which to form a future vision. Careful selection of individuals who reflect the breadth of the health care workforce and market is key to the success of this effort. A skilled leader or outside facilitator is important to lead the process of consensus. The interaction of the group can sometimes lead to the development of new ideas that no one individual would espouse. When these ideas are new and innovative, they enhance the visioning process.

Panels of experts, however, can be unduly influenced by strong opinions held by one or more of the panel members meeting in person. However, the Delphi technique seeks to avoid interaction problems of in-person meetings by conducting rounds of solicited predictions and comments from individuals who form a panel but do not meet. The results of each round are fed back to participants as stimulus to the next round. Each successive round narrows the opinions of the group towards a final prediction. The expectation is that a structured consensus is a better predictor than individual or group predictions. Surveys are a good way to collect opinions about likely futures from a broad-based group of knowledgeable people. Synthesis of this information as part of the planning process allows this data to be used as part of the visioning process.

In common practice, most organizations use a mixture of quantitative and qualitative approaches to develop their environmental assessment. Quantitative projections using internal data sources, data and analysis from trade organizations, and qualitative processes are melded into an organization's vision of the future. The following sections of this chapter look at the various factors that any health care organization should consider as they are developing a vision of the future and a strategic plan.

## SOCIAL, GOVERNMENTAL, AND HEALTH CARE SYSTEM DRIVERS OF CHANGE

There are many forces and trends that will have an impact on the future directions of the health care system in the U.S. Some of the forces and trends are related to overall societal changes and policies that have an impact on health care. These external factors include the changing demographics of the population, federal fiscal policy, including Medicare and Medicaid. Factors internal to the health care system include the preferences and ideology of people, the growing numbers of the uninsured, and emerging advances in information technology and in genomics.

### Changing Demographics

Fundamental to any predictions about the future of health is an understanding of how the users of health care—the American public—will change in the coming years. The two key population changes that are related to health care delivery are the aging of the population and increasing ethnic diversity.

## The Graying of the American Population

At the end of the Second World War, millions of soldiers returned home to wives and loved ones with a resultant explosive increase in birth rates. This postwar generation is called the baby boomers. As the baby boom generation grew and matured, its interests, needs, and concerns have dominated much of the life and culture of this country in the second half of the twentieth century and the beginning of the twenty-first century. As we enter the midpoint of the first decade of this century, the baby boomers are reaching retirement age. The aging of this generation will have a dramatic impact on the age composition of the population as a whole and certainly on the delivery of health care services.

Over the last century, individual life expectancy increased from 49.2 years in 1900 to 76.9 years in 2000. In the early part of the twentieth century the increase in life expectancy was driven by improvements in the public health system. The wholesale adoption of improved sanitation practices, enhanced safety of the food and drug supply, and improved nutrition enabled the United States to dramatically reduce rates of infectious diseases. Pneumonia, tuberculosis, and dysentery as leading causes of death significantly diminished. The last half of the twentieth century witnessed the emergence of chronic illness as the leading cause of death, with heart disease, cancer, and stroke rising to prominence. While advances in prevention services and medical treatment led to a decrease in the death rates due to these diseases, they remain the leading killers in the twenty-first century (U.S. Census Bureau (USCB), 2004).

As the life expectancy of the general population has increased, advances in prevention services and medical treatment for the elderly has resulted in improvements in the quantity and quality of life of those over 65. The increasing life span and dynamics of the baby boom generation has led to a dramatic increase in both the numbers and percentage of the elderly and the frail elderly. The life expectancy of those aged 65 is almost 18 years and for those aged 85, life expectancy is over 6 years. In 2000, some 35 million Americans were aged 65 or older, and 4.2 million were aged 85 or older, representing 12.4% and 1.5% of the U.S. population. By 2030, the number of Americans over age 65 will more than double to 75.7 million, and those aged 85 and over will increase two and half times to 10.1 million (Federal Interagency Forum on Aging Related Statistics (FIFARS), 2004). (See **TABLE 18.1**.)

## TABLE 18.1

### Historic and Projected Age Distribution of U.S. Population

| YEAR | PERCENTAGE 65 OR OLDER | PERCENTAGE 85 OR OLDER |
|------|------------------------|------------------------|
| 1900 | 4.1 | 0.2 |
| 1910 | 4.3 | 0.2 |
| 1920 | 4.7 | 0.2 |
| 1930 | 5.4 | 0.2 |
| 1940 | 6.9 | 0.3 |
| 1950 | 8.2 | 0.4 |
| 1960 | 9.2 | 0.5 |
| 1970 | 9.9 | 0.7 |
| 1980 | 11.3 | 1.0 |
| 1990 | 12.6 | 1.2 |
| 2000 | 12.4 | 1.5 |
| 2010 | 13.2 | 1.9 |
| 2020 | 16.5 | 2.1 |
| 2030 | 20.0 | 2.5 |
| 2040 | 20.5 | 3.5 |
| 2050 | 20.3 | 4.3 |

SOURCE: Federal Interagency Forum on Aging Related Statistics, Appendix A: Detailed Tables, July 2004. http://www.agingstats.gov/tables%202001/Tables-population.html#Indicator%201

The aging of the population will have a dramatic affect on the utilization of health care services over the next decades. Health care resource utilization and cost increase significantly with advancing age. For Medicare beneficiaries, the average cost for care was $9,352 in 1999. The average cost for those aged 65 to 69 was just $6,711. The average costs grew to $16,596 for those over 85. (See FIGURE 18.1.) With increasing age, the likelihood of significant illness increases; 45.5% of those who have reached the age of 85 received nursing home care in 1999. The costs for nursing home care averages over $30,000 per year. Other costs, including medications, are related to more intensive health care services utilization (FIFARS,

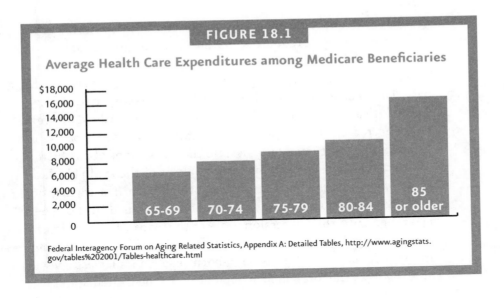

**FIGURE 18.1**

Average Health Care Expenditures among Medicare Beneficiaries

Federal Interagency Forum on Aging Related Statistics, Appendix A: Detailed Tables, http://www.agingstats.gov/tables%202001/Tables-healthcare.html

2004). Therefore, as the population ages, the patterns of cost and utilization can be expected to change. This impact may be mitigated by changes in the long-term care delivery systems as care migrates away from institutional-based care to home- and community-based services. However, even with significant changes as to where the care for the elderly occurs, the portion of the health care dollar devoted to the elderly will increase significantly.

## Increasing Diversity in the Population

The United Sates has been a diverse society since before the American Revolution. The land mass that is now the United States had indigenous populations of Native Americans who greeted the first (culturally mixed) settlers from Europe. In fact, cooperation by these indigenous populations was essential to the survival of many of the first colonies. Since then, the United States has seen numerous waves of immigration from Europe, Africa, Asia, Latin and South America. Many immigrant groups came to the United States to look for economic opportunities and to escape political or economic oppression. Early "immigrants" from West Africa were forcibly removed from their homeland and became the slave labor that drove the economy in the southern states. Each successive group of emigrants added to the cultural richness that makes this country strong. Continued immigration coupled with racial and ethnic variations in population growth are projected to result in a dramatic shift in the demographic character of this country as we move from being a predominantly European-origin population to one of a multi-racial and ethnic make-up.

Data on racial and ethnic groups have not been inclusive in the past. The Census Bureau did not consistently collect data on persons of Hispanic origin until the 1980s. Until recently, data were not collected on subgroups based on ethnic origin of Hispanics or Asians and Pacific Islanders. Despite the limitations of the historical data, clear trends emerge from analysis of the available data. In 1860, 13.2% of the population was foreign-born. The segment of the U.S. population that was foreign-born remained in the 13% to 14% range until the Depression years of the 1930s when large numbers of unemployed Americans led to curtailment of immigration. In 1970, the percentage of foreign-born reached its lowest level at 4.7%. By 1990, the foreign-born population in the United States was 7.9%. This evidence indicates that most of the racial and ethnic diversity in this country is due to population patterns of people born here rather than to immigration (Gibson, 1999).

The European-origin population of the United States changed little, from 80.7% in 1790 to 80.3% 200 years later. The Black population in 1790 and 1990 was 19.3% and 12 % respectively. In 1940, the population of people from European ancestry peaked at 89.8% of the total population, and the Black population was at its lowest level at 9.8% (Gibson, 2002). After almost 200 years of relative stability in the ratios of the racial and ethnic groups in the United States, projections based on current trends indicate a dramatic change will occur over the next few decades. TABLE 18.2 displays the population estimates by the U.S. Census Bureau for the racial and ethnic make-up of future U.S. populations. By the year 2050, only half of the population will be of European ancestry; 24.4% will be Hispanic, 14.6% Black, 8% Asian, and 5.3% other races. (Note: Hispanic is an ethnic designation, not a racial one. Hispanics are predominantly White and Black. Hispanics who are predominantly from the indigenous Native American populations are self-classified as White or Black) (USCB, 2004)

Some groups of people share a more common genetic background because of a common ancestry, or originate from an isolated population. This is true of groups like the Central and Eastern European Ashkenazi Jews. They migrated from the Near East within the last two millennia and dispersed throughout central and eastern Europe. Because of religious and other cultural factors, there was

**TABLE 18.2**

Projected U.S. Population Make-Up

| PERCENTAGE OF POPULATION | 2000 | 2010 | 2020 | 2030 | 2040 | 2050 |
|---|---|---|---|---|---|---|
| White | 81 | 79.3 | 77.6 | 75.8 | 73.9 | 72.1 |
| Black | 12.7 | 13.1 | 13.5 | 13.9 | 14.3 | 14.6 |
| Asian | 3.8 | 4.6 | 5.4 | 6.2 | 7.1 | 8.0 |
| Other | 2.5 | 3.0 | 3.5 | 4.1 | 4.7 | 5.3 |
| Hispanic | 12.6 | 15.5 | 17.8 | 20.1 | 22.3 | 24.4 |
| Non-Hispanic White | 69.4 | 65.1 | 61.3 | 57.5 | 53.7 | 50.1 |

SOURCE: U.S. Census Bureau, 2004, U.S. Interim Projections by Age, Sex, Race, and Hispanic Origin, http://www.census.gov/ipc/www/usinterimproj/ (accessed April 2004)

little intermarriage with host European populations. When they migrated to the United States, they shared a number of common genetic characteristics, which unfortunately included 20 recessive disease genes, including Tay-Sachs (Behar et al., 2004). Except in those rare circumstances, race and ethnicity are not good indicators of common genetic background. The genetic variation within a race is greater than the variation across races, and the variation within general populations with a common national origin is greater than the variation across national origins (Disotell, 2000).

The impact of the increasingly diverse U.S. population on the future of health care is dependent on a number of factors. Racial and ethnic minority groups in the United States have poorer health status than does the majority White population. They have higher rates of death due to heart disease, stroke, cancer, and the other leading causes of death. Racial and ethnic minorities within the United States also have poorer outcomes when they are treated by the health care system. Much of the racial and ethnic disparities in health care and health status are explainable by differences in socioeconomic position. The rate of poverty for nonHispanic Whites has ranged between 9.1% and 14.4% over the last 40 years. For minority populations the poverty rates have been uniformly higher with African Americans ranging from 22.5% to 39.4% and Hispanics from 21.4% to 30.7% during the same time period. (Proctor, 2003) Without a significant redistribution of wealth between the White and minority populations, the expected demographic shift will result in greater disparities and increased poverty rates. These shifts will have an adverse affect on the economic viability of the health care providers who predominantly serve minority populations. If the current disparities continue into the future, then the burden of illness will increase as the minority populations increase. These adverse trends may be mitigated by organized efforts to reduce racial and ethnic disparities currently being developed as public-private partnerships between the United States Department of Health and Human Services, Health Plans, and others.

With the changing racial and ethnic composition of the United States, health care providers will have an increasingly diverse patient population. To assure quality care, caregivers and their staff will need to communicate with patients who have low English proficiency. Further, caregivers and their staff will have to improve their cultural proficiency skills and access to appropriate translation services to achieve the best outcomes. While the predominate language translations services will be in Spanish, shifting patterns of immigration will require that services be available in Polish and other Eastern-European languages, African languages, and the many languages of Asia and the Pacific Islands.

## Changing Trends in Medicare and Medicaid

The government is the largest payer for health care services in the United Sates. Medicare, Medicaid, and the State Child Health Insurance Program (SCHIP) account for over 45% of health care expenditures (Heffler et al., 2003). The Medicare program, which pays for many of the health care services received by the elderly and some of the disabled, has been in existence since 1966 with coverage for the elderly and since 1973 for coverage of eligible people with disabilities. Enrollment in the Medicare program reached 40.5 million in 2002, which is expected to double as the baby boom generation begins to retire (Centers for Medicare & Medicaid Services (CMS), 2004). Medicare currently constitutes 12% of the federal budget (Office of Management and Budget, OMB, 2001).

The Medicaid program, which funds services for many low-income Americans, had 36.6 million enrollees in 2003 (CMS, 2003). Also, 2003 was the first year that the Medicaid and SCHIP enrollment exceeded the Medicare enrollment (41.4 million versus a projected 41.0 million). Incremental improvements in health care insurance coverage for children occurred with the original authorization of SCHIP. This was achieved through a blend of increased income eligibility for Medicaid and enrollment in a state specific coverage plan for the working poor. Expansions since 2000 have included families of eligible children in some states. Medicaid and SCHIP are financed jointly by the federal government and by individual states.

Medicaid has played an increasing role in each State's budget, from 10.2% in 1987 to 20.5% in 2002. The economic downturn that began in 2000 resulted in sharp decreases in available revenue for states. At the same time, increases in enrollment and pharmacy costs resulted in double digit increases in Medicaid costs from state fiscal years 2000 to 2005. Despite the general recovery in the economy, the budget restrictions for states are expected to extend well into the middle of the first decade of the twenty-first century. Mounting spending pressures, resistance to increased state taxes, use of one-time budget balancers, and the "jobless recovery" combine to create an environment where state budgets will continue to face shortfalls without additional reductions in state operations and programs. In response, states have been taking steps to control the growth of the Medicaid program, including prescription drug cost controls, freezing or reducing payments rates to providers, reducing or restricting eligibility, or increasing beneficiary copayments for services (Smith, Ellis, Gifford, Ramesh, & Wachino, 2002; Boyd & Washino, 2004).

As states have made significant changes in response to restrictive financial climates, the federal budget has also been impacted by recent events and policy decisions. The wars in Afghanistan and Iraq, the fiscal legacy of the terrorist attacks on the United States in 2001, the economic down turn at the beginning of the twenty-first century, and federal tax reductions have created a dramatic shift in the federal budget balance. In 2001, the Congressional Budget Office predicted a surplus of $353 billion for the federal fiscal year ending in 2003. In stark contrast to that projection, the federal fiscal year ending in 2003 closed out with a deficit of $374 billion. This represents a drop of over $700 billion. Federal budget deficits are predicted to continue through out the decade, forcing a federal policy response. Political considerations make a tax increase unlikely, meaning that the deficit can only be controlled by reductions in spending. Social Security, Medicare, Medicaid, and other entitlement programs make up 54% of the national budget. Defense spending and interest payments make up another 27% for a total of 81%. The remainder, $494 billion in federal Fiscal Year 2003, funds the bulk of federal programs. With projected budget shortfalls of about $500 billion per year for the rest of the decade, significant budget reduction cannot occur without reductions in entitlement programs such as Medicare and Medicaid.

The impact on health care providers of state and federal budgetary pressures and the policies that will have to be adopted to address them will be far ranging and dramatic. Changes in Medicare, Medicaid, and SCHIP will have an impact on the entire health care marketplace. Those policy changes will impact sectors of the health care delivery system differentially. The more than 80 million Medicare and Medicaid enrollees represent 27% of the population of the United States. However, the two programs combined account for 36% of personal health expenditures, 48% of hospital expenditures, 33% of physician and professional expenditures, 61% of nursing home care, and 32% of home health care (Kaiser, 2004). The balance of this decade will see continued efforts by the states and the Centers for Medicare & Medicaid Services to reduce reimbursement rates and utilization. This will include continued pressure to move surgical and other invasive procedures out of more expensive hospital settings into less expensive ambulatory surgery centers and outpatient clinics. Efforts will continue to move care from nursing homes to home- and community-based services. In addition, the Centers for Medicare & Medicaid Services will continue to push incentives for improving quality and adoption of information technology.

### The U.S. Public's Health Beliefs

The views of the public concerning their health and the actions that they take based on those views play an important role in the health of the nation. How the public views the health care system also has an impact on policymakers and the issues that get addressed in the public policy debate. A person's health beliefs and behaviors are the result of a complex constellation of factors. The foundation of those beliefs is based in the nature of their upbringing and the culture that they come to maturity in. The twentieth century witnessed a dramatic shift in the leading causes of death and disability in the United States. In 1890, the leading causes of death were pneumonia, tuberculosis, and dysentery. In 1938, that pattern shifted and heart disease, cancer, and stroke became the leading causes of death—a pattern that persists until the present time (National Center for Health Statistics (NCHS), 2003). Looking beyond the diseases that lead to death to the health behaviors and risk factors that result in those diseases gives a different view of the causes of death in this nation. From that perspective, the use of tobacco products and alcohol containing products are revealed as the true leading causes of death. Inadequate exercise and unhealthy diet have become the third leading cause of death (McGinnis & Foege, 1993). With the control of many infectious diseases, our modern society has advanced to the point that health improvements become dependent on creating the conditions in which people can make healthy choices, but also requiring that they make them.

The future of health care delivery and public health will be influenced by how Americans respond to the changing nature of the causes of illness. Increased understanding of the roles of behavioral factors in determining health status could influence the types of services and advice Americans seek from health care providers. The growing prevalence of chronic illnesses also will shape the services needed by Americans. More attention to "coordination" and "management" rather than to "procedures" is required to adequately care for chronic conditions.

One noteworthy interaction of services and behavior has been emerging from survey data (Harris Interactive, 2001). Surveys suggest that many times it takes a tragic event to achieve change in attitude and behavior. Survivors of serious illness report improvements in getting regular preventive care (79%), eating a healthy diet (70%), getting up-to-date information about their disease (67%), getting regular exercise (42%), and keeping their weight at a healthy level (36%). This enlightened response appears to have an impact on their family as 80% report that they are more concerned about what family members are doing to prevent disease, injury, and disability (Harris Interactive, 2001).

Just as public opinion beliefs and behaviors drive personal health practices, they also play a role in driving public policy. Public concern about the state of the health care system expressed at the electoral polls in 1991 and 1992 drove the health care reform efforts of 1993 and 1994. Public concern about the direction of the reforms developed by the Administration of President Bill Clinton, however, led to the end of health care reform for the rest of the twentieth century. Yet, once again public concern is placing health care reform on the national agenda. During the 2004 presidential election campaign, more Americans were personally worried about health care costs than about losing jobs, paying rent, or being a victim of a terrorist attack; 87% of the public were very worried or somewhat worried about having to pay more for health care or health insurance, and 64% were worried about not being able to afford the health care services they think that they need, or that their health plan was more concerned about saving money than what was best for them. In addition, 52% of Americans were worried about losing health insurance coverage (Kaiser, 2004).

In 2004, there also was a significant gap in trust between people and their health plans. Polls showed that more than 60% of people trusted doctors and nurses in general and their doctors and nurses who treat them in particular. On the other hand, only 9% trusted managed care companies and only 8% trusted their health insurance company. Yet despite these concerns, people tend to be satisfied with their own health insurance. Two thirds would give their plans an "A" or "B" grade and 76% would recommend their health plan to family members who are healthy (Harris Interactive, 2004).

The contradictory opinions of people concerning health plans and health care insurance in general and their personal health care provider and health plans in particular have been a barrier to fundamental change in the health care system. Thus, it is difficult to develop the collective will to change the health care system when people don't feel a personal stake in the change process.

## Increasing Rates of the Uninsured

The earlier chapter on access in this volume by Billings and Cantor describes the problems faced by the more than 40 million uninsured Americans. The lack of insurance coverage affects access to health care and leads to worse health status for the actual people uninsured and causes financial strains on providers who deliver emergency services to the uninsured and causes financial strains on providers who deliver at least emergence services to the uninsured.

Understanding the future of the health care delivery system in America requires some sense of what happens to the insurance system. If employer-based insurance coverage becomes increasingly less common and if the number of people covered by private insurance continues to decrease, pressure likely will grow to change our financing system. As became clear during debates about the unsuccessful Clinton health reform, many strategies to address the problems with the American approach to insuring health care may greatly affect the "futures" experienced by health care providers.

The future of the uninsured is unclear at this time. One scenario is that no major public action will focus on reducing the number of people without insurance coverage. In that future, communities with large numbers of residents who lack insurance coverage can expect increasing problems with access as individual providers and hospitals either close their doors or refuse to treat the uninsured. The current trend for the uninsured to increasingly utilize hospital emergency departments for nonemergent care will continue. Hospital emergency departments will continue to face overcrowding as patients arrive sicker because of foregone preventive and curative care.

An alternative scenario would see the adoption of reforms in the health care system to assure health care insurance coverage for all or a substantial proportion of the uninsured. In this scenario, health care costs may stabilize as all sectors of the population have access to preventive services and early curative services, thus preventing much of the avoidable illness, disability, or death currently seen in the uninsured. Safety net providers would see a stabilization of their financial bases and might be able to begin competing on quality of service delivery rather than rely on the payer mix of their patients. The uninsured per-capita health care expenditures would be expected to increase as they seek care to prevent illness or treat it earlier. However, because the uninsured are younger, the costs should stabilize over time if there are payoffs from these preventive services.

## Health Information Technology

The future will see expansion of health information technology into all aspects of health and health care. The impact will be seen in hospitals, long-term care settings, caregiver's offices, homes, and communities. However, obstacles and barriers exist that could delay the adoption of these innovations and the associated improvements in quality, safety, efficiency, and effectiveness. These obstacles include clinical information standard development and adoption, financial incentives and disincentives, and clinicians' aversion to information technology. Much progress has been made on the standards front as discussed in chapter 14. Further work will be necessary in developing a robust standards development apparatus to assure that clinical standards, code sets, and medical terms can keep up with the rapid advances in health care implementation. Initiatives by payers to enhance reimbursement to providers who have electronic health records and reduce reimbursement to those who do not could speed up the adoption of information technology. Some components of the incentive system are being considered by CMS and some private payers. Despite the slow adoption of information technology in the late 1990s, clinicians are increasingly adopting mobile computing devices. A 2003 survey found that 46% of surveyed physicians own and use handheld computing devices in clinical settings (iHealthbeat, 2003). As the technology advances and the utility becomes clearer, many more clinicians will convert to the new technology.

President George Bush called for population-wide utilization of electronic health records by 2014. The middle part of the 2000s witnessed an unprecedented pace of adoption of clinical information system standards by the U.S. Department of Health and Human Services. Through DHHS's partnership with the U.S. Department of Veterans Affairs and the U.S. Department of Defense in the Consolidated Health Informatics Initiative, the nation's largest purchasers of health care have adopted clinical data standards that will become the de facto standards for the health care industry. Pressure by groups of private sector purchasers through "pay for performance" arrangements and public reporting through organizations like the Leapfrog Group will help to accelerate the adoption of this new technology.

Improvements in quality, efficiency, and effectiveness associated with information technology will position early and mid-adopters in a more competitive position in the health care market place. The institutions, organizations, and practices that adopt this technology will be more attractive partners in care arrangements and for selection to participate in closed panel relationships. The provider's decision to adopt this technology will need to be based on an assessment of risks related to the lack of full maturity in clinical data standards and the potential to select deadend systems versus the immediate improvements in quality, safety, and competitive position. However, competitive factors and payer incentives will require that most health care providers adopt electronic health records by the end of the decade.

By the beginning of the twenty-first century, a leading use of the Internet was to find health-related information (Fox & Fellows, 2003). As a result, individuals had access to information about new drugs and treatments soon after their development or adoption. In many instances, patients had earlier and more complete information on new diagnostic techniques and therapeutic modalities before their information technology adverse provider. More recent studies have indicated that clinicians are closing the gap in the use of the Internet for keeping current with health information.

In summary, the future of health care delivery will be greatly shaped by how fast information technology is adopted. Although there is not much uncertainty that electronic medical records will emerge as the norm, the impacts of this improved approach to managing information on quality of care are more difficult to predict. But, information technology is a "driver" of the future with much potential to improve our ability to manage and restore health.

### Genomics

An emerging driver of future change in the health care system is the emerging field of genomics. With the sequencing of the human genome in 2003, the genomic era had arrived (National Human Genome Research Institute, 2004). Spurred on by that Herculean effort, and supported by the technology that made it possible, great advances should emerge in linking human diseases with variations in specific genes. A number of diseases have been identified as being phenotypically similar, but genotypically diverse. Genetic markers have been identified that are associated with an increased risk for a number of chronic diseases including lung cancer, breast cancer, and heart disease.

The bio-ethical impact of this new technology has been a matter of great debate. The ease with which genetic testing can now be performed has raised concern about the potential to discriminate based on a person's genetic code in hiring, firing, access to health care, and insurance.

Advances in genomics also will greatly shape the future of the pharmaceutical industry. Recognition of the genetic variability that exists within disease categories leads to the potential for designer medications tailored to fit an individual's genetic makeup. Given the high cost of research, development, marketing and distribution of new pharmaceutical agents, this technology has the potential to substantially raise the costs of health care as it enhances the refinement of treatment regimens. In the past, the pharmaceutical industry has been hesitant to develop drugs for many rare conditions, because the potential market was too small to assure a return on investment. The same financial pressures could also lead to the development of pharmaceuticals that are effective only for the largest genetic subgrouping for treatable illnesses. Legislation and inducement programs to support the development of "orphan drugs" may need to be extended from rare diseases to cover people with rare genotypes.

As with the case of information technology, genomics represents a driver of change that has much potential to improve the effectiveness of health care. However, the many perhaps unintended side effects of advances in genomics will need to be anticipated and managed by health lenders.

## IMPACT OF HEALTH TRENDS ON THE FUTURE OF HEALTH CARE IN AMERICA

Owen's Epigrammata printed in 1605 included the anonymous Latin proverb "Times change and we change with them." In the preceding pages, many of the factors that will change the future of the health care system are discussed. The impact of all of these factors and more is difficult to predict. It is difficult to look at all of the challenges facing organizations in the health care system and not predict that the system is rapidly approaching a collapse. Yet, the health care system is a complex system which responds in ways that only seem logical in retrospect. And, there are some promising aspects of the future—information technology and genomics, for example—that could greatly improve health and health care.

In 2004, Harris Interactive polled health care leaders about the future of the U.S. health care system as it responds to multiple pressures. Their responses reflect one vision of the future of the health care system. They predicted that by 2014 the number of the uninsured would increase to 18% of the United States population. They also predicted that out-of-pocket health care spending could reach as high as a quarter of the health care costs as health expenses approach 18% of GDP. As a result, the majority of those polled predicted that there will be an increase in the proportion of hospital beds provided by for-profit hospitals as well as an increase in the proportion of health care coverage that is provided by investor-owned companies. Coupled with a predicted decrease in the number of employed workers who will have health insurance covered by their employer, they envisioned that the tiering of the health care system will increase (Harris, 2004).

William H. Foege, MD, a leader in the worldwide eradication of smallpox and a former Director of the Centers for Disease Control and Prevention (CDC), said at a 2003 meeting, "There are two kinds of futurists, those that predict the future and those that change the future. We need both." This is true of society as a whole and also true in a health care organization. A manager must be able to use multiple sources of information to make the best possible prediction of the future. Careful analysis and planning of possible futures by a management team is essential for every successful organization. A strategic plan must identify opportunities created by potential, future developments and areas of risk that must be protected. Through rigorous planning and monitoring of external factors and their impact on an organization, a manager can not only predict but also change the future.

## DISCUSSION QUESTIONS

1. What is the relationship of future forecasting to strategic planning, and why are they both important?
2. What are the advantages and disadvantages to quantitative and qualitative forecasting approaches?
3. What are the most important drivers for change in today's health

## CASE STUDY

You have just been appointed to direct the state health agency of a newly elected governor. The governor ran on a campaign promise to reform the health care system. You responsibility is to identify, appoint, and lead a commission to determine the future of the health care system in your state and make recommendations to improve the quality, effectiveness, and efficiency of the system.

1. What kind of people would you appoint to the commission?
2. How would you go about developing the forecast? What methods and approaches would you use?
3. What would be the kind of staff you would hire to support the work of the commission?
4. Outline the elements that should be in the commission's final report.

care system? What other factors would you add to the ones in the book?

4. What changes in the health care system will be most important to consumers? Hospitals? Insurers?

5. What are ways that managers can shape the future for their health care organization and the health care system?

6. Take a topic covered in one of the preceding chapters in this book and discuss the impact of major health care trends on its future.

## REFERENCES

American College of Emergency Physicians, survey conducted by Public Opinion Strategies, Alexandria, VA, released May 13, 2004. http://covertheuninsuredweek.org/media/research/ERSurvey.pdf (accessed July 2004).

Behar, D. M., Hammer, M. F., Garrigan, D., Villems, R., Bonne-Tamir, B., Richards, M., et al. (2004). MtDNA evidence for a genetic bottleneck in the early history of the Ashkenazi Jewish population. *Eur J Hum Genet.*, 12(5), 355–364. http://www.nature.com/cgi-taf/DynaPage.taf?file=/ejhg/journal/v12/n5/abs/5201156a.html&dynoptions=doi 1082935901 (accessed July 2004).

Boyd, D., Washino, V., & Kaiser Commission on Medicaid and the Uninsured. Is the state fiscal crisis over? A 2004 state budget update, 2004. http://www.kff.org/medicaid/loader.cfm?url=/commonspot/security/getfile.cfm&PageID=30459 (accessed May 2004).

Centers for Disease Control, Behavior Risk Factor Surveillance System: Trends Data—Nationwide, June 2004 http://www.cdc.gov/brfss/ (accessed May 2004).

Centers for Medicare & Medicaid Services, Medicare Enrollment: National Trends 1966–2002, June 2004. http://www.cms.hhs.gov/statistics/enrollment/natltrends/hi_smi.asp (accessed May 2004).

Centers for Medicare & Medicaid Service. (2003). CMS Statistics, June 2003. http://www.cms.hhs.gov/researchers/pubs/03cmsstats.pdf (accessed May 2004).

Disotell, T. R. (2000). Human genomic variation. *Genome Biol.*, 1(5) Comment 2004. (Electronic Version: Nov 10, 2000). http://genomebiology.com/2000/1/5/COMMENT/2004 (accessed July 2004).

Federal Interagency Forum on Aging Related Statistics (FIFARS), Appendix A: Detailed tables (accessed July 2004) http://www.agingstats.gov/tables%202001/Tables-population.html#Indicator%201, http://www.agingstats.gov/tables%202001/Tables-healthcare.html

Fox, S., & Fellows, D. Pew Internet and American Life Project, Internet Health Resources, July 16, 2003. http://www.pewtrusts.org/pdf/pew_internet_health_resources_0703.pdf

Gibson, C. J., & Lennon, E., U.S. Census Bureau, Population Division, Historical census statistics on the foreign-born population of the United States: 1850–1990, February 1999. http://www.census.gov/population/www/documentation/twps0029/twps0029.html (accessed April 2004).

Gibson, C., & Jung, K., U.S. Census Bureau, Population Division, Historical census statistics on population totals by race, 1790 to 1990, and by Hispanic origin, 1970 to 1990, for the United States, regions, divisions, and states, September 2002. http://www.census.gov/population/www/documentation/twps0056.html (accessed April, 2004).

Harris Interactive. Elite views on the future of the health care system, February 3, 2004, http://www.harrisinteractive.com/news/allnewsbydate.asp?NewsID=756 (accessed July 2004).

Harris Interactive. Harris Health Care Poll: Disease prevention and health promotion: It often takes a serious illness to get people's attention, March 2001. http://www.harrisinteractive.com/news/allnewsbydate.asp?NewsID=246 (accessed May 2004).

Harris Interactive. Harris Health Care Poll: Too little exercise, rather than eating too much, seen as biggest cause of obesity, April 2004. http://www.harrisinteractive.com/news/newsletters/wsjhealthnews/WSJOnline_HI_Health-CarePoll2004vol3_iss07.pdf (accessed May 2004).

Harris Interactive Health Care Research. Health care poll: Health care professionals, pharmacies, hospitals gain the public's trust, January 28, 2004. http://www.harrisinteractive.com/news/newsletters/wsjhealthnews/WSJOnline_HI_Health-CarePoll2004vol3_iss02.pdf (accessed May 2004).

Harris Interactive Health Care Research. Health care poll: Satisfaction with own health insurance remarkably stable, March 2004. http://www.harrisinteractive.com/news/allnewsbydate.asp?NewsID=781 (May 2004).

Heffler, S., Smith, S., Keehan, S., Clemens, M. K., Won, G., & Zezza, M. (2003, January–June). Office of the Actuary, Centers for Medicare & Medicaid Services, Baltimore, USA. Health spending projections for 2002–2012. *Health Aff* (Millwood). Suppl:W3–54–65 http://content.healthaffairs.org/cgi/reprint/hlthaff.w4.79v1.pdf (accessed May 2004).

iHealth Beat, One third of docs use mobile technology, survey finds, January 7, 2003. http://www.ihealthbeat.org/index.cfm?Action=dspItem&itemID=100423 (accessed July 2004).

Institute of Medicine (IOM). (2004). Hidden costs, value lost. Washington, DC: National Academy Press; Miller, Wilhelmine, Elizabeth Vigdor, & Willard Manning, 2004. Covering The Uninsured: What is it Worth? Health Affairs Web Exclusive, available at content.healthaffairs.org/cgi/reprint/hlthaff.w4.157v1 (accessed July 2004).

Kaiser Family Foundation. Medicaid at a Glance 2004, January 2004.

http://www.kff.org/medicaid/upload/30463_1.pdf (accessed May 2004).

Kaiser Family Foundation. Medicare at a Glance 2004, March 2004. http://www.kff.org/medicare/upload/33319_1.pdf (accessed May 2004).

The Kaiser Family Foundation, Kaiser Health Poll Report: Health Security Watch, March/April 2004. http://www.kff.org/healthpoll report/CurrentEdition/security/index.cfm

Kaufman, D. R., Patel, V. L., Hilliman, C., Morin, P. C., Pevzner, J., Weinstock, R. S., Goland, R., Shea, S., & Starren, J. (2003). Usability in the real world: Assessing medical information technologies in patients' homes. *J Biomed Inform.*, 36(1–2), 45–60.

Informan 2000+, Performance and innovation unit—Understanding best practice in strategic futures work, October 2001. http://www.cam bridgeuniversityfutures.co.uk/Understanding_Best_Practices_Of_ Futures_Work.pdf (accessed July 2004).

McGinnis, J. M., & Foege, W. H. (1993). Actual causes of death in the United States. *Journal of the American Medical Association*, 270, 2207–2212.

Millman, M. (Ed.). (1993). Institute of Medicine Committee on Monitoring Access to Personal Health Care Services. *Access to Health Care in America* (pp. 19–20). National Academy Press.

National Center for Health Statistics (NCHS)—Centers for Disease Control. Deaths and death rates for leading causes of death: Death registration states, 1900–1998, 2004. http://www.cdc.gov/nchs/data/ statab/lead1900_98.pdf (accessed May 2004).

National Committee on Vital and Health Statistics, Information for Health: A Strategy for Building the National Health Information Infrastructure, November 2001. http://www.ncvhs.hhs.gov/nhi ilayo.pdf (accessed July 2004).

National Human Genome Research Institute, An overview of the Human Genome Project, June 2004. http://www.nhgri.nih.gov/12011238 (accessed July 2004).

Office of Management and Budget, Executive Office of the President of the United States, Budget of the United States, 2001. http://w3. access.gpo.gov/usbudget/fy2001/guide02.html (accessed May 2004).

Office of Management and Budget, Executive Office of the President of the United States, 2003 Financial Report of the United States Government, Feb 24, 2004. http://www.whitehouse.gov/omb/pubpress /fy2004/2003_financial_rpt.pdf (accessed May 2004).

Proctor, B. D., & Dalaker, J. U.S. Census Bureau, Poverty in the United States: 2002—Current population reports consumer income, September 2003. http://www.census.gov/prod/2003pubs/p60–222.pdf (accessed May 2004).

Robert Wood Johnson Foundation, Cover the Uninsured Worker Fact

Sheet, May 2004. http://covertheuninsuredweek.org/factsheets/display.php?FactSheetID=109 (accessed May 2004).

Smith, V., Ellis, E., Gifford, K., Ramesh, R., & Wachino, V. Kaiser Commission on Medicaid and the Uninsured: Medicaid spending growth: Results from a 2002 survey, The Henry J. Kaiser Family Foundation, Sept 2002. http://www.kaisernetwork.org/health_cast/uploaded_files/ACF73C4.pdf (accessed May 2004).

U.S. Census Bureau (USCB), U.S. Interim projections by age, sex, race, and Hispanic origin, May 2004. http://www.census.gov/ipc/www/usinterimproj/

Wagner, E. H. (1998). Chronic disease management: What will it take to improve care for chronic illness? *Effective Clinical Practice, 1,* 2–4.

Walonick, D. S. An overview of forecasting methodology, http://www.statpac.com/research-papers/forecasting.htm (accessed June 2004).

# PART V
# APPENDICES

# A

# GLOSSARY

access: An individual's ability to obtain medical services on a timely and financially acceptable basis. Factors determining ease of access also include availability of health care facilities and transportation to them, and reasonable hours of operation.

accreditation: A decision made by a recognized organization that an institution substantially meets appropriate standards.

activities of daily living (ADL): Tasks people can do which are required for normal functioning.

acute care: Medical care of a limited duration, provided in a hospital or outpatient setting, to treat an injury or short-term illness.

administrative costs: Nonmedical expenditures related to the delivery of health care services, including billing, claims processing, marketing, and overhead.

advanced practice nurse: Registered nurse such as a clinical nurse specialist, nurse practitioner, nurse anesthetist, and nurse midwife with a master's or doctoral degree concentrating on a specific area of practice.

adverse selection: Occurs when a population characteristic such as age (e.g., a larger number of persons age 65 or older in proportion to younger persons) increases the potential for higher utilization than budgeted, and increases costs above those of the capitation rate.

ambulatory care: Health care services that patients receive when they are not an inpatient or home in bed.

assisted living: Services provided to individuals who need assistance with activities of daily living.

average daily census: The average number of patients counted in a health care institution, usually over a 1-year period.

behavioral risk factor: An element of personal behavior, such as unbalanced nutrition, use of tobacco products, leading a secondary lifestyle, or the abuse of alcoholic beverages, that leads to an increased risk of developing one or more diseases or negative health conditions.

beneficiary: Any person, either a subscriber or a dependent, eligible for service under a health plan contract.

benefits: Specific areas of plan coverage or services provided, such as outpatient visits and hospitalization, that make up the range of medical services marketed under a health plan.

biotechnology: The application of a technology such as computer science, mechanical engineering, economics, or electronic imaging of one sort or another, to the prevention, diagnosis, evaluation, treatment, or management of a disease or negative health condition.

*NOTE: Several of these definitions have been adapted from terms defined in Healthcare Acronyms & Terms for Boards and Medical Leaders, published by the Governance Institute, 6333 Greenwich Drive, Suite 200, San Diego, CA 92122, June 2004.

*capitation:* A payment method in which a physician or hospital is paid a fixed amount per patient, per year, regardless of the volume or cost of services each patient requires.

*carrier:* An insurer; an underwriter of risk that is engaged in providing, paying for, or reimbursing all or part of the cost of health services under group insurance policies or contracts, medical or hospital services agreements, membership or subscription contracts, or similar group arrangements, in exchange for premiums or other periodic charges.

*case management:* Often utilized as part of a managed care system; a practitioner known as a "gatekeeper" makes decisions regarding the type and volume of services to which the patient may have access.

*case manager:* An individual who coordinates and oversees other health care workers in finding the most effective methods of caring for specific patients.

*catastrophic coverage:* A type of insurance that pays for high-cost health care, usually associated with accidents and chronic illnesses and diseases, such as cancer and AIDS.

*census:* In the U.S., refers to the count of members of the national population and their demographic characteristics undertaken by the U.S. Census Bureau every 10 years on the 10th year, and in the health care delivery system specifically, the number of patients in a hospital or other health care institution at any one time.

*Centers for Medicare & Medicaid Services (CMS):* Administers Medicare, Medicaid, and the State Child Health Insurance Program (SCHIP). Formerly called Health Care Financing Administration (HCFA).

*certificates of need:* Franchises for new services and construction or renovation of hospitals or related facilities, as issued by states.

*chronic care:* Treatment or rehabilitative health services provided to individuals on a long-term basis (over 30 days), in both inpatient and ambulatory settings.

*clinical nurse practitioner:* Nurse with extra training who accepts additional clinical responsibility for medical diagnosis or treatment.

*clinical trials:* The testing on patients in a clinical setting of a diagnostic, preventive, or therapeutic intervention, using a study design that will provide for a valid estimation of safety and efficiency.

*closed panel:* A managed care plan that contracts with physicians on an exclusive basis for services and does not allow those physicians to see patients for another managed care organization.

*coinsurance:* A provision in a member's coverage that limits the amount of coverage by the plan to a certain percentage, commonly 80%. Any additional costs are paid out-of-pocket by the member.

*community hospital:* A hospital offering short-term general and other special services, owned by a corporation or agency other than the federal government.

*community rating:* The rating system by which a plan or an indemnity carrier takes the total experience of the subscribers or members within a given geographic area or "community" and uses these data to determine a reimbursement rate that is common for all groups regardless of the individual claims experience of any one group.

*complementary and alternative medicine:* Refers to a series of diagnostic and treatment interventions that fall outside of the realm of state-licensed medical practice as it is defined by the privileges to use certain restricted diagnostic regimens, prescribe drugs from a restricted list, and practice surgery. Such disciplines include: chiropractic, acupuncture, homeopathy, herbal medicine, naturopathy, therapeutic touch, and the like.

*Consolidated Omnibus Budget Reconciliation Act of 1985 (COBRA):* A federal law (P.L. 99–272), that requires that all employer-sponsored health plans offer certain employees and their families the opportunity to continue, at their personal expense, health insurance coverage under the group plan for up to 18, 24, or 36 months, depending on the qualifying event, after their coverage normally would have ceased (e.g., due to the death or retirement of the employee, divorce or legal separation, resignation or termination of employment, or bankruptcy of the employer).

*Continuous Quality Improvement (CQI):* A systematic approach to improve processes of health care, such as admission to the hospital, or delivery of meals to a patient.

*co-payment:* A specified amount that the insured individual must pay for a specified service or procedure (e.g., $8 for an office visit).

*comprehensive coverage:* A health insurance system that pays for a broad range of services.

*cost sharing:* A provision that requires individuals to cover some part of their medical expenses (e.g., copayments, coinsurance, deductibles).

*cost-shifting:* Refers to passing the cost of one group onto another group. For example, if the rate one group of health plan enrollees pays for services is less than the actual cost of those services, the difference can be made up based on charges higher than cost paid by another group.

*credentialing:* The most common use of the term refers to obtaining and reviewing the documentation of professional providers.

*critical pathway:* The mapping out of day-to-day recommendations for patient care based on best practice and scientific evidence.

*data:* In health, an event, condition, or disease occurrence that is counted. In health services, an episode of care, costs of care, expenditures, quantification of manpower and facilities and their characteristics, and the like.

*deductible:* The amount a patient must pay out-of-pocket, usually annually on a calendar-year basis, before insurance will begin to cover costs.

*defined contribution plan:* Benefits plan which gives employees a certain amount of total compensation to allocate among various benefits, rather than providing employees with the specific benefits, such as hospitalization.

*demographic characteristics:* Refers to such characteristics of an individual or a population group (averages in the latter case) as: age, sex, marital status, ethnicity, geographic location, occupation, and income.

*denominator:* For health care, the total number of people among whom numerator items are being counted (see "numerator").

*diagnosis-related groups (DRGs):* Groups of inpatient discharges with final diagnoses that are similar clinically and in resource consumption; used as a basis of payment by the Medicare program, and as a result, widely accepted by others.

*discharge planning:* A part of the patient management guidelines and the nursing care plan that identifies the expected discharge date and coordinates the various services necessary to achieve the target.

*disproportionate share hospital (DSH):* A hospital that provides a large amount (or disproportionate share) of uncompensated care and/or care to Medicaid and low-income Medicare beneficiaries.

*drug:* A therapeutic drug is a chemical compound used in treating or managing a disease or negative health condition. A recreational drug is a chemical compound that alters the user's mood by providing diversion, relaxation, heightened sensation, or other enjoyment or pleasure.

*Emergency Medical Treatment and Labor Act (EMTALA):* Federal law setting forth requirements for hospitals participating in Medicare to provide emergency care so that patients who cannot pay are not "dumped" to other hospitals.

*Employee Retirement Income Security Act (ERISA):* A 1974 federal law (P.L. 93–406) that set the standards of disclosure for employee benefit plans to ensure workers the right to at least part of their pensions. The law governs most private pensions and other employee benefits, and overrides all state laws that concern employee benefits, including health benefits; therefore, ERISA preempts state laws in their application to self-funded, private employer-sponsored health insurance plans.

*encounter:* A patient visit to a provider. The term often refers to visits to providers by patients in capitated health plans.

*enrollment:* The process by which an individual and family become a subscriber(s) for coverage in a health plan. This may be done either through an actual signing up of the individual or through a collective bargaining agreement on the employer's conditions of employment. A result, therefore, is that the health plan is aware of its entire population of beneficiary eligibles. As a usual practice, individuals must notify the health plan of any changes in family status that affect the enrollment of dependents.

*entitlements:* Government benefits (e.g., Medicare, Medicaid, Social Security, food stamps) that are provided automatically to all qualified individuals, and are therefore part of mandatory spending programs.

*evidence-based medicine (EBM):* That portion of medical practice, estimated at much lower than 50%, which is based on established scientific findings.

*experience rating:* A method used to determine the cost of health insurance premiums, whereby the cost is based on the previous amount a certain group (e.g., all the employees of a particular business) paid for medical services.

*Federal Employee Health Benefits Program (FEHBP):* Also referred to as Federal Employee Plan or FEP. The health plans made available to federal employees as part of their employment benefits.

*fee schedule:* A listing of accepted fees or established allowances for specified medical procedures as used in health plans; it usually represents the maximum amounts the program will pay for the specified procedures.

*fee-for-service:* A billing system in which a health care provider charges a patient a set amount for a specific service.

*fixed costs:* Costs that do not change or vary with fluctuations in enrollment or in utilization of services.

*for-profit hospitals:* Those owned by private corporations that declare dividends or otherwise distribute profits to individuals. Also called "investor—owned," many are also community hospitals.

*formulary:* A listing of drugs prepared by, for example, a hospital or a managed care company, that a physician may prescribe. The physician is requested or required to use only formulary drugs unless there is a valid medical reason to use a nonformulary drug.

*full-time equivalent (FTE):* Refers to the number of hours employees must work to be regarded as full time; thus two half-time employees working 20 hours a week equals one full-time equivalent.

*gatekeeper:* A health care practitioner who makes decisions regarding the type and volume of services to which a patient may have access, generally used by health maintenance organizations (HMOs) to control unnecessary utilization of services.

*generics:* A therapeutic drug, originally protected by a patent, the chemical composition of which meets the standards for that drug set by the

Food and Drug Administration, made by a company other than the company that originally developed and patented the drug. Generics are usually not manufactured and made available until after the original patent has expired.

governance: The activity of an organization that monitors the outside environment, selects appropriate alternatives, and negotiates the implementation of these alternatives with others inside and outside the organization.

governing board: A group of individuals, who under state law own an organization, whether or not they can obtain any financial advantage through such ownership.

graduate medical education: The education and training of physicians beyond the 4 years of medical school, in positions that may be termed internship, residency, fellowship, postgraduate year (PGY) 1, 2, 3, and so on. Although one can enter medical school only with an undergraduate degree of some sort at the baccalaureate level, in the United States, the 4 years of medical school leading to the MD or DO (doctor of osteopathy) degrees are customarily referred to as "undergraduate medical education."

group model: An HMO that contracts with a medical group for the provision of health care services. The relationship between the HMO and the medical group is generally very close, although there are wide variations in the relative independence of the group from the HMO. A form of closed panel health plan.

group practice: Three or more physicians who deliver patient care, make joint use of equipment and personnel, and divide income by a prearranged formula.

health care delivery: The provision of preventive treatment, or rehabilitative health services, from short-term to long-term, to individuals as well as groups of people, by individual practitioners, institutions, or public health agencies.

Health Care Financing Administration (HCFA): A part of the U.S. Department of Health and Human Services. In addition to its many other functions, HCFA is the contracting agency for HMOs that seek direct contract/provider status for provision of the Medicare benefits package. The name has recently been changed to Centers for Medicare & Medicaid Services (CMS).

health care providers: Usually refers to professional health service workers—physicians, dentists, psychologists—who are licensed to practice independently of any other health service worker.

health care workforce: All of the people, professional and nonprofessional alike, who work in the health care services industry.

Health Insurance Portability and Accountability Act of 1996 (HIPAA):

The key provision of this federal law improves health coverage for workers and their families when they change or lose jobs.

*health maintenance organization (HMO):* A managed care company that organizes and provides health care for its enrollees for a fixed prepaid premium.

*Health Plan Employer Data and Information Set (HEDIS):* A standard set of performance measures to measure the quality and performance of health plans, sponsored by the National Committee for Quality Assurance (NCQA).

*health promotion (personal):* Personal health promotion is the science and art of helping people change their lifestyle to move toward a state of optimal health. Optimal health is defined as a balance of physical, emotional, social, spiritual, and intellectual health.

*health systems:* Organizations that work together in predictable ways because of contractual relationships. The systems may or may not be commonly owned.

*Healthy People 2010:* Formal goals and objectives for the nation's health status, updated every 10 years by the federal government.

*home health care:* Health services provided in an individual's home.

*Hospice care:* Programs providing pain relief and supporting services to dying patients in different settings. Hospice care is reimbursable under Medicare.

*hospitalist:* Physicians, usually employed by hospitals, who practice only in acute care settings to provide inpatient care otherwise provided by attending physicians.

*hospitalization:* The admission of a patient to a hospital.

*hospitalization coverage:* A type of insurance coverage that covers most inpatient hospital costs (e.g., room and board), diagnostic and therapeutic services, care for emergency illnesses or injuries, laboratory and x-ray services, and certain other specified procedures.

*human genome:* Projects to develop a draft of the human genetic code, involving billions of pairs of letters in the DNA sequence of 26,000–40,000 genes in the 23 human chromosomes.

*incidence:* The number of new events, disease cases, or conditions, counted in a defined population during a defined period of time.

*indemnity insurance:* Benefits paid in a predetermined amount in the event of a covered loss; differs from reimbursement, which provides benefits based on actual expenses incurred. There are fewer restrictions on what a doctor may charge and what an insurer may pay for a treatment and generally there are also fewer restrictions on a patient's ability to access specialty services.

*Independent Practice Association (IPA):* Association of independent physicians formed as a separate legal entity for contracting purposes with health plans. Physicians see fee-for-service patients as well as those enrolled in HMOs.

*infant mortality:* The death of a child born alive before he or she reaches 1 year of age.

*information technology:* Electronic systems for communicating information. Health care organizations want information technology that is accessible—with privacy safeguards—to multiple users within an organization.

*integrated delivery system (IDS):* A group of health care organizations that collectively provides a full range of health-related services in a coordinated fashion to those using the system.

*integration, horizontal:* Affiliations among providers of the same type (e.g., a hospital forming relationships with other hospitals).

*integration, vertical:* Affiliations among providers of different types (e.g., a hospital, clinic and nursing home forming an affiliation).

*international medical school graduate:* A U.S. citizen or noncitizen physician who has graduated from a medical school not located in the United States that is also not accredited by the U.S. medical school accrediting body, the Liaison Committee on Medical Education.

*investor-owned hospital:* A hospital owned by one or more private parties or a corporation, for the purpose of generating a profitable return on investment.

*Joint Commission on Accreditation of Healthcare Organizations (JCAHO):* A national organization of representatives of health care providers: American College of Physicians, American College of Surgeons, American Hospital Association, American Medical Association, and consumer representatives. The JCAHO offers inspection and accreditation on quality of operations to hospitals and other health care organizations.

*length of stay:* Days billed for a period of hospitalization.

*licensure:* A system established by a given state recognizing the achievement of a defined level of education, experience, and examination performance as qualifying the person or organization meeting those standards to work or operate in a defined area of practice, prohibited to any person or organization that has not met those standards.

*life expectancy:* The predicted average number of years of life remaining for a person at a given age.

*long-term care:* A general term for a range of services provided to chronically ill, physically disabled, and mentally disabled patients in a nursing home or long-term home health care setting.

*loss ratio:* A term used to describe the amount of money spent on health care. A company with a loss ratio of .85, for instance, spends 85 cents of every premium dollar on health care and the remaining 15 cents on administrative costs, such as marketing and profits.

*major medical:* A precursor of "catastrophic coverage," it is coverage characterized by larger maximum limits, which is intended to cover the cost associated with a major illness or injury.

*managed care:* A system of health care delivery that influences or controls utilization of services and costs of services. The degree of influence depends on the model used. For example, a preferred provider organization charges the patients lower rates if they use the providers in the preferred network. HMOs, on the other hand, may choose not to reimburse for health services received from providers with whom the HMO does not contract.

*mandated benefits:* Benefits that a health plan are required to provide by law. This is generally used to refer to benefits above and beyond routine insurance-type benefits, and it generally applies at the state level (where there is high variability from state to state). Common examples include in vitro fertilization, defined days of inpatient mental health or substance abuse treatment, and other special condition treatments. Self-funded plans are exempt from mandated benefits under ERISA.

*Medicaid:* A joint federal/state/local program of health care for individuals whose income and resources are insufficient to pay for their care, governed by Title XIX of the federal Social Security Act, and administered by the states. Medicaid is the major source of payment for nursing home care of the elderly.

*medical savings account:* Accounts similar to individual retirement accounts (IRAs) into which employers and employees can make tax-deferred contributions and from which employees may withdraw funds to pay covered health care expenses.

*medically indigent:* Those who do not have and cannot afford medical insurance coverage and who are not eligible financially for Medicaid.

*Medicare:* A federal entitlement program of medical and health care coverage for the elderly and disabled, and persons with end-stage renal disease, governed by Title XVIII of the federal Social Security Act, and consisting of two parts: Part A—for institutional and home care, and Part B—for medical care.

*Medicare Prescription Drug, Improvement, and Modernization Act (MMA):* Federal law signed in 2004 that offers a discount card at a nominal fee to Medicare beneficiaries for drugs and that will offer a prescription drug benefit starting in 2006 for those on Medicare who enroll and pay a premium.

*Medi-Gap:* Also known as Medicare Supplement Insurance, a type of private insurance coverage that may be purchased by an individual enrolled in Medicare to cover certain needed services that are not covered by Medicare Parts A and B (i.e., "gaps").

**morbidity:** An episode of sickness, as defined by a health professional. A morbidity rate is the number of such episodes occurring in a given population during a given period of time.

**mortality:** A death. A mortality rate is the number of deaths (either the "crude rate," which is all deaths, or a "specific rate," which is by, for example, specific cause, specific location, or specific age group) occurring during a given period of time.

**natality:** A live birth. The natality rate is the number of live births occurring in a given population during a given period of time.

**national health insurance:** A system for paying for one or more categories of health care service, that is organized on a nationwide basis, established by law and usually operated by a government agency.

**National Health Service (NHI):** In the United States and Great Britain NHI refers specifically to the comprehensive, government funded and operated system such as that found in Great Britain.

**network:** An arrangement of several delivery points (i.e., medical group practices affiliated with a managed care organization; an arrangement of HMOs, either autonomous and separate legal entities, or subsidiaries of a larger corporation) using one common insuring mechanism such as Blue Cross/Blue Shield; a broker organization (health plan) that arranges with physician groups, carriers, payer agencies, consumer groups, and others for services to be provided to enrollees.

**nonprofit or not-for-profit plan:** A term applied to a prepaid health plan under which no part of the net earnings accrues, or may lawfully accrue, to the benefit of any private shareholder or individual. An organization that has received 501-C-3 or 501-C-4 designation by the Internal Revenue Service.

**numerator:** For health care, a number of events, disease occurrences, or conditions that are counted, over some defined period of time.

**nurse practitioner (NP):** registered nurses who have been trained at the master's level in providing primary care services, expanded health care evaluations and decision making, and prescriptions under a physician's supervision.

**office visit:** A formal, face-to-face contact between the physician and the patient in a health center, office, or hospital outpatient department.

**open enrollment period:** A requirement that all possible customers for a particular health insurance policy be accepted at all times for coverage and, once accepted, not to be terminated by the insurer due to claims experience.

**outcomes:** Measures of treatments and effectiveness in terms of access, quality, and cost.

**outlier:** Under a DRG system of payment, additional per diem payments are made to the hospital for cases requiring a patient to stay in the hospital beyond a threshold length of stay. Such cases are referred to as "long-stay outliers."

*per diem payment:* Reimbursement rates that are paid to providers for each day of services provided to a patient, based on the patient's illness or condition.

*per member per month (PMPM):* Payment a health plan or provider receives per person every month under capitation arrangements.

*perspective, provider and patient:* The two different vantage points from which the same health services event can be counted, over time. For example, visits by patients to physician offices can be counted as the number of patient visits a physician sees in a year (provider perspective) or the number of visits to the physicians office a patient makes in a year (patient perspective).

*physician assistant (PA):* A specially trained and licensed worker who performs certain medical procedures under the supervision of a physician. Physician assistants are usually not registered nurses.

*point-of-service plan (POS):* A managed care plan that offers enrollees the option of receiving services from participating or nonparticipating providers. The benefits package is designed to encourage the use of participating providers, through higher deductibles and/or partial reimbursement for services provided by nonparticipating providers.

*policy:* Guidelines adopted by organizations and governments that promote or constrain decision-making and action, and limit subsequent choices.

*preexisting condition:* A physical and/or mental condition of an insured that first manifests itself prior to issuance of a policy or that exists prior to issuance and for which treatment was received.

*preferred provider organization (PPO and PPA):* A limited grouping (panel) of providers (doctors and/or hospitals) who agree to provide health care to subscribers for a negotiated and usually discounted fee and who agree to utilization review. The arrangement created among the providers and others (employers, unions, commercial insurers, HMOs, etc.) is called the PPA or preferred provider arrangement.

*premium:* A periodic payment required to keep an insurance policy in force.

*prepayment:* A method of providing, in advance, for the cost of predetermined benefits for a population group through regular periodic payments in the form of premiums, dues, or contributions, including those contributions that are made to a health and welfare fund by employers on behalf of their employees, and payments to HMOs and CMPs made by federal agencies for Medicare eligibles.

*prescription:* An order, usually made in writing, from a licensed physician or his or her authorized designee, to a pharmacy, directing the latter to dispense a given drug, with written orders for its use.

*prevalence:* The total number of events, disease cases, or conditions existing in a defined population, counted during a defined period of time, or at a given point in time (known as "point-prevalence").

*primary care:* The general health care that people receive on a routine basis, that is not associated with an acute or chronic illness or disability, and may be provided by a physician, nurse practitioner, or physician assistant. Definitions of primary care physicians usually include those who practice family medicine, pediatrics, and internal medicine; other physicians often included in this definition are obstetricians and gynecologists, as well as practitioners of preventive and emergency medicine.

*primary care practitioners:* Doctors in family practice, general internal medicine, or pediatrics; nurse practitioners and midwives; and may also include psychiatrists and emergency care physicians.

*privileges:* Rights granted annually to physicians and affiliate staff members to perform specified kinds of care in the hospital.

*public hospital:* A hospital operated by a government agency. In the United States, the most common are the federal government's Department of Veterans Affairs; state governments' mental hospitals; and local governments' general hospitals for the care of the poor and otherwise uninsured.

*public psychiatric hospital:* A hospital devoted to the treatment and management of mental illness and disorders, owned and operated by a government agency (in the United States, most commonly at the state level).

*quality assurance:* A formal set of activities to measure the quality of services provided; these may also include corrective measures.

*quality of care:* Referring to the measurement of the quality of health care provided to individuals or groups of patients, against a previously defined standard.

*rates, crude and specific:* A rate is a measure of some event, disease, or condition occurring in members of a defined population, divided by the total number in that population. For crude rates, the whole population is the denominator. A specific rate defines the denominator by one or more demographic characteristics.

*registered nurse:* A nurse who is a graduate of an approved education program leading to diploma, an associate degree, or a bachelor's degree, who has also met the requirements of experience and exam passage to be licensed in a given state.

*reinsurance:* Insurance purchased by a health plan to protect it against extremely high cost cases.

*relative value system (RVS):* A method of valuing medical services, especially physician services. The federal government changed to an RBRVS (resource-based relative value scale) physician payment system in early 1992, an RVS payment system for physician services to Medicare recipients. Each service is assigned a given number of relative value units based on, for example, how long it takes to do a procedure, which is multiplied by a national conversion factor to determine a dollar amount for payment of that service.

*reserves:* A fiscal method of withholding a certain percentage of premiums to provide a fund for committed but undelivered health care and such uncertainties as higher hospital utilization levels than expected, overutilization of referrals and accidental catastrophes.

*resource-based relative value scale (RBRVS):* As of January 1, 1992, Medicare payments are based on a resource-based relative value scale, replacing the customary and prevailing charge mechanism for fee-for-service providers participating in the Medicare program. The objective is that physician fees should reflect the relative value of work performed, their practice expense, and malpractice insurance costs.

*risk:* Any chance of loss, or the possibility that revenues of the health plan will not be sufficient to cover expenditures incurred in the delivery of contractual services.

*risk contract:* A contract to provide services to beneficiaries under which the health plan receives a fixed monthly payment for enrolled members, and then must provide all services on an at-risk basis.

*risk management:* Identification, evaluation, and corrective action against organizational behaviors that would otherwise result in financial loss or legal liability.

*Sarbanes-Oxley Act (SOA):* 2002 federal legislation that affects corporate governance, financial disclosure, and the practice of public accounting.

*self-insurance:* A program for providing group insurance with benefits financed entirely through the internal means of the policyholder, in place of purchasing coverage from commercial carriers. By self-insuring, firms avoid paying state taxes on premiums and are largely exempt from state-imposed mandates.

*skilled nursing facility (SNF):* Facility providing care for patients who no longer require treatment in the hospital but who do require 24-hour medical care or rehabilitation services.

*socialized health service:* Usually an epithet used by opponents of any type of national government involvement in either the financing or operation of a health care delivery system on a nationwide basis, to describe any such system, regardless of whether such a government could itself be defined as "socialist" or not.

*solo practice:* Individual practice of medicine by a physician who does not practice in a group or does not share personnel, facilities, or equipment with three or more physicians.

*staff model:* An HMO that employs providers directly, who see members in the HMO's own facilities. A form of closed panel HMO.

*stakeholders:* Persons with an interest in the performance of an organization. Examples of hospital stakeholders are physicians and nurses, payers, managers, patients, and government.

*Stark legislation:* Federal laws that place limits on physicians referring patients to facilities in which they have a meaningful ownership stake.

*strategic planning:* A process reviewing the mission, environmental surveillance, and previous planning decisions used to establish major goals and nonrecurring resource allocation decisions.

*surveillance:* Ongoing observation of a population for rapid and accurate detection of events, conditions, or diseases.

*teaching hospital:* A hospital in which undergraduate and/or graduate medical education takes place.

*tertiary care:* Highly specialized medical care or procedures which are performed by specialized physicians in some but not all hospitals.

*third-party administrator:* An organization that acts as an intermediary between the provider and consumer of care but does not insure care.

*underwriting:* This refers to bearing the risk for something (i.e., a policy is underwritten by an insurance company); also the analysis that is done for a group to determine rates or to determine whether the group should be offered coverage at all.

*uninsured:* In the United States, a person who is not the beneficiary of any third-party source of payment for health care services.

*universal health insurance:* Usually refers to a national health insurance system that provides for comprehensive coverage for all permanent residents of a country.

*utilization:* Quantity of services used by patients, such as hospital days, physician visits, or prescriptions.

*utilization review:* A system for measuring and evaluating the utilization by physicians for their patients of various health services ranging from diagnostic tests to admission to hospital, against a preestablished standard of "good" or "appropriate" utilization of such services.

*vertical integration:* The affiliation of organizations providing different kinds of service, such as hospital care, ambulatory care, long-term care, and social services.

*vital statistics:* Numbers and rates for births, deaths, abortions, fetal deaths, fertility, life expectancy, marriages, and divorces.

*volunteers:* People who are not paid for giving their time to the health care organization, their only compensation being the satisfaction they achieve from their work.

*wraparound plan:* Commonly used to refer to insurance or health plan coverage for copayments and deductibles that are not covered under a member's base plan, such as Medicare.

# B

# A GUIDE
# TO SOURCES
# OF DATA

Jennifer A. Nelson and
Mary Ann Chiasson

Portions of the information about sources of health and health care data for the United States were adapted from a previous edition of this appendix, compiled by Steven Jonas and Christine T. Kovner.

THIS APPENDIX IS a guide to the principal sources of health and health services data for the United States as of 2004. It contains up-to-date descriptions of these sources, indicates how frequently each is published, lists the categories of data and other information they contain, and gives information for ordering and downloading. Also included is a brief introduction to sources of international data.

Almost all federal sources of data are available for purchase through the U.S. Government Printing Office (USGPO), Superintendent of Documents, P.O. Box 371954, Pittsburgh, PA 15250–7954; Web site: bookstore.gpo.gov; tel. (866) 512–1800, FAX: (202) 512–2250.

Health data are available not only in print form, but also on the Internet. Many of the publications indicated in this appendix are available in whole or in part via the Internet; others may be ordered using the Internet. Basic statistical tables are often included on government and organization Web sites, sometimes via an interactive database that allows the user to design tables with variables of interest. In addition, many data sets are available for public use and can be downloaded from the Internet or ordered on CD-Rom. Most of the data available online, particularly data from federal sources, are free.

## COMPREHENSIVE GUIDES TO DATA SOURCES

There are two comprehensive guides to sources of data that are published annually. The first appears in the Statistical Abstract of the United States (see item B.1, below). Its Appendix I, "Guide to Sources of Statistics, State Statistical Abstracts and Foreign Statistical Abstracts," contains an extensive listing of sources of health data (as well as the sources of all other data appearing in the Statistical Abstract). It also includes a list of telephone and Internet contacts for federal agencies with statistical programs. Appendix III, "Limitations of the Data," presents brief descriptions and analyses of the limitations of the major sources of data listed in Appendix I.

The second regularly published comprehensive guide to sources appears in Health, United States (see item A.1.a, below). Its Appendix I contains very useful, detailed descriptions of all the common health data sources published by the several branches of the federal government, the United Nations, and some private agencies.

In addition, the AHA Guide, published regularly by the American Hospital Association (see item D.1, below), lists in its Part C the major national, international, U.S. government, state and local government, and private "Health Organizations, Agencies, and Providers" with addresses, telephone numbers, and Web site addresses.

## USING THE INTERNET TO ACCESS DATA

The Internet is changing the way that we seek and retrieve data. Information and statistics on almost any topic can be easily obtained with a few clicks of a computer mouse. However, the volume of information available can be overwhelming, and it can be difficult to know where to begin to look for the particular bit of information needed. The following are a few places to begin a search for health and health services data. Specific Internet addresses relating to the principal sources listed in the following sections are noted in those sections.

The federal government is a major source of health data. Each department of the U.S. government has an Internet address; some of them are listed in the sections below. All federal government department and agency Web sites can be accessed through **www.firstgov.gov**. In addition, access to federal data produced by more than 70 agencies in the U.S. government can be obtained via **www.fedstats.gov**. Two agencies that are responsible for a large amount of population, health and health services data are the U.S. Census Bureau (**www.census.gov**) and the Centers for Disease Control and Prevention (**www.cdc.gov**). Exploring their Web sites is a good way to become familiar with the data available.

Most states and professional organizations have Web sites as well. Links to state sites, which can be excellent sources of state and local data, are available at **www.statelocalgov.net** or through **www.firstgov.gov**. The Web sites of state departments of health and other agencies can also be reached via state homepages.

The National Association of Health Data Organizations Web site (**www.nahdo.org**) includes a Health Website Search Module, which includes links to the sites of federal and state agencies as well as numerous health care associations and nonprofit organizations that have health information and data. It provides an overview of health information sources available via the Internet as well as access to those sources. Internet search engines such as Yahoo and Google can be used to locate the sites of other organizations.

## PRINCIPAL SOURCES OF U.S. HEALTH AND HEALTH CARE DATA

### A. Centers for Disease Control and Prevention (CDC)
Web site: www.cdc.gov

### 1. National Center for Health Statistics (NCHS)
Web site: www.cdc.gov/nchs/

Part of the Centers for Disease Control and Prevention in the U.S. Department of Health and Human Services, the National Center for Health Statistics (NCHS) is the federal government's primary agency for vital and health statistics. Through its data systems, the NCHS collects data on health status, health behavior, and the use of health care; it also serves as the repository for data from the nation's vital statistics systems. Data are collected through national population surveys such as the National Health and Nutrition Examination Survey (NHANES), the National Health Interview Survey (NHIS), the National Survey of Family Growth (NSFG), and the National Immunization Survey (NIS). Health services data are collected through a family of surveys of health care providers, collectively known as the National Health Care Surveys (NCHS), which include the National Hospital Discharge Survey (NHDS), the National Ambulatory Medical Care Survey (NAMCS), the National Hospital Ambulatory Medical Care Survey (NHAMCS), the National Survey of Ambulatory Surgery (NSAS), the National Nursing Home Survey (NNHS), the National Home and Hospice Care Survey (NHHCS), the National Employer Health Insurance Survey (NEHIS), and the National Health Provider Inventory (NHPI).

Data from the Vital Statistics System and the health surveys are published in a series of regular and periodic reports (see items a-d, below). The center's Web site serves as an entry to a great deal of information about these data systems and to data in tabular form, as well as publication lists and downloadable versions of many publications. In addition, many of these data sets are available for public use and can be downloaded from the Web site.

### a. Health, United States

*Health, United States* is published annually. A wide variety of health and health care delivery systems data are presented, primarily in tabular form, under categories such as population, fertility and natality, mortality, determinants and measures of health, utilization of health resources, health care resources, and health care expenditures, and health insurance. *Health, United States* also contains useful appendices describing sources and limitations of the data (described above), as well as a glossary (Appendix II: Definitions and Methods). It is a boon to students and researchers in health care delivery systems analysis because it provides one-stop shopping for the most important health and health care data.

*To order:* USGPO
*To download:* www.cdc.gov/nchs/hus.htm.

### b. National Vital Statistics Report (NVSR)

The *NVSR* publishes several types of reports. "Provisional Data," published monthly, contains the most recent figures for the traditional vital statistics—births, deaths, marriages, and divorces. The *NVSR* publishes preliminary and final data on each of these vital statistics for each year. In addition, special analyses on related topics using vital statistics data appear periodically. These reports were formerly published as *Monthly Vital Statistics Reports*.

> *To order:* To receive this publication regularly, contact NCHS: tel. (866) 441–6247; email: nchsquery@cdc.gov
> *To download:* www.cdc.gov/nchs/products/pubs/pubd/nvsr/nvsr.htm (individual reports)
> www.cdc.gov/nchs/nvss.htm (entry page for vital statistics reports and data)

### c.  Vital Statistics of the United States (VSUS)
These are the full, highly detailed annual reports on vital statistics from the NCHS, the summary versions of which are published in the supplements of the NVSR. Data are available for years from 1890 to the present.

> *To order:* Reports for some years are available from USGPO.
> *To download:* www.cdc.gov/nchs/products/pubs/pubd/vsus/vsus.htm

### d.  Vital and Health Statistics
These publications of the NCHS, distinct from the Vital Statistics reports described in items b and c above, appear at irregular intervals. As of 2004, there were 18 series, not numbered consecutively. Most of them report data from ongoing studies and surveys that the NCHS carries out, such as NHIS, NSFG, and others listed above. Also published are *Advance Data from Vital and Health Statistics*, which provide early data from many of the surveys, detailed reports on which are often later published in the following 18 series: Series 1, Programs and Collection Procedures; Series 2, Data Evaluation and Methods Research; Series 3, Analytical and Epidemiological Studies; Series 4, Documents and Committee Reports; Series 5, International Vital and Health Statistics Reports; Series 6, Cognition and Survey Measurement; Series 10, Data from the National Health Interview Survey; Series 11, Data from the National Health Examination Survey, the National Health and Nutrition Examination Surveys, and the Hispanic Health and Nutrition Examination Survey; Series 12, Data from the Institutionalized Populations Surveys; Series 13, Data from the National Health Care Survey; Series 14, Data on Health Resources: Manpower and Facilities; Series 15, Data from Special Surveys; Series 16, Compilations of Advance Data from Vital and Health Statistics; Series 20, Data on Mortality; Series 21, Data on Natality, Marriage, and Divorce; Series 22, Data from the National Mortality and Mortality Natality Surveys; Series 23, Data from the National Survey of Family Growth; Series 24, Compilations of Data on Natality, Mortality, Marriage, and Divorce.

> *To order:* USGPO
> *To download:* www.cdc.gov/nchs/products/pubs/pubd/series/ser.htm

2.  National Center for Chronic Disease Prevention and
    Health Promotion (NCCDPHP)
    Web site: www.cdc.gov/nccdphp/

Charged with preventing and controlling chronic disease and promoting healthy behaviors, the National Center for Chronic Disease Prevention and Health Promotion not only supports and administers programs, but also collects data to monitor the progress of those efforts and to measure the prevalence of health risk behaviors. The surveillance systems listed below are a major part of these efforts and are collaborations with state health and education departments and other agencies.

a.  *Behavioral Risk Factor Surveillance System (BRFSS)*
    Web site: www.cdc.gov/brfss/

The Behavioral Risk Factor Surveillance System (BRFSS) is an ongoing data collection program designed to serve a dual purpose: to meet the need for behavioral health data, necessary for designing preventive programs to reduce morbidity and mortality, and to meet the need for that data at the state level where the activities and targeting of resources generally occur. States use a CDC-developed standard core questionnaire to conduct telephone surveys collecting data on health risks and behaviors. BRFSS data files for 1990–2002 are available to download free in several formats. In addition, *BRFSS Summary Prevalence Reports* are published annually. Topics covered include general health status, quality of life, health insurance, smoking status, alcohol consumption, immunization, HIV/AIDS, overweight/obesity, and screening for diabetes, cholesterol, hypertension, and colorectal, breast, and cervical cancer. These reports are available to download from the BRFSS Web site. Prevalence and trends data, much of it accessed through an interactive database, are also available directly from the Web site. In addition, the Web site includes searchable databases of published work that uses BRFSS data.

b.  *Youth Behavioral Risk Surveillance System (YBRSS)*
    Web site: www.cdc.gov/yrbss/

The Youth Behavioral Risk Surveillance System was designed to monitor health risk behaviors, such as tobacco, alcohol, and drug use; unhealthy diet and inadequate physical activity; sexual risk behaviors; and behaviors related to unintentional injury and violence, among the nation's youth. The YBRSS includes a national survey conducted by CDC as well as state and local surveys conducted by local health and education departments, all directed toward 9th through 12th grade students. Representative samples of public and private high school students are surveyed every two years using a standard questionnaire. Data files, fact sheets, a bibliography, and data tables created through an interactive database are available on the YRBSS Web site.

### c. Pregnancy Risk Assessment Monitoring System (PRAMS)

Web site: www.cdc.gov/reproductivehealth/srv_prams.htm

The Pregnancy Risk Assessment Monitoring System is a state-specific surveillance system surveying a population-based sample of women who have recently delivered a live infant, about maternal attitudes and behaviors during and immediately following pregnancy. Thirty-one states and New York City participate in PRAMS as of 2004. The PRAMS Web site includes Surveillance and Special Reports, which can be downloaded, as well as a list of publications that use PRAMS data.

### d. Cancer Registries

Web sites: www.cdc.gov/cancer/npcr/seer.cancer.gov

State cancer registries collect data on incidence, stage of disease at diagnosis, treatment, and outcomes for the different cancer types and body locations. The CDC supports these registries and promotes the use of data collected through its National Program of Cancer Registries (NPCR). In conjunction with the National Cancer Institute's Surveillance, Epidemiology, and End Results (SEER) Program, NPCR periodically produces *United States Cancer Statistics* (most recently in 2000), a compilation of data collected by the registries. Additional state and national data are available from the NPCR and SEER Web sites.

### 3. Morbidity and Mortality Weekly Report (MMWR)

Web site: www.cdc.gov/mmwr/

This is a weekly publication of the Centers for Disease Control and Prevention. It is available free via the Internet or email subscription. It is also available by annual subscription from the USGPO. However, following a large subscription price increase in 1982, *MMWR*, in the public domain, has also been made available at a much lower cost by other organizations, such as the Massachusetts Medical Society. In the past, *MMWR* was concerned primarily with communicable disease reporting, and it continues to provide reports on infectious disease surveillance. However, *MMWR* now also regularly presents brief reports on chronic diseases and special studies of such diverse health topics as alcohol consumption among pregnant and childbearing-age women, human rabies, progress toward global poliomyelitis eradication, rubella syndrome in the United States, adult blood lead epidemiology and surveillance, prevalence of arthritis, state-specific prevalence of cigarette smoking among adults, and many other topics. In addition to articles, *MMWR* publishes weekly the numbers by state of reported provisional cases of selected notifiable diseases (from the National Notifiable Disease Surveillance System), including (as of 2004) AIDS, chlamydia, coccidiodomycosis, cryptosporidiosis, encephalitis/meningitis, West Nile, *Escherichia coli*, giardiasis, gonorrhea, *H. influenzae* (invasive), viral hepatitis (acute, by type), Legionellosis, Listeriosis,

Lyme disease, malaria, meningococcal disease, pertussis, animal rabies, Rocky Mountain spotted fever, salmonellosis, shigellosis, streptococcal disease (invasive, group A), *Streptococcus pneumoniae* (invasive); primary, secondary, and congenital syphilis, tuberculosis, typhoid fever, and varicella. *MMWR* also reports deaths in 122 U.S. cities on a weekly basis and periodically publishes "Recommendations and Reports" of various governmental and nongovernmental health agencies and organizations, and the results of "CDC Surveillance Summaries" on various diseases, conditions, and procedures.

> *To order:* www.cdc.gov/mmwr/ (email); USGPO (print); Massachusetts Medical Society, P.O. Box 9120, Waltham, MA 02454–9120 (print)
>
> *To download:* www.cdc.gov/mmwr/ (editions from 1982 to the present are available)

## B. United States Census Bureau
Web site: www.census.gov

### 1. Statistical Abstract of the United States
Web site: www.census.gov/statab/www/

Published annually by the U.S. Census Bureau, the *Statistical Abstract* contains a vast collection of tables reporting information and data collected by many different government (and in certain cases nongovernment) agencies. The principal health and health services data are found under the headings Population, Vital Statistics, and Health and Nutrition.

> *To order:* USGPO; www.ntis.gov/product/statistical-abstract.htm; a CD-Rom version is available from Customer Services, Census Bureau, tel.
> (301) 763-INFO (4636); FAX: (888) 249–7295 (toll-free) or (301) 457–3842
> *To download:* www.census.gov/statab/www/

### 2. U.S. Census of Population
Web site: www.census.gov/main/www/cen2000.html (2000 census)

The U.S. Constitution requires that a census be taken every 10 years, at the beginning of each decade. The original purpose of the census was to apportion seats in the House of Representatives. Since it was first taken, the census and the voluminous amount of data it produces—going well beyond a simple count—have come to serve many other purposes as well. Many reports on the decennial censuses, as well as interim special counts and analyses known as *Current Population Reports* (see item B.3, below), are published by the Census Bureau (a part of the U.S. Department of Commerce). A good place to begin is in Section 1 of the *Statistical Abstract* (see item B.1, above). Much highly detailed information drawn from the decennial national census data is published periodically in hardcover compendia. Also available are special analyses for a wide variety of geographical subdivisions of the country. In addition, much data, including tables created through interactive databases, can be accessed through the Census Bureau Web site. A Census Bureau Product Catalog is available on the Census Bureau Web site.

> *To order:* Various publications are available from: USGPO; U.S. Department of Commerce, Bureau of the Census (MS 0801), P.O. Box 277943, Atlanta, GA 30384–7943, tel. (301) 763-INFO (4636), FAX: (310) 457–3842
> *To download:* Various data and publications may be downloaded from www.census.gov/main/www/cen2000.html.

### 3. Current Population Reports

> Web site: www.census.gov/main/www/cprs.html

In addition to reports from the decennial censuses, the Census Bureau regularly publishes *Current Population Reports (CPRs)*. They present estimates, projections, sample counts, and special studies of selected segments of the population. Reports in the following series are available: P-20, Population Characteristics; P-23, Special Studies; P-25, Population Estimates and Projections; P-60, Consumer Income; and P-70, Household Economic Studies. Information on the content of each series is available from the Census Bureau Web site. CD-Roms with data files and reports can be ordered through the Census Bureau. Additional information about the data and methodology is available from **www.bls.census.gov/cps/cpsmain.htm** or by calling survey staff at (301)763–3806.

> *To order:* USGPO; www.census.gov/mp/www/rom/msrom5fb.html
> *To download:* www.census.gov/main/www/cprs.html

## C. Centers for Medicare & Medicaid Services (CMS)

> Web site: www.cms.hhs.gov

### 1. Health Care Financing Review

> Web site: www.cms.hhs.gov/review/

*The Health Care Financing Review* is a quarterly publication of the Centers for Medicare & Medicaid Services (CMS), formerly the Health Care Financing Administration (HCFA), in the U.S. Department of Health and Human Services. It annually publishes the official CMS reports, "National Health Expenditures" and "Health Care Indicators." It also publishes an extensive and wide-ranging series of academic articles, reports, and studies. The emphasis is on Medicare/Medicaid (for which CMS is directly responsible), but "a broad range of health care financing and delivery issues" are also covered. CMS also publishes an annual Medicare and Medicaid Statistical Supplement to the Health Care Financing Review.

> *To order:* USGPO (subscription)
> *To download:* www.cms.hhs.gov/review/

## 2. Other data available from CMS

CMS makes available additional data on health care financing, particularly Medicare and Medicaid. It publishes an annual *Data Compendium*, which includes historic, current, and projected data about these programs. In addition, CMS data and statistics, including data tables and data files from the Medicaid and Medicare systems, can be accessed at **www.cms.hhs.gov/researchers/**.

## D. American Hospital Association (AHA)

Web site: www.aha.org

*1. American Hospital Association Guide to the Health Care Field*

The *AHA Guide*, available in print or on CD-Rom, lists and profiles U.S. hospitals and healthcare organizations, including systems, networks, and alliances. It includes basic data on size, location, type, ownership, and services as well as information on utilization and expenses. It also contains the comprehensive lists of health and health care organizations referred to in an earlier section of this appendix.

*To order:* Tel. (800) 242–2626; FAX: (312) 422–4505; www.ahaonline store.com

*To download:* Not available

## 2. Hospital Statistics

AHA also publishes *Hospital Statists*, based on an annual survey of over 5,000 hospitals. It contains a great deal of summary descriptive, utilization, and financial data on U.S. hospitals, presented in many different cross-tabulations. It can also be purchased on a CD-Rom, which includes Microsoft Excel data tables and allows users to customize tables.

*To order:* Tel. (800) 242–2626; FAX: (312) 422–4505; www.ahaonline store.com

*To download:* Not available

## E. Physician and Nursing Organizations

### 1. Center for Health Policy Research of the American Medical Association

Web site: www.ama-assn.org

The Center for Health Policy Research produces a variety of useful data on the physician work force and related subjects. The Center regularly conducts a survey of physicians, the Patient Care Physician Survey (previously the Socioeconomic Monitoring System). Titles appearing on a regular basis include *Physician Socioeconomic Statistics, Physician Compensation and Production Report, State Medical Licensure Requirements and Statistics, Physician*

*Characteristics and Distribution in the U.S.*, and *Practice Patterns*, a series of specialty-specific socioeconomic studies.

> *To order::* Tel. (800) 621–8335; catalog.ama-assn.org/Catalog/home.jsp
>
> *To download:* Very little is available for free download

### 2. National Council of State Boards of Nursing

> Web site: www.ncsbn.org

The National Council of State Boards of Nursing is a source of data about the licensing and employment of nurses. The Council regularly compiles *Licensure and Examination Statistics* and publishes a series of reports on findings from the Practice Analysis Studies. Information, abstracts, executive summaries, and limited data are available online, while these and other publications may be purchased. Links to other nursing and nursing statistics sites are available as well.

> *To order:* National Council of State Boards of Nursing, Dept. 77–3953, Chicago, IL 60678–3953; www.ncsbn.org/resources/publications.asp
>
> *To download:* Very little is available for free download

## INTERNATIONAL HEALTH AND HEALTH SERVICES DATA

What follows is not a comprehensive guide to sources of international population and health data, but an accounting of several major sources, which are good places to begin. Many of the Web sites listed below also include links to other sites where international health data may be found, including foreign government Web sites and statistical and health agencies in countries around the world.

### A. United States Census Bureau International Programs Center

> Web site: www.census.gov/ipc/www/

The International Programs Center (IPC) of the U.S. Census Bureau produces a publication entitled *Global Population Profile* (formerly *World Population Profile*). The most recent edition is for 2002. It includes data on population growth, fertility, mortality, migration, population aging, and contraceptive use for the world, regions, development categories, and some specific countries. The International Programs Center also produces other reports on various related topics. In addition, it administers an online International Database that has statistical tables of demographic and socio-economic data for all countries of the world.

> *To order:* USGPO
>
> *To download:* www.census.gov/ipc/www/publist.html

## B. United Nations (UN)

Web site: www.un.org

The United Nations system is comprised of a host of agencies and organizations devoted to a wide variety of topics of international relevance; many of these collect and compile population and health data.

Most UN publications can be ordered through the UN Publications Department (United Nations Publications, Room DC2-0853, Dept. I004, 2 UN Plaza, New York, NY 10017; tel. (800) 253-9646; (212) 963-8302; FAX: (212) 963-3489; email: publications@un.org) or online at www.un.org/Pubs/. An online catalog of UN publications is available through the publications Web site, or a copy can be requested by emailing booknews @un.org. Specific ordering information for some publications can be found on individual agency Web sites.

Links to the Web sites of all UN agencies can be found at **www.unsys tem.org**. Some UN offices and agencies to consider when looking for international health data are World Health Organization (WHO), United Nations Population Fund (UNFPA), United Nations Statistics Division (UNSD), United Nations Children's Fund (UNICEF), Joint United Nations Program on HIV/AIDS (UNAIDS), and the Population Division of the United Nations Department of Economic and Social Affairs (UNPD).

### 1. World Health Organization (WHO)

Web site: www.who.int

The World Health Organization is the principal UN source for health and health care data. WHO publishes an annual *World Health Report* that includes a number of population health indicators as well as a narrative discussion of world health, each year examining one additional topic in more depth. For example, the 2004 *Report* focuses on the global HIV/AIDS epidemic. The WHO Statistical Information System (www.who.int/who-sis/) includes core health indicators from the *Report* as well as links to a variety of other information and data, to other world health sites, and to the Department of Health or Statistical Bureau Web sites for many countries.

*To order:* www.who.int/pub/; WHO Publications Center USA, 49 Sheridan Ave, Albany NY 12210, tel. (518) 436-9686, FAX: (518) 436-7433
*To download:* www.who.int/whr/

### 2. United Nations Statistics Division (UNSD)

Web site: unstats.un.org/unsd/

The United Nations Statistics Division provides statistics on numerous topics including demographics and vital statistics. It publishes a *Monthly Bulletin of Statistics (MBS)* and a quarterly journal, *Population and Vital Statistics Report,* that reports population estimates, birth and mortality statistics for the world, regions, and 229 countries or areas. Both are available by subscription in online and print editions. The UNSD also publishes annually the *Demographic Yearbook* and two general statistical references: *Statistical Yearbook* and *World Statistics Pocketbook*. Limited data are freely available online and a number of data files are available for purchase on CD-Rom.

*To order:* UN Publications Department
*To download:* Not available

### 3. United Nations Population Fund (UNFPA)
Web site: www.unfpa.org

UNFPA produces an annual report entitled *The State of the World Population*, which includes statistics. It can be downloaded from UNFPA or ordered through the UN Publications Department. Additional data and policy information are available in *Country Profiles for Population and Reproductive Health*, published biennially. Data from the report are also available online (www.unfpa.org/profile/), where they are updated annually. This publication can be downloaded or requested directly from UNFPA.

*To order:* UN Publications Department (*State of the World Population*)
www.unfpa.org/profile/ (*Profiles*)
*To download:* www.unfpa.org/swp/ (*State of the World Population*)
www.unfpa.org/publications/ (*Profiles*)

### 4. United Nations Children's Fund (UNICEF)
Web site: www.unicef.org

Basic indicators related to child health, organized by country, can be accessed via the UNICEF Web site. In addition, information from UNICEF's key statistical databases can be accessed at **www.childinfo.org**, including data on child survival and health, nutrition, maternal health, and immunization, among other topics. UNICEF also produces an annual report, *The State of the World's Children*, which includes many child health statistics.

*To order:* UN Publications Department
*To download:* www.unicef.org/publications/

### 5. United Nations Population Information Network (POPIN)
Web site: www.un.org/popin/

The United Nations Population Information Network is a guide to population information on UN system Web sites. It provides links to statistics and publications on population-related data such as fertility, mortality, and migration produced by agencies and organizations throughout the UN system, including many of those listed above.

## C. Demographic and Health Surveys

Web site: www.measuredhs.com

The Demographic and Health Survey program, also known as MEASURE DHS+, is funded by the United States Agency for International Development (USAID) and implemented by Macro International, Inc., and is a source of population and health data for developing countries. MEASURE DHS+ provides developing countries with assistance in undertaking surveys to collect data on population, family planning, maternal and child health, child survival, sexually transmitted infections, and reproductive health. These data are available for public use in a number of formats. Basic country statistics are available on the DHS+ Web site. Publications with comprehensive survey results for individual countries can be downloaded or ordered. Other publications available include comparative, analytic, and trend reports. Data sets are available to authorized researchers. The DHS STATcompiler (www.measuredhs.com/statcompiler/) is an online database, which allows users to create custom tables drawing on hundreds of surveys from numerous countries and including hundreds of indicators.

*To order:* www.measuredhs.com/pubs/; tel. (301) 572–0958

*To download:* www.measuredhs.com/pubs/

# C

# A LISTING OF USEFUL HEALTH CARE WEB SITES

Kelli Hurdle

This version of Appendix C builds on that of the previous edition, by Leslie Reis.

# CATEGORIES OF ONLINE RESOURCES

1. Web site finders and links
2. Government Web site finders and links
3. Bibliographical search
4. Statistics and databases
5. Government agencies
6. Trade associations
7. Professional associations
8. Other health-related organizations
9. International health and health services data
10. Consulting firms
11. Online industry news
12. Magazines and journals online
13. Job search
14. General information resources
15. Glossaries

## 1.  WEB SITE FINDERS AND LINKS

| | |
|---|---|
| www.achoo.com | Achoo Internet health care directory; search engines and links |
| www.aha.org/resources | American Hospital Association Resource Center; links to other health care related Web sites |
| www.auburn.edu/~burnsma/ha.html | Auburn University's director of health administration and policy links |
| www.healthfinder.gov | Health Finder; search engine and links to other health sites |
| www.movingideas.com | Idea Central; health policy links |
| www.google.com | Google; generic Internet directory with hundreds of thousands of different subject categories |
| medworld.Stanford.edu | Independent Stanford Medical Student Web site; medical and health Web page search engine |
| www.medweb.emory.edu/medweb | MedWeb; Emory University's medical and health information search engine |
| www.health.gov.NHIC | National Health Information Center; links to Web sites of 1,200 health organizations |
| www.understandinghealthcare.com | Understanding Healthcare; answers hundreds of key questions related to health and medical care, and provides links to other resources and Web sites |

## 2. GOVERNMENT WEB SITE FINDERS AND LINKS

| | |
|---|---|
| www.fedworld.gov | FedWorld; links and information search engine for the federal government |
| firstgov.gov | The U.S. Government Official Web Portal |
| www.statelocalgov.net/index.cfm | State and local government on the Internet; directory of official state, county, and city government Web sites |
| www.loc.gov/global/state/stategov | State and local governments; maintained by the Library of Congress |
| www.hhs.gov/agencies | U.S. Department of Health and Human Services; links to all HHS agencies |
| www.nttc.edu/gov_res.html | Virtual library; U.S. government sources; legislative, executive, agencies, and states |

## 3. BIBLIOGRAPHICAL SEARCH

| | |
|---|---|
| igm.nlm.nih.gov | Grateful Med; health care bibliographical search engine |
| www.ipl.org | Internet Public Library |
| lcweb.loc.gov | Library of Congress |
| www.medscape.com | Medscape; medical search engine; access to online journals and current news |
| www2.ari.net/chrc/oldchrc/nhirc | National Health Information Resources Center; clearinghouse and communications hub for health information |
| www.nlm.nih.gov | National Library of Medicine, National Institutes of Health |
| www.ncbi.nlm.nih.gov/PubMed | Pub Med; National Library of Medicine's search engine that accesses citations in MedLine and Pre-MedLine and other related databases |
| www.amedeo.com | Amedeo; Medical literature guide; links to Web sites on various health topics |
| www.ovid.com | Ovid; access to thousands of health journals, texts, and databases |

## 4. STATISTICS AND DATABASES

| | |
|---|---|
| www.ahcpr.gov/data | Agency for Healthcare Research and Quality; access to the Healthcare Cost and Utilization Project, the National Medical Expenditure Study, the Safety Net Monitoring Initiative, and other governmental data and studies |
| www.ahd.com | American Hospital Directory; online data for most U.S. hospitals constructed from claims data, cost reports, and other public use files obtained from CMS; includes hospital characteristics, financial data, inpatient utilization, outpatient utilization, and links to the hospitals' Web sites |
| stats.bls.gov/iif | Bureau of Labor Statistics; Injuries, Illnesses, and Fatality program data |
| oshpd.cahwnet.gov | California Office of Statewide Health Planning and Development; utilization and financial data for California hospitals and long-term care facilities |
| www.fedstats.gov | FedStats; links to federal data and statistics produced by government agencies |
| www.cms.hhs.gov | Centers for Medicare & Medicaid (formerly the Health Care Financing Administration); data and statistics, including utilization, financial, and monthly reports |
| www.hsls.pitt.edu/inters/guides/statcbw.html | Health Sciences Library System; guide to locating hospitals |
| www.health.gov/healthypeople | Healthy People; access to Healthy People 2010, of HHS, prevention agenda and national health objectives information |
| www.hospitallink.com | Hospital Link; provides basic information on all hospitals in the United States |
| www.healthgrades.com | Health Grades, The Healthcare Quality Experts; source of hospital quality ratings and advisory services |
| www.nahdo.org | National Association of Health Data Organizations; links to the sites of federal and state agencies, other health care associations, and nonprofit organizations that have health information and data |
| www.cdc.gov/nchs | National Center for Health Statistics; basic source of data in the health care field |
| www.nlm.nih.gov/databases | National Library of Medicine; databases and electronic information sources |
| www.census.gov/prod | *Statistical Abstract of the United States/Healthcare*; complete publications with over 1,000 tables and charts for years 2001–2003 |
| www.census.gov/dmd | U.S. Census Bureau; Census 2000 data |

## 5. FEDERAL GOVERNMENT AGENCIES

| | |
|---|---|
| www.ahcpr.gov | Agency for Healthcare Research and Quality |
| stats.bls.gov | Bureau of Labor Statistics |
| www.census.gov | Census Bureau |
| www.cdc.gov | Centers for Disease Control and Prevention |
| www.cms.hhs.gov | Centers for Medicare & Medicaid (formerly HCFA) |
| www.cbo.gov | Congressional Budget Office |
| www.ha.osd.mil | Department of Defense, Health Affairs |
| www.ed.gov | Department of Education |
| www.dhhs.gov | Department of Health and Human Services |
| www.usdoj.gov | Department of Justice |
| www.dhs/gov/dhspublic | Department of Homeland Security |
| www.dol.gov | Department of Labor |
| www.va.gov | Department of Veterans Affairs |
| www.epa.gov | Environmental Protection Agency |
| www.uscourts.gov | Federal Judiciary |
| www.ftc.gov | Federal Trade Commission |
| www.fda.gov | Food and Drug Administration |
| www.gao.gov | Government Accounting Office |
| www.gpo.gov | Government Printing Office |
| www.hrsa.gov | Health Resources and Services Administration |
| www.house.gov | House of Representatives |
| www.ihs.gov | Indian Health Service |
| www.medpac.gov | Medicare Payment Advisory Commission |
| www.nih.gov | National Institutes of Health |
| www.nlm.nih.gov | National Library of Medicine |
| www.ophs.dhhs.gov/ophs | Office of Public Health and Science |
| www.senate.gov | Senate |
| www.ssa.gov | Social Security Administration |
| www.whitehouse.gov | White House |

## 6. TRADE ASSOCIATIONS

| | |
|---|---|
| www.himanet.com | Advanced Medical Technology Association; organizations that manufacture health care products and equipment |
| www.aahp.org | American Association of Health Plans; information and statistics regarding managed health care plan enrollment, benefits, utilization, and prices |
| www.aahc.net | American Association of Healthcare Consultants; consulting firms focusing on the health care industry |
| www.aaihds.org | American Association of Integrated Healthcare Delivery Systems |
| www.abms.org | American Board of Medical Specialties; medical specialty and subspecialty societies |
| www.his.com/~afhha/usa.html | American Federation of Home Health Agencies; home health organizations |
| www.ahca.org | American Health Care Association; assisted living, nursing facility, and subacute care providers |
| www.aha.org | American Hospital Association; hospital and health systems |
| www.ambha.org | American Managed Behavioral Healthcare Association; health plans focused exclusively on behavioral (mental) health |
| www.amia.org | American Medical Informatics Association; dedicated to the development and application of medical informatics in support of patient care, teaching research, and health care administration |
| www.aphanet.org | American Pharmaceutical Association; drug manufacturers and pharmacists |
| www.aslme.org | American Society of Law, Medicine and Ethics; provides information for professionals working with law, health care, policy and ethics; access to journals, newsletters, and research projects |
| www.ahcnet.org | Association of Academic Health Centers; medical and other health sciences schools in addition to their teaching hospitals |
| www.aamc.org | Association of American Medical Colleges; medical schools, academic societies, and teaching hospitals |
| www.aupha.org | Association of University Programs in Health Administration; graduate and undergraduate programs in health administration |
| www.chausa.org | Catholic Health Association; Catholic hospitals and health systems |
| www.fahs.com | Federation of American Health Systems; investor-owned hospitals and health systems |
| www.ahip.org | America's Health Insurance Plans; health insurance companies and managed care organizations |

| | |
|---|---|
| www.nahc.org | National Association for Home Care; home health provider |
| www.nacds.org | National Association of Chain Drug Stores; represents views and policy positions of member drug chains |
| www.naph.org | National Association of Public Hospitals and Health Systems; provides legislative and public policy information publications |
| www.ncsbn.org | National Council of State Boards of Nursing; source of data about the licensing and employment of nurses; annual statistics and publications |
| www.nhpco.org | National Hospice and Palliative Care Organization; represents organizations that provide hospice and palliative care |

## 7. PROFESSIONAL ASSOCIATIONS

| | |
|---|---|
| www.aameda.org | American Academy of Medical Administrators; chief medical officers in hospitals and health systems |
| www.achca.org | American College of Health Care Administrators; managers of long-term care, assisted living, and subacute facilities |
| www.ache.org | American College of Health Care Executives; executives/managers in all types of health care organizations |
| www.acpe.org | American College of Physician Executives; physician executives in all segments of the health care industry |
| www.healthlawyers.org | American Health Lawyers Association |
| www.ama-assn.org | American Medical Association; physicians |
| www.ana.org | American Nurses' Association; registered nurses |
| www.am-osteo-assn.org | American Osteopathic Association; osteopathic physicians |
| www.apha.org | American Public Health Association; public health professionals |
| www.aone.org | Association of Nurse Executives; nurse managers |
| www.aanp.org | American Academy of Nurse Practitioners; nurse practitioners |
| www.cmsa.org | Case Management Society of Manager; case manager |
| www.hfma.org | Health care Financial Management Association; financial management professionals in health care organizations |
| www.mgma.com | Medical Group Management Association; physician practice and medical group managers |
| www.nahq.org | National Association for Healthcare Quality; quality management professionals |
| www.nahse.org | National Association of Health Services Executives; African American health care executives |

| | |
|---|---|
| www.NLN.org | National League for Nursing; provides information on nursing education programs and publications |
| www.phrma.org | Pharmaceutical Researchers and Manufacturers of America; research-based pharmaceutical and biotechnology companies |
| www.nmha.org | National Mental Health Association |
| www.aapa.org | American Academy of Physician Assistants |
| www.naemt.org | National Association of Emergency Medical Technicians |
| www.apta.org | American Physical Therapy Association |
| www.certifieddoctor.org | American Board of Medical Specialties Public Education Program; verifies a doctor's certification status |

## 8. OTHER HEALTH-RELATED ORGANIZATIONS: ASSOCIATIONS, ACCREDITING BODIES, CENTERS, INSTITUTES AND FOUNDATIONS

| | |
|---|---|
| www.aarp.org | American Association of Retired Persons |
| www.ahsr.org | Association for Health Services Research; membership organization of individuals involved in policy and management research |
| www.astho.org | Association of State and Territorial Health Officials; links to public health agencies in all states; state initiatives and publications |
| www.bluecares.com | Blue Cross/Blue Shield Association; represents Blue Cross and Blue Shield associations throughout the country |
| www.chcs.org | Center for Health Care Strategies; a health policy research and resource center affiliated with the Woodrow Wilson School of Public and International Affairs at Princeton University |
| www.futurehealth.ucsf.edu | Center for Health Professions; University of California, San Francisco health manpower policy research center sponsored by the Pew Foundation |
| www.hschange.com | Center for Studying Health System Change; Washington-based research organization dedicated to studying how the country's health care system is changing and how these changes are affecting communities |
| www.tcf.org | The Century Foundation; research foundation undertaking analyses of major economic, political, and social institutions and issues |
| www.cmwf.org | The Commonwealth Fund; a nonprofit foundation engaged in independent research on health and social policy issues |
| www.ebri.com | Employee Benefit Research Institute; conducts research on employee benefits provided by commercial corporations |

| | |
|---|---|
| www.iom.edu | Institute of Medicine; a component of the National Academy of Sciences that studies health policy issues |
| www.iha.org | Integrated Health Association; California-based group of health plans, physician groups, and health systems, plus academic, purchaser, and consumer representatives involved in policy development and special projects focused on integrated health care and managed care |
| www.jcaho.org | Joint Commission on the Accreditation of Healthcare Organizations; accrediting body for health systems, hospitals, and other providers |
| www.kff.org | Kaiser Family Foundation; foundation supporting health services research and demonstration projects |
| www.markle.org | The Markle Foundation; addresses critical public needs, specifically in the areas of health and national safety |
| www.mathematica-mpr.com | Mathematica Policy Research; conducts health and social policy research |
| www.nashp.org | National Academy for State Health Policy; disseminates information designed to assist states in the development of practical, innovative solutions to complex health policy issues |
| www.nchc.org | National Coalition on Health Care; the nation's largest and most broadly representative alliance working to improve America's health care; research and education about emerging health trends and policy studies |
| www.ncsl.org/program/health/forum | National Conference of State Legislatures; Forum for State Health Policy Leadership |
| www.ncqa.org | National Committee for Quality Assurance; accrediting body for managed health care plans and designers of HEDIS |
| www.projecthope.org | Project Hope; a nonprofit organization that conducts research and policy analysis on both United States and foreign health care systems |
| www.rand.org | RAND Corporation; a nonprofit institution that helps improve policy and decision-making through research and analysis |
| www.rwjf.org | Robert Wood Johnson Foundation; foundation that funds health services research and demonstration projects |
| www.uhfnyc.org | United Hospital Fund; health services research and philanthropic organization that addresses issues affecting hospitals and health care in New York City |
| www.urban.org | Urban Institute; a nonprofit policy and research organization |
| www.wbgh.com | Washington Business Group on Health; national nonprofit organization devoted to the analysis of health policy and related worksite issues from the perspective of large public sector employers |
| www.wkkf.org | W.K. Kellogg Foundation; a foundation that funds health services research and demonstration projects |

| | |
|---|---|
| www.healthprivacy.org | Health Privacy Project; provides health care stakeholders with the information needed to work more effectively toward greater protection of health information through research studies, policy analyses, Congressional testimony, extensive work with the media, and a Web site |
| www.wellspouse.org | Well Spouse Foundation; offers support to husbands, wives, and partners of people with chronic illnesses and disabilities |

## 9. INTERNATIONAL HEALTH AND HEALTH SERVICES DATA

| | |
|---|---|
| www.bls.gov/bls/other.htm | Bureau of Labor Statistics; national and international statistical agencies |
| www.census.gov/ipc/www | International Programs Center of the U.S.Census Bureau; *World Population Profile* last published in 2002; online International Database |
| www.unsystem.org | United Nations; links to the Web sites of all UN agencies |
| www.unicef.org | United Nations Children's Fund; basic indicators related to child health; *The State of the World's Children*, published annually |
| www.un.org/popin | United Nations Population Information Network; a guide to population information on UN system Web sites |
| www.un.org/Depts/unsd | United Nations Statistics Division; *Population and Vital Statistics Report* published quarterly |
| www.census.gov/main/www/ stat_int.html | U.S. Census Bureau; international statistics agencies |
| www.who.int/en | World Health Organization |
| www.who.int/whosis | World Health Organization Statistical Information System |
| www.measuredhs.com | Demographic and Health Survey Program; source of demographic and health data for developing countries |

## 10. CONSULTING FIRMS

| | |
|---|---|
| www.aahc.net | American Association of Healthcare Consultants |
| www.arthurandersen.com | Arthur Andersen, LLP |
| www.chpsconsulting.com | Center for Health Policy Studies |
| www.ey.com | Ernst and Young, LLP |
| www.kpmg.com | KPMG Consulting |
| www.lewin.com | The Lewin Group; health and human service consulting firm |
| www.pwc.global.com | PricewaterhouseCoopers |

## 11. ONLINE INDUSTRY NEWS: HEALTH NEWS UPDATED DAILY OR WEEKLY

| | |
|---|---|
| www.ahanews.com | AHA News; daily reports for health care executives |
| www.cnn.com/HEALTH | CNN; health news updated daily |
| www.nytimes.com/pages/health.index | New York Times; health news updated daily |
| www.hhnmag.com | Health and Hospitals Network; health industry news updated daily |
| www.newsrx.net | News Rx Network; current news stories; reports on bioscience, biotech/pharma, health, and medicine |
| www.individual.com | Free customized news service; index of online news stories on a variety of topics; updated weekly; can select health care news page |
| kaisernetwork.org/ | Kaiser Network of the Kaiser Family Foundation; provides daily updates on health and health policy news, as well as webcasts, interviews, and public opinion |

## 12. MAGAZINES AND JOURNALS ONLINE

| | |
|---|---|
| www.apha.org/journal | *American Journal of Public Health and The Nation's Health*; published by the American Public Health Association; article archives |
| www.healthaffairs.org | *Health Affairs*; health policy articles and abstracts |
| www.cms.hhs.gov/Review/ | *Health Care Financing Review*; source of Medicare and Medicaid data and national health statistics and expenditures |
| www.healthforum.com | *Health Forum Journal*; selected articles available for the past five years |
| www.jama.ama-assn.org | *Journal of the American Medical Association* |
| www.trusteemag.com | *Magazine for Health Care Governance*; article archive |
| www.managedcaremag.com | *Managed Care Magazine*; access to current articles and analyses |
| www.Milbank.org/quarterly.html | *The Milbank Quarterly: Journal of Public Health and Health Care Policy*; access to current articles and archives |
| www.modernhealthcare.com | *Modern Healthcare*; weekly news journal for health care management professionals |
| www.cdc.gov/mmwr | *Morbidity and Mortality Weekly Report*; weekly publication of the Centers for Disease Control and Prevention |
| www.nejm.org | *New England Journal of Medicine* |

## 13. JOB SEARCH

| | |
|---|---|
| www.ache.org/career.html | American College of Healthcare Executives; career page; employment opportunities listing |
| www.futurestep.com | Future Step, a Korn/Ferry Company; Web-based job search/finding site for jobs in health administration |
| www.h-s.com | Heidrick and Struggles; executive search firm |
| www.kornferry.com | Korn/Ferry International; executive search firm |
| www.mcol.com/emp.htm | Managed Care On-Line; employment opportunities listing |
| www.tylerandco.com | Tyler and Company; executive search firms |

## 14. GENERAL INFORMATION RESOURCES: REPOSITORIES OF GUIDES, STUDIES, PAPERS, INFORMATION, AND MORE

| | |
|---|---|
| http://hippo.findlaw.com | Health Hippo |
| www.healthonline.com | Health OnLine |
| www.heatlhhero.com | Health Hero Network; helps patients and providers communicate via the Web; involves patients in the management of their illnesses |
| www.healthweb.com | HealthWeb |
| www.medconnect.com | MedConnect; online resource for medical professionals |
| www.refdesk.com/health/html | Refdesk; virtual encyclopedia for health and medicine |
| www.vh.org | The Virtual Hospital; University of Iowa Hospitals and Clinics; a digital library of health information |
| www.hopkinsmedicine.com | Johns Hopkins Medicine; extensive online access to medical research and general health information |
| www.understandinghealthcare.com | Understanding Healthcare; answers hundreds of key questions related to health and medical care, and provides links to other resources and Web sites; a virtual encyclopedia |

## 15. GLOSSARIES

| | |
|---|---|
| www.medterms.com | Medicine Net; online medical dictionary |
| www.who.ch/pll/ter/dicfair.html | World Health Organization; medical terminology search engine and dictionary |
| www.webmd.com | Web MD; online medical information source |

# INDEX

# A

## H

# Q

quality improvement, 579
risk adjusted outcomes, 563
risk-adjusted quality outcomes, 561–564
risk adjustment, 562
  methodologies, 562–563
strategies for managing quality, 565–580
uneven nature of, 4
Quasi-economic barriers to care, 604–609

# R

Race, 217
  access to health care, 598–600
Racial make-up of United States population,
  change in, 672
Radio Frequency Identification tags, 488
Randomized controlled clinical trials,
  conducting of, 400
Range of service options, availability of, 314
Rate, defined, 18
Reference pricing, use of, 647–648
Registered nurse, 434–435
Reimbursement, 73–77
  costs, 79–80
  diagnostic related groups, 75–76
  doctors, payment, 73–77
  government, 238
  health insurance, structure of, 78–79
  hospitals, payment, 75
  managed care, 75
  per diem hospital reimbursement, 76–77
  physician payment rates, government
    regulation of, 74–75
  prospective payment, 75–76
  quality, incentives for, 80
Research and development, 381–382, 397–398
  investment in, 376
Residency training, 440
  specialties, 441
Residential population, average age of, 297
Resident retention, issue of, 303
Resource allocation
  efficiency of, 183
  equity of, 183
Resource availability/performance, 603–604
Resource-Based Relative Value Scale,
  Medicare, 74
Resources, efficient use of, 486–488
Resource use tradeoffs, assessment of, 650
Responsibilities, overlap of, 107–108
Revenue cycle, 651
Revenue sources, limits on, 617
Risk-adjusted quality outcomes, 561–564
Risk adjustment, 562
  methodologies, 562–563
Risk communication, problem of, 123
Risk factor-specific mortality, 29–30
Rural areas, 603
Rural hospital, 229
  defined, 229

# S

Safety net hospitals, 228
Safety net system, 70
SCHIP. See State Children's Health Insurance
  Program
Secondary prevention, 100–101
Secular nonprofit systems, 232
Self-efficacy, positive health impacts of, 314
Self-employment, 73
Self-insure exemption, ERISA simply from
  state regulation, 149
Self-management, 266
  skill training, 336–337
Self-monitoring nature of, 452
Service level model, cost of, 302
Service quality, 479–482
Short-stay patients, 281
Short-term side effects, detection of, 378
Sliding scale payments, 242
Small employers, 615
Small medical technology firms, vulnerability
  of, 397
Smoking cessation, significant improvements
  in, 331
Social Darwinism, 193
Social ecological models, 346–352
Social insurance model, 316
Social justice, 97
Social learning theory, 336–337
Social marketing strategies, emergence of,
  339
Social science approach, 169
Social Security financing, 167
Societal goals, 288–289
Societal-level forces, health determined by,
  98–100
Socioeconomic status, 217–218
Soft savings, defined, 483
Solo-based private practice physicians, 177
Solo practitioners, 214–215
Sources of financing
  government, 166
  out of pocket, 166
  private insurance, 166
  social security, 166
Sources of health care data, 708–716
Specialized functional managers, 527
Specialty care, 223–224
  defined, 223
Stacey's Zone of Complexity, 544–548
Stages of change model, 337–339
Stakeholder, 522
  competing interests of, 7
  positions, 533–534
Standardization, lack of, 496–497
Standards for services, 105
Standards of medical practice, problems
  meeting, 230–231
State authority, infrastructure, 114–119